The **BIOMEDICAL ENGINEERING** Series

Series Editor Michael R. Neuman

# An Introduction
# to Biomaterials

# Biomedical Engineering Series

*Edited by* Michael R. Neuman

## Published Titles

*Electromagnetic Analysis and Design in Magnetic Resonance Imaging,* Jianming Jin

*Endogenous and Exogenous Regulation and Control of Physiological Systems,* Robert B. Northrop

*Artificial Neural Networks in Cancer Diagnosis, Prognosis, and Treatment,* Raouf N.G. Naguib and Gajanan V. Sherbet

*Medical Image Registration,* Joseph V. Hajnal, Derek Hill, and David J. Hawkes

*Introduction to Dynamic Modeling of Neuro-Sensory Systems,* Robert B. Northrop

*Noninvasive Instrumentation and Measurement in Medical Diagnosis,* Robert B. Northrop

*Handbook of Neuroprosthetic Methods,* Warren E. Finn and Peter G. LoPresti

*Signals and Systems Analysis in Biomedical Engineering,* Robert B. Northrop

*Angiography and Plaque Imaging: Advanced Segmentation Techniques,* Jasjit S. Suri and Swamy Laxminarayan

*Analysis and Application of Analog Electronic Circuits to Biomedical Instrumentation,* Robert B. Northrop

*Biomedical Image Analysis,* Rangaraj M. Rangayyan

*An Introduction to Biomaterials,* Scott A. Guelcher and Jeffrey O. Hollinger

The **BIOMEDICAL ENGINEERING** Series
Series Editor Michael R. Neuman

# An Introduction to Biomaterials

Edited by
## Scott A. Guelcher
## Jeffrey O. Hollinger

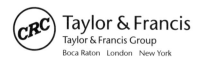

Taylor & Francis
Taylor & Francis Group
Boca Raton   London   New York

A CRC title, part of the Taylor & Francis imprint, a member of the
Taylor & Francis Group, the academic division of T&F Informa plc.

Published in 2006 by
CRC Press
Taylor & Francis Group
6000 Broken Sound Parkway NW, Suite 300
Boca Raton, FL 33487-2742

International Standard Book Number-10: 0-8493-2282-0 (Hardcover)
International Standard Book Number-13: 978-0-8493-2282-2 (Hardcover)
Library of Congress Card Number 2005051086

---

**Library of Congress Cataloging-in-Publication Data**

---

An introduction to biomaterials / edited by Scott A. Guelcher, Jeffrey O. Hollinger.
    p. ; cm. -- (Biomedical engineering series)
  Includes bibliographical references and index.
  ISBN 0-8493-2282-0 (alk. paper)
  1. Biomedical materials. I. Guelcher, Scott A. II. Hollinger, Jeffrey O. III. Biomedical engineering series (Boca Raton, Fla.)
  [DNLM: 1. Biocompatible Materials. 2. Equipment Design. 3. Prostheses and Implants. QT 37 I6183 2005]

R857.M3I68 2005
610'.28'4--dc22                                           2005051086

---

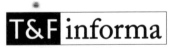

Taylor & Francis Group
is the Academic Division of T&F Informa plc.

**Visit the Taylor & Francis Web site at**
**http://www.taylorandfrancis.com**

**and the CRC Press Web site at**
**http://www.crcpress.com**

# *Preface*

The theme for this book emphasizes applications of biomaterials for patient care. The book is directed to upper level undergraduates and graduate students in the biomedical disciplines.

The editors recognize the complexity of biological systems and, especially, the challenges for design and development of biomedical therapies to address clinical needs.

We have assembled chapters prepared by authorities on key types of biomaterials. Moreover, we have included chapters underscoring the process of biomaterial design, a development directed toward clinical application as well as testing that will lead to a therapy for a clinical target. Consequently, several chapters have been dedicated to a clinical focus. This approach is unique and will be a helpful tool in the educational process of biomedical students.

It was not the goal for the editors to produce a comprehensive tome covering either all biomaterials or all aspects of biomaterial design, development, testing, and clinical applications. Chapter authors have provided key citations and directions for students to pursue when more comprehensive details on a topic are necessary.

It was our goal to provide a lucid perspective on the standards available and the logic for those standards where biomaterials can address clinical needs. Therefore, the book has been formatted with that theme. There are chapters on consensus standards and regulatory approaches to testing paradigms followed by chapters on specific classes of biomaterials and with closing chapters on clinical topics that integrate materials sciences and patient applications.

As editors, we are especially grateful to the authors of each chapter who committed considerable time and energy to the work.

We hope the students for whom this book has been specially crafted will be guided and inspired and that it will be an invaluable resource in the exciting and rewarding biomaterials field.

# Editors

**Scott A. Guelcher, Ph.D.** is an assistant professor of chemical engineering at Vanderbilt University. From 2003 to 2005, Dr. Guelcher was an NIH.NRSA post-doctoral fellow in the Bone Tissue Engineering Center at Carnegie Mellon University. In 1999, he joined Bayer Corporation's Polyurethanes Division (South Charleston, West Virginia), performing product and process development for the polyols business. Dr. Guelcher received his Ph.D. (on the aggregation of colloidal particles during electrophoretic deposition) from Carnegie Mellon University in 1999 and his M.S. degree from the University of Pittsburgh in 1996. Before this, while working for Eastman Chemical Company's Chemical Process Research group (Kingsport, Tennessee), Dr. Guelcher provided product and process development, including nutraceutical products, polyesters, and cellulose esters, for a number of businesses. In 1992, he received his B.S. degree in chemical engineering from Virginia Tech. Dr. Guelcher is an inventor on several U.S. patents and is an author of several research publications

**Jeffrey O. Hollinger, D.D.S., Ph.D.** is the director, Bone Tissue Engineering Center (BTEC), Carnegie Mellon University (CMU) and is a tenured professor of biomedical engineering and biological sciences. He has been at CMU since June 2000.

Dr. Hollinger also holds adjunct professorial-level appointments in orthopedics and plastic surgery at the University of Pittsburgh Medical School and serves on the scientific boards of several companies.

Dr. Hollinger had been at the Oregon Health Sciences University from 1993 to 2000 as a tenured professor of surgery, anatomy, and developmental biology at the School of Medicine. He was also the president and director for research for the Northwest Wound Healing Center.

Prior to 1993, Dr. Hollinger was in the United States Army at the United States Army Institute of Dental Research in Washington, D.C. where he headed the physiology department and directed the bone program. He retired as a colonel after 20 years of active military duty.

Dr. Hollinger's training in dentistry at the University of Maryland School of Dentistry was followed by a residency program in the United States Army and postgraduate work in physiology at the University of Maryland resulting in a Ph.D.

Dr. Hollinger's research focuses on bone tissue engineering and includes polymers, gene therapy, cells, signaling molecules, and surgical models to test bone regenerative therapies. He has been funded through the NIH, NIST.ATP, DOD, and several corporate sponsors. Dr. Hollinger has published over 150 peer-reviewed articles, abstracts, chapters in texts, and texts and is on the editorial board and is a reviewer for many clinical and scientific journals.

# Contributors

**Gregory H. Altman**  Department of Biomedical Engineering, Tufts University, Medford, Massachusetts

**James M. Anderson**  Department of Pathology, Case Western Reserve University, Cleveland, Ohio

**Thomas W. Braun**  School of Dental Medicine, University of Pittsburgh, Pittsburgh, Pennsylvania

**John H. Brekke**  Tissue Engineering Consultants, Inc., Duluth, Minnesota

**Constance R. Chu**  Department of Orthopaedic Surgery, University of Pittsburgh Physicians, Pittsburgh, Pennsylvania

**Mark Citron**  Regulatory Affairs & Quality Systems, BioMimetic Pharmaceuticals, Inc, Franklin, Tennessee

**Bradford L. Currier**  Department of Orthopedic Surgery, and Tissue Engineering and Polymeric Biomaterials Laboratory, Mayo Clinic College of Medicine, Rochester, Minnesota

**Kay C. Dee**  Department of Applied Biology and Biomedical Engineering, Rose-Hulman Institute of Technology, Terre Haute, Indiana

**Bruce A. Doll**  School of Dental Medicine, University of Pittsburgh, Pittsburgh, Pennsylvania

**Edward J. Dormier**  Ethicon, Inc., Somerville, New Jersey

**Michael Dornish**  FMC BioPolymer/NovaMatrix, Oslo, Norway

**Thomas A. Einhorn**  Department of Orthopaedic Surgery, Boston University Medical Center, Boston, Massachusetts

**David W. Grainger**  Department of Chemistry, Colorado State University, Fort Collins, Colorado

**Scott A. Guelcher**  Department of Chemical Engineering, Vanderbilt University, Nashville, Tennessee

**Joshua C. Haarer**  Department of Applied Biology and Biomedical Engineering, Rose-Hulman Institute of Technology, Terre Haute, Indiana

**Gregory M. Harbers**  Department of Chemistry, Colorado State University, Fort Collins, Colorado

**Jeffrey O. Hollinger**  Bone Tissue Engineering Center, Carnegie Mellon University, Pittsburgh, Pennsylvania

**Rebecca L. Horan**  Department of Biomedical Engineering, Tufts University, Medford, Massachusetts

**Dennis D. Jamiolkowski**  Ethicon, Inc., Somerville, New Jersey

**Sanjeev Kakar**  Department of Orthopaedic Surgery, Boston University Medical Center, Boston, Massachusetts

**Yusuf M. Khan**  Departments of Orthopaedic Surgery and Biomedical Engineering, University of Virginia, Charlottesville, Virginia

**Joachim Kohn**  Rutgers University, Piscataway, New Jersey

**Ash Kukreja**  School of Dental Medicine, University of Pittsburgh, Pittsburgh, Pennsylvania

**Prashant N. Kumta**  Department of Materials Science and Engineering, Carnegie Mellon University, Pittsburgh, Pennsylvania

**James W. Larson III**  Department of Orthopaedic Surgery, University of Pittsburgh Medical Center, Pittsburgh, Pennsylvania

**Cato T. Laurencin**  Departments of Orthopaedic Surgery, Biomedical Engineering, and Chemical Engineering, University of Virginia, Charlottesville, Virginia

**Philip LeDuc**  Department of Mechanical Engineering, Carnegie Mellon University, Pittsburgh, Pennsylvania

**Kam W. Leong**  Department of Biomedical Engineering, Johns Hopkins University School of Medicine, Baltimore, Maryland

**Yihua Loo**  Department of Biomedical Engineering, Johns Hopkins University School of Medicine, Baltimore, Maryland

**Lichun Lu**  Departments of Orthopedic Surgery and Biomedical Engineering, and Tissue Engineering and Polymeric Biomaterials Laboratory, Mayo Clinic College of Medicine, Rochester, Minnesota

**Jonathan Mansbridge**  Smith and Nephew, Memphis, Tennessee

**Kacey G. Marra**  Division of Plastic Surgery, Department of Bioengineering, University of Pittsburgh, Pittsburgh, Pennsylvania

**Antonios G. Mikos**  Department of Bioengineering, Rice University, Houston, Texas

**John Mitchell**  Department of Restorative Dentistry, Oregon Health & Science University, Portland, Oregon

**Lakshmi S. Nair**  Department of Orthopaedic Surgery, University of Virginia, Charlottesville, Virginia

**Henry R. Piehler**  Departments of Engineering and Public Policy, Materials Science and Engineering, and Biomedical Engineering, Carnegie Mellon University, Pittsburgh, Pennsylvania

**Priya Ramaswami**  Department of Biomedical Engineering, University of Pittsburgh, McGowan Institute for Regenerative Medicine, Pittsburgh, Pennsylvania

**Frank Rauh**  FMC BioPolymer, Princeton, New Jersey

**Lizzie Y. Santiago**  Departments of Surgery and Bioengineering, Pittsburgh, Pennsylvania

**Jaap Schut**  Rutgers University, Piscataway, New Jersey

**Ali Seyedain**  School of Dental Medicine, University of Pittsburgh, Pittsburgh, Pennsylvania

**Xinfeng Shi**  Department of Bioengineering, Rice University, Houston, Texas

**Bill Tawil**  Baxter BioSurgery, Westlake Village, California

**Kipling Thacker**  Life Core Biomedical, Chaska, Minnesota

**Hasan Uludağ**  Department of Chemical and Materials Engineering, University of Alberta, Edmonton, Alberta, Canada

**William R. Wagner**  McGowan Institute of Regenerative Medicine, University of Pittsburgh, Pittsburgh, Pennsylvania

**Shanfeng Wang**  Departments of Orthopedic Surgery and Biomedical Engineering, and Tissue Engineering and Polymeric Biomaterials Laboratory, Mayo Clinic College of Medicine, Rochester, Minnesota

**Yadong Wang**  Wallace H. Coulter Department of Biomedical Engineering, Georgia Institute of Technology, Atlanta, Georgia

**Shelley R. Winn**  Division of Plastic and Reconstructive Surgery, Oregon Health & Science University, Portland, Oregon

**Michael J. Yaszemski**  Departments of Orthopedic Surgery and Biomedical Engineering, and Tissue Engineering and Polymeric Biomaterials Laboratory, Mayo Clinic College of Medicine, Rochester, Minnesota

# Contents

# 1

## *Introduction*

**Scott A. Guelcher and Jeffrey O. Hollinger**

The scope of *An Introduction to Biomaterials* relates to materials, both synthetic and natural, that are implanted in the human body for the purposes of promoting improved human health. A consensus definition of a "biomaterial" developed in 1986 and frequently referenced in the literature is (Williams, 1986; Ratner et al., 2004):

> A biomaterial is a nonviable material used in a medical device, intended to interact with biological systems.

The recent development of materials containing living cells (e.g., artificial organs and tissue-engineered scaffolds) challenges the inclusion of the word "nonviable" in the traditional definition of a biomaterial. However, this book will focus on the properties and applications of biomaterials as defined above.

The book is divided into three parts. Part I (Chapters 2–6) emphasizes the assessment of biological performance and compatibility where the important concepts of biocompatibility, cell-material interactions, protein adsorption, *in vitro* testing and *in vivo* testing paradigms are presented. These concepts enable the design and development of biomaterials from the bench to the bedside. Part II (Chapters 7–18) describes the synthesis, characterization, properties, and applications of specific classes of clinically significant biomaterials, including natural and synthetic materials for both hard and soft tissue applications. These chapters are intended to introduce the reader to biomaterials that are either in clinical use or the subject of current research. Part III (Chapters 19–27) relates to clinical applications of biomaterials with an emphasis on tissue engineering and implants. These chapters demonstrate the significance of biomaterials in improving human health, particularly in the area of regenerative medicine.

Successful design and development of biomaterials requires expertise in a broad range of subjects, as described below. A wide array of skills and disciplines are necessary to bring a biomaterial from the bench to the bedside.

*Biocompatibility.* A consensus definition has also been developed for the term "biocompatibility", which is an important aspect of biomaterials science:

> Biocompatibility is the ability of a material to perform with an appropriate host response in a specific application (Williams, 1986).

Examples of "an appropriate host response in a specific application" could include attachment, proliferation, and differentiation of osteoprogenitor cells to a degradable bone void filler; minimal protein adsorption onto a cardiovascular stent; or a mild inflammatory response. There is no precise definition for biocompatibility; it is typically defined in terms of performance related to a specific application (Ratner et al., 2004). The concept of biocompatibility is expanded upon in more detail in Chapter 2.

*Materials science.* Successful design and development of biomaterials also requires materials synthesis and characterization of physical and mechanical properties, which is typically an area of expertise for chemists, materials scientists, and chemical engineers. Examples of important physical and mechanical properties include porosity, protein adhesion, contact angle, elastic modulus, tensile strength, elongation at break, durability, and *in vivo* stability. Ideally, the properties of a biomaterial incorporated in an implant or device are tuned to the requirements of the application. For example, a hip prosthesis must be strong, rigid, durable, and nondegradable *in vivo*. In contrast, a bone void filler must be porous, osteoconductive, and must degrade at a rate in register with that of fracture healing. Synthesis strategies and characterization techniques for specific biomaterials are presented in Chapters 7 to 18.

*Biological function.* Functional biology must guide the design of a clinical therapy that is either a biomaterial or a combination biomaterial and biological. While it may seem a great deal is known about functional biology of cells, tissues, organs and systems, in truth, we recognize that tremendous voids exist in our knowledge. It therefore becomes a daunting challenge to design and develop either a biomaterial or biomaterial and biological that will address specific biological — that is, clinical — needs. Despite the many voids that exist in our current biological knowledge base, the chapters on biologic performance and the chapters dedicated to biomaterials, provide key instructional guidance. Moreover, these chapters inspire us to learn more and explore biology more comprehensively.

*Clinical practice.* Biomaterials formatted as devices and implants and combined with biologicals must also be designed to be compatible with clinical practice. Moreover, the design must be clinically practical, not complex. Multistage complex therapeutics are daunting regulatory challenges, manufacturing nightmares and, in the operating room, are highly susceptible to problems. Consequently, the clinical chapters in this textbook emphasize practical, rational approaches to clinical targets.

*Regulatory issues.* In the United States, the Food and Drug Administration (FDA) regulates devices implanted into the human body to ensure that they are safe and effective. Typically, a number of biological and clinical tests must be performed to demonstrate that the device is safe. Therefore, commercialization of a new medical device requires a significant investment to comply with regulatory requirements. Regulatory issues are discussed in greater detail in Chapter 6.

---

## References

Ratner, B., Hoffman, A., Schoen, F., and Lemons, J., Introduction: biomaterials science: a multi-disciplinary endeavor, In: *Biomaterials Science: An Introduction to Materials in Medicine*, Ratner, B., Hoffman, A., Schoen, F., and Lemons, J., Eds., Elsevier, Boston (2004).

Williams, D.F., *Definitions in Biomaterials, Proceedings of a Consensus Conference of the European Society for Biomaterials. 1987 March 3–5*, Elsevier, Chester (1986).

# 2

# Fundamental Biological Requirements of a Biomaterial

James M. Anderson

## CONTENTS

## 2.1   Introduction

In identifying fundamental biological requirements of a biomaterial, numerous approaches may be taken. The approach presented in this chapter is a practical approach, based to a great extent on regulatory requirements and standards. The goal of this chapter is to provide a pathway or roadmap for the practical approach to the identification of fundamental biological requirements for biomaterials, medical devices or prostheses. Therefore, the chapter is compartmentalized into five sections: biocompatibility, materials for medical devices, *in vitro* tests for biocompatibility, *in vivo* tests for biocompatibility, and summary. Perspectives are presented throughout the chapter to provide insight into how regulatory agencies may view certain aspects and issues regarding the various topic areas. Numerous caveats are presented to provide perspective on how fundamental biological requirements of a biomaterial, medical device or prosthesis might be viewed by regulatory agencies.

As the intended use of a biomaterial, either alone or in combination with other biomaterials in medical devices or prostheses, is to assist in the health and welfare of humans, governmental regulation of the biomaterial or medical device is required to ensure appropriate and adequate safety and efficacy of the biomaterial or medical device. In this regard, it is noteworthy that the Food and Drug Administration (FDA) does not regulate biomaterials, but rather regulates the "as used" medical device or product intended for clinical application in humans. It is important to understand that the FDA does not regulate nor approve biomaterials, but rather, the FDA regulates the use of biomaterials in the final end-stage "as used" medical device, i.e., product.

In considering the fundamental biological requirements of a biomaterial for clinical application, it must be remembered that the biological requirements for a material in one application may be different than those required in another application, even though the same biomaterial is being used. From this perspective, the intended application of the biomaterial or medical device dictates the biological requirements necessary to ensure safety and efficacy of the medical device or product.

## 2.2  Biocompatibility

The most commonly used term to describe appropriate biological requirements of a biomaterial or biomaterials used in a medical device is biocompatibility. A simplistic definition of biocompatibility is that materials do not create any adverse tissue reactions. A more helpful definition of biocompatibility is the ability of a material to perform with an appropriate host response in a specific application (Williams, 1987). This definition is helpful in that it links material properties or characteristics with performance, i.e., biological requirements, with a specific application, a specific medical device or biomaterial used as a medical device. The "appropriate host response" implies identification and characterization of tissue reactions and responses that could prove harmful to the host and/or lead to ultimate failure of the biomaterial, medical device or prosthesis through biological mechanisms. Viewed from another perspective, the "appropriate host response" implies identification and characterization of the tissue reactions and responses critical for the successful use of the biomaterial or medical device. Biocompatibility assessment is considered to be a measure of the magnitude and duration of the adverse alterations in homeostatic mechanisms that determine the host response (Anderson, 2001). Safety assessment or biocompatibility assessment of a biomaterial or medical device is generally considered to be synonymous.

## 2.3  Materials for Medical Devices

In the selection of biomaterials to be used in device design and manufacture, the first consideration must be the fitness for purpose with regard to characteristics and properties of the biomaterial(s). These include chemical, toxicological, physical, electrical, morphological, and mechanical properties. Relevant to the overall *in vivo* assessment of tissue compatibility of a biomaterial or medical device is knowledge of the chemical composition of the materials, including the conditions of tissue exposure as well as the nature, degree, frequency, and duration of exposure of the device and its constituents to the intended tissues in which it will be used. Table 2.1 presents a list of biomaterial components and

**TABLE 2.1**

Biomaterials and Components

| |
|---|
| The material(s) of manufacture |
| Intended additives, process contaminants, and residues |
| Leachable substances |
| Degradation products |
| Other components and their interactions in the final product |
| The properties and characteristics of the final product |

characteristics that may affect the overall biological response of the medical device. Knowledge of the presence and quantity of these components in the medical device, i.e., final product, is necessary. The range of potential biological hazards is broad and may include short-term effects, long-term effects, or specific toxic effects, which should be considered for every material and medical device. However, this does not imply that testing for all potential hazards will be necessary or practical.

While the biomaterials and components listed in Table 2.1 are only superficially, if at all, considered in the research and development of new biomaterials, they become exceedingly important as the biomaterial moves from the R&D stage to the product stage of development. The components of biomaterials may play unexpected roles in the biocompatibility of the material or materials under consideration for a given medical device. Low molecular weight materials such as intended additives, process contaminants, residues, leachable substances, and degradation products may migrate and diffuse from the material and coat the surface of the material, potentially leading to different biological interactions than that intended with the original material. Examples of this that have been identified in the past include processing aids that have coated the metal components of heart valves and wax extrusion aids that have ultimately coated the surfaces of polyurethane pacemaker leads. These examples illustrate how the material surfaces at the tissue/implant interfaces were of different chemistry than that intended by the manufacturer. Thus, knowledge of the components and composition of the materials of manufacture are important in predicting biological responses, both intended and unintended responses. The possibility also exists that these low molecular weight components, having diffused to the surface of the material in contact with tissue, may ultimately be released into the tissue leading to modified or undesirable tissue reactions. Short-term biological assessment of the biomaterial may not identify these possibilities as the diffusion from the bulk of a material to its surface requires time. Therefore, long-term *in vivo* assessment and accelerated *in vitro* procedures to identify these possibilities may be necessary.

As final product or "as-used" medical devices are generally made available in the sterilized state, the effect of sterilization and sterilization technique must also be considered. Steam sterilization, radiation sterilization, or ethylene oxide sterilization may lead to modifications in the surface and bulk properties of the material and this may have a potential impact on the biocompatibility. Radiation sterilization may crosslink or degrade polymers leading to property changes. Ethylene oxide residuals are known to have an adverse reaction on *in vitro* toxicity tests. For these reasons, characterization of the final product following sterilization is necessary.

As stated earlier, testing for all potential hazards may not be necessary or practical. If a material and its components are well known and its manufacturing, processing, and sterilization procedures have been characterized in regard to potential changes in the materials or biocompatibility, testing may not be necessary.

## 2.4  *In Vitro* Tests for Biocompatibility

The most common type of biocompatibility assay is the use of cell culture systems to identify cytotoxicity, cell adhesion, cell activation, or cell death. Cell culture assays are used extensively in biocompatibility studies of new biomaterials as well as being required in biocompatibility assessment programs for products, i.e., biomaterials, medical devices, and prostheses (Johnson et al., 1985; Northup, 1986; U.S. Pharmacopeia, 2004).

Three types of cell culture assays are commonly used for evaluating biocompatibility. These are: direct contact, agar diffusion, and extract dilution. Direct contact cell culture is most commonly used by investigators studying the biocompatibility of new biomaterials. In this type of assay, the investigator can use the cell type for which the biomaterial under investigation is intended for clinical use. For example, biomaterials intended for devices such as prosthetic heart valves, vascular grafts, and other cardiovascular devices will use human or animal endothelial cells to investigate biocompatibility as well as to investigate the capability of this cell type to proliferate and present the appropriate endothelial cell phenotype when in contact with the biomaterial. Studies involving inflammation and the foreign body response will use primary cells from blood or macrophage cell lines available through biological suppliers or cell banks. Materials intended for hard tissue or orthopedic application are commonly studied with osteoblasts or osteoblast cell lines. This type of assay permits the investigator to use the specific cell type in investigating the cell interaction and biocompatibility of the biomaterial for an intended application in an organ or tissue. This is a distinct advantage of this type of assay. Using appropriate negative and positive control materials as well as other biomaterials intended for similar application, new biomaterials can be assayed for a wide variety of types of cell interactions using this assay system.

The extract dilution type of cell culture assay requires a solvent extraction of the biomaterial under consideration and testing of this extract, most commonly at various dilutions, for evidence of cytotoxicity and cellular interaction. This type of cell culture assay finds its most common use in providing information for regulatory compliance. As identified in the previous section (Materials for Medical Devices) and in Table 2.1, small molecular weight extractables are of concern regarding biocompatibility. The extraction assay, carried out with a series of solvents that are hydrophilic and hydrophobic, permits examination of the potential cytotoxicity of extracts and the identification of materials within a biomaterial that may be cytotoxic. These types of assay ultimately permit identification and characterization of cytotoxic materials within biomaterials or the lack of cytotoxicity, as well as providing correlation with *in vivo* assays such as sensitization, irritation, intracutaneous (intradermal) reactivity, and other tests where the *in vivo* injection of extracts is required.

For regulatory purposes, the direct contact test commonly involves the development of a near-confluent monolayer of L-929 mammalian fibroblast cells on a culture plate. Biomaterial specimens under investigation are carefully placed on these cell layers with fresh culture medium and incubated for 24 h at 37°C. The culture medium and specimens are removed, the cells are fixed and stained with appropriate histological stains. Light microscopic evaluation is then used to identify cells adherent to the culture plate. Other cellular morphological characteristics can also be identified using this technique. Unlike those used for research purposes, regulatory cell culture assays most commonly use established cell lines. The use of established cell lines such as the L-929 mammalian fibroblast cell line offers the advantage of less assay repeatability, reproducibility, and efficiency. In addition, cell lines are more commonly available than are primary cells. For research, the most common practice is to directly culture cells on the new biomaterial surface.

*In vitro* cytotoxicity assays are the initial biocompatibility screening tests for a wide variety of biomaterials used in medical devices and prostheses. After the cytotoxicity profile of a candidate biomaterial has been determined, more application-specific tests may be performed to assess the biocompatibility of the biomaterial under end-use conditions. In general, biomaterials identified as being nontoxic *in vitro* will be nontoxic in *in vivo* assays. Biomaterials identified as toxic in *in vitro* assays must be further investigated for clinical acceptability. There are examples where low levels of toxicity are present with biomaterials but this does not preclude or obviate their use in medical devices. An excellent example of this is with glutaraldehyde-fixed porcine valves that produce adverse effects *in vitro* due to low residues of glutaraldehyde. In spite of the negative *in vitro* findings, this material is still used in the development of prosthetic heart valves for clinical use. This is an example of where the risk of low levels of toxicity is outweighed by the clinical advantage of the use of this material.

## 2.5  *In Vivo* Tests for Biocompatibility

From a practical perspective, the *in vivo* assessment of the biocompatibility of biomaterials and medical devices is carried out to determine that the device performs as intended, i.e., designed, and presents no significant harm to the patient or user. Thus, the goal of the *in vivo* assessment of biocompatibility is to predict whether a medical device presents potential harm to the patient or user by evaluation under conditions simulating clinical use.

Recently, extensive efforts have been made by government agencies, i.e., FDA, and regulatory bodies, i.e., ASTM, ISO, USP, to provide procedures, protocols, guidelines and standards which may be used in the *in vivo* assessment of the tissue compatibility of medical devices (FDA, 1995; Chapekar, 1996; AAMI, 1997; Langone, 1998; ISO and ASTM, 1999). This chapter draws heavily on the ISO 10,993 standard, Biological Evaluation of Medical Devices, in presenting a systematic approach to the *in vivo* assessment of tissue compatibility of medical devices (AAMI, 1997).

*In vivo* tests for assessment of biocompatibility are chosen to simulate end-use applications. To facilitate the selection of appropriate tests, medical devices with their component biomaterials can be categorized by the nature of body contact of the medical device and by the duration of contact of the medical device. Table 2.2 presents medical device categorization by body contact and contact duration. The tissue contact categories and subcategories as well as the contact duration categories have been derived from standards, protocols, and guidelines utilized in the past for safety evaluation of

**TABLE 2.2**

Medical Device Categorization by Tissue Contact and Contact Duration

*Tissue contact*
  Surface devices
    Skin
    Mucosal membranes
    Breached or compromised surfaces
  External communicating devices
    Blood path, indirect
    Tissue/bone/dentin communicating
    Circulating blood
  Implant devices
    Tissue/bone
    Blood

*Contact duration*
  Limited, ≤24 h
  Prolonged, >24 h and <30 days
  Permanent, >30 days

medical devices. Certain devices may fall into more than one category, in which case testing appropriate to each category should be considered.

Two perspectives may be considered in the *in vivo* assessment of the biocompatibility of biomaterials and medical devices. The first perspective involves the utilization of *in vivo* tests to determine the general biocompatibility of newly developed biomaterials for which some knowledge of the tissue compatibility is necessary for further research and development. In this type of situation, manufacturing and other processes necessary to the development of a final product, i.e., medical device, have not been carried out. However, the *in vivo* assessment of biocompatibility at this early stage of development can be used to evaluate the general tissue responses of the biomaterial as well as to provide additional information relating to the proposed design criteria in the production of a medical device. While it is generally recommended that the identification and quantification of extractable chemical entities of a medical device should precede biological evaluation, it is quite common to carry out preliminary *in vivo* assessments to determine if there may be unknown chemical entities which produce adverse biological reactions. Utilized in this fashion, early *in vivo* assessment of a biomaterial may provide insight into the biocompatibility of a material and may facilitate further development of a biomaterial into a medical device. Obviously, adverse reactions observed at this stage of development for a biomaterial would require further efforts to improve the biocompatibility of the biomaterial and identify the agents responsible for the adverse reactions.

The second perspective regarding the *in vivo* assessment of medical devices focuses on the biocompatibility of the final product, that is, the medical device and its component materials in the condition in which it is implanted. While medical devices in their final form and condition are commonly implanted in carefully selected animal models to determine function as well as biocompatibility, it may not be appropriate to carry out all of the recommended tests necessary for regulatory approval on the final device. In these situations, some tests may be carried out on biomaterial components of devices which have been prepared under manufacturing and sterilization conditions and other processes utilized in the final product development.

In this section, brief perspectives on the general types of *in vivo* tests are presented (Table 2.3). Details regarding these tests are found in the references. The ultimate selection of tests for *in vivo* biocompatibility assessment is based on the characteristics and end-use application of the device or biomaterial under consideration.

*Sensitization, Irritation, and Intracutaneous (Intradermal) Reactivity.* Exposure to or contact with even minute amounts of potential leachables in medical devices or biomaterials can

**TABLE 2.3**

*In Vivo* Tests for Biocompatibility

---

Sensitization
Irritation
Intracutaneous reactivity
Systemic toxicity (Acute toxicity)
Subchronic toxicity (Subacute toxicity)
Genotoxicity
Implantation
Hemocompatibility
Chronic toxicity
Carcinogenicity
Reproductive and developmental toxicity
Biodegradation
Immune responses

---

result in allergic or sensitization reactions. Sensitization tests estimate the potential for contact sensitization of medical devices, materials and/or their extracts; they are usually carried out in guinea pigs, and should reflect the intended route (skin, eye, mucosa) and nature, degree, frequency, duration and conditions of exposure of the biomaterial in its intended clinical use. Emphasis is placed on utilizing extracts of the biomaterials to determine the irritant effects of potential leachables. Intracutaneous (intradermal) reactivity tests determine the localized reaction of tissue to extracts of medical devices, biomaterials, or prostheses in the final product form. Irritation and intracutaneous tests may be applicable where determination of irritation by dermal or mucosal irritation tests is not appropriate — albino rabbits are most commonly used.

Since these tests focus on determining the biological response of leachables which may be present in biomaterials, their extracts in various solvents are utilized to prepare the injection solutions. Critical to the conduct of these tests is the preparation of the test material and/or extract solution and the choice of solvents that must have physiological relevance.

*Systemic Toxicity (Acute Toxicity) and Subacute and Subchronic Toxicity.* Systemic toxicity tests estimate the potential harmful effects of either single or multiple exposures, during a period of less than 24 h, to medical devices, biomaterials and/or their extracts. These tests evaluate the systemic toxicity potential of medical devices which release constituents into the body. These tests also include pyrogenicity testing.

In these tests, the form and area of the material, the thickness, and the surface area to extraction vehicle volume are critical considerations in the testing protocol. Appropriate extraction vehicles, i.e., solvents, should be chosen to yield a maximum extraction of leachable materials to conduct the testing. Mice, rats, or rabbits are the usual animals of choice for the conduct of these tests and depending on the intended application of the biomaterial, oral, dermal, inhalation, intravenous, intraperitoneal, or subcutaneous application of the test substance may be used. Acute toxicity is considered to be the adverse effects that occur after administration of a single dose or multiple doses of a test sample given within 24 h. Subacute toxicity (repeat dose toxicity) focuses on adverse effects occurring after administration of a single dose or multiple doses of a test sample per day given during a period of from 14 to 28 days. Subchronic toxicity is considered to be the adverse effects occurring after administration of a single dose or multiple doses of a test sample per day given during a part of the lifespan, usually 90 days but not exceeding 10% of the lifespan of the animal.

Pyrogenicity (fever producing) tests are also included in the systemic toxicity category to detect material-mediated pyrogenic reactions of extracts of medical devices or materials. It is noteworthy that no single test can differentiate pyrogenic reactions that are material-mediated from those due to endotoxin contamination.

*Genotoxicity. In vivo* genotoxicity tests are carried out if indicated by the chemistry and/or composition of the biomaterial (see Table 2.1) or *in vitro* test results indicate potential genotoxicity. Initially, at least three *in vitro* assays should be used and two of these assays should utilize mammalian cells. The initial *in vitro* assays should cover the three levels of genotoxic effects: DNA effects, gene mutations, and chromosomal aberrations. *In vivo* genotoxicity tests include the micronucleus test, the *in vivo* mammalian bone marrow cytogenetic tests — chromosomal analysis, the rodent dominant lethal tests, the mammalian germ cell cytogenetic assay, the mouse spot test and the mouse heritable translocation assay. Not all of the *in vivo* genotoxicity tests need be performed and the most common test is the rodent micronucleus test. Genotoxicity tests are performed with appropriate extracts or dissolved materials using appropriate media as suggested by the known composition of the biomaterial.

*Implantation.* Implantation tests assess the local pathological effects on living tissue of a sample of a material or final product that is surgically implanted or placed into an implant site or tissue appropriate to the intended application of the biomaterial or medical device. Evaluation of the local pathological effects is carried out at both the gross level and the microscopic level. Histological (microscopic) evaluation is utilized to characterize various biological response parameters. For short-term implantation evaluation out to 12 weeks, mice, rats, guinea pigs, or rabbits are the usual animals utilized in these studies. For longer term testing in subcutaneous tissue, muscle or bone, animals such as rats, guinea pigs, rabbits, dogs, sheep, goats, pigs, and other animals with relatively long life expectancy are suitable. If a medical device is to be evaluated, larger species may be utilized. For example, substitute heart valves are usually tested in sheep, while calves are usually the animal of choice for ventricular assist devices and total artificial hearts.

*Hemocompatibility.* Hemocompatibility tests evaluate effects on blood and/or blood components by blood-contacting medical devices or materials. *In vivo* hemocompatibility tests are usually designed to simulate the geometry, contact conditions, and flow dynamics of the device or material in its clinical application. From the ISO standards perspective, five test categories are indicated for hemocompatibility evaluation: thrombosis, coagulation, platelets, hematology, and immunology (complement and leukocytes).

Two levels of evaluation are indicated: Level 1 (required), and Level 2 (optional). Regardless of blood contact duration or time, hemocompatibility testing is indicated for external communicating devices — blood path, indirect; external communicating devices — circulating blood; and blood-contacting implant devices.

Several issues are important in the selection of tests for hemocompatibility of medical devices or biomaterials. While *in vivo* testing in animals may be convenient, species differences in blood reactivity must be considered and these may limit the predictability of any given test in the human clinical situation. While blood values and reactivity between humans and nonhuman primates are very similar, European community law prohibits the use of nonhuman primates for blood compatibility and medical device testing. Hemocompatibility evaluation in animals is complicated by the lack of appropriate and adequate test materials; for example, appropriate antibodies for immunoassays. Use of human blood in hemocompatibility evaluation implies *in vitro* testing, which usually requires the use of anticoagulants which are not usually present with the device in the clinical situation, except for perhaps the earliest implantation period. While species differences may complicate hemocompatibility evaluation, the utilization of animals in short- and long-term testing is considered to be appropriate for evaluating thrombosis and tissue interaction.

*Chronic Toxicity.* Chronic toxicity tests determine the effects of either single or multiple exposures to medical devices, materials, and/or their extracts during a period of at least 10% of the lifespan of the test animal, e.g., over 90 days in rats. Chronic toxicity tests may be considered an extension of subchronic (subacute) toxicity testing and both may be evaluated in an appropriate experimental protocol or study.

*Carcinogenicity.* Carcinogenicity tests determine the tumorigenic potential of medical devices, materials, and/or their extracts from either single or multiple exposures or contacts over a period of the major portion of the lifespan of the test animal. A new carcinogenicity test using a transgenic mouse assay is currently under investigation (Yamamoto et al., 1998). This assay is less time-consuming and less expensive than the two animal life-time assay. Carcinogenicity tests should be conducted only if data from other sources suggest a tendency for tumor induction. In addition, both carcinogenicity (tumorigenicity) and chronic toxicity may be studied in a single experimental study. With biomaterials, carcinogenicity studies focus on the potential for solid-state carcinogenicity, i.e., the Oppenheimer effect. In carcinogenicity testing, controls of a comparable form and shape should be included; polyethylene implants are a commonly used control material. The use of appropriate controls is imperative as animals may spontaneously develop tumors and statistical comparison between the test biomaterial/device and the controls is necessary.

*Reproductive and Developmental Toxicity.* These tests evaluate the potential effects of medical devices, materials, and/or their extracts on reproductive function, embryonic development (teratogenicity), and prenatal and early postnatal development. The application site of the device must be considered and tests and/or bioassays should only be conducted when the device has potential impact on the reproductive potential of the subject.

*Biodegradation.* Biodegradation tests determine the effects of a biodegradable material and its biodegradation products on the tissue response. They focus on: the amount of degradation during a given period of time (the kinetics of biodegradation), the nature of the degradation products, the origin of the degradation products (e.g., impurities, additives, corrosion products, bulk polymer, etc.), and the qualitative and quantitative assessment of degradation products and leachables in adjacent tissues and in distant organs. The biodegradation of biomaterials may occur through a wide variety of mechanisms, which in part are biomaterial dependent, and all pertinent mechanisms related to the device and the end-use application of the device must be considered. Test materials comparable to degradation products may be prepared and studied to determine the biological response of degradation products anticipated in long-term implants. An example of this approach is the study of metallic and polymeric wear particles, which may be present with long-term orthopedic joint prostheses.

*Immune Responses.* Immune response evaluation is not a component of the standards currently available for *in vivo* tissue compatibility assessment. However, ASTM, ISO, and the FDA currently have working groups developing guidance documents for immune response evaluation where pertinent. An example of the need for immune response evaluation is with modified natural tissue implants such as collagen that has been

**TABLE 2.4**

Potential Immunological Effects and Responses

---

*Effects*
  Hypersensitivity
    Type I — anaphylactic
    Type II — cytotoxic
    Type III — immune complex
    Type IV — cell-mediated (delayed)
  Chronic inflammation
  Immunosuppression
  Immunostimulation
  Autoimmunity

*Responses*
  Histopathological changes
  Humoral responses
  Host resistance
  Clinical symptoms
  Cellular responses
    T cells
    Natural killer cells
    Macrophages
    Granulocytes

---

utilized in a number of different types of implants. The Center for Devices and Radiological Health of the FDA has released a draft immunotoxicity testing guidance document whose purpose is to provide a systematic approach for evaluating potential adverse immunological effects of medical devices and constituent materials (Langone, 1998). Immunotoxicity is any adverse effect on the function or structure of the immune system or other systems as a result of an immune system dysfunction. Adverse or immunotoxic effects occur when humoral or cellular immunity needed by the host to defend itself against infections or neoplastic disease (immunosuppression) or unnecessary tissue damage (chronic inflammation, hypersensitivity, or autoimmunity) is compromised. Potential immunological effects and responses that may be associated with one or more of these effects are presented in Table 2.4.

## 2.6  Summary

The identification of the fundamental biological requirements of a biomaterial first requires an identification of how the biomaterial is to be used and in what type of implant, medical device or prosthesis the biomaterial is to be used. Having identified the intended application of the biomaterial, the identification of the tissues that will contact the biomaterial and the implant duration of the biomaterial, medical device or prosthesis is necessary. Once these parameters have been defined, appropriate *in vitro* and *in vivo* assays can be selected to identify the success or failure of the biomaterial and its intended application. A broad perspective in the selection of *in vitro* and *in vivo* biocompatibility assays is necessary to not only identify adverse reactions but also to identify reactions that indicate the successful function of the biomaterial in its intended application. Adverse tissue responses do not necessarily reject a biomaterial from use in a medical device or prosthesis. Adverse tissue responses do require a risk assessment evaluation in which the risks are weighed against the benefits in the use of the biomaterial. A risk assessment program may involve additional biocompatibility testing in addition to the development of a rationale and justification for continued use of a biomaterial that may present with adverse tissue reactions. Finally, it must be remembered that appropriate and adequate biocompatibility evaluation requires testing of the material, medical device or prosthesis in its "end-use" state, that is, as a product in which manufacturing processes and sterilization procedures have been considered.

## References

AAMI Standards and Recommended Practices, Biological evaluation of medical devices, Association for the Advancement of Medical Instrumentation, Vol. 4. 1998. Vol. 4S, Supplement, (1997).

Anderson, J.M., Biological responses to materials, *Annu. Rev. Mater. Res.*, **31**, 81–110 (2001).

ASTM, American Society for Testing and Materials, *Annual book of ASTM standards*, ASTM F-619-97, Practice for Extraction of Medical Plastics; ASTM F-720-96, Practice for Testing Guinea Pigs for Contact Allergens: Guinea Pig Maximization Test; ASTM F-748-95, Practice for Selecting Generic Biological Test Methods for Materials and Devices; ASTM F-749-98, Practice for Evaluating Material Extracts by Intracutaneous Injection in the Rabbit; ASTM F-981-93, Practice for Assessment of Compatibility of Biomaterials (Nonporous) for Surgical Implants with Respect to Effect of Materials on Muscle and Bone; ASTM F-1439-96, Guide for the Performance of Lifetime Bioassay for the Tumorigenic Potential of Implant Materials; ASTM F-763-93, Practice for Short-Term Screening of Implant Materials (1999).

Chapekar, M.S., Regulatory concerns in the development of biologic–biomaterial combinations, *J. Biomed. Mater. Res. Appl. Biomater.*, **33**, 199–203 (1996).

FDA Blue Book Memorandum G95-1: FDA-modified version of ISO 10,993 — Part 1, *Biological evaluation of medical devices — Part 1: evaluation and testing* (1995).

ISO 10,993, *Biological evaluation of medical devices*, International Standards Organization, Geneva, Switzerland: ISO 10,993-1, Evaluation and testing; ISO 10,993-2, Animal welfare requirements; ISO 10,993-3, Tests for genotoxicity and reproductive toxicity; ISO 10,993-4, Selection of tests for interactions with blood; ISO 10,993-5, Tests for cytotoxicity: in vitro methods; ISO 10,993-6, Tests for local effects after implantation; ISO 10,993-7, Ethylene oxide sterilization residuals; ISO 10,993-9, Framework for the identification and quantification of potential degradation products; ISO 10,993-10, Tests for irritation and sensitization; ISO 10,993-11, Tests for systemic toxicity; ISO 10,993-12, Sample preparation and reference materials; ISO 10,993-13, Identification and quantification of degradation products from polymers; ISO 10,993-14, Identification and quantification of degradation products from ceramics; ISO 10,993-15, Identification and quantification of degradation products from metals and alloys; ISO 10,993-16, Toxicokinetic study design for degradation products and leachables.

Johnson, H.J., Northup, S.J., Seagraves, P.A., Atallah, M., Garvin, P.J., Lin, L., and Darby, T.D., Biocompatibility test procedures for materials evaluation *in vitro*. II. Objective methods of toxicity assessment, *J. Biomed. Mater. Res.*, **19**, 489–508 (1985).

Langone, J.J., *Immunotoxicity Testing Guidance*, Draft Document, Office of Science and Technology, Center for Devices and Radiological Health, Food and Drug Administration (1998).

Northup, S.J., Mammalian cell culture models, In: *Handbook of Biomaterials Evaluation: Scientific, Technical and Clinical Testing of Implant Materials*, von Recum, A.F., Ed., Macmillan, New York, pp. 209–225 (1986).

U.S. Pharmacopeia, *Biological reactivity tests in-vitro*, *U.S. Pharmacopeia 23*, Vol. 27. United States Pharmacopeial Convention, Inc., Rockville, MD (2004), 2173–2175.

Williams, D.F., Definitions in biomaterials, In: *Proceedings of a Consensus Conference of the European Society for Biomaterials*, Chester, England, March 3–5, 1986, Vol. 4. Elsevier, Amsterdam (1987).

Yamamoto, S., Urano, K., Koizumi, H., Wakana, S., Hioki, K., Mitsumori, K., Kurokawa, Y., Hayashi, Y., and Nomura, T., Validation of transgenic mice carrying the human prototype c-Ha-ras gene as a bioassay model for rapid carcinogenicity testing, *Environ. Health Perspect.*, **106** (Suppl. 1), 57–69 (1998).

# 3

# Cell–Material Interactions: Fundamental Design Issues for Tissue Engineering and Clinical Considerations

Gregory M. Harbers and David W. Grainger

## CONTENTS

## 3.1  Introduction

As discussed in accompanying chapters, all materials implanted into the human body, whether synthetic or natural, are instantly barraged with thousands of surface-active proteins, saccharides, lipids, and smaller molecule solutes found in all physiological fluids: multiple interfacial forces are involved in this adsorption, and several thousand known serum proteins participate in this response. Cells, as larger, slower diffusing species, arrive on an implant surface at later times, when smaller molecule adsorption processes are well-advanced kinetically and thermodynamically. In short, control of this biological adsorption response to biomaterials has proven extremely challenging. To date, all biomaterials developed or implanted react with physiological fluids to greater or lesser extents; none is "inert," none fully rejects this biological adsorption *in vivo*. Therefore, the biocompatible properties of all implanted biomaterials, however defined, are currently inseparable from ubiquitous adsorption of this interfacial protein film that directly apposes the host tissue. The surface competition eventually produces an adherent conditioning film of surface-adsorbed species of mixed composition and heterogeneity on all biomaterials. Biomaterials surface chemistry influences the kinetics and thermodynamics of this response, but often is observed empirically to exhibit a disappointing result *in vivo*: biomaterials integration with host cells and tissues, and desired biocompatibility performance requirements (i.e., healing) are often sub-optimal in many tissue compartments and surgical applications. Implanted surfaces cannot yet be reliably endowed with one of two frequently desired bio-performance endpoints to improve host integration: (1) biased, noncommensurate, selective uptake of extracellular matrix proteins found in trace quantities in serum to surfaces in order to promote reliable long-term cell adhesion, or (2) complete repulsion of all protein adsorption to render the surface nonbiologically reactive and perhaps noninflammatory.

A popular approach to improving the interface between materials and physiological systems, including blood and tissues, is to promote rapid and direct attachment of different cell types to the implanted biomaterial, either prior to (*ex vivo*) or immediately after (*in vivo*) implantation. In general, this can provide several desired responses, including biomaterial stabilization via cell attachment and tissue fixation, mitigating possible infection by reducing bacterial-surface attachment sites, and reduced thrombogenicity via biomaterial coverage with nonactivating cell surfaces. Two general surface properties are exploited for this purpose: (1) surface attachment of cell-specific adhesion ligands for cell receptor engagement, and (2) limited nonspecific protein adsorption that might interfere with cell-surface recognition. Many different approaches are reported towards these ends, including chemical grafting of known cell adhesion peptide sequences and motifs, direct, selective adsorption of extracellular matrix proteins containing cell adhesion domains from purified matrix solutions, and simultaneous repulsion of nonspecific protein adsorption complicating this response by using surface modification. To date, only limited success has been reported toward achieving these goals beyond simple *in vitro* studies. While this general strategy facilitates cell-surface contact and adhesion, it does not guarantee further steps essential to clinical utility of implantable cell-biomaterials constructs. These requirements include the biomaterial's continual maintenance of cell phenotype, proliferative and differentiation cues, recruitment and stability of multiple cell phenotypes in co-culture, potential to recapitulate tissue-like constructs, and synergy of cell behavior in coordinated ways with properties of the supporting biomaterial scaffolds.

## 3.2 Materials Requirements in Tissue Engineering

As an interdisciplinary approach combining life and biological sciences with materials science, transport and structural considerations, and surgical utility, tissue engineering seeks to develop suitable material-cell hybrid living constructs suitable to regenerate function for diseased and damaged tissues (Figure 3.1) (Atala and Lanza, 2002; Guilak et al., 2003; Saltzman, 2004). The approach attempts to overcome long-standing, classic limitations in less-complex implantation of biomaterials alone in engaging host cells and tissues to re-grow absent, compromised, or damaged tissues. Native tissue contains multiple cell types working together synergistically using constant tactile and biochemical communication, and organized in space to both optimally communicate in concert as well as with nerves and essential microvasculature (capillaries) to produce tissue function. Tissue engineering seeks to reproduce both form and function. In contrast to simpler precedent biomaterials designs, tissue engineering attempts the development of new materials or strategies directly combining living components (cells, tissue fragments) or their recruitment agents (chemokines, cytokines, drugs) into implantable delivery systems. Critically, the approach seeks device integration and functional tissue regeneration improvements to circumvent major clinical problems with biomaterials healing, donor tissue/organs that include organ scarcity, difficulty in matching donor organs with individual patients, chronic rejection, and cell/tissue morbidity.

Various tissue engineering approaches to regenerating form and function have been pursued, including: (1) injection of tissue-specific viable cells directly into damaged tissue (i.e., for Parkinson's or Alzheimer's mitigation), (2) encapsulation of specific cell types (i.e., pancreatic islets for diabetes) within synthetic permeable matrices that allow release of specific, therapeutic small molecules (i.e., insulin, dopamine) but prevent either host cytokines or immune cells from either entering, or encapsulated cells from escaping, and (3) to seed materials scaffolds with living cells *in vitro*, and then implant those hybrid cultured constructs within tissues or allow their maturation within artificial, well-controlled physiological surrogate environments prior to implantation (i.e., bioreactor culture). Materials scaffolds, or three-dimensional polymer matrices facilitating these behaviors with cells, have been developed in numerous initiatives, including the regeneration of skin, bone, cartilage, blood vessels, and peripheral nerves (Lanza et al., 2000). By strategy, the bulk scaffold architecture guides the organization and development of seeded or recruited cells to regenerate tissue mass and function, both *in vitro* and *in vivo*. This offers clinical utility beyond current limitations imposed by simpler biomaterials devices. As opposed to classic clinical biomaterials that fully supplant all native tissue function (primarily mechanical or structural) in surgical replacement or augmentation, tissue engineering scaffolds must exhibit an array of more complex, sophisticated properties to facilitate full and reliable recapitulation of tissue functional restoration. Beyond structural function, tissue engineering scaffolds designed as artificial bulk templates serve to mimic certain developmental aspects of the *in vivo* environment of the native extracellular matrix (ECM), providing more natural and controllable substrata and milieu to promote cell proliferation, differentiation, maintenance of natural phenotype, and ultimately function as a viable tissue-like living mass. Additional versatility to the approach includes incorporation of released bioactive substances and cellular cues within the scaffold for timed release at desired sites and times, controlled degradation of the scaffold over time to eliminate both undesired healing complications around permanent biomaterials and mass transport limitations for bulk tissue products, and some ability to control morphology and shape of the biomaterial and its co-habitating cellular fraction to duplicate tissue mass and dimensions *de novo*. These capabilities then mandate certain sophisticated materials requirements beyond conventional "biocompatibility" to be reliably coordinated and complementary to accomplish these performance goals combining living systems and implantable devices.

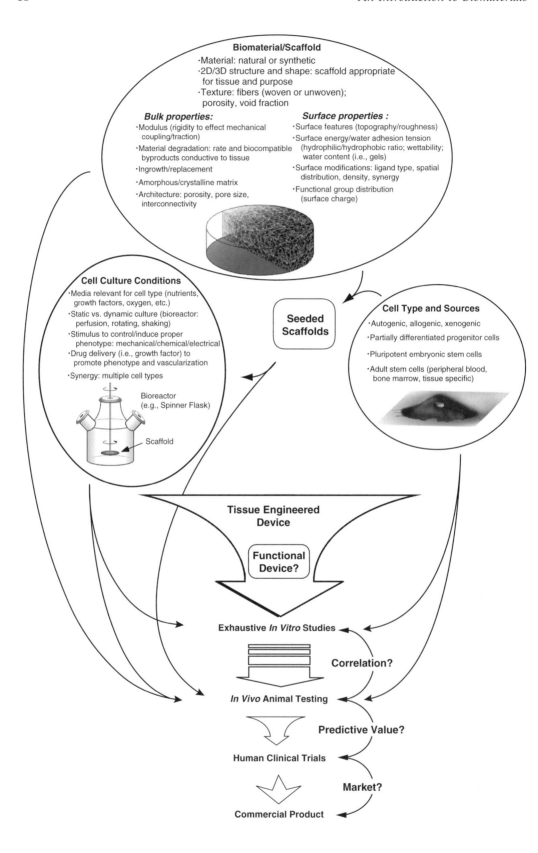

### 3.2.1 Scaffold Bulk Fabrication Issues

Tissue engineering scaffolds have been fabricated from both natural and synthetic materials using various methods including both conventional techniques used for decades with classical biomaterials (typically polymer molding, casting, foaming and leaching strategies, and network or gel formation methods), and more recently, more precise, bulk form-fidelity using rapid prototyping to help gain more control over critical design features using layer-by-layer computer-aided construction (Yeong et al., 2004). Beyond tissue-matched structural and mechanical requirements, other important tissue engineering-specific materials parameters to consider include: (1) a bulk, low-density material's porous, fibrillar or webbed macrostructure suitable to promote complete and homogeneous cell infiltration, adhesion, proliferation, and rapid endogenous matrix production; (2) suitable three-dimensional (3-D) (highly porous) surface with open geometry (interconnectivity) to facilitate mass transport (oxygen and metabolites in, catabolites out); (3) adequate surface morphology and materials physiochemical properties to encourage intracellular signaling, phenotypic expression, and further host cell recruitment; (4) mitigation of ubiquitous host inflammatory responses and chronic healing issues (see later chapters) that complicate tissue recapitulation *in situ*; (5) materials selection of natural or synthetic scaffold materials based on ease of processing, predictable degradation rates, nontoxic by-products, adequate mechanical properties (both surface and bulk), and host protein interactions, and (6) cell seeding techniques that ensure uniform distribution and sufficient cell density (Leong et al., 2003). Several of these considerations will be discussed in later chapters.

### 3.2.2 Bioactive Agents and Controlled Release in Tissue Engineering

An important set of design distinctions of the tissue engineering approach over conventional biomaterials implants is the ability to directly accommodate and implant living cells as tissue precursors, and the ability to release bioactive agents locally from the scaffold to the living components to prompt specific physiological responses in both space and time. Bioactive agent release is used to prompt interactions between the matrix and biological environment (i.e., cells and ECM components) as well as accelerate differentiation and tissue regeneration. Enhancements with this approach include the ability to control cell differentiation and morphology using known native mitogens and morphogens (Kirker-Head, 2000; Seeherman et al., 2002). Various bioactive molecules (e.g., signaling peptides, recombinant growth factors, synthetic drugs) have been released to improve materials interactions with cells (Gittens and Uludag, 2001; Chen and Mooney, 2003). Of particular current interest are the potent mitogens and morphogens, including PTH, VEGF, ILGF-1, BMPs, PDGF, NGF, TGF-beta 1, 2, and 3, KGF, EGF, FGF, and insulin, released locally from device surfaces. To date, only single-component release has been reported using selected biologically active substances with single kinetic regimes. This does not approximate the native physiological growth factor behavior in which multiple, interactive (pleiotropic) factors are produced or inhibited in tissue regenerative scenarios, using complex phasic patterns, both spatially and temporally, to control tissue form and function. Future scaffold designs will anticipate this complexity more accurately through

---

**FIGURE 3.1**
Tissue engineering as a hybrid discipline involving materials science and engineering, bioreactor conditions, biotechnology and cell biology, and functional assessments, resulting in combinations of *in vitro*, *in vivo* (preclinical animal work followed by human clinical studies), and product validation trials.

the use of multiple released bioactive agents chosen for specific functions at select temporal control points in endogenous tissue regeneration, and released in coordinated, perhaps synergistic, kinetic regimes.

### 3.2.3   Scaffold Design and Surface Chemistry

As summarized above in the Introduction and in later chapters, surface chemistry, as the initial and ultimate interface apposing implant material with host physiology, plays an important role in scaffold biomaterials design. The biological response to any implanted material is highly dependent on multiple temporal and distance-dependent interactions between the implant material's outermost surface atoms/molecules with physiological ions, molecular water, solutes, lipids and colloidal particles, proteins, and other macromolecules present in the complex biological milieu surrounding every implant (Andrade, 1973). This instant (initiated within microseconds upon implant exposure *in vivo*) interaction produces many different adsorption events and mechanisms related to the biomaterials chemistry that then redefines the interface as a heterogeneous biological conditioning film (Andrade, 1985; Malmsten, 1998). This adsorbed biological surface layer in turn then determines how cells that arrive at later times due to slower transport and diffusivity interact with the implanted surface (see later chapters). At the molecular level, both the scaffold micro-architecture and its surface chemical composition influence biomolecular adsorption interactions. Ultimately, these continuous, dynamic interfacial interactions determine the chemical and physiological reactivity and stability of the implant material *in vivo*, and its ability to function in the desired tissue engineering application. Because the scaffold surface characteristics determine the nature of the adsorbed interfacial layer, the acceptance, integration, and durability of an implant depend on these surface characteristics and their initial and eventual equilibrium behavior *in vivo* at the biomaterial–tissue interface.

While few strategies pretend to claim complete control over interfacial adsorption from full physiological solutions, several material methods attempt to modify or bias protein adsorption behavior to favor specific properties. Generally, these are categorized as adsorption of a conditioning film that either (1) eliminates (limits) cell recognition and reactivity (including platelet/blood coagulation activation) at the surface, or (2) promotes rapid cell integration and colonization of the scaffold. Certain limited surface chemistries (Figure 3.2) passively adsorb trace (from $\mu$g/ml serum concentration) ECM proteins from serum at sufficient density, with sufficient conformational accessibility, and sufficient tractability among more plentiful adsorbed non-ECM proteins (at mg/ml concentration, e.g., albumin, globulins, lipoproteins) to permit cell receptor access, engagement, and mechanical tension on surfaces. *These surfaces are considered "cell conducive" in serum, an important, distinguishing characteristic unfortunately found only on a minority of biomaterials.* Most other scaffold surfaces are not spontaneously cell conducive upon exposure to physiological milieu, possessing surface chemistries that adsorb conditioning films that

- passively drown adsorbed ECM protein access to cell receptors through excess adsorption of non-ECM proteins (e.g., albumin, $\sim 40$ mg/ml in serum, high diffusivity, highly surface active, ubiquitously adsorbed to all materials), resulting in surface densities of ECM components insufficient to support cell adhesion, or

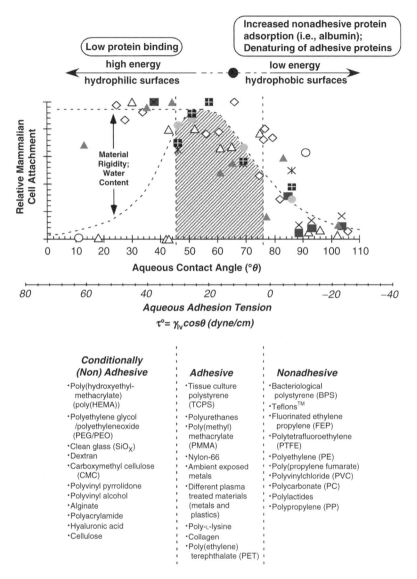

**FIGURE 3.2**
Empirically derived correlations between cell adhesion in serum cultures versus substrate surface water adhesion tension. Several studies have observed optima in this relationship where moderate surface polarity is associated with maximal cell adhesion. Substrate chemistries can be arbitrarily grouped into categories based on their surface water adhesion tension, interactions with serum proteins, and abilities to support cell adhesion. An aqueous contact angle of 65° has been defined as one possible division between hydrophilic and hydrophobic surfaces (Vogler, 1998), although such a division is meant to be correlative here. For water, $\gamma_{lv} = 72.8$ dyne/cm (Vogler, 1998). Data were compiled from van Wachem et al. (1985), Vogler and Bussian (1987), Tamada and Ikada (1994), Lee et al. (1998), and Vogler (1998). For comparison, each individual data set was normalized to one.

- denature key ECM proteins upon adsorption to limit their bioactivity and cell receptor recognition, or
- lack the necessary ECM adhesion strength (i.e., tractability or surface/bulk modulus coupling) to elicit or maintain the necessary mechanical traction forces produced by attached, spread cells critical for adhesion and ultimately matrix production and phenotypic expression.

Depending on the intended device application, (i.e., vascular blood-contacting, soft tissue, endocrine, or connective tissue replacement), several clinical considerations make *a la carte* selection of all of these surface properties and interactions with proteins possibly desirable. For example, highly albuminated surfaces exhibit low bacterial adhesion, low blood coagulation, and low cell attachment reactivity attractive to blood-contact applications. Tissue culture polystyrene retains sufficient fractions of tightly adsorbed ECM on this stiff polymer support to optimally culture cells *in vitro*. Significantly, most clinically approved biomaterials may possess attractive bulk properties (e.g., fatigue durability, bulk modulus, elasticity), but frequently lack surface properties suitable for the desired application (i.e., highly activating to blood coagulation, highly denaturing to proteins, or noncell conducive): many bulk materials used in clinical applications are often not cell conducive. Transforming the surfaces of these clinically interesting biomaterials with surface modification techniques to elicit selective cell adhesion and phenotypic expression for the tissue of interest provides value in improving noncell conducive, but otherwise clinically attractive biocompatible materials, into cell-conducive clinical materials. Such a transformation approach requires a rationale and strategy directed to tissue engineering requirements. Modifying the scaffold material surface throughout its bulk with cell-recognition ligands (i.e., known ECM peptide fragments, truncated or full ECM proteins, or recombinant growth factors) that facilitate ready cell receptor engagement for specific cell types, or exploitation of certain limited surface chemistries that facilitate selective, sufficient ECM adsorption from complex milieu *in situ* are most commonly pursued in this context. Both require careful manipulation and chemical control over surface properties prior to implantation to elicit cell-surface interactions. The former approach places the biochemical requirements for cell recognition and attachment on the scaffold surface, hoping that the ubiquitous adsorbed conditioning film does not bury them to approaching cells, while the second approach seeks to bias natural uptake of sufficient ECM from host fluids to impart cell-conducive behavior both in culture and postimplantation. To fully appreciate requirements to effectively interface cells, scaffolds and biomolecules together in viable tissue engineering constructs, more performance aspects of the material's chemistry, physiological environment in which the material/scaffold resides and extracellular matrix requirements for regenerating the tissue of interest is imperative. Other essential design considerations, including mass transport, bulk structural needs, drug release, and degradation considerations, are not further addressed in this chapter.

Tissue engineering scaffold materials are selected for cell culture capabilities based on both their bulk and surface properties. Bulk properties define the material's modulus, elasticity, mechanical and structural properties. As described below, these mechanical properties are important to cell culture efficiency: adhesion, proliferation, and phenotypic expression. Surface properties have been empirically correlated to cell attachment efficiency for decades. Figure 3.2 shows an important correlation between surface energy (most readily described by the aqueous contact angle, or degree of surface wetting by water) and cell attachment from serum-containing cultures. The classical interfacial energy descriptor, the Young equation (Adamson and Gast, 1997; Morra, 2001), is often applied to use experimentally determined contact angles (wetting) to calculate resulting surface energies. However, this equation best applies to HOMOGENEOUS/SMOOTH/RIGID material surfaces where surface disparities are sub-micron in size. This treatment does not apply to heterogeneous biomaterials where porosity, chemical surface heterogeneity, roughness from topology, fiber weaves, or etching, surface rearrangement or softness, elasticity, or release of active agents are encountered. Unfortunately, most biomaterials do not suit these ideal requirements, mandating approximations from idealized methods and model materials.

At higher surface energy (reduced contact angle, increased aqueous wetting) on rigid surfaces, cell attachment is generally enhanced, compared to very low surface energy (more hydrophobic) surfaces. This can be rationalized as an intrinsic ability of the surface to promote adsorption of ECM proteins from culture milieu at sufficient density and adsorptive strength and with maintenance of adhesion motif integrity to both promote cell receptor engagement and facilitate cell-induced traction forces and tension to produce a spread phenotype. This cell attachment trend on more rigid materials is consistent across most of the higher surface energy spectrum (for water contact angles $0° < \theta < 75°$). By contrast, on polymeric bulk materials an optimum in the surface energy for cell attachment is frequently observed in serum-containing culture. In this case, high polymer surface energy correlates with high wetting but also increased solubility in water. To prevent dissolution, high surface energy polymers are cross-linked into insoluble biomaterial networks (hydrogels). However, despite being cross-linked, this thermodynamically favored interaction with water remains: gel bulk matrix swelling, reduced mechanical modulus, and increased surface elasticity all combine with increased gel water content to both reduce protein adsorption necessary for cell recognition and attachment, and reduce mechanical force transduction elicited by attaching cells on these matrices. The combined result is that attaching cells on swollen hydrogels cannot find sufficient matrix, and in locations where matrix proteins are present (e.g., by pre-adsorption from pure solutions) cell receptors cannot produce sufficient mechanical transduction to promote cell spreading and proliferation. As substrate surface energy decreases, both mechanical properties (from reduced hydration and bulk swelling) and serum protein adsorption properties increase, eventually producing the optimal cell culture surface observed in this figure. At highest contact angles (lowest surface energies, most hydrophobic surfaces), interfacial tension in aqueous media is high, and surface hydration energy is low and unfavorable, producing minimal swelling and therefore minimal loss in surface mechanical properties, and promoting serum protein adsorptive replacement of interfacial surface water in a protein-denaturing response that unfolds interior, hydrophobic protein domains onto the biomaterial surface to exchange solvation water (Andrade, 1985; Adamson and Gast, 1997; Malmsten, 1998; Morra, 2001). Globular non-ECM proteins (e.g., albumins, globulins), the most abundant in serum, lack cell-recognition sites. Hence, these low energy surfaces typically exhibit low cell-conducive behavior.

Surface energies for solids as defined by the empirical factor, critical surface tension (Andrade, 1985; von Recum, 1994; Adamson and Gast, 1997), are frequently correlative to the onset of biologically interesting parameters (e.g., cell adhesion). Critical surface tensions near $40\,\text{mN/m}$ ( $=$ dynes/cm) define an empirical threshold between cell attachment and nonattachment. For example, PTFE (Teflon™) exhibits a critical surface tension of $18.5\,\text{mN/m}$, and an aqueous contact angle of $\sim108°$) and in serum exhibits substantial protein uptake but very little cell attachment. By contrast, tissue culture polystyrene, a cell adhesion standard, has a critical surface tension value of $\sim64\,\text{mN/m}$ (value estimated from Vogler, 1998). Empirical correlations argue for using water adhesion tension ($\tau°$) as a possible metric in predicting how materials will behave in response to protein adsorption and subsequent long-term biological response (Vogler, 1998; 1999). That is, measured critical surface tensions and their comparison with aqueous water adhesion tension are long-time foci for predicting biological reactivity (Andrade, 1985; Malmsten, 1998; Morra, 2001). Figure 3.2 categorizes some materials into classes that fit this simplistic empirical relationship between *aqueous adhesion tension and cell adhesion from serum milieu*. This relationship has some notable exceptions: water's interaction with polar, nonswelling, rigid surfaces produces distinct cellular behavior from that resulting from water's more complex behavior with swellable, nonrigid surfaces. Well-known differences between significant cell adhesion to hydrophilic clean glass (rigid, contact angle $\sim0°$)

contrasted to poor cell adhesion observed for hydrophilic swollen polymer surfaces (compliant hydrogels, contact angle $\sim 20°$) is a prominent example of these differences where substrate effects beyond simple energy interpretations, but involving more complex effects of interfacial hydration, must be considered.

Typically, as polymer hydrogels are generally benign and practical materials for several implant and controlled drug release applications, they must be chemically grafted with cell adhesion motifs, either within the network or on their surface, in order to interact reliably with cells, especially in tissue engineering strategies (Mann et al., 2001; Sakiyama-Elbert and Hubbell, 2001; Schmidt and Leach, 2003). Grafting very hydrophilic, water-swollen substrates with cell adhesion peptides exploits both the properties of a low-background material (i.e., minimal nonspecific protein adsorption) with high cell specificity (grafted adhesion domains), a unique trait not found in many biomaterials. Newer matrix fabrication methods are incorporating cell-recognized and enzyme-cleavable protein domains, creating hybrid materials that respond to local cellular reactions.

## 3.3 ECM Molecules as Essential Determinants of Cell Adhesion and Expression

The ECM comprises a multitude of different proteins and proteoglycans mixed into an intricate network of macromolecules expressed, secreted, deposited, and processed by, and also fully surrounding, cells within tissues. ECM is initially produced as a soluble mix of biopolymers that are processed and enzymatically assembled into an organized network lattice structure by cell membrane-based enzymes and receptors. Cells surround themselves by this matrix, anchoring and orienting using membrane-based receptors that engage and couple to ECM both mechanically and chemically. In connective tissues such as bone, skin, and cartilage, ECM comprises a larger portion, by volume, of the tissue compared with the cells. Additionally, different tissue types exhibit ECM of different biochemical compositions and perhaps different mechanical properties to accommodate or guide cell expression and tissue function. Attachment-dependent cell types must interact with the ECM to ensure proper development, migration, proliferation, shape and function (Alberts et al., 1994; Grzesik and Robey, 1994). Proteoglycans and other glycoproteins bearing specific saccharide sequences, and fibrous proteins, either structural (collagen, elastin) or adhesive (fibronectin, laminin) (Alberts et al., 1994), somehow select for specific cell types. Saccharide units comprise the minority mass component, but because of their substantial hydration volume, represent most of the ECM volume fraction. For this brief ECM discussion, the matrix proteins are classified as either collagenous or noncollagenous biopolymers.

### 3.3.1 Components of the ECM

The collagens, the major component of skin and bone, represent a family of 15 structural proteins constituting roughly 25% of the total protein mass in mammals. Fibrillar collagens (types I, II, III, V, and XI, with type I as most abundant) are found in connective tissues. Once secreted into the ECM, collagen aggregates to form "rope-like" triple helix (10 to 300 nm diameter) fibrils that often further aggregate to form collagen fibers. Other types of collagens have been grouped into the fibril-associated and network-forming collagens (Alberts et al., 1994).

Glycosaminoglycans (GAGs) are nonproteinaceous (hence, noncollagenous) ECM components comprising unbranched polysaccharide chains of repeating disaccharide units. Each disaccharide typically contains an amino sugar (N-acetylglucosamine or N-acetylgalactosamine), often sulfated, and a uronic acid (glucuronic or iduronic) pairing. Due to the high sulfate and carboxyl content, GAGs are highly negatively charged and thus extremely hydrophilic, producing extended hydrated GAG chains forming networks and gels. This swelling or gel-like behavior ensures that GAGs occupy most of the extracellular space even though they only comprise about 10% by weight of all the ECM proteins (Alberts et al., 1994). Chondroitin sulfates, heparans, and hyaluronic acids are the three most abundant GAGs in ECM.

GAGs generally covalently bind ECM proteins to form brush-like, highly hydrated *proteoglycans*, a specific class of *glycoproteins*. In addition to providing hydrated space around and between cells, proteoglycans are thought to be involved in intercellular signaling. Additionally, GAGs on proteoglycans or alone can bind and regulate other secreted proteins like proteases, protease inhibitors, and growth factors (Alberts et al., 1994). A consequence of this binding is the formation of local tissue-bound reservoirs of enzyme inhibitors and potent cell signaling growth factors or other cytokines (for a review of proteoglycans, see Hardingham and Fosang, 1992). Importantly, the cell surface is densely decorated with a variety of glycoproteins, GAGs and proteoglycans, providing a diverse biochemical matrix of unique hydration and binding capability. This property, combined with the actions of membrane-spanning cell ECM-specific receptors (i.e., integrins, see below) endow the cell membrane surface with multiple capabilities to interact with the ECM surrounding each cell. Faithful recapitulation of this chemical and bio-structural ECM environment appears to be important in tissue-engineered devices to produce cell responses desired for functional devices. However, due to their intrinsic chemical and architectural complexity, proteoglycans represent the least understood and poorest mimicked aspect of ECM in tissue engineered products.

Interactions between cell-surface proteoglycans and glycoproteins (e.g., heparin and heparin-like carbohydrates) and ECM proteins are electrostatic by nature. Cardin and Weintraub identified consensus heparin-binding sequences found in adhesive ECM proteins (e.g., vitronectin, fibronectin, laminin, and bone sialoprotein) of the form XBBXBX and XBBBXXBX (X: hydrophobic amino acid; B: positively charged amino acid) (Cardin and Weintraub, 1989; Hubbell, 1995). The positively charged basic amino acids (B) located in the ECM heparin-binding domains interact with the negatively charged sulfate and carboxylate groups found in proteoglycans. These electrostatic interactions are powerful in physiology, allowing general cell surface attachment with certain basic protein domains in ECM, independent of receptor engagement. Recently, these interactions have been exploited in tissue engineering applications to make biomedical hydrogels based on heparin-binding domains (Sakiyama et al., 1999). Surfaces grafted with both heparin-binding cofactors and integrin-binding peptides (i.e., RGD containing peptides), exhibit a more complete cellular response (e.g., cell attachment, spreading, focal contact formation, and cytoskeletal organization) (Laterra et al., 1983; Woods et al., 1986; Dalton et al., 1995; Rezania and Healy, 1999).

More specific cell attachment and interaction with ECM noncollagenous proteins, including osteopontin (OPN), bone sialoprotein (BSP), fibronectin (FN), vitronectin (VN), osteonectin (OSN), and thrombospondin (TS), or with other cells, requires cell surface adhesion receptors. Receptor sub-families include the integrins, the Ig superfamily, the selectins, the cadherins, leucine-rich glycoproteins (LRG) (i.e., decorin, biglycan), mucins, and CD44 (Horton, 1995). Each receptor type recognizes and binds specific protein domains present on ECM proteins, including collagens. The ECM noncollagenous proteins (see Table 3.1) exhibit conserved motifs in their sequence that engage with

**TABLE 3.1**

Extracellular Matrix (ECM) Adhesion Proteins and Their Known Cell-Binding Domains Paired with Specific Cell Membrane Integrin Receptors with which They Interact (Receptor–Ligand Pair) (Hynes, 1987, 1992, 2002; Albelda and Buck, 1990; Komoriya et al., 1991; Ruoslahti, 1991; Staatz et al., 1991; Aota et al., 1994; Haas and Plow, 1994; Akiyama et al., 1995; Hubbell, 1995; Elbert and Hubbell, 1996; Flores et al., 1996; Bhatnagar et al., 1997; Rezania et al., 1997; Bayless et al., 1998; Denda et al., 1998; Huber et al., 1998; Krutzsch et al., 1999; Rezania and Healy, 1999; Anselme, 2000; Barry et al., 2000; Calzada et al., 2003; Podolnikova et al., 2003; Yamamoto et al., 2003; Bamdad et al., 2004; Lishko et al., 2004; Mercado et al., 2004)

| ECM Protein | Peptide Binding Sites | Integrin Receptors | Proteoglycan Binding Region |
|---|---|---|---|
| Collagen | RGD, DGEA, GFOGER (Helical), GTPGPQGIAGQRGVV (P15) | $\alpha_1\beta_1, \alpha_2\beta_1, \alpha_{10}\beta_1, \alpha_{11}\beta_1, \alpha_3\beta_1, \alpha_{IIb}\beta_3$ | |
| Laminin | RGD, IKVAV, YIGSR, PDSGR, RNIAEIIKDA | $\alpha_1\beta_1, \alpha_2\beta_1, \alpha_3\beta_1, \alpha_6\beta_1, \alpha_7\beta_1, \alpha_6\beta_1, \alpha_{IIb}\beta_3$ | PRRARV |
| Fibronectin | RGD, EILDV, REDV, PHSRN | $\alpha_3\beta_1, \alpha_4\beta_1, \alpha_5\beta_1, \alpha_V\beta_1, \alpha_{IIb}\beta_3,$ $\alpha_V\beta_3, \alpha_V\beta_6, \alpha_8\beta_1, \alpha_4\beta_7, \alpha_V\beta_5$ | |
| Vitronectin | RGD | $\alpha_V\beta_1, \alpha_V\beta_3, \alpha_V\beta_5, \alpha_V\beta_8, \alpha_8\beta_1, \alpha_{IIb}\beta_3$ | |
| Osteopontin | RGD, SLAYGLR, SVVYGLR, LDV | $\alpha_V\beta_3, \alpha_4\beta_1, \alpha_8\beta_1, \alpha_9\beta_1, \alpha_V\beta_1, \alpha_V\beta_5, \alpha_5\beta_1$ | |
| Bone Sialoprotein (BSP) | RGD, NGEPRGDTYRAY | $\alpha_V\beta_3, \alpha_{IIb}\beta_3$ | FHRRIKA |
| Thrombospondin Superfamily | RGD, FQGVLQNVRFVE, VTXG | $\alpha_V\beta_3, \alpha_1\beta_1, \alpha_3\beta_1, \alpha_4\beta_1, \alpha_6\beta_1, \alpha_{IIb}\beta_3$ | |
| Tenascin C | RGD, VFDNFVLK | $\alpha_7\beta_1, \alpha_8\beta_1, \alpha_9\beta_1, \alpha_V\beta_6$ | |
| Fibrinogen | RGD | $\alpha_M\beta_2, \alpha_{IIb}\beta_3, \alpha_5\beta_1$ | |

cell receptors. These receptors represent the second, powerful, yet more specific cell attachment mechanism to matrix surrounding them, as well as to ECM deposited by adsorption, onto biomaterials surfaces. The integrin receptor family has been studied extensively for over two decades and continues to attract considerable research attention for its importance in cell–substratum adhesion, and to a lesser extent cell–cell adhesion and aggregation (Hynes, 2002, 2004).

### 3.3.2 Cell-Surface Integrin Receptors

The integrin superfamily is the cell's central interaction and control feature with extracellular matrix adhesion proteins, maintaining the integrity of cells and tissues while integrating cellular function and the many diverse signals that impinge on cells (Hynes, 1987, 1992; Hubbell, 1995; Horwitz, 1997). Integrins are essential to many biological phenomena and disorders including embryonic development, thrombosis, blood clotting, wound healing, inflammation, rheumatoid arthritis, cancer, and osteoporosis (Hynes, 1992; Horwitz, 1997). Most mediate cell–substratum adhesion using ECM protein engagement, although some mediate cell–cell adhesion as well as cell–cell aggregation (Hynes, 1992; Horwitz, 1997). Since integrins are membrane-spanning proteins, they establish a two-way communication between inside and outside the cell. Within the cell, depending on integrin-coupled signals from the cytoplasm, integrins become recruited and concentrated to certain membrane locations by lateral diffusion, and active or inactive through a conformational change (Hynes, 1992; Horwitz, 1997; Calderwood, 2004). Outside the cell, integrin binding to ECM sites, and associated stimuli from this cell mechanical coupling to its local environment, transduce signals into the cell to set off potent signaling cascades towards the nucleus, resulting in regulation of genome, protein expression and phenotypic modulation (see Figure 3.3). These outside-in integrin-mediated signals constantly feedback environmental factors to cellular responses, ultimately determining the fate of a cell as shown in Figure 3.3 by converting mechanical stimuli into biochemical signaling (e.g., mechanotransduction). Resulting gene expression regulates normal cell functions such as cell motility, proliferation, cytoskeletal organization, cell survival (e.g., apoptosis), and protein production that cues signals to other cells upon release (Horwitz, 1997). As a critical cellular environmental sensing element and molecular "glue" to ECM, integrins are *integral* to the signal transduction pathways necessary for normal cell phenotypic expression and maintenance.

The active integrin receptor consists of carefully paired transmembrane subunit heterodimers comprising noncovalently associated α and β glycoprotein subunits linked through their extracellular globular domains in a calcium ion-dependent manner, forming a single hydrophobic transmembrane sequence (Sato et al., 1994). Currently, as shown in Figure 3.4, 18 α and 8 β subunits combine to form 26 known α/β receptor combinations, each with slightly different ECM site specificity (Albelda and Buck, 1990; Hubbell, 1995). Figure 3.4 shows the association of the different integrin subunit combinations and the major ECM proteins with which they are known to interact. Structurally, the α subunits (120 to 180 kDa) are larger than the β subunits (90 to 110 kDa) (Hynes, 1992). with short cytoplasmic domains ($\leq 50$ amino acids), and longer extracellular domains ($\alpha > 100$ kd; $\beta > 75$ kd). The ECM motif ligand binding site is located within the fold created from α/β dimerization. Importantly, the cytoplasmic portion of the integrin must be anchored to the cytoskeleton through formation of complexes between focal adhesion plaques composed of numerous cytoplasmic proteins found (focal adhesion kinases, paxillin, tensin, vinculin, talin, α-actinin, etc.) and the integrin cytoplasmic tails (Horwitz, 1997). Integrin clustering affects the strength of ECM adhesion, hence developing interactive biomaterials with spatially defined clusters

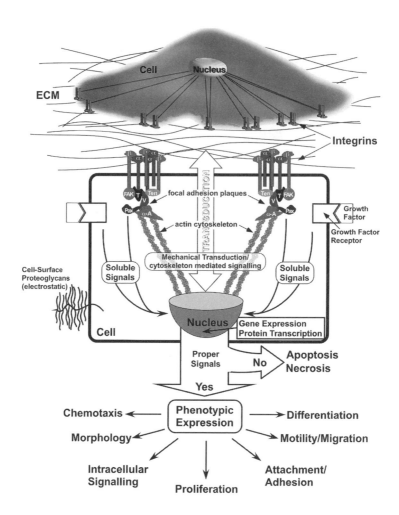

**FIGURE 3.3**
Global "outside-in" signaling pathways for cells interacting with extracellular matrix (ECM). Signaling routes — haptotactic receptor-mediated or soluble signal-induced — proceed from extracellular receptor engagement through the membrane to the cytoplasm and eventually to the nucleus. Abbreviations: FAK (focal adhesion kinase), T (talin), V (vinculin), Ten (tensin), Pax (paxillin), α-A (α-actinin). (Adapted from Figure 4–12 in Cotran, 1999 with permission from Elsevier.)

of cell adhesion ligands recognized by adhesion receptors may promote cell adhesion and ultimately phenotype (Koo et al., 2002). However, evidence also exists to suggest that if cells are too adherent, unable to detach, no migration or proliferation will ensue, resulting in cell senescence, and apoptosis (Truskey and Proulx, 1993).

## 3.4  Peptide and Protein Ligand Surface Density and Accessibility Effects

### 3.4.1  Ligand Density

As previously addressed, a critical goal of tissue engineering is to control and guide the attachment, proliferation, and phenotypic expression of cells from the cell–material interface into the scaffold, ultimately to produce a viable and functional tissue surrogate.

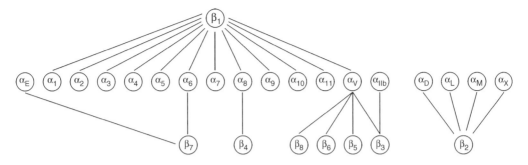

| Cell Receptor | ECM Ligands |
|---|---|
| $\alpha_1\beta_1$ | Col-I, -IV, LM, TSP |
| $\alpha_2\beta_1$ | Col-I, -IV, LM, FN, Cha |
| $\alpha_3\beta_1$ | FN, LM, VN, Col-I, EP, Nid, Ent |
| $\alpha_4\beta_1$ | FN, VCAM-1, IN, TSP |
| $\alpha_5\beta_1$ | FN, FB |
| $\alpha_6\beta_1$ | LM-1, -2, -4, -5 (*in vitro* only), TSP |
| $\alpha_7\beta_1$ | LM-1, TN-C |
| $\alpha_8\beta_1$ | FN, TN-C, VN, OP |
| $\alpha_9\beta_1$ | TN-C, OP |
| $\alpha_{10}\beta_1$ | Col, FN |
| $\alpha_{11}\beta_1$ | Col |
| $\alpha_v\beta_1$ | FN, VN |
| $\alpha_D\beta_2$ | VCAM-1 |
| $\alpha_L\beta_2$ | ICAM-1 to –3 |
| $\alpha_M\beta_2$ | C3bi, ICAM-1, FX, FB |
| $\alpha_X\beta_3$ | C3bi(?), FB |
| $\alpha_v\beta_3$ | VN, FB, FN, vWF, TSP, OP, BSP, cytotactin/tenascin, HIV Tat Protein |
| $\alpha_{IIb}\beta_3$ | FN, FB, VN, vWF, Col, TSP, LM |
| $\alpha_6\beta_4$ | LM-1, BM |
| $\alpha_v\beta_5$ | VN, FN, HIV Tat protein, BSP, OP |
| $\alpha_v\beta_6$ | FN, cytotactin/tenascin |
| $\alpha_E\beta_7$ | E-Cad |
| $\alpha_4\beta_7$ | VCAM-1, ACAM-1, MadCAM, FN |
| $\alpha_v\beta_8$ | VN |

Fibronectin (FN), laminin (LM), vitronectin (VN), collagen (Col), epiligrin (Ep), nidogen (Nid), entactin (Ent), invasin (IN), addressin cell adhesion molecule (ACAM), fibrinogen (FB), thrombospondin (Tsp), Von Willebrand factor (vWF), osteopontin (OP), bone sialoprotein (BSP), factor X (FX), basement membrane (BM), mucosal addressin cell adhesion molecule (MadCAM), vascular cell adhesion molecule (VCAM), tenascin C (TN-C), intercellular cell adhesion molecule (ICAM), condroadherin (Cha), E cadherin (E-Cad) and complement peptide (C3bi).

**FIGURE 3.4**
Cell integrin receptor subunit pairings and biological specificity for adhesion motifs on cell types. (Hynes, 1987, 2002; Albelda and Buck, 1990; Ruoslahti, 1991; Haas and Plow, 1994; Milner et al., 1999; Anselme, 2000; Wehrle-Haller and Imhof, 2003; Lai and Cheng, 2005; see additional Refs. in Table 3.1).

Ideally, such cell–materials behavior should be reliable and predictable by device design and construction. One parameter known to significantly affect cell-proliferation kinetics and function is the density of surface attachment motifs (i.e., ligands), whether short synthetic peptides or whole proteins from the ECM. Direct physisorption of entire, native ECM adhesive proteins (e.g., plasma, serum, or purified fibronectin, vitronectin, collagen, or mixtures) to biomaterials surfaces remains a popular route to modify materials to improve cell–material interactions. Exposure to complete plasma is most relevant because it closely (although not exactly) duplicates what happens when surfaces are placed in a corporeal environment (uncontrolled protein adsorption). This is an important distinction when performing *in vitro* controlled culturing conditions. However, simple physisorption from serum often denatures many proteins, causing conformational changes that can alter their cell receptor affinity or availability (i.e., to cell integrins). Orientation of the adsorbed protein can make the active cell-binding domain inaccessible to cell receptors, thus preventing ligand–receptor engagement and subsequent cell attachment or signaling (Grainger et al., 2003). Furthermore, competitive adsorption from serum often obeys a mass action law (Krishnan et al., 2004), meaning that high mass fraction proteins in plasma (e.g., albumin, globulins, not trace ECM proteins) adsorb at high densities, precluding sufficient adsorbed densities of ECM required for cell attachment. Hence, both surface-adsorbed protein composition and conformation must support cell attachment. This is difficult to predict and reliably accomplish on most biomaterial scaffolds used for tissue engineering from serum. Hence, purified or compositionally biased ECM proteins can be directly pre-adsorbed to biomaterials prior to surgical placement in order to encourage cell attachment. However, to elicit favorable cellular responses, required surface densities of adsorbed proteins need to be substantially higher than when short ECM protein fragments, or cell adhesion peptides, are grafted to surfaces (Massia and Hubbell, 1991). For grafted adhesion peptides, the orientation of the grafted peptide and hence the active integrin binding-site are known and more accessible compared with physisorbed full proteins with unknown surface conformations and orientations. Consequently, ever since the pioneering work of Pierschbacher and Ruoslahti (1984) who first identified the ubiquitous integrin-binding Arg–Gly–Asp (RGD) peptide domain in fibronectin and demonstrated that minimal amino acid sequences possess binding affinities similar to that of the parent full protein, substantial work has focused on identifying and studying the minimal peptide sequences from a number of the adhesive ECM proteins sufficient to encourage cell binding (see Table 3.1). These motifs have been exploited in surface modification strategies to control cell–material interactions as well as for use in developing new peptide drugs (e.g., eptifibatide, Integrilin™). Short protein fragment immobilization is attractive since surface density, orientation, and accessibility can all be controlled, thus yielding cell-conducive materials with more predictable, reliable interfacial behavior. This is an essential performance feature for tissue engineering. Cell adhesion peptides are also easily synthesized, purified and sterilized, they are relatively inexpensive, do not rely on tertiary structure for bioactivity, are less susceptible to enzymatic degradation, more readily chemically immobilized on surfaces, less likely to elicit an immunogenic response, and do not denature.

The RGD sequence found within many adhesion proteins (see Table 3.1) and recognized by many integrin receptors has been most often studied (Hersel et al., 2003). However, functional substitution of short peptides to mimic entire ECM proteins must also consider amino acids flanking the known binding site. Cell receptor affinity and specificity are optimized by accounting for amino acids surrounding the binding site, possibly introduced by some secondary structure. Hence, ECM components from the tissue of interest are best inspected for "helper" sequences found within those proteins to include in ECM peptide surrogates. Numerous studies have demonstrated the importance of the flanking amino acids in determining the activity and specificity of RGD and other ligands. Slight changes adjacent to the ligand diminish or abolish cell-binding activity (Pierschbacher and Ruoslahti, 1984; Hautanen et al., 1989; Maeda et al., 1991; Bogusky et al., 1992; Horton et al., 1993; Sato et al., 1994). For example, the sequence GRGDSP was shown to have a much higher binding affinity compared to the reduced sequence RGDS, and when the central Gly was replaced with a Val, integrin activity was abolished. Similarly, replacement of the flanking Asp with a Phe (RGDD → RGDF) required a 200-fold increase in ligand concentration to produce similar inhibition effects from the snake venom, echistatin (Sato et al., 1994). Often, peptides with scrambled binding sites (e.g., RGD → RDG) or with Glu (E) substituted for Asp (D) (RGD → RGE) are used as negative experimental controls since such changes abolish integrin activity. Secondary peptide structure can be important as well, as evidenced by the greater activity of cyclic peptides containing the RGD sequence compared to their linear counterparts (Horton et al., 1993; Cardarelli et al., 1994; Yamada et al., 1994). Taken together, it is imperative that the flanking amino acids are considered when designing new peptides to elicit specific biological activities.

A substantial body of literature exists reporting the effects of peptide adhesion ligand density on both short-term (cell attachment, spreading, adhesion plaque formation (e.g., focal contacts), and cell migration) and long-term (e.g., cell differentiation and phenotypic expression) cellular events on model biomaterials (Brandley and Schnaar, 1988; Danilov and Juliano, 1989; Massia and Hubbell, 1990; Massia and Hubbell, 1991; Rezania and Healy, 2000; Hersel et al., 2003). For example, Massia and Hubbell (1991) showed that cell adhesion, spreading and focal contact formation *in vitro* was dependent on immobilized RGD ligand density. Using fibroblasts, they demonstrated that cell spreading required a minimum RGD ligand density of 1 fmol/cm$^2$, while cell spreading and focal contact formation required a minimum density of 10 fmol/cm$^2$ on rigid surfaces modified with RGD-containing peptides. Surface rigidity or elasticity changes these minimum required densities dramatically (see Section 3.6). Hence, peptide immobilization strategies must consider both the material and tissue-derived cells of interest.

In addition to cell spreading and focal adhesion formation, cell adhesion ligand density as well as integrin–ligand binding affinities and the degree of integrin expression (i.e., number of available cell receptors) affect both the strength of attachment and the extent of cell migration and thus cell phenotype (DiMilla et al., 1992, 1993; Palecek et al., 1997). At low ligand densities, cell motility is limited due to the lack of available binding sites, but that at high ligand densities, the surface is too adhesive, or "sticky," so that cell locomotion is severely restricted. For example, with increasing concentrations of physisorbed fibronectin on glass, the attachment strength of smooth muscle cells increased linearly, but a biphasic relationship was shown to exist for migration speed due to the "stickiness" of the surface (DiMilla et al., 1992, 1993). Additionally, at high ligand densities, both the rate of cell spreading and the strength of detachment were shown to plateau, thus demonstrating possible saturation of available surface receptors. In fact, cell migration influences proliferation, and it has been theorized that an optimal ligand density exists for cell migration and ultimately phenotypic expression (Zygourakis et al., 1991a,b; Mooney et al., 1995; Ward et al., 1995; Lauffenberger and Horwitz, 1996; Saterbak and Lauffenburger, 1996). Because the ability of cells to proliferate and differentiate depends on the ability to disengage their cell-surface connections, cell capability to develop phenotypically and ultimately form viable tissue is intimately intertwined with properties of receptor–ligand engagement. As one example, longer-term events such as osteoblast-like cells expressing their proper phenotype and developing a mineralized matrix has been shown to depend on ligand densities on RGD-modified materials (Rezania et al., 1999; Rezania and Healy, 2000) as well as on surfaces preadsorbed with different concentrations of whole bone sialoprotein, a major noncollagenous ECM protein found within bone ECM (Zhou et al., 1995).

### 3.4.2 Ligand Accessibility

Intuitively, the ability of a cell contacting an engineered surface to readily find and effectively engage the adsorbed or grafted ligand (ECM protein or surrogate peptide) is critical for developing effective biomimetic materials for tissue engineering. Ligand accessibility depends on two factors; namely, the ligand must extend a sufficient distance from the surface and must not be masked (buried) by adsorbing proteins in the culture milieu. The latter requirement, not described here in further detail, has been addressed by developing surface modification methods and film coatings that attempt to minimize nonspecific protein adsorption (i.e., surface grafting polyethylene glycol (PEG) or dextran (Ratner et al., 2004)). This problem remains a formidable challenge for all materials immersed in physiological milieu. The former technical requirement has been most often addressed by using different tether chemistries and chain lengths to graft active ligands (Francis et al., 1998; Hern and Hubbell, 1998; Dori et al., 2000; Houseman and Mrksich, 2001). For example, Hern and Hubbell incorporated an RGD peptide with and without a 3400 MW PEG spacer into a photopolymerized cross-linked hydrogel network of PEG-diacrylate. After 24 h in serum-containing media (important!), hydrogels without RGD peptide only supported spreading of 5% of seeded foreskin fibroblasts. When RGD or RDG (inactive control) peptides were incorporated into the hydrogels without the spacer chain, these scaffolds supported only ~50 and 15% of cell spreading, respectively. However, when the RGD or RDG peptides were coupled to the 3400 MW spacer chain and then incorporated into the network, the hydrogels supported 70 and 0% spreading, respectively. Gels without spacer chain tethers supported minimal nonspecific cell spreading, presumably only through contact with trace amounts of adsorbed serum proteins expected on this hydrogel surface. Addition of the spacer chain produced specific receptor–ligand engagement as evidenced by the active versus inactive control comparisons. In another study, Houseman and Mrksich (2001) used RGD peptides grafted to different oligo(ethylene glycol) (EG) units (i.e., tri, tetra, penta, and hexa EG oligomers) on gold supports as nonfouling bioactive surfaces. As EG chain length increased, 3T3 fibroblast attachment, spreading, and adhesion strength decreased even though peptide density remained constant. Presumably, this can be related to both surface mechanical properties (i.e., modulus) as well as ligand accessibility and altering steric hindrance. In another demonstration of accessibility effects, Dori et al. (2000) created Langmuir–Blodgett lipid membranes on mica composed of either PEG lipids with different length head groups or binary mixtures (50:50) of collagen-like peptide amphiphiles and PEG lipids. On surfaces with only the PEG lipids, human melanoma cells neither attached nor spread. On mixed surfaces where the PEG lipids were approximately twice the length of the amphiphile (e.g., adhesive ligand not accessible) no attachment or spreading was observed. When the PEG moiety and amphiphile were approximately the same length, cells attached but did not spread. In contrast, on mixed surfaces where the adhesion amphiphile was longer than the PEG head group, and hence fully accessible, cells not only attached but they also spread. These results demonstrate that the cell adhesion motif must be accessible to the cell surface receptors. Therefore, accessibility is a critical component of any engineered product for controlling cell–material interactions if the device is to be successful.

## 3.5  Topography and Surface Heterogeneity

A wide variety of cell types respond to both microtopography (0.11 to 100 $\mu$m features) and nanotopography (1 to 100 nm features) in what has become known as *contact guidance* (see Curtis and Wilkinson, 1998; Abrams et al., 2002 for reviews). This behavior is partially explained by dimensions of cells ($\mu$m), cellular adhesion apparatus (i.e., protein aggregates such as integrin clusters; nm–$\mu$m scale), and individual proteins (nm). Materials for tissue engineering can exploit surface topography or texture/roughness at dimensions that enhance cell haptotaxis. Cellular response (adhesion, spreading, protein production, alignment, cytoskeletal organization, morphology) to topography has used fabricated surfaces with well-defined features (i.e., islands, pillars, grooves, ridges), typically generated using photolithography or electron beam lithography methods (Curtis and Wilkinson, 1998; Folch and Toner, 2000). Cellular response to random topography/ roughness (i.e., grit blasted, simple abrasion, solution etching of metals) is difficult to interpret because it is impossible to isolate specific features responsible for the response. However, regular control of nano- and micro-topographical features on/within biomaterials or pore size (for polymeric scaffolds) has not typically been a design criteria and consequently, most surface topography used is random, except in model investigative cases. However, use of macro-sized features (i.e., super-micron pores, stamped patterns, sintered beads) has been more thoroughly studied for cell behavior. This is especially true for orthopedic implants to promote tissue on- and in-growth and subsequent mechanical fixation. As more complex devices are tissue-engineered, incorporation and consideration of these factors with reliable, large-scale fabrication techniques suitable for multiple materials types will be critical for success.

Topographic or surface heterogeneous feature effects have been studied using micropatterned surfaces developed with numerous features including, but not limited to, well-defined islands or stripes of varying area and shape (Singhvi et al., 1994; Chen et al., 1997; Thomas et al., 1999), surfaces containing ridges and grooves (square or V-shaped) of varying width and height/depth, as well as stepped substrates (van Kooten and von Recum, 1999) (see Table 2 in Abrams et al. (2002) for a comprehensive listing with references of the effects of feature, feature size, and spatial frequency on the behavior of numerous cell types). Chen et al. (1997) demonstrated that the survival of capillary endothelial cells could be modulated by confining cells to adhesive islands of varying size. They showed that apoptosis decreased and DNA synthesis increased with increasing island size (75 to 3000 $\mu$m$^2$). On surfaces with evenly spaced adhesive islands (3, 5, or 20 $\mu$m diameter with 6, 10, or 40 $\mu$m spacing), cells bridged the closely spaced islands (6 and 10 $\mu$m spacing), but not the 40 $\mu$m spacing, to form stable focal contacts and induce cell spreading. By keeping cell–ECM contact area constant in this study, it was shown that cell projected area (cell shape) was the critical determinant responsible for cell survival as well as switching between proliferation and quiescence. Thomas et al. (1999) employed micropatterned surfaces with multiple island shapes and sizes to selectively control osteoblast attachment and spreading. Cells on islands <900 $\mu$m$^2$ were unable to organize their cytoskeleton independent of island shape, whereas after long-term culture (21 days), cell cytoskeletal organization on larger islands was dictated by shape (circles, ovals, squares, rectangles). Analogous cell responses to island spacing are observed in parallel grooves and ridges (Clark et al., 1987).

Although interpretation of random topographical effects on cellular surface behavior is difficult, these conventional surfaces are important for implant biomaterials use and are more prevalent currently than customized surfaces with precisely controlled sub-micron features. Gross cellular behavior, including matrix protein production and phenotypic expression, on textured surfaces compared to control "smooth" surfaces is readily studied. Acid-etched "nanotexturing" (random topography) influences on osteogenic cell production of matrix proteins cultured on titanium surfaces (machined or acid etched) showed that early expression of noncollagenous bone matrix proteins (osteopontin and bone sialoprotein) was upregulated on nanotextured surfaces compared to machined surfaces or glass controls (de Oliveira and Nanci, 2004). This behavior is important for osteogenic implants and can be extended to other cell types.

---

## 3.6   Surface Rigidity/Mechanical Coupling

In addition to surface architecture, topography, ligand type, density, and accessibility affecting cellular behavior, substrate mechanical properties (how cells respond to material surface elasticity) (surface modulus) are now becoming recognized as an important parameter. In particular, cell focal adhesions associated with integrin cytoplasmic regions act as mechanosensors that convert mechanical forces into biochemical signaling (Schwarz et al., 2003). Consequently, cells are very tactile, constantly applying forces via mechanically active structures (i.e., cytoskeletal features) by pushing or pulling to actively probe the mechanical properties of their surroundings and respond accordingly (i.e., degree of spreading) in a process called durotaxis (Lo et al., 2000). In this way, durotaxis is similar to cell haptotactic response; cells spread more on surfaces with higher ligand densities. However, as previously mentioned, once ligand density surpasses a critical threshold, cell motility is hindered, with subsequent reduction in spreading and differentiation. For this reason, ligand density and substrate stiffness are significantly coupled variables that together determine average cell behaviors, such as extent of cell spreading, shape, and molecular organization (Engler et al., 2004). Therefore, if the substrate is too soft, cells do not respond to increases in adhesion ligand density: pliable or water-swollen, soft substrates (i.e., hydrogels) require substantial ligand densities ($\sim 1000$-fold higher) to elicit similar responses to more rigid substrates (Elbert and Hubbell, 2001). Additionally, depending on the elastic properties of the matrix, cells respond by orienting in the direction of the greatest effective stiffness with subsequent strengthening of their adhesion contacts and cytoskeleton (Bischofs and Schwarz, 2003). In essence, cells are guided by elasticity gradients, preferring regions of greater stiffness (Schwarz et al., 2003). This has profound implications for use of soft gel materials (alginates, acrylates, etc.) in tissue engineering.

Cell motility, adhesion, and proliferation all involve the generation of physical forces, most often in tension across the cell. For cells to attach and spread on surfaces, a force balance between the substrate tension and cell traction forces must be possible. If the substrate is unable to withstand the tractional forces generated by cell cytoskeletal actin stress fibers connected to the ECM via focal adhesion plaques (i.e, material is too soft or pliable), then cells will detach due to their inability to establish stable focal adhesions. Similarly, the substrate must be able to resist contractile pre-stresses within the cell that, in addition to traction forces generated by the cell, have been shown to be proportional to cell stiffness (Wang et al., 2002). Once detached and rounded on these pliable materials, anchorage-dependent cells will apoptose. Given that focal adhesions are the primary physical link between the cell and external environment, they can dynamically alter size in response to external forces to re-establish force equilibrium. For stationary fibroblasts, typical forces at mature focal contacts (10 to 60 h postplating) are in the range of 10–30 nN with a linear relationship between the size of the focal adhesion and the magnitude of the force (Schwarz et al., 2003). These forces are reasonable given that focal adhesions contain hundreds of integrin adhesion molecules acting in concert. Single molecule-associated forces are on the order of pN (i.e., biotin–avidin has a static rupture force of 5 pN; Merkel et al., 1999) so, within focal adhesions, this pN scale is amplified to the nN scale by multiple cell-surface bonds (Schwarz et al., 2003).

In the first study using collagen-coated polyacrylamide gels formed with varying cross-linking densities, Pelham and Wang (1997) examined the effect of elasticity on the behavior of rat kidney epithelial and NIH 3T3 fibroblasts. By varying the cross-linking density, they were able to produce substrates of similar chemical composition but different moduli. They showed that, compared to cell behavior on rigid substrates, cells on more flexible substrates exhibited reduced spreading, increased motility, increased lamellipodia ruffling, and differences in focal contact formation. On flexible surfaces, focal contacts were irregularly shaped and tended to experience more dynamic turnover while those on rigid substrates showed a normal wedge-shaped morphology and greater stability. When cells on flexible substrates were treated with a tyrosine phosphatase inhibitor to artificially increase tyrosine phosphorylation, they formed focal adhesions indistinguishable from those formed on stiff or rigid substrates. Similarly, when they disrupted the cytoskeleton by inhibiting myosin light chain kinase activity or myosin motor activity in cells on rigid substrates, the focal adhesions reverted to what was observed on the most flexible substrates. These results demonstrate the role of substrate stiffness in regulating tyrosine phosphorylation of proteins found within focal adhesions leading to more stable focal contacts as well as the critical role of the cytoskeleton in aiding cellular response to substrate mechanical properties.

## 3.7 Mechanical Stress and Cell Signaling: Effects of Shear, Cyclic Shear, Hydrodynamic Shear, and Mechanical Loading

Few tissues develop or function in quiescent culture absent of forces or shear stresses. However, cell culture and seeding in tissue engineering devices is often performed in static culture conditions, without mechanical stress effects shown to be important for cell phenotypic development and maintenance. Long-known effects of culture conditions and substrate chemistry on cell attachment mechanisms and their implications for stimulating natural receptor-mediated pathways should also include selected mechanical stimuli, including shear stresses, to activate important signaling pathways that influence many cell functions (Figure 3.5). Hence, conditions more relevant to physiological environments under continuous or cyclical flow, tension or flexure (e.g., vascular endothelium, lung tissue, bone tissues) are shown *in vitro* to influence in significant ways the behavior and phenotypic properties of cells (Torday and Rehan, 2003; Huang et al., 2004). These stimuli are known to activate specific stress-activated signaling pathways involving the protein kinase family in cells. Culture requirements are moving away from quiescent static culture on rigid plastic supports to contextual, tissue-specific requirements using mechanical and fluid cyclical stresses applied in sophisticated bioreactors, to prompt specific tissue-like cell functional development.

Blood under flow behaves as a Newtonian fluid (shear rate and shear stress are directly proportional). Physiological shear stresses can range from 1 to 30 dynes/cm$^2$ for stable laminar flow, with higher ranges under turbulence or branch points. Fluid shear stress and shear rates are well-known to influence or even control the behavior of cells in vascular tissues (Girard and Nerem, 1995; McIntire et al., 1998; Nerem et al., 1998). Vascular shear stress has been shown to change cell cytoskeletal morphology (Girard and Nerem, 1995), alter growth factor expression (Frangos et al., 1985; Liu, 1999), regulate cell proliferation (Liu, 1998; Frangos et al., 1999), and apoptosis (Dimmeler and Zeiher, 1999; Frangos et al., 1999). Recent work has implicated a connection between shear stress effects on vascular endothelial cells and resulting migration behavior of smooth muscle cells (Liu and Goldman, 2001). Such shear stress could result in mechanically

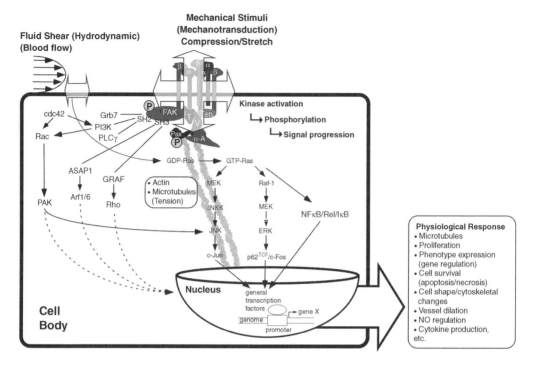

**FIGURE 3.5**

Cell signals and cell outside-in signal pathways modulated by mechanical stimuli. Pathway redundancy is evident: all terminate at the nuclear gene expression level. Many pathways still have not been fully elucidated and this scientific picture is a "work in progress". Nonetheless, mechanics have a profound effect on cell behavior and are an important consideration in culture and signal assays for tissue engineering systems (Hynes, 2002; Li et al., 1996; Schwartz and Assoian, 2001; Parsons, 2003; Ingber, 2003). Abbreviations: FAK (focal adhesion kinase), T (talin), V (vinculin), Ten (tensin), Pax (paxillin), α-A (α-actinin), P (phosphorylated), PAK (p21-activated kinase), ASAP1 (a GAP, GTPase-activating protein, for Arf1 and Arf6), GRAF (a GAP for Rho), PI3K (phospatidylinositol 3 kinase), PLCγ (phospholipase C-γ), SH2 (Src homology domain 2), SH3 (Src homology domain 3), MEK (a MAPKK, mitogen-activated protein kinase kinase), MEKK (a MAPKKK, mitogen-activated protein kinase kinase kinase), JNK (c-Jun NH2-terminal kinase), JNKK (a JNK kinase), ERK (extracellular signal-regulated kinase).

transduced effects on cell populations located in adjacent radial layers in the vascular tissue. Additionally, protein kinase-mediated signaling from endothelial cells, directly exposed to blood fluid shear, to smooth muscle cells peripheral and adjacent to them, is also possible.

Interestingly, bacterial colonization of implants and tissues occurs under shear as well, with different microbes preferring different shear environments. As tissue engineered constructs are designed as perfect "homes" for cells to grow, they also represent significant infection potential. Fluid dynamics should also be incorporated into infection models as well.

## 3.8   Cell Seeding and Nutrient Transport in Scaffolds

Tissues are organized 3-D masses of confluent highly differentiated cell bodies highly perfused with capillary networks to provide mass transport. Nutrient-related exchange and transport parameters in tissue are known (Levick, 2000). Scaffold designs often reproduce bulk form (3-D shape and volume) but lack requisite transport networks to replicate native perfusion and mass transport properties of real tissue. Significantly, this also affects the ability to recruit cell types, either seeded or from the host post-implant, into the tissue engineered device to stimulate effective cell colonization and tissue regeneration. Without this capability, most tissue engineering strategies are doomed to small size scales over which diffusion-mediated exchange and transport function. Hence, cell recruitment, viability and mass transport to maintain these cells are essential features. Methods that ensure uniform cell seeding throughout the construct are an important point of design focus. Cells simply seeded onto the exterior of a construct tend to penetrate only a few hundred microns, leaving the majority of the scaffold interior devoid of cells and ultimately devoid of any potential to serve as a functional tissue replacement. This has profound implications for functional regeneration as well as programmed, often desired degradation of the scaffold, which are very dependent upon cell density and intrinsic metabolic activity.

To circumvent this problem and provide a more uniform seeding density, techniques such as "drop on" and low-pressure centrifugation have been introduced (Halbleib et al., 2003). With hydrogels, or more pliable scaffolds, direct injection of cells into the scaffold attempts to impose homogeneous seeding. However, this technique also tends to create localized cell micro-aggregates at the point of injection. The ability of cells to penetrate throughout the scaffold bulk during the seeding process will ultimately depend on the scaffold's density, void fraction or porous architecture, as well as its tortuosity. Similarly, scaffold architecture will help determine cell migration and redistribution abilities within the scaffold over time. Additionally, seeded cells can simply pass through or migrate out of gel or porous scaffolds with gravitational forces (settling), depending on the scaffold architecture, cell-adhesive character of the scaffold material, and how quickly infiltrating cells form stable cell attachments to counter either gravity or dynamic flow conditions in the culturing system. However, even if homogeneous seeding is accomplished, defining the culture conditions for encouraging specific phenotypes and growth requirements within each scaffold design is critical (Godbey and Atala, 2002; Barron et al., 2003).

Cell encapsulation studies pre-dating tissue engineering have shown the importance of efficient, effective mass transport and adverse effects of transient hypoxia on cells in biomaterials (Uludag et al., 2000; Orive et al., 2004). The ability to produce transport networks within engineered biomaterials as efficient as capillary beds is in fact primitive and currently rate limiting to progress. Recognizing that each cell within any tissue is only 1 to 2 cell diameters away from a blood supply, current passive mass transport strategies within bulk polymer matrices are drastically insufficient to produce effective, requisite transfer of metabolites and dissolved gasses. Cells not within 200 microns of a blood vessel suffer from nutrient transport limitations and hypoxia, producing immediate phenotypic alterations and ultimately cell apoptosis. Artificial 3-D constructs must ensure proper transport of nutrients, oxygen, growth factors, cell chemotactic factors, cell–cell signaling molecules, and metabolic wastes (Botchwey et al., 2003). Without sufficient transport throughout the matrix, cells within the interior of the scaffold will not remain viable, or at best, fail to express their proper phenotype, due to lack of appropriate nutrients or chemical stimuli. Early cell encapsulation work has documented large spatial hetero-geneities in bulk cell–materials hybrid devices, typically showing viable cells within a few hundred microns of the device interface with the host, and decreasing cell densities beyond that distance, with large interior areas completely devoid of viable cells, despite culture or fabrication methods originally producing homogeneous cell density prior to implant. Additionally, transient acute hypoxic stress upon implantation is known to permanently alter cell phenotype (de Vos et al., 2002). Overcoming transport limitations in large tissue engineering constructs remains a significant hurdle in developing viable organs. Without functional surrogate capillary beds to deliver both nutrients and stimuli as well as remove metabolic wastes or possible cytotoxic degradation products from scaffold degradation, large tissue engineered organs will remain elusive. For these reasons, various dynamic culturing systems (bioreactors) are being developed to actively control fluid flow, reliable mass transport and controlled exchange. However, even with dynamic systems including spinning flasks, rotating bioreactors, or direct perfusion chambers, defining the optimal conditions for individual cell types within scaffolds intended for diverse implant applications remains a challenge. Not only are dynamic systems used to overcome transport limitations, but also to elicit proper phenotype since cells respond dynamically to moderate fluid shear (i.e., with gene regulation). In addition, culture systems that also provide mechanical stimuli are being examined for connective tissues such as bone and cartilage that respond directly to mechanical loading.

## 3.9   Angiogenesis and Neovascularization

Certain tissue-engineered structures (avascular cartilage and cornea that need no blood supply, heart valves and bladder sufficiently thin to survive on diffusion-limited transport, and skin that obtains its nutrients from surrounding vascular beds) have proven functional without providing an exogenous blood supply. However, beyond these selected cases, biomaterials and scaffold fabrication sophistication alone can never effectively address diffusion-limited problems with mass transfer in bulk, living tissue engineered devices larger than a few hundred microns. Facilitated and active transport systems might possibly overcome these issues if carefully incorporated into scaffold designs. The problem is "how?" Focus currently lies in *de novo* growth of new microvascular networks into and within biomaterials to connect the host blood supply into and develop a neovascular network directly within the device (Sieminski and Gooch, 2000; Cassell et al., 2002; Zisch et al., 2003; Patel and Mikos, 2004; Kannan et al., 2005). Vascularized structures are created in two primary strategies: (1) stimulation of endogenous angiogenic responses to grow new vessels using both vasculogenic and angiogenic cues, and (2) fabricating tubular networks that duplicate the vascular tree in the tissue-engineered structure. Because acute local hypoxia upon implantation can permanently alter cell phenotype (or worse, kill most cells) within a bulk device, design considerations must consider the time necessary for host response to accomplish sufficient therapeutic angiogenesis into the device to accommodate cell survival, or pre-endow the scaffold with sufficient perfusion capability prior to cell seeding and growth to eliminate acute hypoxic risks. Review of the different diverse approaches for neovascularization and therapeutic angiogenesis in the context of tissue-engineered devices is beyond the scope of this chapter. References provided should give adequate direction for a more thorough understanding of the current issues and challenges in this area that remains an important roadblock to bulk implant success (Ennett and Mooney, 2002).

## 3.10   Conclusions

In order to prove clinically useful, tissue engineering designs must consider many molecular-scale parameters to impart properties necessary to maintain cell densities, viabilities and phenotypes required in these devices to really legitimize their value to regenerative medicine. Molecular understanding and control of the scaffold interface, bulk and surface mechanics and transport properties, cellular biology, signaling pathways, and long-term functional recapitulation are essential.

Clinical research is also demonstrating the value of nearly identical molecular-based physiological and pathological approaches to validating the impact of these same parameters on *in vivo* therapies: recent research in disease and interventional surgery has begun linking apoptosis and necrosis pathways to tissue development, ischemic injury and heart failure (Elsasser et al., 2000; Martinez-Lemus et al., 2003; Armstrong and Bischoff, 2004) and device reactions (Indolfi et al., 2003; Mongiardo et al., 2004) and will likely continue to use signal pathway correlations to assess progress in tissue engineering as much as they are used now in studies of disease (Vogel and Baneyx, 2003; Lutolf and Hubbell, 2005).

One closing note: significantly, while both tissue engineering and clinical research currently converge on novel molecular biological approaches promising to innovate and direct new implant device strategies, *in vitro* testing models and their *in vivo* evaluations continue to suffer from poor correlations. A frequent complaint from the clinical side is that bench-scale *in vitro* results are not often corroborated by clinical device behaviors. Despite many improvements and success stories with *in vitro* device performance (i.e., low protein adsorption, high cell viability, and phenotypic retention), results with the same device designs *in vivo* frequently produce disappointing performance. This is a pattern of poor predictability that has plagued biomaterials development for decades, throwing into question the value of *in vitro* testing methods as well as the true level of understanding of the complexity of host-implant response. New device design methods developed *in vitro* should continually seek validation with *in vivo* results. After all, the host *in vivo* implant environment is the ultimate testing ground for true biological response and therapeutic assessment. Limitations in current abilities to reproduce these conditions *in vitro* should not serve as active distraction from the true performance issues, but rather to spur greater understanding of the *in vitro–in vivo* disconnections.

## Acknowledgment

The authors are grateful for support from NIH grants EB000473 and EB000796. Ongoing discussions with E. Vogler and M. Yamato are greatly appreciated.

## References

Abrams, G.A. et al., Effects of substratum topography on cell behavior, In: *Biomimetic Materials and Design*, Dillow, A.K. and Lowman, A.M., Eds., Marcel Dekker, Inc., New York, pp. 91 (2002).

Adamson, A.W. and Gast, A.P., Eds., *Physical Chemistry of Surfaces*, 6th ed., Wiley, New York (1997).

Akiyama, S.K., Olden, K., and Yamada, K.M., Fibronectin and integrins in invasion and metastasis, *Cancer Metastas. Rev.*, **14** (3), 173 (1995).

Albelda, S.M. and Buck, C.A., Integrins and other cell adhesion molecules, *FASEB J.*, **4**, 2868 (1990).

Alberts, B. et al., Cell junctions, cell adhesion, and the extracellular matrix, In: *Molecular Biology of the Cell*, 3rd ed., Garland Publishing, Inc., New York. pp. 971 (1994).

Andrade, J.D., Interfacial phenomena and biomaterials, *Med. Instrum.*, **7** (2), 110 (1973).

Andrade, J.D., Ed., *Surface and Interfacial Aspects of Biomedical Polymers: Surface Chemistry and Physics*, Vol. 1. Plenum, New York (1985).

Andrade, J.D., Ed., *Surface and Interfacial Aspects of Biomedical Polymers: Protein Adsorption*, Vol. 2, Plenum, New York (1985).

Anselme, K., Osteoblast adhesion on biomaterials, *Biomaterials.*, **21** (7), 667 (2000).

Aota, S., Nomizu, M., and Yamada, K.M., The short amino acid sequence pro–his–ser–arg–asn in human fibronectin enhances cell-adhesive function, *J. Biol. Chem.*, **269** (40), 24756 (1994).

Armstrong, E.J. and Bischoff, J., Heart valve development: Endothelial cell signaling and differentiation, *Circ. Res.*, **95** (5), 459 (2004).

Atala, A. and Lanza, R.P., Eds., *Methods of Tissue Engineering*, Academic Press, San Diego, CA (2002).

Bamdad, M. et al., Alpha1beta1-integrin is an essential signal for neurite outgrowth induced by thrombospondin type 1 repeats of sco-spondin, *Cell Tissue Res.*, **315** (1), 15 (2004).

Barron, V. et al., Bioreactors for cardiovascular cell and tissue growth: a review, *Ann. Biomed. Eng.*, **31** (9), 1017 (2003).

Barry, S.T. et al., Analysis of the alpha4beta1 integrin–osteopontin interaction, *Exp. Cell Res.*, **258** (2), 342 (2000).

Barry, S.T. et al., A regulated interaction between alpha5beta1 integrin and osteopontin, *Biochem. Biophys. Res. Commun.*, **267** (3), 764 (2000).

Bayless, K.J. et al., Osteopontin is a ligand for the alpha4beta1 integrin, *J. Cell Sci.*, **111** (Pt 9), 1165 (1998).

Bhatnagar, R.S., Qian, J.J., and Gough, C.A., The role in cell binding of a beta-bend within the triple helical region in collagen alpha 1 (i) chain: structural and biological evidence for conformational tautomerism on fiber surface, *J. Biomol. Struct. Dyn.*, **14** (5), 547 (1997).

Bischofs, I.B. and Schwarz, U.S., Cell organization in soft media due to active mechanosensing, *Proc. Natl. Acad. Sci. U.S.A.*, **100** (16), 9274 (2003).

Bogusky, M.J. et al., Nmr and molecular modeling characterization of rgd containing peptides, *Int. J. Pept. Protein Res.*, **39** (1), 63 (1992).

Botchwey, E.A. et al., Tissue engineered bone: measurement of nutrient transport in three-dimensional matrices, *J. Biomed. Mater. Res. A*, **67** (1), 357 (2003).

Brandley, B.K. and Schnaar, R.L., Covalent attachment of an arg–gly–asp sequence peptide to derivatizable polyacrylamide surfaces: Support of fibroblast adhesion and long-term growth, *Anal. Biochem.*, **172**, 270 (1988).

Calderwood, D.A., Integrin activation, *J. Cell Sci.*, **117** (Pt 5), 657 (2004).

Calzada, M.J. et al., Recognition of the n-terminal modules of thrombospondin-1 and thrombospondin-2 by alpha6beta1 integrin, *J. Biol. Chem.*, **278** (42), 40679 (2003).

Cardarelli, P.M. et al., Cyclic rgd peptide inhibits alpha-4 beta-1 interaction with connecting segment 1 and vascular cell adhesion molecule, *J. Biol. Chem.*, **269** (28), 18668 (1994).

Cardin, A.D. and Weintraub, H.J.R., Molecular modeling of protein–glycosaminoglycan interactions, *Arteriosclerosis*, **9**, 21 (1989).

Cassell, O.C. et al., Vascularisation of tissue-engineered grafts: the regulation of angiogenesis in reconstructive surgery and in disease states, *Br. J. Plast. Surg.*, **55** (8), 603 (2002).

Chen, R.R. and Mooney, D.J., Polymeric growth factor delivery strategies for tissue engineering, *Pharm. Res.*, **20** (8), 1103 (2003).

Chen, C.S. et al., Geometric control of cell life and death, *Science*, **276** (5317), 1425 (1997).

Clark, P. et al., Topographical control of cell behaviour. I. Simple step cues, *Development*, **99** (3), 439 (1987).

Cotran, R.S., Tissue repair: cellular growth, fibrosis, and wound healing, In: *Pathologic Basis of Disease*, 6th ed., Cotran, R.S., Kumar, V., and Collins, T., Eds., Elsevier Saunders, Philadelphia, pp. 89 (1999).

Curtis, A.S. and Wilkinson, C.D., Reactions of cells to topography, *J. Biomater. Sci. Polym. Ed.*, **9** (12), 1313 (1998).

Dalton, B.A. et al., Role of the heparin binding domain of fibronectin in attachment and spreading of human bone-derived cells, *J. Cell Sci.*, **108** (5), 2083 (1995).

Danilov, Y.N. and Juliano, R.L., (arg–gly–asp)n-albumin conjugates as a model substratum for integrin-mediated cell adhesion, *Exp. Cell Res.*, **182** (1), 186 (1989).

Denda, S., Reichardt, L.F., and Muller, U., Identification of osteopontin as a novel ligand for the integrin alpha8 beta1 and potential roles for this integrin–ligand interaction in kidney morphogenesis, *Mol. Biol. Cell*, **9** (6), 1425 (1998).

de Oliveira, P.T. and Nanci, A., Nanotexturing of titanium-based surfaces upregulates expression of bone sialoprotein and osteopontin by cultured osteogenic cells, *Biomaterials*, **25** (3), 403 (2004).

de Vos, P., Hamel, A.F., and Tatarkiewicz, K., Considerations for successful transplantation of encapsulated pancreatic islets, *Diabetologia*, **45** (2), 159 (2002).

DiMilla, P.A. et al., Measurement of cell adhesion and migration on protein-coated surfaces, *Mater. Res. Soc. Symp. Proc.*, **252**, 205 (1992).

DiMilla, P.A. et al., Maximal migration of human smooth muscle cells on fibronectin and type iv collagen occurs at an intermediate attachment strength, *J. Cell Biol.*, **122** (3), 729 (1993).

Dimmeler, S. and Zeiher, A.M., Nitric oxide-an endothelial cell survival factor, *Cell Death Differ.*, **6** (10), 964 (1999).

Dori, Y. et al., Ligand accessibility as means to control cell response to bioactive bilayer membranes, *J. Biomed. Mater. Res.*, **50** (1), 75 (2000).

Elbert, D.L. and Hubbell, J.A., Surface treatments of polymers for biocompatibility, *Annu. Rev. Mater. Sci.*, **26**, 365 (1996).

Elbert, D.L. and Hubbell, J.A., Conjugate addition reactions combined with free-radical cross-linking for the design of materials for tissue engineering, *Biomacromolecules*, **2** (2), 430 (2001).

Elsasser, A., Suzuki, K., and Schaper, J., Unresolved issues regarding the role of apoptosis in the pathogenesis of ischemic injury and heart failure, *J. Mol. Cell Cardiol.*, **32** (5), 711 (2000).

Engler, A. et al., Substrate compliance versus ligand density in cell on gel responses, *Biophys. J.*, **86** (1 Pt 1), 617 (2004).

Ennett, A.B. and Mooney, D.J., Tissue engineering strategies for in vivo neovascularisation, *Expert Opin. Biol. Ther.*, **2** (8), 805 (2002).

Flores, M.E. et al., Bone sialoprotein coated on glass and plastic surfaces is recognized by different beta 3 integrins, *Exp. Cell Res.*, **227** (1), 40 (1996).

Folch, A. and Toner, M., Microengineering of cellular interactions, *Annu. Rev. Biomed. Eng.*, **2**, 227 (2000).

Francis, G.E. et al., Pegylation of cytokines and other therapeutic proteins and peptides: the importance of biological optimisation of coupling techniques, *Int. J. Hematol.*, **68** (1), 1 (1998).

Frangos, J.A. et al., Flow effects on prostacyclin production by cultured human endothelial cells, *Science*, **227** (4693), 1477 (1985).

Frangos, S.G., Gahtan, V., and Sumpio, B., Localization of atherosclerosis: role of hemodynamics, *Arch. Surg.*, **134** (10), 1142 (1999).

Girard, P.R. and Nerem, R.M., Shear stress modulates endothelial cell morphology and f-actin organization through the regulation of focal adhesion-associated proteins, *J. Cell Physiol.*, **163** (1), 179 (1995).

Gittens, S.A. and Uludag, H., Growth factor delivery for bone tissue engineering, *J. Drug Target.*, **9** (6), 407 (2001).

Godbey, W.T. and Atala, A., In vitro systems for tissue engineering, *Ann. NY Acad. Sci.*, **961**, 10 (2002).

Grainger, D.W. et al., Assessment of fibronectin conformation adsorbed to polytetrafluoroethylene surfaces from serum protein mixtures and correlation to support of cell attachment in culture, *J. Biomater. Sci. Polym. Ed.*, **14** (9), 973 (2003).

Grzesik, W.J. and Robey, P.G., Bone matrix rgd glycoproteins: immunolocalization and interaction with human primary osteoblastic bone cells in vitro, *J. Bone Miner. Res.*, **9** (4), 487 (1994).

Guilak, F. et al., Eds., *Functional Tissue Engineering*, Springer, New York (2003).

Haas, T.A. and Plow, E.F., Integrin-ligand interactions: a year in review, *Curr. Opin. Cell Biol.*, **6**, 656 (1994).

Halbleib, M. et al., Tissue engineering of white adipose tissue using hyaluronic acid-based scaffolds. I: In vitro differentiation of human adipocyte precursor cells on scaffolds, *Biomaterials*, **24** (18), 3125 (2003).

Hardingham, T.E. and Fosang, A.J., Proteoglycans: many forms and many functions, *FASEB*, **6**, 861 (1992).

Hautanen, A. et al., Effects of modification of the rgd sequence and its context on recognition by the fibronectin receptor, *J. Biol. Chem.*, **264** (3), 1437 (1989).

Hern, D.L. and Hubbell, J.A., Incorporation of adhesion peptides into nonadhesive hydrogels useful for tissue resurfacing, *J. Biomed. Mater. Res.*, **39** (2), 266 (1998).

Hersel, U., Dahmen, C., and Kessler, H., Rgd modified polymers: biomaterials for stimulated cell adhesion and beyond, *Biomaterials*, **24** (24), 4385 (2003).

Horton, M.A., Interaction of connective tissue cells with the extracellular matrix, *Bone*, **17** (2), 51S (1995).

Horton, M.A. et al., Modulation of vitronectin receptor-mediated osteoclast adhesion by arg–gly–asp peptide analogs: a structure-function analysis, *J. Bone Miner. Res.*, **8** (2), 239 (1993).

Horwitz, A.F., Integrins and health, *Sci. Am.*, **276** (5), 68 (1997).

Houseman, B.T. and Mrksich, M., The microenvironment of immobilized arg–gly–asp peptides is an important determinant of cell adhesion, *Biomaterials*, **22** (9), 943 (2001).

Huang, H., Kamm, R.D., and Lee, R.T., Cell mechanics and mechanotransduction: Pathways, probes, and physiology, *Am. J. Physiol.—Cell Physiol.*, **287** (1), C1 (2004).

Hubbell, J.A., Biomaterials in tissue engineering, *Biotechnology*, **13** (6), 565 (1995).

Huber, M. et al., Modification of glassy carbon surfaces with synthetic laminin-derived peptides for nerve cell attachment and neurite growth, *J. Biomed. Mater. Res.*, **41** (2), 278 (1998).

Hynes, R.O., Integrins: a family of cell surface receptors, *Cell*, **48**, 549 (1987).

Hynes, R.O., Integrins: versatility, modulation, and signaling in cell adhesion, *Cell*, **69**, 11 (1992).

Hynes, R.O., Integrins: bidirectional, allosteric signaling machines, *Cell*, **110** (6), 673 (2002).

Hynes, R.O., The emergence of integrins: a personal and historical perspective, *Matrix Biol.*, **23** (6), 333 (2004).

Indolfi, C. et al., Molecular mechanisms of in-stent restenosis and approach to therapy with eluting stents, *Trends. Cardiovasc. Med.*, **13** (4), 142 (2003).

Ingber, D.E., Tensegrity ii. How structural networks influence cellular information processing networks, *J. Cell Sci.*, **116** (Pt 8), 1397 (2003).

Kannan, R.Y. et al., The roles of tissue engineering and vascularisation in the development of micro-vascular networks: a review, *Biomaterials*, **26** (14), 1857 (2005).

Kirker-Head, C.A., Potential applications and delivery strategies for bone morphogenetic proteins, *Adv. Drug Delivery Rev.*, **43** (1), 65 (2000).

Komoriya, A. et al., The minimal essential sequence for a major cell type-specific adhesion site (cs1) within the alternatively spliced type iii connecting segment domain of fibronectin is leucine-aspartic acid-valine, *J. Biol. Chem.*, **266** (23), 15075 (1991).

Koo, L.Y. et al., Co-regulation of cell adhesion by nanoscale rgd organization and mechanical stimulus, *J. Cell Sci.*, **115** (7), 1423 (2002).

Krishnan, A., Siedlecki, C.A., and Vogler, E.A., Mixology of protein solutions and the vroman effect, *Langmuir*, **20** (12), 5071 (2004).

Krutzsch, H.C. et al., Identification of an alpha(3)beta(1) integrin recognition sequence in thrombospondin-1, *J. Biol. Chem.*, **274** (34), 24080 (1999).

Lai, C.F. and Cheng, S.L., Alphavbeta integrins play an essential role in bmp-2 induction of osteoblast differentiation, *J. Bone Miner. Res.*, **20** (2), 330 (2005).

Lanza, R.P., Langer, R.S., and Vacanti, J., Eds., *Principles of Tissue Engineering*, 2nd ed., Academic Press, San Diego (2000).

Laterra, J., Silbert, J.E., and Culp, L.A., Cell surface heparan sulfate mediates some adhesive responses to glycosaminoglycan-binding matrices, including fibronectin, *J. Cell Biol.*, **96** (1), 112 (1983).

Lauffenberger, D.A. and Horwitz, A.F., Cell, migration: A physically integrated molecular process, *Cell*, **84**, 359 (1996).

Lee, J.H. et al., Interaction of different types of cells on polymer surfaces with wettability gradient, *J. Colloid Interface Sci.*, **205** (2), 323 (1998).

Leong, K.F., Cheah, C.M., and Chua, C.K., Solid freeform fabrication of three-dimensional scaffolds for engineering replacement tissues and organs, *Biomaterials*, **24** (13), 2363 (2003).

Levick, J.R., Haemodynamics: pressure, flow and resistance, In: *An Introduction to Cardiovascular Physiology*, 3rd ed., Levick, J.R., Ed., Arnold, London, p. 118 (2000).

Li, Y.S. et al., The ras-jnk pathway is involved in shear-induced gene expression, *Mol. Cell Biol.*, **16** (11), 5947 (1996).

Lishko, V.K. et al., Multiple binding sites in fibrinogen for integrin alphambeta2 (mac-1), *J. Biol. Chem.*, **279** (43), 44897 (2004).

Liu, S.Q., Influence of tensile strain on smooth muscle cell orientation in rat blood vessels, *J. Biomech. Eng.*, **120** (3), 313 (1998).

Liu, S.Q., Focal expression of angiotensin ii type 1 receptor and smooth muscle cell proliferation in the neointima of experimental vein grafts: relation to eddy blood flow, *Arterioscler. Thromb. Vasc. Biol.*, **19** (11), 2630 (1999).

Liu, S.Q. and Goldman, J., Role of blood shear stress in the regulation of vascular smooth muscle cell migration, *IEEE Trans. Biomed. Eng.*, **48** (4), 474 (2001).

Lo, C.M. et al., Cell movement is guided by the rigidity of the substrate, *Biophys. J.*, **79** (1), 144 (2000).

Lutolf, M.P. and Hubbell, J.A., Synthetic biomaterials as instructive extracellular microenvironments for morphogenesis in tissue engineering, *Nat. Biotechnol.*, **23** (1), 47 (2005).

Maeda, T. et al., Artificial cell adhesive proteins engineered by grafting the arg−gly−asp cell recognition signal: factors modulating the cell adhesive activity of the grafted signal, *J. Biochem.*, **110**, 381 (1991).

Malmsten, M., Ed., *Biopolymers at Interfaces*, 2nd ed., M. Dekker, New York (1998).

Mann, B.K. et al., Smooth muscle cell growth in photopolymerized hydrogels with cell adhesive and proteolytically degradable domains: synthetic ecm analogs for tissue engineering, *Biomaterials*, **22** (22), 3045 (2001).

Martinez-Lemus, L.A. et al., Integrins as unique receptors for vascular control, *J. Vasc. Res.*, **40** (3), 211 (2003).

Massia, S.P. and Hubbell, J.A., Covalent surface immobilization of arg−gly−asp- and tyr−ile−gly− ser−arg-containing peptides to obtain well-defined cell-adhesive substrates, *Anal. Biochem.*, **187**, 292 (1990).

Massia, S.P. and Hubbell, J.A., An rgd spacing of 440 nm is sufficient for integrin $\alpha_v\beta_3$-mediated fibroblast spreading and 140 nm for focal contact and stress fiber formation, *J. Cell Bio.*, **114** (5), 1089 (1991).

McIntire, L.V. et al., Effect of flow on gene regulation in smooth muscle cells and macromolecular transport across endothelial cell monolayers, *Biol. Bull.*, **194** (3), 394 (1998).

Mercado, M.L. et al., Neurite outgrowth by the alternatively spliced region of human tenascin-c is mediated by neuronal alpha7beta1 integrin, *J. Neurosci.*, **24** (1), 238 (2004).

Merkel, R. et al., Energy landscapes of receptor-ligand bonds explored with dynamic force spectroscopy, *Nature*, **397** (6714), 50 (1999).

Milner, R. et al., Distinct roles for astrocyte alphavbeta5 and alphavbeta8 integrins in adhesion and migration, *J. Cell Sci.*, **112** (Pt 23), 4271 (1999).

Mongiardo, A. et al., Molecular mechanisms of restenosis after percutaneous peripheral angioplasty and approach to endovascular therapy, *Curr. Drug Targets Cardiovasc. Haematol. Disord.*, **4** (3), 275 (2004).

Mooney, D.J., Langer, R., and Ingber, D.E., Cytoskeletal filament assembly and the control of cell spreading and function by extracellular matrix, *J. Cell Sci.*, **108(Pt 6)** (5), 2311 (1995).

Morra, M., Ed., *Water in Biomaterials Surface Science*, Wiley, New York (2001).

Nerem, R.M. et al., The study of the influence of flow on vascular endothelial biology, *Am. J. Med. Sci.*, **316** (3), 169 (1998).

Orive, G. et al., History, challenges and perspectives of cell microencapsulation, *Trends Biotechnol.*, **22** (2), 87 (2004).

Palecek, S.P. et al., Integrin-ligand binding properties govern cell migration speed through cell-substartum adhesiveness, *Nature*, **385**, 537 (1997).

Parsons, J.T., Focal adhesion kinase: The first ten years, *J. Cell Sci.*, **116** (Pt 8), 1409 (2003).

Patel, Z.S. and Mikos, A.G., Angiogenesis with biomaterial-based drug- and cell-delivery systems, *J. Biomater. Sci. Polym. Ed.*, **15** (6), 701 (2004).

Pelham, R.J. Jr and Wang, Y., Cell locomotion and focal adhesions are regulated by substrate flexibility, *Proc. Natl. Acad. Sci. U.S.A.*, **94** (25), 13661 (1997).

Pierschbacher, M.D. and Ruoslahti, E., Cell attachment activity of fibronectin can be duplicated by small synthetic fragments of the molecule, *Nature*, **309**, 30 (1984).

Podolnikova, N.P. et al., Identification of a novel binding site for platelet integrins alpha iib beta 3 (gpiibiiia) and alpha 5 beta 1 in the gamma c-domain of fibrinogen, *J. Biol. Chem.*, **278** (34), 32251 (2003).

Ratner, B.D. et al., Eds., *Biomaterials Science: an Introduction to Materials in Medicine*, 2nd ed., Elsevier Academic Press, London (2004).

Rezania, A. and Healy, K.E., Biomimetic peptide surfaces that regulate adhesion, spreading, cytoskeletal organization, and mineralization of the matrix deposited by osteoblast-like cells, *Biotechnol. Progr.*, **15** (1), 19 (1999).

Rezania, A. and Healy, K.E., The effect of peptide surface density on the mineralization of matrix deposited by osteogenic cells, *J. Biomed. Mater. Res.*, **52** (4), 595 (2000).

Rezania, A. et al., The detachment strength and morphology of bone cells contacting materials modified with a peptide derived from bone sialoprotein, *J. Biomed. Mater. Res.*, **37** (1), 9 (1997).

Rezania, A. et al., Bioactivation of metal oxide surfaces: I. Surface characterization and cell response, *Langmuir*, **15** (20), 6931 (1999).

Ruoslahti, E., Integrins, *J. Clin. Invest.*, **87** (1), 1 (1991).

Sakiyama-Elbert, S.E. and Hubbell, J.A., Functional biomaterials: design of novel biomaterials, *Ann. Rev. Mater. Res.*, **31**, 183 (2001).

Sakiyama, S.E., Schense, J.C., and Hubbell, J.A., Incorporation of heparin-binding peptides into fibrin gels enhances neurite extension: an example of designer matrices in tissue engineering, *Faseb. J.*, **13** (15), 2214 (1999).

Saltzman, W.M., *Tissue Engineering: Engineering Principles for the Design of Replacement Organs and Tissues*, Oxford University Press, Oxford (2004).

Saterbak, A. and Lauffenburger, D.A., Adhesion mediated by bonds in series, *Biotechnol. Progr.*, **12** (5), 682 (1996).

Sato, M. et al., Structure-activity studies of s-echistatin inhibition of bone resorption, *J. Bone Miner. Res.*, **9** (9), 1441 (1994).

Schmidt, C.E. and Leach, J.B., Neural tissue engineering: strategies for repair and regeneration, *Annu. Rev. Biomed. Eng.*, **5**, 293 (2003).

Schwartz, M.A. and Assoian, R.K., Integrins and cell proliferation: regulation of cyclin-dependent kinases via cytoplasmic signaling pathways, *J. Cell Sci.*, **114** (Pt 14), 2553 (2001).

Schwarz, U.S. et al., Measurement of cellular forces at focal adhesions using elastic micro-patterned substrates, *Mat. Sci. Eng. C—Bio. S.*, **23** (3), 387 (2003).

Seeherman, H., Wozney, J., and Li, R., Bone morphogenetic protein delivery systems, *Spine*, **27** (16 Suppl 1), S16 (2002).

Sieminski, A.L. and Gooch, K.J., Biomaterial-microvasculature interactions, *Biomaterials*, **21** (22), 2232 (2000).

Singhvi, R. et al., Engineering cell shape and function, *Science*, **264** (5159), 696 (1994).

Staatz, W.D. et al., Identification of a tetrapeptide recognition sequence for the alpha 2 beta 1 integrin in collagen, *J. Biol. Chem.*, **266** (12), 7363 (1991).

Tamada, Y. and Ikada, Y., Fibroblast growth on polymer surfaces and biosynthesis of collagen, *J. Biomed. Mater. Res.*, **28** (7), 783 (1994).

Thomas, C.H. et al., Surfaces designed to control the projected area and shape of individual cells, *J. Biomech. Eng.*, **121** (1), 40 (1999).

Torday, J.S. and Rehan, V.K., Mechanotransduction determines the structure and function of lung and bone: A theoretical model for the pathophysiology of chronic disease, *Cell Biochem. Biophys.*, **37** (3), 235 (2003).

Truskey, G.A. and Proulx, T.L., Relationship between 3t3 cell spreading and the strength of adhesion on glass and silane surfaces, *Biomaterials*, **14** (4), 243 (1993).

Uludag, H., De Vos, P., and Tresco, P.A., Technology of mammalian cell encapsulation, *Adv. Drug Delivery Rev.*, **42** (1-2), 29 (2000).

van Kooten, T.G. and von Recum, A.F., Cell adhesion to textured silicone surfaces: the influence of time of adhesion and texture on focal contact and fibronectin fibril formation, *Tissue Eng.*, **5** (3), 223 (1999).

van Wachem, P.B. et al., Interaction of cultured human endothelial cells with polymeric surfaces of different wettabilities, *Biomaterials*, **6** (6), 403 (1985).

Vogel, V. and Baneyx, G., The tissue engineering puzzle: a molecular perspective, *Annu. Rev. Biomed. Eng.*, **5**, 441 (2003).

Vogler, E.A., Structure and reactivity of water at biomaterial surfaces, *Adv. Colloid Interface Sci.*, **74**, 69 (1998).

Vogler, E.A., Water and the acute biological response to surfaces, *J. Biomater. Sci., Polym. Ed.*, **10** (10), 1015 (1999).

Vogler, E.A. and Bussian, R.W., Short-term cell-attachment rates: a surface-sensitive test of cell-substrate compatibility, *J. Biomed. Mater. Res.*, **21** (10), 1197 (1987).

von Recum, A.F., Ed., *Handbook of Biomaterials Evaluation*, 2nd ed., Macmillan, New York (1994).

Wang, N. et al., Cell prestress. I. Stiffness and prestress are closely associated in adherent contractile cells, *Am. J. Physiol.—Cell Physiol.*, **282** (3), C606 (2002).

Ward, M.D., Dembo, M. and Hammer, D.A., Kinetics of cell detachment — effect of ligand density, *Ann. Biomed. Eng.*, **23** (3), 322 (1995).

Wehrle-Haller, B. and Imhof, B.A., Integrin-dependent pathologies, *J. Pathol.*, **200** (4), 481 (2003).

Woods, A. et al., Adhesion and cytoskeletal organisation of fibroblasts in response to fibronectin fragments, *EMBO J.*, **5** (4), 665 (1986).

Yamada, T. et al., Functional analysis and modeling of a conformationally constrained arg–gly–asp sequence inserted into human lysozyme, *Biochemistry-us*, **33** (39), 11678 (1994).

Yamamoto, N. et al., Essential role of the cryptic epitope slayglr within osteopontin in a murine model of rheumatoid arthritis, *J. Clin. Invest.*, **112** (2), 181 (2003).

Yeong, W.Y. et al., Rapid prototyping in tissue engineering: challenges and potential, *Trends Biotechnol.*, **22** (12), 643 (2004).

Zhang, W.M. et al., Alpha 11beta 1 integrin recognizes the gfoger sequence in interstitial collagens, *J. Biol. Chem.*, **278** (9), 7270 (2003).

Zhou, H.Y. et al., Stimulation by bone sialoprotein of calcification in osteoblast-like mc3t3-e1 cells, *Calcif. Tissue Int.*, **56** (5), 403 (1995).

Zisch, A.H., Lutolf, M.P., and Hubbell, J.A., Biopolymeric delivery matrices for angiogenic growth factors, *Cardiovasc. Pathol.*, **12** (6), 295 (2003).

Zygourakis, K., Bizios, R., and Markenscoff, P., Proliferation of anchorage-dependent contact-inhibited cells: I. Development of theoretical models based on cellular automata, *Biotechnol. Bioeng.*, **38** (5), 459 (1991).

Zygourakis, K., Markenscoff, P., and Bizios, R., Proliferation of anchorage-dependent contact-inhibited cells: Ii. Experimental results and validation of the theoretical models, *Biotechnol. Bioeng.*, **38** (5), 471 (1991).

# 4

## Protein Adsorption at the Biomaterial/Tissue Interface

**Philip LeDuc and Yadong Wang**

## CONTENTS

## 4.1 Introduction

Novel technologies that are based upon material science applications in medical regimes are producing a renaissance in improving human health. Unfortunately, foreign materials introduced into the body inherently induce responses that are deleterious to normal physiological functions. Therefore, understanding and controlling material properties to eliminate or minimize these reactions are critical to continuing to advance biomaterials technology. One of these critical response pathways to foreign materials is intricately linked to the interactions between material surface properties and the adsorption of proteins. To understand this complex interplay, one must delve into the realms of multi-disciplinary science and applications that cross the boundaries of biology, engineering, and chemistry simultaneously. The ultimate results in mastering these interconnected fields will be products that are able to diagnose and treat diseases in applications ranging from tissue engineering to drug delivery for improving human lives.

The temporal set of events that occurs for biomaterials *in vivo* initiates with the material being introduced into the body where it contacts body fluid (BF). A myriad of solutes in the BF such as ions, lipids, carbohydrates, and proteins begin to adsorb on the surface of the material. Among these, protein deposition and adsorption are critical to understand because of their important role in biology. To accurately understand the interface between these organic and inorganic arenas, one must first define the systems to explore, i.e., the biomaterials and the proteins. A biomaterial is often described as a nonviable material intended to interact with biological systems in medicine. Early biomaterials included many natural materials while their modern counterparts encompass man-made materials such as metals, ceramics, and synthetic polymers. These foreign materials elicit responses from the body, which have been the subject of research for thousands of years. Proteins play an important role in this response as a protein layer is deposited at the interfacial surfaces within seconds of material introduction (Ratner et al., 1996). This response is not necessarily an active response of the body to the material, but often due to the presence of an abundance of proteins in the BFs that leads to an attachment of proteins at the surface. Over long time periods though, protein adsorption can lead to inflammatory responses including foreign body giant cell formation and fibrous encapsulation of the biomaterial. This temporally separated reaction is common in many biological systems where a short-term response is followed by a long-term solution. For example, in sensory mechanisms of nerves, contact between a hot surface and a human hand elicits an immediate reflex response through the reflex arc that does not involve the brain (Lippold, 1969). Over a longer duration, the nervous impulses from sensory nerve cells are sent to the brain causing a final reaction of the body to this heat through burn treatment steps including localized repair mechanisms. This is analogous to the type of response found in an aforementioned biomaterials scenario where short and long term responses are specifically targeted for minimizing damage to the body.

After the initial protein reaction to a foreign material in the physiological environment, the responses evolve into a more controlled sequence of events to accept or reject the biomaterial as cells are integrated into the cascading scenarios (Andrade and Hlady, 1986; Anderson, 2001). This response includes the recruitment of many cell types, which are known to be present at the interface of this foreign material and plays an active role as they adapt the local environment through secretion and digestion of proteins including remodeling the extracellular matrix (ECM) environment (Alberts et al., 1994). An invasion of cells is initiated as a response to a foreign material and furthermore a subsequent recruitment of additional cells may occur, which will lead to encapsulation of the biomaterial as the body isolates it from the physiological environment. This scenario is exhibited by an event as simple as a splinter in the human hand. The splinter is a foreign material that the body will attempt to isolate from the internal body. Swelling occurs in adjacent areas due to the response of the cells organizing into an encapsulation scheme. As common materials induce this reaction, one challenge in biomaterials is to deceive the body into not recognizing materials being introduced into the body as a foreign material and thus preventing the physiological response from initiating. One must understand the initiation events and the associated long term response of protein adsorption to develop methods to combat the physiological response. If these sequential events are identified then an upstream event (i.e., protein interactions with biomaterials) can be targeted to attempt to circumvent the downstream issues (i.e., physiological response).

In this chapter, the relationship of proteins and their adsorption in the field of biomaterials will be discussed. The structure and properties of proteins that are involved with specific biomaterials will be described. Next, the adsorption of proteins will be explained with respect to the various constraints including solid–liquid interfaces, diffusion, and protein types. Also, the specific interactions of these protein-adsorbed biomaterials will be elaborated on with respect to cell attachment. Finally, applications for these advanced biomaterials including fields such as tissue engineering and drug delivery will be presented.

---

## 4.2 Proteins (Structure, Properties)

### 4.2.1 Structure

Proteins are natural polymers made from L-α-amino acids with the general structure shown in Figure 4.1. There are 20 common natural amino acids, yet proteins exhibit a diverse range of properties and functions. The amino acids can be divided into different categories including hydrophilicity, aliphatic or aromatic side chains, and acidic or basic side chains. The structure of a protein can be deciphered at four levels: primary, secondary, tertiary, and quaternary. The primary structure refers to the amino acid sequence in the linear polypeptide chain of a protein. The secondary structures are formed by folding of polypeptide chains into regular structures such as α-helix, β-sheet, and turns and loops. The tertiary structure of a protein is formed by further folding of its polypeptide chains that results in a compact three-dimensional structure. A multisubunit structure assembled from several folded polypeptide chains is referred to as the quaternary structure of a protein.

The primary structure of a protein determines its higher order of structures along with its properties and functions. Covalent bonds assemble the amino acids to form the backbone of a protein, although certain posttranslational modifications that crosslink polypeptide chains such as disulfide bridges and desmosine involve covalent bonds as well. Because proteins are macromolecules containing a large number of functional groups, the weak noncovalent interactions aggregate into a dominant force that determines how a protein folds into its three-dimensional structure. These interactions include electrostatic, hydrogen bonding, van der Waals, and hydrophobic interactions. Because these interactions are inherently much weaker than covalent bonds, the folded protein structure is usually metastable, thus proteins, especially those in mammals, denature at or below approximately 60°C.

Proteins are tightly compacted molecules as evidenced by their high density of 1.4 (the density of most synthetic polymers is about 1.1). The majority of proteins are in an aqueous environment, thus the preponderance of the exposed residues are polar or ionic, whereas the nonpolar ones form the core of a protein. On the contrary, certain membrane bound proteins such as porins exhibit the opposite structural characteristics where the outer is hydrophobic, and the inner is hydrophilic within a water filled channel; this is because they function as channels facilitating diffusion of polar molecules in a hydrophobic environment provided by the alkyl chains of the lipid bilayer.

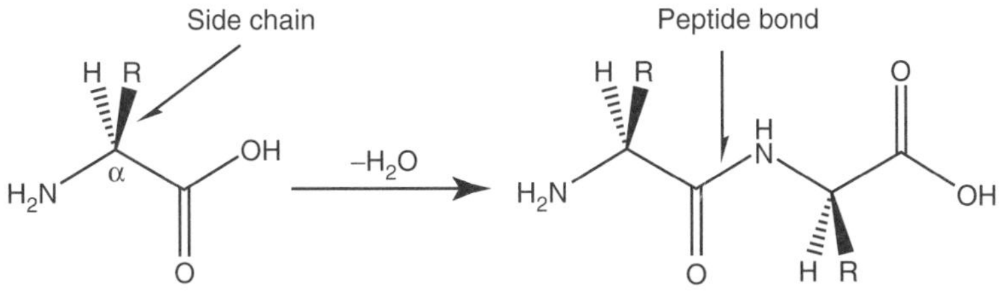

**FIGURE 4.1**
General structure of L-α-amino acids and peptide bond formation.

From a surface perspective, proteins differ greatly with respect to hydrophobicity while being observed to be highly active at surfaces. Distinctions need to be made for describing the characteristics of proteins based on their spatial organization: fibrous and globular. First, molecules can be randomly distributed and highly soluble along with flexible chains. These proteins are often disordered or can be led into this state through denaturing with chemicals or heat treatment. Fibrous proteins are largely comprised of α-helices and β-sheets in an ordered and regular structure. These fibrous proteins are often insoluble in water and assume structural roles in cells and tissues. Proteins can contain the same constituents as the fibrillar proteins in the helices and sheets, but conversely exist in a highly disordered organization. When these proteins are compacted into a localized region of high density with an approximately spherical shape, they are known as globular proteins. These proteins comprise a significant percentage of the protein species yet they are only a minority of the available protein mass. This wide spectrum of manifestations contributes to their diversity of biological function, which includes classes of proteins such as antibodies, immunoglobins, collagens, and enzymes.

## 4.2.2   Properties

The three-dimensional structure of a protein dictates its properties and functions, which differ across a broad spectrum. This is illustrated by decomposing their structures into their elementary building blocks: the amino acids. The name and codes (one- and three-letter) of the 20 common amino acids are listed along with their molecular weight and side chain p$K$a when appropriate (Figure 4.2). The name of each category reflects the property of each subgroup of amino acids. The functional groups in amino acid side chains include amine, imidazole, guanidine, carboxylic acid, alcohol, phenol, thiol, thioether, indole, and carboxamide. Proteins assemble their appropriate functional groups and arrange them in an optimal configuration to yield a wide range of properties and functions. For example, collagens and elastins provide structural and mechanical stability of the human body; enzymes maintain the metabolic equilibrium of the tissue; antibodies help the immune systems recognize foreign substances; cadherins assemble neighboring cells together; ion channel and aquaporins facilitate transport through cell membranes; hemoglobins are specialized to carry $O_2$; myoglobins stores $O_2$ in tissues; albumins solubilize substances in the blood; and fibrinogen plays a key role in blood clotting.

These proteins can then form complex assemblies by association with other biomolecules including complementary proteins, carbohydrates, and nucleic acids to accomplish a multitude of critical functions. For example, integrins in cell membranes interact with ECM molecules (fibronectin) and intracellular proteins (talin and vinculin) that further link to cytoskeleton protein (actin). This integrated network provides a direct link across the cell membrane. Interactions with carbohydrates include proteoglycans, which are molecules formed between proteins and glycosaminoglycans, a form of carbohydrates. One example of proteoglycans is chondroitin sulphate proteoglycans that lubricate joints. Finally, nucleic acids and histones form a tight complex and compact the greater than 1000 $\mu$m long DNA strands to a few $\mu$m, preserving organizational structures in the nucleus.

Proteins exhibit different mechanical properties as well with variations in their structural rigidity. The rigid proteins usually fulfill structural roles in the body. For example, cytoskeleton proteins such as filamentous actin, keratin, nuclear laminin, vimentin, and tubulin establish shape. They also provide mechanical strength and locomotion to cells as well as facilitating intracellular transport. Alternatively, relatively flexible proteins are critical to the assembly of proteins with other biopolymers and the conformational change of proteins in basic biological processes such as enzyme catalysis

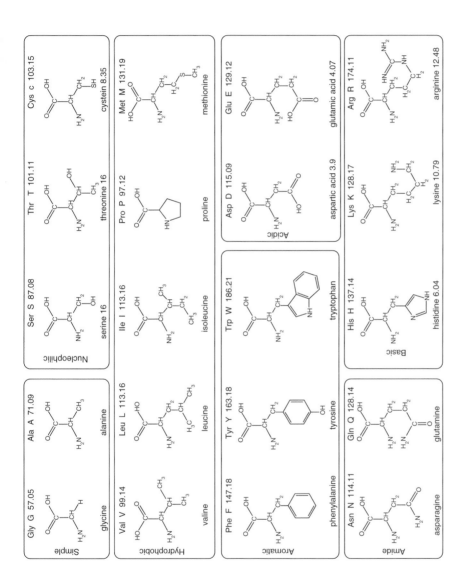

**FIGURE 4.2**

Structure and selected properties of common natural amino acids. The three- and one-letter code of each amino acid is followed by its residue weight (molecular weight with a water molecule removed). When appropriate, side chain pKa follows the full name.

and information transmission. For example, when a subunit in hemoglobin binds $O_2$, the $Fe^{2+}$ is oxidized to $Fe^{3+}$, and shrinks into the plane of the porphyrin. This results in the entire protein reorganizing into a shape that eases the subsequent binding of $O_2$ to the other three subunits in hemoglobin.

Finally, proteins differ in size, shape, charge, and hydrophilicity, all of which affect their affinity with a particular biomaterial. For example, protein adsorption on a biomaterial surface is a dynamic process. The Vroman effect reflects the dynamic profile of adsorbed proteins at the surface of a material and it reflects the interplay of kinetics and thermodynamics. Initially, proteins of high concentration (usually smaller ones such as albumin in plasma) dominate the adsorbed species, yet over the long term, proteins with higher affinities to the surface (usually larger ones such as kininogen) will gradually replace the more abundant but lower affinity proteins. Eventually the surface will reach a thermodynamically steady-state.

## 4.3   Types and Properties of Biomaterials for Adsorption

The second player in protein adsorption is the biomaterial. Current biomedical materials include metals, ceramics, and polymers. The temporal response of these materials to the physiological environment is essential to understand. Although all materials in the biological systems degrade over time, metals and some ceramic materials erode very slowly and are considered nonbiodegradable. Commonly used metals are alloys of iron, titanium, and cobalt and are found in orthopedic, dental, and cardiovascular implants. Ceramic materials include glass, ceramics, and glass–ceramics and are used also in orthopedic and dental applications (Hench and Polak, 2002).

Polymers represent one of the most diverse groups of biomaterials and include both natural and synthetic biopolymers. Examples of natural biomaterials are collagen, hyaluronic acid, chitosan, alginate, fibrin, and agrose. Synthetic biomaterials include variations of poly(methacrylate)s, poly(alkene)s, poly(siloxane)s, poly(amide)s, poly(carbonate)s, poly(ester)s, poly(urethane)s, and synthetic polypeptides. Certain crosslinked polymers swell significantly in water, and are further classified as hydrogels. Biodegradable polymers have attracted increasing attentions in biomaterials research recently. Examples of biodegradable polymers are poly(lactic acid), poly(glycolic acid), poly($\varepsilon$-caprolactone)s, polydioxanone, poly(hydroxyacid)s, polyanhydrides, polyfumerates, polysebacates, polyurethanes, polyethylene glycol (PEG) based polymers, and a wide range of copolymers made from these.

Surface properties of biomaterials such as hydrophilicity, charge, elemental composition, and morphology are all important determinants in protein adsorption. The diversity of proteins means it is challenging to determine universal rules that govern protein adsorptions, however, there are some general observations that are useful for estimating protein adsorption on biomaterials: (1) extremely hydrophilic or hydrophobic materials usually inhibit protein adsorption; (2) charged surfaces often interact favorably with proteins as most proteins are charged; (3) higher surface roughness generally promotes interactions with proteins, thus enhancing protein adsorption. The surface of biomaterials though can be modified to alter protein adsorption. Depending on the application, protein adsorption can be desirable or inhibitory due to the elicited physiological response. Protein adsorption on cardiovascular grafts is generally considered negative thus polytetrafluoroethylene, which inhibits adsorption, has been relatively successful as a graft material. Protein adsorption is generally not advantageous in certain drug delivery methods. PEG has been widely used to bestow "stealthness" upon drugs circulating in the blood because it renders the surface resistant to protein adsorption, thus delaying the clearance by liver and kidney. Conversely, in specific tissue engineering applications, protein adsorption is encouraged. Numerous tissue engineering efforts employ the modification of a biomaterial's surface with proteins such as collagen, fibronectin, and laminin. Both drug discovery and tissue engineering applications with respect to protein adsorption will be discussed later.

## 4.4 Adsorption

Adsorption includes "the accumulation of gases, liquids, or solutes on the surface of a solid or liquid" for protein adsorption at a biomaterial interface. The focus here will be on the accumulation of proteins on a solid within a liquid environment (American Heritage Dictionary, 2000). There are two types of proteins in biological fluids, soluble and insoluble, related to this adsorption. The soluble proteins are involved in adsorption to biomaterials in the body and can be affected by a variety of parameters including the rate of their spreading (Figure 4.3). They have a less regular structure than their insoluble counterparts and thus characterizing their properties and behaviors is challenging (Blanch and Clark, 1996). Furthermore, these proteins can have similar functions but with a conspicuously different sequence and associated characteristics. The insoluble proteins are usually constrained by their structural incorporation within tissue and are often related to scaffolding function. Due to this immobilization, they normally do not freely diffuse or interact with biomaterials. However, they can interact with implanted materials in other manifestations such as cells depositing molecules during foreign body encapsulation at a later stage.

Overall, in protein interactions with biomaterials, a diversity of processes governs accumulation. The concentration is one factor that dictates this interplay although it is deceptive in protein adsorption as the surface protein layer is not simply a reflection of a thick layer of a bulk protein solution. Due to this complex process, the density of molecules at the surface, which is known to be much greater than the density in the aqueous solution, implicates alternative mechanisms that are contributing to the adsorption process beyond pure concentration effects (MacRitchie, 1990). In the following sections, the adsorption processes involving energy barriers of diffusion, surface adsorption, and solid–liquid interface issues will be described although there are also other contributors including electrical charge and dehydration of the surface.

### 4.4.1 Diffusion

In one of the initial steps in protein adsorption, molecules must move into the local proximity of the surface. The ability of a molecule to arrive at a surface while residing in a homogenous aqueous environment is related to the random movement of the molecules, which is also known as diffusion (Figure 4.4). The behavior of proteins related to biomaterial adsorption with respect to diffusion is often challenging to capture using classic theories and representations. Diffusion based upon rigid solids or spheres can be described with the Stokes–Einstein equations, yet these can fail to capture the

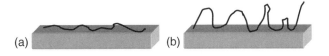

(a)   (b)

**FIGURE 4.3**
Schematic of protein adsorbed to surface in (a) fast spreading or (b) slow spreading.

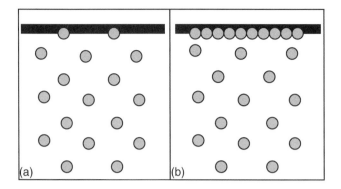

**FIGURE 4.4**
Drawing of molecules near the surface at (a) an initial time point with minimal adsorption and (b) a later time with a higher surface concentration of adsorbed proteins.

characteristics of proteins, which have the ability to swell and also exist in a soluble form. Further, the rigidity of molecules in solution with respect to mobility can be quite different from a solid material exhibiting behaviors of semi-flexible chains or the hydrodynamic behavior of a polymer. For this reason, molecules are often described in terms of their radius of gyration (de Gennes, 1997). This radius of gyration is analogous to the dimensions of a sphere, but the distribution of the atoms in the proteins is not repeatable thus requiring this alternate parameter for an approximate description. This radius of gyration, $r_g$, is correlated to the hydrodynamic radius, $r_e$, through the assumption of a randomly coiled chain behavior in Equation 4.1:

$$r_g = \xi r_e \tag{4.1}$$

Using this relationship and the Stokes–Einstein equation for molecules, Equation 4.2 relates its diffusion coefficient, $D$, to the radius of gyration:

$$D = \frac{kT}{6\pi\mu\xi r_g} \tag{4.2}$$

where $T$ is the temperature in Kelvin, $\mu$ is the solution viscosity, $r_g$ is in Angstroms, and $k$ is the Boltzmann constant. This approach though is not satisfactory for all proteins as the characteristics of rod-like proteins are captured through an approximation of one-tenth of their length in lieu of $r_g$. For molecular weight above $10^6$ Da, representing these molecules as spheres is a more accurate approximation where their length can be correlated to the radius of gyration through

$$L = \sqrt{12r_g} \tag{4.3}$$

Determining the radius of gyration is in general challenging relative to measuring the diameter of a sphere and thus various methods are currently utilized including quasi-elastic laser-light and small angle x-ray scattering. Table 4.1 includes representative diffusion coefficients and radii of gyration for various molecules.

While this is important to understand molecular motion, this activity is the behavior of individual proteins. For adsorption to biomaterials, the process is characterized by the activity of thousands of proteins and thus is the average property of the motion of many of these individual molecules. On a further note, desorption is a reverse process of adsorption which involves the release of protein attachments from the surface. As the system comes to equilibrium, the net change is the sum of the adsorption and desorption

**TABLE 4.1**

Characteristics of Molecules Including Molecular Weight, Diffusion
Coefficients, and Radii of Gyration Based on Blanch and Clark (1996)

| Molecule | Molecule Weight | Diffusion ($\times 10^{-7}$ cm$^2$ sec$^{-1}$) | Radius of Gyration (Å) |
|---|---|---|---|
| Hemoglobulin | 64,500 | 6.3 | 24.8 |
| Bovine serum albumin | 66,000 | 5.9 | 29.8 |
| Myosin | 570,000 | 1.0 | 468.0 |
| Ovalbumin | 45,000 | 7.3 | 24.0 |
| DNA | 4,000,000 | 0.1 | 1170.0 |

rates; in a significant number of cases, desorption can be ignored. Due to the intricate
nature of diffusion involved with protein adsorption, theories of diffusion are
implemented in a more complex representation.

### 4.4.2 Surface Adsorption

For attachment of molecules to biomaterials at solid/fluid interfaces, there are often no
fixed adsorption sites. (There are exceptions though for specific site attachment including
the adsorption of molecules onto self-assembled monolayers of alkanethiols.) A number of
theories describe the effects relating to the adsorption of proteins once they arrive at the
surface through initial diffusion based approaches. During adsorption molecules often
experience an interfacial pressure at the interface and thus an inherent energy barrier must
be overcome for attachment. This adsorption characteristic is independent of the type of
films and only resides in the magnitude of the pressure if the effects of electrical charge are
minimal. Thus for the transition from a bulk fluid with molecules in an aqueous
environment to an interfacial film, the interfacial pressure contributes to the molecular
adsorption with a biomaterial.

One of the current critical challenges in surface adsorption is in the development of
molecular engineered biomaterials with respect to nonfouling surfaces (Hoffman, 1999;
Morra and Cassineli, 1999; Emoto et al., 2000). While surface adsorption is critical for many
biomaterials, uncontrolled adhesion of molecules can also lead to deleterious reactions in
the body. Nonfouling surfaces have the ability to resist the random adsorption of proteins
and thus increase the specificity of the precise type and quantity of proteins for material
applications. This is especially relevant in the biomaterials community as having
a prescribed formula for molecules on the surface can be the controlling parameter for
acceptance or rejection by the human body. The presence of cell signaling molecules in
engineered materials will often lead to the activation of specific pathways leading to
uncontrolled cellular and ultimately pathogenic response. Thus one must have confidence
not only in the presence of beneficial molecules, but also in the absence of nonspecific
inhibitory molecules.

From an experimental and practical standpoint, understanding surface concentrations
of the adsorbed proteins is often misleading. With surface adsorption, the concentration of
the molecules is usually in the range of 1–10 $\mu$g/ml, but this is deceptive as the characteristic unit for this surface event should be in terms of mass per unit area not unit volume.
A simplistic assumption for determination of this concentration per unit area
is made through the height of a given molecular layer. If the layer is assumed to be
100 Å with a 1 mm$^2$ area containing 1 $\mu$g of protein, a local concentration of
1 $\mu$g/(1 mm$^2$ * 100 Å) = 1 mg/mm$^3$ is found. As a point of comparison, a value of the

density for a pure protein is 1.4 mg/mm$^3$ thus the concentration of the protein at this surface layer is extremely high. When comparing the surface concentration to the bulk solution concentration, a three order of magnitude increase is revealed and thus careful consideration must be exhibited when examining surface protein concentrations.

### 4.4.3  Protein Types for Adsorption

A wide range of molecules exhibit adsorption characteristics that are involved in biomaterial interactions including molecules that are blood-based, oxygen carriers, enzymes, and ECM proteins, which can affect a diversity of biological functions (Table 4.2). Specific proteins that are blood-based include albumin and fibrinogen, which are both found in the blood and are known to adsorb to polymers including polyethylene. Albumin can be coagulated with heat and other chemicals while fibrinogen is converted to fibrin when blood clots. Proteins that are oxygen carriers include hemogloblin and hemoglobin S. These adsorb to biomaterials and are involved in the transport of oxygen to the tissue in the body from the lungs. Further, tryptophan synthase is a 27 kDa protein that interacts with biomaterials and is important in the catalysis of the conversion of serine. Finally, ECM proteins are known to interact with cells through attachment to transmembrane proteins through the formation of adhesion complexes. The ECM proteins include fibronectin, vitronectin, laminin, and collagen, which are often scaffolding for the formation of tissue such as basement membranes; these are discussed in more detail later. The stability and structure of these proteins are related to an array of factors including conformational entropy, hydrophobicity, Coulomb interactions, van der Waals interactions, hydrogen bonds, and bond lengths/angles. The characteristics of individual proteins in combination with the surface properties of the biomaterial interact to define the final interface.

### 4.4.4  Behavior and Control at Solid–Liquid Interface

Protein adsorption onto surfaces is a complex set of competing events that give rise to final surface properties (Malmsten, 1998). This process of biomaterial adsorption is generally governed by electrostatic interactions between the protein and surface, the dispersion interactions, the state of hydration of the surface and the protein molecules, and the structural adaptations of the protein. There are a number of other factors though that contribute to the overall elements including biomolecule molecular weight, number of atoms, number of residues, surface area, positive surface charge, positively charged area, negative surface charge, negatively charged area, charges on the surface hydrophobic surface area, total surface hydrophobicity, hydrophilic surface area, total surface hydrophilicity isoelectric point, dipole moment, solution protein concentration, pH, buffer surface, and surface tension.

**TABLE 4.2**

Surface Activity, Function, and Location of Molecules Based on Horbett et al. (1996)

| Protein | Function | Location | Surface Activity |
|---|---|---|---|
| Collagen | Extracellular matrix | Tissue | Good coating to multiple polymers |
| Hemoglobin S | Oxygen carrier | Sickle red cells | Air–water activity better than hemoglobin |
| Albumin | Carrier | Blood | Low on polyethylene |
| Fibrinogen | Clotting | Blood | High on polyethylene |

While this is a complicated set of interactions and each material has different surface characteristics, there are methods to help modify the protein adsorption behavior and thus exert a modest amount of control over this process. One example is PEG modified surfaces, which are used to produce a dense and strongly attached molecular layer at biomaterial–aqueous solution layers. This inhibits protein adsorption as well as cellular attachment, which are important characteristics to control for biocompatibility of materials in mammals. In this, PEG has been shown to significantly reduce the attachment of plasma proteins and platelets *in vitro* and *in vivo*. Conversely, PEG is also used in a reverse process for the immobilization of proteins. This is accomplished through modifying the free end of the polymer chain into a free reactive group through thermal activation methods as well as incorporating microemulsions. Thus PEG is an example of a relatively robust tool for tailoring protein surface interactions.

Finally, proteins must be characterized along with their counterpart material to understand and reproduce beneficial protein adsorbed biomaterials. Most surface analysis techniques can be adapted to analyze the interactions of proteins and biomaterials surfaces. For example, if protein adsorption evokes a change in elemental composition of the surface, x-ray photoelectron spectroscopy can be used to analyze this adaptation. Additionally, functional group information of the surface can be obtained by Fourier transform infrared spectroscopy methods. Ellipsometry is useful in assessing the thickness of the adsorbent. Atomic force microscopy can be used to observe changes in surface morphology after protein adsorption. These are a brief illustration of techniques, which are implemented in characterizing samples.

## 4.5 Protein Adsorption and Interactions with Cells

The ability of cells to interact with materials that are coated with proteins influences their biocompatibility. Engineered cell interactions in the human body can be influenced by the attachment of cells to artificial scaffolding such as a biomaterial. This applies to a diversity of systems including regrowth of bone through osteogenic activity to tissue engineering artificial vasculature through the utilization of endothelial and smooth muscle cell attachment and proliferation. The ability for cells to attach to these substrates resides directly with the cell–ECM interactions, and these interactions can allow local control of the attachment and spreading of cells on biomaterials (Figure 4.5).

The binding of a cell to the ECM can occur through the formation of protein links extending from the intra- to the extra-cellular domains. One of these connections is the focal adhesion complex (FAC), which is a heterocomplex of proteins including integrins, paxillin, vinculin, and talin. Integrins (or "integrators") play a key role in the FACs. Integrins are transmembrane heterodimers comprised of glycoprotein subunits $\alpha$ and $\beta$. The $\alpha$ chain is terminated on the cytosolic side by the HOOC and

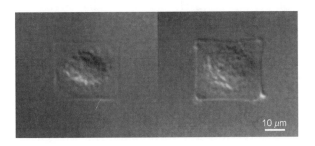

**FIGURE 4.5**
Cells patterned in square geometries through a self-assembled monolayer with square adhesive regions for cell attachment and nonadhesive regions in the surrounding areas to inhibit cell attachment.

the β chain by COOH. One end of the integrin is exposed from the exterior of the cell and binds to the ECM; while the cytoplasmic end of the β chain binds to both talin and α-actinin. Thus integrins link the ECM with the cytoskeleton of a cell. Many different types of ECM proteins feature an important arg-gly-asp (RGD) peptide sequence that is the recognized by integrins. There are many types of these families of heterodimers that bind to a diversity of ECM including the more common ECMs, fibronectin and laminin, which bind to over 10 different sets of integrins. The surface density of the molecules can also cause issues with biological activity through conformational changes (Michael et al., 2003). The FACs are connected to the internal cell structure of the actin cytoskeleton in most cases except circumstances including hemidesmosomes where $\alpha_6\beta_4$ connects to the intermediate filaments, which is another cytoskeletal filament. These filament systems provide structural and organizational support for the entire cell thus the FACs directly link the extracellular world (i.e., the ECM) to the intracellular architecture (i.e., the cytoskeleton).

Through these surface interactions, the ability of cells to form stable structures is found. The structural behavior in mammalian cells such as osteoblasts, osteoclasts, endothelial, smooth muscle, and cardiovascular cells are known to be heavily influenced by the filaments systems of the aforementioned cytoskeleton (Li et al., 1997; Small and Gimona, 1998; Bellin et al., 1999; Kaibuchi et al., 1999; Tamm, 1999; Krol et al., 2000; Bellin et al., 2001; de Curtis, 2001; Schweitzer et al., 2001; Hasezawa and Kumagai, 2002; Ilsley et al., 2002; van Niel and Heyman, 2002). This complex and highly organized structure plays a major role in not only cell shape, but also in motility (Rivero et al., 1996; Soll, 1997; Machesky and Cooper, 1999; Small et al., 1999; Casanova, 2002), division (Sanger and Sanger, 1979; Streiblova and Hasek, 1987; Izutsu, 1991; Bogre et al., 2000; de Castro et al., 2000), and polarity (Fleming et al., 1986; Ishikawa, 1989; Nelson et al., 1990; Parry et al., 1990; Fath et al., 1993; Hable and Kropf, 1998; Svoboda et al., 2001). Aside from the structural interactions, cells have the ability to modulate the activity of the integrins through biochemical activation. For example, this occurs in the response of platelets where $\beta_3$ integrin is activated in the membrane in order to bind to the protein fibrinogen that induces blood clot formation as well as the accumulation of platelets. Thus the binding of proteins to material surfaces for cell attachment can affect the behavior of cells in both a structural and biochemical form; this alters its utility as a plausible biomaterial.

## 4.6 Applications for Protein Adsorption

### 4.6.1 Tissue Engineering

Tissue engineering is the application of "the principles of biology and engineering to the development of viable substitutes that restore, maintain or improve the function of human tissues" (Lanza et al., 2000). Biomaterials research and tissue engineering are closely related as one key concept in tissue engineering is to reconstitute tissues by culturing appropriate cells or cell mixtures in a biomaterial scaffold. Cell adhesion is crucial to the success of tissue engineering constructs, which is closely related to protein adsorption.

One of the critical properties in tissue engineering is the biocompatibility of materials for a specific application. This is especially important as the material scaffolding has to support the growth of biologically functional tissues. Despite the diverse surface properties of biomaterials studied in the past several decades, the immune system seems to respond similarly. Most biomaterials implanted will elicit an acute inflammatory response, which is followed by chronic inflammation signaled by foreign body giant cell formation and fibrous encapsulation. One possible mechanism for this apparent independence of biocompatibility to the nature of the material is that the materials are perceived as foreign by the body as protein adsorbs on the biomaterial surfaces nonspecifically. In comparison, native tissue expresses specific cell surface markers that results in an identifiable proteinous surface pattern that the immune system perceive as "self."

Biomaterial surface modifications should ideally result in a surface that encourages specific protein adsorption patterns. The list of engineered tissues is growing rapidly, covering most tissue types in the body, and the type of protein adsorption profiles varies greatly among the different applications. There are numerous potential modifications to bridge this relationship between protein adsorption and tissue engineering, which include modifying the entire surface with a natural protein. For example, fibronectin can be coated in the lumen of tubular biomaterial scaffolds to facilitate endothelialization of the lumen. Furthermore, one can pattern the surface with functional groups to achieve a desirable protein adsorption pattern. The hydrophilicity and charge of a surface can be altered with functional groups such as $CH_3$, $OH$, $NH_3^+$, and $COO^-$ to control the protein adsorption pattern and therefore the cell adhesion pattern. Also, scientists can tether oligopeptides comprising the active site of the proteins of interest to the surface of biomaterials. Surfaces patterned with molecules that enhance and inhibit cell adhesion have been used to regulate cell adhesion pattern and to spatially control co-culture of different types of cells (Figure 4.5).

### 4.6.2 Drug Delivery

The ability to deliver drugs to general and specific locations inside the body is another application of biomaterials with respect to protein adsorption (McGrath and Kaplan, 1997). There are various delivery schemes, but a common form is intravenous administration. This delivery elicits a variety of physiological responses and thus the material of interest must be tailored to combat the natural defenses of the body. One system that is used is colloidal carriers due to a minimal response with respect to macrophage encapsulation. Proteins in these carrier systems, which are adsorbed at the phospholipids interfaces, are known to increase the efficacy of the drug delivery. This behavior has been attributed to a number of factors including the fluidity of the carrier surface. There are numerous carriers with respect to colloidal arrangements including micelles, liposomes, and emulsion droplets. Micelles are composed of block copolymers and are thermodynamically stable to allow for positive characteristics in storage and preparation. One well characterized system of micelles is a PEG–polyaspartate conjugate containing adriamycin. Liposomes are another colloid, which have shown much promise in drug discovery over the past several decades due to their ability to solubilize both oil and water soluble materials. Liposomes are phospholipids filled with fluid in which chemicals or pharmaceutical agents are encapsulated. Due to their phospholipid bilayers they are believed likely to be more comparable to cell structures in the composition of the plasma membrane; thus they exhibit more biologically compatible characteristics. Finally, an emulsion droplet is the most common colloid method in use as a product. Emulsions are a mixture of different liquid solutions that will not normally mix, but are controlled to self-organize into colloidal systems such as in oil–water emulsions. These are select examples of molecular based drug delivery systems although there are many others that are discussed in other chapters including protein release schemes with adsorption to or encapsulation within materials.

In summary, protein adsorption plays a significant role in the biomaterial interface. Understanding adsorption though is complicated by the variety of interconnected characteristics, yet progress has been made in a number of significant areas. The further exploration of the governing processes related to adsorption will help guide scientists in the future to make advances in numerous and diverse arenas including tissue engineering and drug discovery. Diverse skill sets are needed in these integrated fields including knowledge in chemistry, biology, and engineering simultaneously. Ultimately, through these interdisciplinary efforts, scientific as well as technological advances will be expanded; these will have a significant impact on human health for many years into the future.

## References

Alberts, B. et al., *Molecular Biology of the Cell*, 3rd ed., Garland Publishing, New York (1994).
*American Heritage Dictionary*, Houghton Mifflin, Boston (2000).
Anderson, J.M., *Annu. Rev. Mater. Res.*, **31**, 81 (2001).
Andrade, J.D. and Hlady, V., *Adv. Polym. Sci.*, **79**, 1 (1986).
Bellin, R.M. et al., *J. Biol. Chem.*, **274**, 29493 (1999).
Bellin, R.M., Huiatt, T.W., Critchley, D.R., and Robson, R.M., *J. Biol. Chem.*, **276**, 32330 (2001).
Blanch, H.W. and Clark, D.S., *Biochemical Engineering*, Marcel Dekker, New York (1996).
Bogre, L., Calderini, O., Merskiene, I., and Binarova, P., *Results Probl. Cell Differ.*, **27**, 95 (2000).
Casanova, J.E., *Am. J. Physiol. Gastrointest. Liver Physiol.*, **283**, G1015 (2002).
de Castro, R.D., van Lammeren, A.A., Groot, S.P., Bino, R.J., and Hilhorst, H.W., *Plant Physiol.*, **122**, 327 (2000).
de Curtis, I., *EMBO Rep.*, **2**, 277 (2001).
de Gennes, P.G., *Soft Interfaces*, Cambridge University Press, Cambridge (1997).
Emoto, K., Nagasaki, Y., Iijima, M., Kato, M., and Kataoka, K., *Colloids Surf. B Biointerfaces*, **18**, 337 (2000).
Fath, K.R., Mamajiwalla, S.N., and Burgess, D.R., *J. Cell Sci. Suppl.*, **17**, 65 (1993).
Fleming, T.P., Cannon, P.M., and Pickering, S.J., *Dev. Biol.*, **113**, 406 (1986).
Hable, W.E. and Kropf, D.L., *Dev. Biol.*, **198**, 45 (1998).
Hasezawa, S. and Kumagai, F., *Int. Rev. Cytol.*, **214**, 161 (2002).
Hench, L.L. and Polak, J.M., *Science*, **295**, 1014 (2002).
Hoffman, A.S., *J. Biomater. Sci. Polym. Ed.*, **10**, 1011 (1999).
Horbett, T.A., Ratner, B.D., and Schakenraad, J.M., In: *Biomaterials Science*, Ratner, B.D., Ed., Academic Press, San Diego, CA (1996).
Ilsley, J.L., Sudol, M., and Winder, S.J., *Cell Signal.*, **14**, 183 (2002).
Ishikawa, H., *Tanpakushitsu Kakusan Koso*, **34**, 1742 (1989).
Izutsu, K., *Hum. Cell*, **4**, 100 (1991).
Kaibuchi, K., Kuroda, S., and Amano, M., *Annu. Rev. Biochem.*, **68**, 459 (1999).
Krol, A.Y., Grinfeldt, M.G., Vereninov, A.A., and Malev, V.V., *Membr. Cell Biol.*, **14**, 69 (2000).
Lanza, R.P., Langer, R., and Vacanti, J.P., *Principles of Tissue Engineering*, Academic Press, San Diego, CA (2000).
Li, Y.Q., Moscatelli, A., Cai, G., and Cresti, M., *Int. Rev. Cytol.*, **176**, 133 (1997).
Lippold, O.C., *J. Physiol.*, **202**, 55P (1969).
Machesky, L.M. and Cooper, J.A., *Nature*, **401**, 542 (1999).
MacRitchie, F., *Chemistry at Interfaces*, Academic Press, San Diego, CA (1990).
Malmsten, M., Ed., *Biopolymers at Interfaces*, Marcel Dekker, New York (1998).
McGrath, K. and Kaplan, D., Eds., *Protein-Based Materials*, Birkhauser, Boston (1997).
Michael, K.E. et al., *Langmuira*, **19**, 8033 (2003).
Morra, M. and Cassineli, C., *J. Biomater. Sci. Polym. Ed.*, **10**, 1107 (1999).
Nelson, W.J., Hammerton, R.W., Wang, A.Z., and Shore, E.M., *Semin. Cell Biol.*, **1**, 359 (1990).

Parry, G., Beck, J.C., Moss, L., Bartley, J., and Ojakian, G.K., *Exp. Cell Res.*, **188**, 302 (1990).

Ratner, B.D., Hoffman, A.S., Schoen, F.J., and Lemons, J.E., *Biomaterials Science*, Academic Press, San Diego, CA (1996).

Rivero, F. et al., *J. Cell Sci.*, **109** (Pt 11), 2679 (1996).

Sanger, J.W. and Sanger, J.M., *Methods Achiev. Exp. Pathol.*, **8**, 110 (1979).

Schweitzer, S.C. et al., *J. Cell Sci.*, **114**, 1079 (2001).

Small, J.V. and Gimona, M., *Acta Physiol. Scand.*, **164**, 341 (1998).

Small, J.V., Kaverina, I., Krylyshkina, O., and Rottner, K., *FEBS Lett.*, **452**, 96 (1999).

Soll, D.R., *Cell Motil. Cytoskeleton*, **37**, 91 (1997).

Streiblova, E. and Hasek, J., *Izv. Akad. Nauk. SSSR Biol.*, 353 (1987).

Svoboda, A., Slaninova, I., and Holubarova, A., *Acta Biol. Hung.*, **52**, 325 (2001).

Tamm, S.L., *Microsc. Res. Tech.*, **44**, 293 (1999).

van Niel, G. and Heyman, M., *Am. J. Physiol. Gastrointest. Liver Physiol.*, **283**, G251 (2002).

# 5

## In Vitro *Testing of Biomaterials*

Shelley R. Winn, John Mitchell, and Hasan Uludağ

## CONTENTS

## 5.1  Introduction

A biomaterial can be defined as any natural or synthetic material used in a medical device that is intended to interact with a biological system (Black, 1982; von Recum and LaBerge, 1995). *In vitro* assay systems have historically been utilized as the initial screening methods to determine if biomaterials exhibit cytotoxicity or compatibility with living cells. Early procedures for assessing cytotoxicity were based on morphological changes leading to cell death and were utilized by many laboratories. Several tests have achieved widespread use and are currently used as internationally recognized standardized *in vitro* tests for biocompatibility. Biocompatibility is a performance index; a qualitative descriptor indicating how well living systems interact with a material and how the interaction meets

**TABLE 5.1**
Advantages and Limitations of Biocompatibility Tests

| Test/Assay | Advantages | Limitations |
|---|---|---|
| *In vitro* tests | Quick turnover (days), low cost, high throughput screening, standardized with appropriate controls | Relevance to *in vivo* outcome inconsistent |
| *In vivo* tests | Provides multi-system interactions, more comprehensive than *in vitro* tests | Relevance to clinical use questionable, low turnover (weeks to months), high cost and low throughput, animal use concerns, variable and control assurance difficult, outcome can be difficult to interpret |
| Usage tests | Relevance to clinical use assured | Low turnover (weeks to months), high cost and low throughput, animal use concerns, variable and control assurance difficult, outcome can be difficult to interpret |

the designed expectations for a targeted purpose and implantation site (von Recum et al., 1999). The *in vitro* systems can provide rapid and cost-effective means of predictive behaviors on biological interactions, but the relevance to the more complex *in vivo* environment must be kept in perspective (Table 5.1).

When discussing the relevance of *in vitro* assays to the *in situ* biocompatibility of a medical device, several issues have been discussed. In the 1993 *Tests for cytotoxicity: in vitro methods*, the proposed cell culture assays were presented as *in vitro* correlates to local *in situ* tissue toxicity assays, such as the irritation and implantation assays. Because the actions of potential chemical toxins that produce adverse effects in animals or humans exert their damage at the cellular level, it was reasoned that the cellular response is the foundation for establishing biological responses to foreign materials or substances. In addition, three interfaces between *in vitro* assays and animal toxicology have been proposed: screening tests, mechanistic studies, and risk assessment. Because screening tests are the most advanced and utilized, they will likely remain the major choice for evaluating *in vitro* toxicity/toxicology (*Sample preparation and reference materials*, 1993).

This chapter will describe the variety of *in vitro* testing systems currently in use to screen biomaterials for cytotoxicity (cellular compatibility). These include routine cytotoxicity tests and mutagenesis assays. In addition, several advanced testing paradigms are presented that provide tissue-specific responses (e.g., bone marrow cultures) that may provide a more representative response similar to that observed in the clinical setting.

## 5.2 Background Concepts

A critical term for the evaluation of biomaterial biocompatibility is toxicity. A toxic material is defined as something that releases a chemical in a quantity sufficient to kill cells directly or indirectly by inhibiting important metabolic pathways. A cytotoxic material is a term used to define an agent that is "cell killing." The percent of cell death is an indication of the potency (dose) of the agent/chemical. Although several factors may contribute to the toxicity of a chemical, the dose of the agent delivered to the cell is the most important factor.

Exposure dose refers to the amount of the cytotoxic agent delivered to a test system. This is in contrast to the delivered dose, the dose of the agent actually absorbed by a cell. In the example of an animal exposed to a noxious or cytotoxic agent contained within the breathable or absorbable atmosphere, only a portion of the agent will be delivered to organs and cells (the delivered dose). Because cells are inherently sensitive to the toxic effects of foreign agents, the most sensitive cells responding to the toxic agent are known as the target cells. Thus, *in vitro* testing of biomaterials evaluates target cell toxicity by a potency of delivered doses of the test substance. This is in contrast to the exposure dose delivered to a whole animal and accounts for the increase in sensitivity of *in vitro* testing methods compared to animal toxicity data. Therefore, over the past two decades, scientists, industry, and the government have recognized that the most accurate, cost-effective, and practical means to assess the biocompatibility of a test biomaterial is a combination of *in vitro*, animal, and usage tests (e.g., teeth). Table 5.1 outlines the advantages and limitations of the *in vitro*, general animal tests (*in vivo*), and usage tests.

In the evolution of biocompatibility testing, some scientists have questioned the usefulness of *in vitro* and toxicity testing in whole-animal experiments. If the outcomes do not correlate with what was expected in usage tests and clinical results, then why are they useful? As previously mentioned, this differential outcome should not be surprising when considering exposure and delivered doses of an agent, and additional barriers, such as the dentin barrier in teeth existing in usage tests and clinical use that are absent with *in vitro* and whole-animal tests. It is therefore important to keep in mind that each type of test is designed to measure a different aspect of a biological response to biomaterials.

Initially, a pyramid scheme for testing biomaterials was proposed to visualize the testing paradigms (Figure 5.1). In this scheme, all of the candidate materials are tested at the bottom of the pyramid, with preferred candidates continuing as the testing continues toward the top of the pyramid. The bottom of the pyramid would be represented by a variety of unspecific *in vitro* toxicity tests. Preferred candidates would be selected and the next tier would evaluate toxicity dealing with conditions more relevant to the materials targeted application (pre-clinical toxicology study). The final tier would be represented by a clinical trial of the material in its intended clinical use. More recently, pyramid schemes have been proposed that divided stages into initial, secondary, and usage tests. In these schemes, the types of tests have been broadened to include biological responses in addition to toxicity, such as mutagenicity and immunogenicity. The concept of a usage test in an animal model was also proposed prior to initiation of a clinical trial. Presumably, safer materials had been developed and unsafe materials screened out. Although

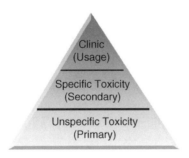

**FIGURE 5.1**
A pyramid strategy for the use of biocompatibility tests to assess the safety of medical devices (and their constituents). The evaluation of materials begins at the bottom of the pyramid and proceeds upward. The number of tests required diminishes upward because unacceptable materials are screened out in the early testing phases. Early strategies proposed unspecific toxicity, specific toxicity, and clinical trials. More recent strategies involve a primary, secondary, and usage schemata (in parentheses).

improved, the inability of *in vitro* and animal usage tests to predict clinical utility has led to the development of refined, modified schemes for biocompatibility testing.

The most recent testing schemes have emphasized the use of biocompatibility tests in combinations to evaluate materials. This emphasis is reinforced by the notion that all of the tests, either alone or in combination, continue to be of value when assessing the biocompatibility of a biomaterial during the developmental phase, and even into clinical applicability. The newer schemes also acknowledge that individual testing methods currently in place cannot absolutely screen in or out a material. Lastly, these latest schemes incorporate a philosophy that assessing biocompatibility of a new or modified biomaterial is an ongoing and evolving process. Certainly, evolving strategies for the future will continue to utilize a combinatorial approach as the technologies and methods for testing improve.

An important consideration in utilizing *in vitro* tests for assessing biocompatibility and cytotoxicity is the soluble components within a biomaterial or medical device. A majority of medical devices are comprised of water-insoluble materials, such as nonresorbable polymers, metals, and ceramics; but other components can be incorporated into the final product to obtain the desired outcome for improvements in physicochemical and manufacturing properties. This could be agents such as antioxidants, antibiotics, fillers, plasticizers, and mold release agents; agents either in the formulation or additives from the manufacturing process. Thus, leachables or surface-layered materials may inadvertently impact the outcome and, thus, the methods for extracting biomaterials have been standardized to improve reproducibility and eliminate unwanted contaminants. In rare instances, complete dissolution of the biomaterial may be warranted; however, this does not simulate the clinical target and may create degradation products that may not otherwise occur in a clinical setting.

## 5.3   Standards That Assess Biocompatibility

Standardization for any process is laborious, lengthy, and can be made more difficult by a lack of agreement on the appropriateness and impact of particular tests. The passage of the Medical Device Bill by the United States Congress in 1976 put an emphasis on biological testing of all medical devices. This law enabled the development of suitable systems to improve and ensure public safety. In 1977, the National Heart, Lung, and Blood Institute (NHLBI) reviewed its status in biomaterials development, determining that more reliable approaches to evaluating and standardizing the study of biomaterials and their interactions with blood was necessary. Two groups, the physicochemical characterization of biomaterials group and a blood–material interaction group, were formed. Following the recommendation of three primary reference materials — namely low-density polyethylene, silica-free polydimethylsiloxane, and fluorinated ethylene propylene — the NHLBI-funded research to establish guidelines, standardized methods, and materials (*Guidelines for blood–materials interactions*, 1980, 1985; *Guidelines for physicochemical characterization for biomaterials*, 1980).

In the early 1990s, the International Union for Pure and Applied Chemistry (IUPAC) formed a group to address "Interactions of Polymers with Living Systems." Although studies were performed by a number of laboratories throughout the world in an effort to standardize testing procedures for polymeric materials, the results were not published (Belanger and Marois, 2001). The three main areas of research focused on the interactions of materials with blood, biocompatibility and inflammation, and *in vivo* studies.

ISO 10993 is the most extensive and standardized document available intended to provide international standards and methodologies for evaluating biomedical materials/devices (www.iso.ch, 1992). Scientists from the International Standards Organization (ISO), as well as several multi-national working groups, were formed to develop these standards. ISO 10993, published in 1992 containing 12 parts (www.iso.ch, 1992), is the most recent standard available and is recognized as the reference guide for biological testing. Guidelines to determine the appropriate selection of tests are provided in part 1. Part 3 describes tests for genotoxicity, carcinogenicity, and reproductive toxicity, while part 4 presents the tests and reference guide for materials intended for interactions with blood. Part 5 describes tests for cytotoxicity: *in vitro* methods. The document divides testing procedures into two categories, initial and supplementary. Initial tests are intended to assess cytotoxicity, sensitization, and systemic toxicity. While it is recommended that some of the tests be performed *in vitro*, others are intended for evaluation in animal models. The supplementary tests are generally performed in animal model systems, with the implant site analogous to the intended clinical use.

## 5.4   General Testing Methods

There are three primary *in vitro* cell culture cytotoxicity assays described in the 2004 U.S. Pharmacopeia; the agar diffusion test, the direct contact test, and the elution, or extract dilution assay (U.S. Pharmacopeia, 2004). In addition, similar standards are published by the American Society for Testing and Materials (ASTM), the British Standards Institute (BSI), and the International Standards Organization (ISO). Assays described in the 2004 U.S. Pharmacopeia are required by regulatory agencies in the United States (Food and Drug Administration), Europe, Australia, Japan, and other countries. The ASTM and BSI standards are consensus standards and it is expected that the ISO standards will soon supplant individual national regulations in most of Europe. These three *in vitro* tests are based on cellular morphology, such that the outcome is measured by observing changes in the shape and structure of the plated cells, as well as the outcome of cell toxicity as assessed by changes in viable cell populations. The differences in the assays are dependent on how the test material is exposed to the cells. The test material can either be placed directly on the cells, or the material or additives can be extracted from the test material in an appropriate solution. The solution containing the extract can then be added into the culture medium that feeds the cells. For example, the recommendation of ISO 10993-5 is to test a portion of a finished device, some of the devices components, or an extract of the components. Each method can be chosen based on the characteristics of the test material and the rationale of the test for assessing compatibility.

### 5.4.1   Agar Diffusion Test

This assay utilizes a monolayer of cells generally plated on a tissue culture-treated plastic dish or multi-well with an agar or agarose overlay (3 to 4 mm). Agarose is generally preferred since the gelling point is generally 30 to 34°C, while most agar products are observed to gel in the 40 to 45°C range, hence contributing to thermal shock during the overlay process. After the agar/agarose has solidified, samples of positive and negative control materials, as well as the test article, are placed on the overlay in tissue culture media and analyzed daily for up to 3 days. Vital or nonvital stains can be incorporated into the agar/agarose to be incorporated into viable (live) cells, such as neutral red, or nonviable (dead) cells, such as trypan blue. Vital dyes are actively recruited and

**TABLE 5.2**
Graded Scale for Agar Diffusion and Direct Contact Tests

| Grade | Type of Reactivity | Comments on Reactivity Zone |
|---|---|---|
| 0 | None | No detectable reactivity zone |
| 1 | Minimal | Very few degenerated or malformed cells next to sample |
| 2 | Mild | Reactive zone limited to area adjacent to sample |
| 3 | Moderate | Zone may extend to 1 cm beyond sample |
| 4 | Severe | Zone extends beyond 1 cm around sample area |

Adapted from USP23-NF18, copyright 1994.

transported into viable cells, where they remain or are retained, provided the cell membrane remains intact and is not permeabolized by cytotoxic events. Nonvital dyes are not actively transported, remaining outside the cell, unless cytotoxic events have permeabolized the cell membrane. Cytotoxicity is generally assessed by semi-quantitative graded scale from 0 (no reaction) to grade 4 (severe) (Table 5.2). The agar diffusion assay has demonstrated validation for dose response, correlation with the direct contact assay, and correlation with the intramuscular implantation assay in the rabbit model (Bultitude and Boocock, 1977). The Agar diffusion test is actually a barrier model because agents must diffuse through the agar before making contact with the plated cells. Other barrier assays include the Millipore® filter assay (Hanks et al., 1996), Transwell® or other porous compartmentalization (Winn and Hollinger, 2000), and dentin barrier tests (Hanks et al., 1996).

## 5.4.2   Direct Contact Test

As the name implies, in contrast to the placement of test articles on an agar overlay (barrier model), the direct contact assay utilizes a monolayer of cells on which the materials are placed in direct contact with the cells. As with the Agar diffusion test, this system is dependent on the diffusion of substances from the test article and into the culture medium. In contrast to barrier models, movement of the test article can potentially disrupt the cellular monolayer. Disturbing the cell layer can result in cellular trauma due to physical interactions, thereby leading to a misinterpretation of cell death as a cytotoxic response. Cultures are generally incubated at 24 and 48 h and cell viability is assessed with vital or nonvital stains, semi-quantified with a graded scale as described in the Agar diffusion section (Table 5.2). Greater sensitivity has been observed for detecting toxic agents in plastic samples with the direct contact assay as compared to the rabbit intramuscular implantation assay. Although sensitive, this technique can be prone to methodological difficulties. The results should be verified with other tests.

## 5.4.3   Extract Dilution (Elution) Test

For the extract dilution test, also known as the elution test, an extract of the material is prepared and evaluated for cytotoxicity. An extract of the material can be prepared by using a physiologic solution, such as 0.9% normal saline, phosphate-buffered saline, other biologic buffers such as Hanks balanced salt solution, or appropriate tissue culture medium with or without serum. Other extraction solvents include dimethyl sulfoxide, vegetable oil, weak acids or bases, etc. Whatever extraction solvent is chosen, it should be compatible with the physicochemical characteristics of the sample. The solvent must not change the crystalline structure, cause hydrolysis, or affect covalent linkages of the test sample. Furthermore, the concentration of the extraction solvent should be compatible with the culture system and obviously not induce toxicity of the plated cells. According to ISO10993-12, (biological evaluation of medical devices), samples prepared for cytotoxicity testing should be adequately cleaned and sterilized to prevent misleading results or contamination of the culture system. An appropriate surface area-to-volume ratio of the test article to the volume of culture medium should also be considered. Guidelines are provided in the 2004 U.S. Pharmacopeia. An extract should be placed within the tissue culture media of a near-confluent monolayer of plated cells. An evaluation of toxicity should be performed 24 and 48 h later. In contrast to focal or localized cell damage that may be observed with the Agar diffusion or direct contact tests, the pattern of toxicity in the elution test will be observed as a consistent pattern throughout the plated cells. Live or dead cells can be assessed with vital/nonvital stains as previously described, or assessed with metabolic assays. Reactivity grades for the elution test are similar (in principle), to the direct contact/Agar diffusion tests, but graded in more general terms (Table 5.3).

### 5.4.4 Endpoints for Assessment

Cellular toxicity leads to progressive cell death. Cell death has historically been divided into two categories: necrosis, or extrinsic factor-induced cell death; and apoptosis, or programmed cell death (Majno and Joris, 1995). These two responses are distinct with regards to the observed morphological differences, as well as the timing of appearance, the type and strength of stimulus necessary for induction of the cascade. The factors that contribute to cellular necrosis are primarily extrinsic, examples include: hypoxia-ischemia (lack of oxygen), thermal insults, exposure to toxic agents, and traumatic insults. A progressive loss of membrane integrity allows the influx of ions and water, resulting in cytoplasmic swelling, nuclear pyknosis (shrinkage), release of lysosomal and granular contents into the surrounding extracellular space, with subsequent inflammation. Apoptosis is highly coordinated, and thought to be linked to intrinsic genetically linked mechanisms. Extrinsic factors, however, are now recognized as contributors to the apoptotic process. Apoptosis is characterized by cytoplasmic and nuclear shrinkage, chromatin margination and fragmentation, and eventual breakdown of the cell into multiple spherical bodies that generally retain membrane integrity. Although once thought to be functionally opposed forms of cell death, the current consensus is that both necrosis and apoptosis constitute two extremes of a continuum.

In addition to the vital and nonvital stains available to monitor cellular viability in the Agar diffusion, direct contact and elution tests, more specific histochemical stains are

**TABLE 5.3**
Graded Scale for Extract Dilution (Elution) Test

| Grade | Type of Cell Response | Comments on Cellular Response |
|-------|----------------------|-------------------------------|
| 0 | None | No detectable adverse cellular response |
| 1 | Minimal | No more than 20% of the cells display adverse response |
| 2 | Mild | No more than 50% of the cells display adverse response |
| 3 | Moderate | No more than 70% of the cells display adverse response |
| 4 | Severe | Cells display near complete adverse response |

Adapted from USP23-NF18, copyright 1994. Adverse cellular response defined as cells that have rounded up, and are loosely attached to the tissue culture substrate; and display cell lysis (detachment and destruction).

available to monitor apoptosis. A nuclear stain such as bisbenzimide (e.g., Hoechst 33258, 33342; ApopTag®) is effective at labeling the morphological changes in nuclear chromatin structure that can be viewed with a fluorescent microscope. The nuclear stain, in conjunction with the "terminal deoxynucleotidyl transferase-mediated dUTP-biotin nick end labeling (TUNEL)" assay, is also a means to detect and quantify apoptotic cell death at single cell levels in tissue culture. However, the sensitivity and selectivity of the TUNEL assay has been less than optimal for distinguishing necrotic, apoptotic and sublethal injured cells in tissue sections.

### 5.4.5   Other Assays for Cell Function

In addition to the standardized Agar diffusion, direct contact and elution tests, other methods are available that characterize the enzymatic or biosynthetic activity (metabolism) of cells to assess a cytotoxic response. The 3-(4,5-dimethylthiazol-2-yl)-2,5-diphenyltetrazolium bromide (MTT) assay is based on the ability of a mitochondrial dehydrogenase enzyme from within living cells to cleave the tetrazolium rings of the yellow MTT to form dark blue formazan crystals (Mosmann, 1983). The number of viable, live cells is proportional to the level of formazan product created; the color of which can be quantified with a simple colorimetric assay (e.g., ELISA plate reader), following solubilization of the cells to liberate the formed crystals (see Figure 5.2). Other formazan generating assays, or assays that measure reduced metabolic activities are available. These include NBT, WST, and XTT — if the dehydrogenases in the cell cultures are not active due to the influence of cytotoxic agents, the formazan product will not be created. AlamarBlue® is another metabolic activity indicator that utilizes an oxidation-reduction system that changes color in response to the chemical reduction of the reagent in the growth medium during cell growth. Other cytotoxicity assays include assays that measure plasma membrane damage/leakage such as 51-Chromium release and the release of lactate dehydrogenase (LDH).

Other tests are available to assess cytotoxic responses of cultured cells that monitor/measure plasma membrane damage and deoxyribonucleic acid (DNA) fragmentation. The synthesis of DNA (or protein) by cells is generally assessed by adding a radioisotope pre-label, such as 3H-thymidine (or 3H-leucine), and quantifying the radioisotope that has been incorporated into DNA or protein. An alternative,

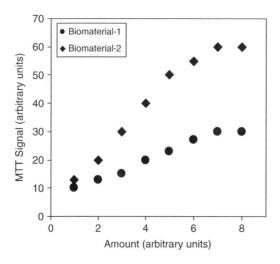

**FIGURE 5.2**
Evaluating the compatibility of biomaterials can be assessed with cellular enzyme activity as depicted in this figure. MTT is a yellow, soluble molecule that when reduced by cellular activity, results in a blue insoluble formazan product deposited within the cell. The quantity of formazan formed is proportional to the enzyme activity, which is proportional to an index such as cell number. Most of the assays assessing cellular enzyme activity are assessed in this manner.

non radioactive pre-label DNA uptake method can utilize bromodeoxyuridine (BrdU), which, under conditions of cell-mediated cytotoxicity, can be released into the cytoplasm of cells or in the culture supernatant due to plasma leakage of damaged cells. The BrdU-labeled DNA can be quantified with an enzyme-linked immunosorbent assay (ELISA).

### 5.4.6 Mutagenesis Assays

Determining the safety of a product, irrespective of whether the product is a pharmaceutical or medical device, should include evaluation of its genotoxic potential. Genotoxic mutagens directly alter the DNA of the cell through several mechanisms, and may be mutagens in their native state, or may require transformation to become active mutagens. One of the basic criteria for developing biomedical devices from biomaterials simply states they should not be carcinogenic (Lyman, 1975). Carcino-genesis is literally the production or origin of cancer, and mutagens may or may not be carcinogens. Once a biomaterial or pharmaceutical is in the body, it should not cause an uncontrolled proliferation of host cells (i.e., induce mitogenic properties) in the tissue as a result of its degradation product, leaching components or corroded materials. The widely used, short-term *in vitro* assay for mutagenesis, which has demonstrated collaborative data with *in vivo* carcinogenicity, is Ames' Salmonella mutation assay (Ames et al., 1975).

Mutagenesis assays determine the effect that a reagent or material has on a cell's genetic make-up; with genotoxicity being defined as an agent that irreversibly binds or interacts with the nucleic acids to alter or change the DNA. The Ames test is a short-term mutagenesis assay that is the most widely used and validated genetic toxicology assay, and utilizes mutant stocks of histidine-dependent *Salmonella typhimurium*. Because native stocks of the bacteria do not require the addition of exogenous histidine for survival, exclusion of histidine from the culture broth has provided a system to determine if an added chemical or material has the ability to convert a mutant strain back to a native strain. When the bacteria are exposed to a genotoxic agent, point mutations occur in the genome, and the mutations can result in bacterial strains that no longer require exogenous histidine. Additives, or extractable chemicals that significantly increase the frequency of revertant colonies to a native state, have demonstrated an increased probability of exhibiting a carcinogenic potential in mammals.

According to ISO 10993 standards, the tests should cover three levels of genotoxicity; namely DNA effects, gene mutations, and chromosomal aberrations. Several of the test systems should preferably be mammalian-derived. The cell transformation test of Styles utilizes the growth potential of mammalian-derived fibroblast cell lines within soft agar gels. The untransformed cells generally will not grow within an agar gel. However, genotoxic agents that genetically-modify to transform the cells will grow below the gel surface. This activity has been correlated with the carcinogenic potential of agents in mammals. Styles originally reported greater than 90% accuracy in determining a carcinogenic activity of an agent or chemical in this system, however, the reproducibility of this system has not been universal. Two other systems of note are the sister chromatid exchange system and the chromosomal aberration assay in Chinese Hamster Ovary (CHO) cells (Phelps, 1999). An increase in the rate of sister chromatid exchange has been correlated with increased rates of DNA damage and mutations. The aberration assay categorizes structural changes observed in the chromosomes or chromatids as: simple, complex, or other. A test material is mutagenic if a statistically significant increase in aberrations is observed when compared to a negative control over a minimum of two increasing dose concentrations.

## 5.5  Specific Model Systems

### 5.5.1  Evaluation of Blood–Materials Interactions (BMIs)

A variety of medical devices — including catheters, blood vessel prostheses, heart valves, hemodialyzers, and oxygenators — are frequently used in humans and represent a class of biomaterials exhibiting BMIs. Current procedures evaluating blood compatibility and toxicity will be reviewed. Control over the biomaterials-tissue interface is the critical component defining the success or failure of a medical device. The dynamic interplay between biological, physical, as well as clinical and other technological factors should be considered when designing and evaluating a medical device and the biomaterials therein.

Blood compatibility can be defined as the inability of a material surface to activate the blood coagulation cascade (thrombosis), or to attract/alter platelets and leukocytes. Most material surfaces exhibit a wide range of thrombogenic responses, varying from complete occlusion to partial consumption of blood clotting factors. Although no materials to date have exhibited an ideal blood–material interface, research has been directed at producing materials that prevent thrombosis. In addition, material substrates have been modified to improve blood compatibility, such as the application or incorporation of therapeutic substances that prevent deposition of fibrin and other formed elements of the blood-material interface. Actual surface modifications of the material have also been undertaken to enhance the blood compatibility of BMIs. Several of the *in vitro* test methods utilized for evaluating the blood compatibility of material surfaces will be presented.

Following the general acute tissue culture toxicity tests previously described, the evaluation of test materials as BMIs are generally carried out to assess hemolysis (destruction of red blood cells with the liberation of hemoglobin), and a variety of thrombogenic potential tests, and platelet function studies. Additional studies on the nature of the protein adsorbed onto the material surface can be helpful in developing strategies to block or absorb critical adhesion factors involved in platelet adhesion, activation of the clotting cascade, and in thrombus (blood clot) formation. Ellipsometry can detect the thickness and refractive index of the absorbed protein layer on the material surface.

*Hemolysis:* The hemolytic potential of a test material can be assessed by the exposure of the appropriate quantity of the test material to oxalated rabbit blood to be incubated, along with positive and negative controls, for a standardized time (e.g., 1 h) at a standardized temperature (e.g., $36 \pm 1°C$). Following centrifugation, the absorbance of the supernatant is determined at a desired wavelength (e.g., 545 nm). The percentage of hemolysis (destruction of red blood cells) is then calculated, and if the hemolysis is less than 5%, the test material can be considered to be nonhemolytic.

*Thrombogenic potential:* A variety of tests are available and utilized to evaluate the thrombogenesis (formation of a blood clot) on material surfaces. Coagulation can occur via the intrinsic pathway (activation of Factor VII) and the extrinsic pathway (activation of tissue factor). The coagulation time test measures the time required for the formation of a firm clot. An enhanced coagulation time in comparison to an uncoated glass substrate is generally acknowledged to be nonthrombogenic. Other clotting tests include the thrombin time test, recalcification time test, an activated partial thromboplastin time test, and Russell's viper clotting time test. Antithrombin III binding studies and assays of various clotting factors, (e.g., V, VIII, XI, and XII) are also useful in assessing the thrombogenic potential of a material. Platelet adhesion, function, and retention with microbeads, are other tests to characterize the thrombogenic potential of a material surface.

Many tests are available to assess the hemocompatibility and evaluations of BMIs. In 1984, low-density polyethylene and polymethylsiloxane became the primary reference materials as tools for the validation of standardized and novel *in vitro* tests for evaluating BMIs (*Guidelines for blood–materials interactions*, 1985). As is the case with other assays and testing paradigms, variable results have occurred with the primary reference materials, and can occur with the methodology chosen to measure the blood cell adhesion or activation at the surface of materials. Caution should be taken when interpreting the results since issues such as the type of sterilization method used or the source of the raw materials can greatly impact the outcome. Continued testing and validation of reference materials for all types of *in vitro* testing paradigms will continue to improve the quality and reproducibility of the assays.

### 5.5.2 Evaluation of Biomaterials with Bone Marrow Cells (BMCs)

Cells derived from bone marrow provide a unique opportunity to evaluate biomaterial properties with a pluripotent cell population (Prockop, 1997). Bone marrow cells (BMC) can differentiate into a variety of cellular phenotypes upon exposure to appropriate stimuli. Phenotypes include hematopoietic, osteogenic, chondrogenic, and adipogenic lineages. This allows better understanding of cellular responses to biomaterials, since more diverse outcomes can be observed as compared to previously described specialized assays that lead to narrow, well-defined outcomes. A more realistic evaluation of biomaterial properties is expected with the use of BMC because *in vivo* responses to biomaterials are better mimicked than the responses obtained from the cell lines (Mankani et al., 2001). Two major classes of cells derived from BMC are bone-forming osteoblasts and bone-resorbing osteoclasts. Hence, evaluating biomaterials with BMC is an obvious benefit when the intended use of the biomaterials is in orthopedic applications. Probing functional outcome is usually attempted for such biomaterials. The end point of the assay often depends on the functional outcome expected from the use of the biomaterial. If the biomaterial is intended for an orthopedic device capable of inducing new bone tissue, evaluation for deposition of new mineralized matrix is appropriate. If the biomaterial is intended to participate in osteoclastic resorption, BMC could be utilized to investigate the cell-mediated resorption reminiscent of the resorption experienced by the mineralized tissue. Table 5.4 summarizes the main outcomes that are used for investigating the osteogenic response of BMC exposed to biomaterials. Particular attention should be paid to evaluation of BMC attachment to biomaterials, given that it might determine both osteoblastic and osteoclastic responses *in vivo* (see Figure 5.3 for possible outcomes from a typical *in vitro* study). Cell attachment on biomaterial surfaces could be quantified by a battery of generic assays, such as direct cell counts, and/or protein and DNA assays. Assays based on cellular enzymatic activities; such as succinate or lactate dehydrogenases, and acid/alkaline phosphatases, might also be useful for this purpose. A time-course of attachment kinetics provide good information for a quantitative comparison among biomaterial surfaces, assuming biomaterials do not elicit a direct cytotoxic response on BMC.

#### 5.5.2.1 Culture Conditions and Cell Source on Cellular Outcomes

As with any primary cell culture, it is important to develop standardized protocols to isolate and expand the cells before biomaterial testing. Small differences in cell preparation

**TABLE 5.4**

BMC Osteoblastic and Osteoclastic Features Displayed *In Vitro*

|  | Parameter | Comments |
| --- | --- | --- |
| Osteoblastic Features | Alkaline phosphatase (ALP) activity | Enzyme believed to be responsible for hydrolysis of inorganic phosphates to accelerate mineralization |
|  | Extracellular matrix (ECM) deposition | Deposition of specific ECM components, such as collagen I, osteocalcin, osteopontin and bone-sialoprotein, could be used as a marker of ECM deposition |
|  | Extracellular mineralization | End result of cumulative osteoblastic activity |
|  | *In vivo* bone formation assay | Given the unpredictable shortcomings of any in vitro assay, in vivo assays for bone induction may be useful. Implantation at a subcutaneous site may represent a convenient format without interference from cells at an orthopedic site (Mankani et al., 2001). |
| Osteoclastic Features | Tartarate-resistant acid phosphatase (TRAP) activity | Not necessarily an osteoclastic marker, but used in combination with multinucleation ($> 3$ nucleus/cell) for osteoclastic-like cell phenotype. |
|  | Matrix metalloproteinases (MMPs) | MMPs are key enzymes in extra-cellular matrix degradation and turnover. |
|  | Resorption pit formation | End result of cumulative osteoclastic activity |

The summarized parameters represent commonly used phenotypic markers.

conditions may influence cellular outcome in the assays (e.g., heparin is sometimes used during the extraction of cells from bone marrow to reduce blood clotting during the isolation procedure. In our hands, eliminating heparin during cell extraction was found to give a more robust cell growth subsequently). An appropriate stimulus is usually employed for transformation of cells if one wishes to utilize BMC for a functional outcome. Dexamethasone in the case of osteoblastic transformation, and GM-CSF/RANKL (Granulocyte Macrophage-Colony Stimulating Factor/Receptor Activator of NFkB (RANK) Ligand) combination in the case of osteoclastic transformation are typical supplements. Dexamethasone, long recognized as a synthetic anabolic steroid capable of increasing the osteoblastic features in BMC cultures (Rickard et al., 1994), has not been beneficial when used by some investigators. A high proportion of human donor-derived BMC did not require dexamethasone supplementation for *in vivo* bone formation in an animal model (Mendes et al., 2002). Dexamethasone was shown to dose-dependently decrease the initial colony establishment in rat (Richard et al., 1995; Dobson et al., 1999) and human BMC (Martin et al., 1997), so that it should be utilized at later stages of BMC culture. Alternatively, morphogenetic growth factors; such as Bone Morphogenetic Protein-2, Growth and Differentiation Factor-5 (Shimaoka et al., 2004), and bFGF (Lisignoli et al., 2002), could be used for osteogenic differentiation to eliminate dexamethasone in culture. Since the presence of dexamethasone can also influence the osteoclast generation, attention must be paid to the dose of dexamethasone exposed to the BMC (Sivagurunathan et al., 2005).

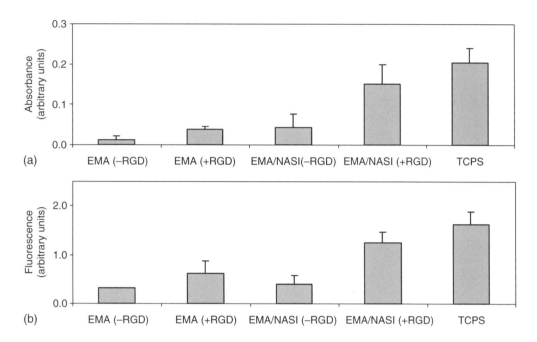

**FIGURE 5.3**

Evaluating the compatibility of arginine–glycine–aspartic acid (RGD) grafted polymer surfaces for attachment of BMC. The polymer surfaces were created on tissue culture polystyrene (TCPS), and consisted of non-peptide reactive *N*-isopropylacrylamide/ethylmethacrylate surfaces (EMA) and peptide-reactive *N*-isopropylacrylamide/ethylmethacrylate/*N*-acryloxysuccinimide (EMA/NASI) surfaces. Each surface was tested for cell attachment either untreated (−RGD) or after treatment with RGD (+RGD). Attachment of BMC was tested 48 h post-seeding by using the MTT assay (a) and a commercially available DNA assay (b). Note that the attachment of BMC to RGD-grafted surfaces, EMA/NASI (+RGD), was equivalent to that of cells added to TCPS.

An important consideration in the development of BMC-based evaluation assays is the age of the BMC donor. It is generally recognized that BMC from aged sources possesses lower osteogenic activity (Dodson et al., 1996; Inoue et al., 1977; Muschler et al., 2001; Justesen et al., 2002; Mendes et al., 2002) due to a lower proportion of pluripotent stem cells and/or decreased ability of BMC to differentiate (i.e., form the mature phenotype). However, this view is challenged in other studies that employed human BMC, which did not indicate an obvious difference between young and aged BMC in a xenograft model (Stenderup et al., 2004). The response of BMC to growth factors, e.g., to basic Fibroblast Growth Factor (bFGF), is also dependent on the age of the BMC source; BMC derived from aged animals was more responsive to bFGF (Kotev-Emeth et al., 2000). in line with our recent results (Varkay et al., 2005). This observation suggests that osteogenic factors might be more beneficial for aged individuals, and that the use of biomaterials for investigating osteogenic response of BMC might be more appropriate with aged cells.

### 5.5.2.2 *Disadvantages of BMC in Bioassays*

The use of BMC and other tissue culture systems that are comprised of multiple cell types, should be expected to exhibit a greater degree of variability when compared to assays performed with cell lines. Previous *in vitro* studies evaluated osteoblast functions isolated from young and aged donors and observed an age-related decrease in osteoblast function. Osteoblasts from older donors appeared to have a reduced capacity to form bone *in vitro*. However, no differences in the bone forming capacity *in vivo* was observed in human-derived osteoblasts isolated from young (24 to 30 years old) and aged (71 to 81 years old) donors (Stenderup et al., 2004). The authors suggested that the age-associated decrease in bone formation observed with *in vitro* bioassays could be due to deficiencies in the bone microenvironment. One would also be careful to avoid changes in the phenotypic features of the cells because BMC exhibit a dynamic phenotype. This was recently noted in studies designed to probe the expression of integrins used for binding to biomaterials (Ter Brugge et al., 2002). The repertoire of integrin receptors was dependent on the source of BMC (i.e., animal-to-animal variation), time of culture, as well as the nature of the substrates on which BMC were cultured. BMC in culture also undergo progressive commitment, based on molecular markers (Banfi et al., 2002). With such a dynamic cell source, extra care is needed to optimize the cell-based assays for quantitative purposes. The current methodologies for the use of BMC are, therefore, mostly restricted to early research activities. Bioassays for biomaterial quality control/assurance are likely to continue to rely on cell lines.

### 5.5.3   Evaluation of Restorative Dental Materials

*In vitro* testing of dental materials represents additional challenges because the intended *in vivo* environment of this class of materials is the oral cavity. Biocompatibility of dental materials depends largely on their composition, location, and their interactions with the body. The wide range of materials used, and the differing environments, require that the materials be tested *in vivo* as much as possible to replicate the complex physiologic environment.

It is not uncommon for a dental restoration to contain metal, ceramic, and polymer materials; each of which elicit a unique biological response due to composition differences. Additionally, the biological response to a material is dependent on whether the materials release components and whether those components are toxic, immunogenic, or mutagenic at the released concentrations. Location within the oral cavity partially determines a material's biocompatibility. In fact, a material that appears to be biocompatible when in contact with the oral mucosa, may cause an adverse reaction if implanted in more specific locations. For example, materials that are in direct contact with tooth pulp may elicit a cytotoxic response. In contrast, the same material may be biocompatible when placed into contact with dentin or enamel.

Because materials may interact with several tissues within the body, this interaction often affects biocompatibility. In addition, application of forces from mastication, changes in pH, and the corrosive breakdown resulting from immersion in biological fluids can alter a materials biocompatibility.

### 5.5.3.1   Tooth Tissue

Dentin tissue forms the greatest bulk of the tooth. The dentin matrix surrounds dentinal tubules that are filled with cell processes. These processes extend from cells (odontoblasts) that reside in the pulp chamber of the tooth. The tubules run the entire length between the dentoenamel junction and the pulp. There are between 20,000 and 50,000 tubules/mm$^2$ in the tooth. Their diameter varies from about 0.5 to 2.5 μm (see Figure 5.4).

Filling the tubules and surrounding the cell processes is a serum-like fluid. It has direct connection to the pulp chamber, and is maintained under an intercellular hydraulic pressure of about 24 mm Hg. The pulpal circulation pressure causes fluid-flow in the

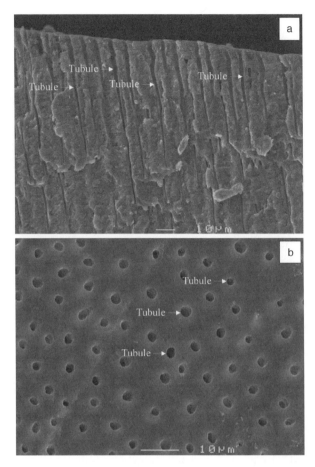

**FIGURE 5.4**
Scanning electron micrographs of human dentin tissue. The variation in tubule width from the pulp chamber to the dentoenamel junction is shown in the longitudinal section in (a). (b) shows the inner surface of the pulp chamber on which the cells reside and the tubule openings through which they extend their processes (arrows).

tubules to be directed from the pulp outward occurring when enamel or cementum surrounding the dentin is removed. Thus, this tissue provides a patent connection and pathway for component diffusion inward to the cells in the pulp.

### 5.5.3.2 *Dentin Barrier Tests*

When restorative materials are placed into teeth, a layer of dentin will generally be interposed between the restorative material and the living cells in the pulp chamber. This barrier of dentin may be as thin as a few tenths of a millimeter thick, yet it is effective in modulating the cytotoxic effects of many dental materials, acting as a barrier through which toxic materials must diffuse to reach pulp tissue. The thickness of the dentin and the directionality of the dentinal tubules correlate directly with the protection provided to pulp cells. Assays have accordingly been developed to incorporate dentin slices between a test sample and the cells in culture, providing directional diffusion between the restoration material and the culture medium.

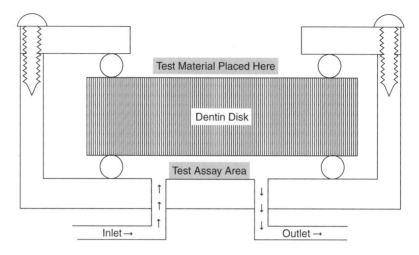

**FIGURE 5.5**
A sliced disk of dentin can be used as a barrier between a test material and cells to assess the biocompatibility of materials placed on dentin. In this test, components of the test material must diffuse through the dentin in order to affect the cells growing on the other side. Additionally, culture media or saline may be added and removed from the assay area through the access ports. This fluid may be collected and analyzed to allow measurement of the diffusion rate, or alternatively may be used to treat cells directly and observe the affect on metabolism and cell growth.

In this test, specific to dental materials testing, the test material is placed on one side of a dentin slab. It is spatially isolated from cells growing in a chamber on the other side of the slab. Only components which release themselves from the material, and successfully diffuse through the dentin thickness, can influence the cells growing on the other side (see Figure 5.5).

The complete biological effect of restorative materials on tooth pulp cells is still unclear. Restorative materials may directly impact pulpal tissues in a cytotoxic manner, or they may play a subsidiary role by causing sub-lethal changes. This may ultimately render those cells more susceptible to bacterial or neutrophil attack. It is clear, therefore, that the design of tests measuring pulp cell irritation *to materials* must include conditions for eliminating bacteria, bacterial products, and other microleakage. An understanding of the major role of dentin tissue in mitigating the negative effects of microleakage remains imprecise.

## 5.6  Summary

The desire to develop high throughput *in vitro* screening systems, as well as to provide alternatives to animal testing, has led to the development and refinement of a variety of *in vitro* assays for assessing biomaterial cytotoxicity and compatibility. Cell culture systems have been useful as a screening method for cytotoxicity and genotoxicity. Moreover, the evolution of tissue specific cell culture systems will continue to develop and should result in an outcome more representative to that observed in the clinical setting.

# References

Ames, B.N., McCann, J., and Yamasaki, E., Methods for detecting carcinogens and mutagens with the Salmonella/mammalian microsome mutagenicity test, *Mutation Res.*, **31**, 347–364 (1975).

Banfi, A., Bianchi, G., Notaro, R., Luzzatto, L., Cancedda, R., and Quarto, R., Replicative aging and gene expression in long-term cultures of human bone marrow stromal cells, *Tissue Eng.*, **8**, 901–910 (2002).

Belanger, M-C. and Marois, Y., Hemocompatibility, biocompatibility, inflammatory and *in vivo* studies of primary reference materials low-density polyethylene and polydimethylsiloxane: a review, *J. Biomed. Mater. Res. Appl. Biomater.*, **58**, 467–477 (2001).

Black, J., The education of the biomaterialist: report of a survey, *J. Biomed. Mater. Res.*, **16**, 159–167 (1982).

Bultitude, F.W. and Boocock, G., *Interlaboratory trial of cell culture methods for BSI technical committee SGS/26-toxicity tests for medical rubber and plastics*, Ministry of Defense, AWRE Chemistry Division, London (1977).

Dobson, K., Reading, L., and Scutt, A., A cost-effective method for the automatic quantitative analysis of fibroblastic colony-forming units, *Calcif. Tissue Int.*, **65**, 166–172 (1999).

Dodson, S.A., Bernard, G.W., Kenney, E.B., and Carranza, F.A., *In vitro* comparison of aged and young osteogenic and hemopoietic bone marrow stem cells and their derivative colonies, *J. Periodontol.*, **67**, 184–196 (1996).

*Guidelines for blood–materials interactions*. National Heart, Lung and Blood Institute, Washington, D.C. (1980).

*Guidelines for blood–materials interactions*. National Heart, Lung and Blood Institute, Washington, D.C. (1985).

*Guidelines for physicochemical characterization for biomaterials*. National Heart, Lung and Blood Institute, Washington, DC 1980.

Hanks, C.T., Wataha, J.C., and Sun, Z., *In vitro* models of biocompatibility: a review, *Dental Mater.*, **12**, 186–193 (1996).

Inoue, K., Ohgushi, H., Yoshikawa, T., Okumura, M., Sempuku, T., Tamai, S., and Dohi, Y., The effect of aging on bone formation in porous hydroxyapatite: biochemical and histological analysis, *J. Bone. Min. Res.*, **12**, 989–994 (1977).

Justesen, J., Stenderup, K., Eriksen, E.F., and Kassem, M., Maintenance of osteoblastic and adipocytic differentiation potential with age and osteoporosis in human marrow stromal cell cultures, *Calcif. Tissue Int.*, **71**, 36–44 (2002).

Kotev-Emeth, S., Savion, N., Pro-Chen, S., and Pitaru, S., Effect of maturation on the osteogenic response of cultured stromal bone marrow cells to basic fibroblast growth factor, *Bone*, **27**, 777–783 (2000).

Lisignoli, G., Fini, M., Giavaresi, G., Nicoli, A.N., Toneguzzi, S., and Facchini, A., Osteogenesis of large segmental radius defects enhanced by basic fibroblast growth factor activated bone marrow stromal cells grown on non-woven hyaluronic acid-based polymer scaffold, *Biomaterials*, **23**, 1043–1051 (2002).

Lyman, D.J., Polymers in medicine and surgery, *Polymer Science and Technology*, Vol. 8. Kronenthal, R.L., Ed., Plenum, New York, pp. 29–49 (1975).

Majno, G. and Joris, I., Apoptosis, oncosis, and necrosis. An overview of cell death, *Am. J. Pathol.*, **146**, 16–19 (1995).

Mankani, M.H., Kuznetsov, S.A., Fowler, B., Kingman, A., and Robey, P.G., *In vivo* bone formation by human bone marrow stromal cells: effect of carrier particle size and shape, *Biotech. Bioeng.*, **72**, 96–107 (2001).

Martin, I., Muraglia, A., Campanile, G., Cancedda, R., and Quarto, R., Fibroblast growth factor-2 supports *ex vivo* expansion and maintenance of osteogenic precursors from human bone marrow, *Endocrinol*, **138**, 4456–4462 (1997).

Mendes, S.C., Tibbe, J.M., Veenhof, M., Bakker, K., Both, S., Platenburg, P.P., Oner, F.C., de Bruijn, J.D., and van Blitterswijk, C.A., Bone tissue-engineered implants using human bone marrow stromal cells: effect of culture conditions and donor age, *Tissue Eng.*, **8**, 911–920 (2002).

Mosmann, T.J., Rapid colorimetric assay for cellular growth and survival: application to proliferation and cytotoxicity assays, *J. Immunol. Methods*, **65**, 55–63 (1983).

Muschler, G.F., Nitto, H., Boehm, C.A., and Easley, K.A., Age- and gender-related changes in the cellularity of human bone marrow and the prevalence of osteoblastic progenitors, *J. Orthop. Res.*, **19**, 117–125 (2001).

Phelps, J.B., Genotoxicity, In: *Handbook of Biomaterials Evaluation: Scientific, Technical and Clinical Testing of Implant Materials*, von Recum, A.F., Ed., Taylor & Francis, Philadelphia, pp. 367–380 (1999).

Prockop, D.J., Marrow stromal cells as stem cells for nonhematopoietic tissues, *Science*, **276**, 71 (1997).

Richard, D.J., Kazhdan, I., and Leboy, P.S., Importance of 1,25-dihydroxyvitamin D3 and the nonadherent cells of marrow for osteoblast differentiation from rat marrow stromal cells, *Bone*, **16**, 671–678 (1995).

Rickard, D.J., Sullivan, T.A., Shenker, B.J., Leboy, P.S., and Kazhdan, I., Induction of rapid osteoblast differentiation in rat bone marrow stromal cell cultures by dexamethasone and BMP-2, *Dev. Biol.*, **161**, 218–226 (1994).

*Sample preparation and reference materials*, Biological Evaluation of Medical Devices, Part 12. International Organization for Standardization, Geneva (1993).

Sivagurunathan, Z.S., Muir, M.M., Brennan, T.C., Seale, J.P., and Mason, R.S., Influence of glucocorticoids on human osteoclast generation and activity, *J. Bone. Min. Res.*, **20**, 390–398 (2005).

Shimaoka, H., Dohi, Y., Ohgushi, H., Ikeuchi, M., Okamoto, M., Kudo, A., Kirita, T., and Yonemasu, K., Recombinant growth/differentiation factor-5 (GDF-5) stimulates osteogenic differentiation of marrow mesenchymal stem cells in porous hydroxyapatite ceramic, *J. Biomed. Mater. Res.*, **68**, 168–176 (2004).

Stenderup, K., Rosada, C., Justesen, J., Al-Soubky, T., Dagnaes-Hansen, F., and Kassem, M., Aged human bone marrow stromal cells maintaining bone forming capacity *in vivo* evaluated using an improved method of visualization, *Biogerontology*, **5**, 107–118 (2004).

Ter Brugge, P.J., Torensma, R., De Ruijter, J.E., Figdor, C.G. and Jansen, J.A., Modulation of integrin expression on rat bone marrow cells by substrates with different surface characteristics, *Tissue Eng.*, **8**, 615–626 (2002).

*Tests for cytotoxicity: in vitro methods*, Biological Evaluation of Medical Devices, Part 5. International Organization for Standardization, Geneva (1993).

www.iso.ch; reference to document ISO 10993-1:1992(E).

U.S. Pharmacopeia, *Biological Reactivity Tests In Vitro*, U.S. Pharmacopeia 23, 27, United States Pharmacopeial Convention, Rockville, MD, pp. 2173–2175 (2004).

Varkay, M., Kucharski, C., Haque, T., Sebald, W., and Uludag, H., *In vitro* osteogenic response of rat bone marrow cells to bFGF and BMP-2 treatment, *Clin. Orthop. Rel. Res.*, (2005), submitted.

von Recum, A.F., Jenkins, M.E., and von Recum, H.A., Introduction: biomaterials and biocompatibility, In: *Handbook of Biomaterials Evaluation: Scientific, Technical and Clinical Testing of Implant Materials*, von Recum, A.F., Ed., Taylor & Francis, Philadelphia, pp. 1–8 (1999).

von Recum, A.F. and LaBerge, M., Educational goals for biomaterials science and engineering: prospective views, *J. Appl. Biomat.*, **6**, 137–144 (1995).

Winn, S.R. and Hollinger, J.O., An osteogenic cell culture system to evaluate the cytocompatibility of Osteoset®, a calcium sulfate bone void filler, *Biomaterials*, **21**, 2413–2425 (2000).

# 6

## *Considerations for the* In Vivo *Testing of Biomaterials*

**Jeffrey O. Hollinger and Mark Citron**

## CONTENTS

## 6.1 Introduction

The process from laboratory to bedside is dynamic and encompasses multiple competencies. While any text on the subject of product development organizes the subject matter in a deliberative and sequential approach, the reality is that product development is an iterative and anything but straightforward effort. In prior chapters, a number of these issues have been identified. This chapter will provide the necessary information to address the fundamental considerations of product life-cycle in the preclinical development phase. Consequently, the two conceptual issues underscored are:

1. Regulatory framework to progress to the clinic
2. Risk and risk mitigation

Chapter 2 and Chapter 5 provided a platform describing biomaterial design and development from the bench to the bedside. Therefore, these chapters highlight a logical, systematic progression of tests involving *in vitro* and *in vivo* biomaterial interactions that will determine suitability (i.e., safety and efficacy) for patient applications. Consequently, it is noteworthy to recap chapter themes and their progression to the preclinical (*in vivo*) emphasis for this chapter.

Chapter 2 described the biological fundamental we recognize as biocompatibility (i.e., safety). Therefore, consistent with a bench to the bedside approach, Chapter 2 provided a Food and Drug Agency (FDA) overlay where biomaterial regulation focused on the "as used" medical device (composed of the biomaterial) that is otherwise presumed safe and efficacious. However, as previously noted, the FDA does not clear or approve biomaterials; they approve devices. As a result, any single device design needs to undergo its own individual developmental process.

Purposefully omitted in Chapter 2 was the integration of biomechanics with biology. The intentional exclusion of biomechanics in a biomaterials discussion does not mean biomechanics subserves biology. Rather, at this time the FDA as a regulatory agency and the standards identified (in Chapter 2), neither offer nor provide biomechanical target values (i.e., biofunctional thresholds) for biomaterials.

Interactions of biomaterials with the host and the host–implant interface (e.g., protein-surface), as well as the blood–biomaterial interaction, are determinants of biocompatibility (i.e., safety). Protein properties such as size, charge, conformation/configuration (structure) and the surface of the biomaterial will impact *in vivo* responses. Surface properties key to materials–host interactions include topography, hydrophobicity, hydrophilicity, heterogeneity and potential. Moreover, the interaction between the implant and blood (i.e., the blood–biomaterial interaction) that produces a unique mechanical environment are underscored by biological principles fluid flow, shear, material compliance, and mechanical fatigue.

In Chapter 5, the specific *in vitro* testing paradigms were described that may be applied to screen biomaterial biocompatibility. The systematic, standardized approach to acquire fundamental biological performance outcome must be antecedent to *in vivo* assays. Chapter 5, consequently, provided a road map approach promulgated by seminal accomplishments of the Medical Device Amendments to the Food, Drug and Cosmetic Act that occurred in 1976, the International Union for Pure and Applied Chemistry (in the early 1990s), as well as the biocompatibility standards as described by the International Standards Organization (ISO) published as ISO 10993 that was first recorded in 1992 and has undergone numerous supplements. There were other key accomplishments established to standardize and unify biomaterials testing that were highlighted in Chapter 3 as well. Moreover, we purposefully used redundancy in Chapter 2 and Chapter 3 when referring to biomaterial biocompatibility, standards and standards testing to provide an instructional bulwark leading *in vivo* biomaterials testing.

Chapter 4 for *in vivo* testing will continue the didactic benefits of consistency in nomenclature and terminology and standards redundancy, as well as underscoring the logic for a targeted clinical correlate in the animal model testing paradigm. Furthermore, the systematic, hierarchal approach to biomaterials testing that will integrate safety and efficacy will be thematic with Chapter 2 and Chapter 5.

Singularly unique in the *in vivo* model system distinguishing this system from other test beds, is the responsibility for humane use of the test system (i.e., the animal model). Regardless of the phylogenetic level of the *in vivo* test system (animal model), vertebrate use must comply with the epochal Animal Welfare Act (1985 and subsequent amendments) and the National Institutes of Health (e.g., The Public Health Service Policy on Humane Care and Use of Laboratory Animals, 1986). Moreover, all animal research protocols must be reviewed and approved by an Institutional Animal Care and Use Committee (IACUC). In response to the biomaterials testing, the IACUC will insist on measurable, quantifiable outcome measures from the *in vivo* experiment.

This chapter consequently, will pay especial attention to regulatory organizations, standards and the *in vivo* preclinical process that will presage the clinic.

## 6.2 Animals Are Key to *In Vivo* Testing

The obviousness that animals are key to *in vivo* testing is of striking importance and readily acknowledged by the community of individuals involved in biomaterials testing. However, the aspect of *in vivo* biomaterials testing protocols that may be overlooked and underappreciated by experimentalists is the humane component.

The fundamental of humane use must be included as an integral hallmark component of the humane care of experimental animals. The procedural details enumerated for animal husbandry policy and policy compliance are daunting. A tremendous amount of coordinated effort, pride and dedication are absolutely necessary to ensure experimentalists treat (i.e., use) animals humanely and that facilities and personnel where animals are housed and used for experiments perform all animal husbandry aspects in a humane manner.

Specific standards and stringent criteria must be fulfilled by vivaria administering animal husbandry that includes veterinary care, record keeping, the actual bricks and mortar of the animal facilities (i.e., dedicated space per animal, known as runs), human interaction, feeding and fluid management, waste disposal, environmental policy and regulations, temperature, air circulation, personnel training, credentialing, record keeping, the operating theatre, methods of restraint and transport to and from the holding facilities to the operating theatre, as well as anaesthesia, euthanasia and disposal.

Only the best of the best vivaria complying with the rigorous level of performance and standards will be approved by the American Association for Accreditation of Laboratory Animal Care (AAALAC) and the American Association for Laboratory Animal Sciences (AALAS).

It is highly noteworthy to recognize the fact that animal testing, especially in higher-order species (for example, dogs and nonhuman primates), is always a challenging expense, with in-life experimentation often protracted. Therefore, outcome measurements must be unambiguous and quantifiable. These two goals can be elusive.

Meticulous, detailed planning and flawless execution of animal studies are absolutes. Lost time and money to redo failures are untenable.

Moreover, adherence to standard protocols for the *in vivo* testing enables correlation of outcome among different facilities. Furthermore, experimental design of the animal tests must enable reproducible and accurate outcome data that can be quantitated. And of course, the animal selected must be a preclinical correlate of the clinical target of the biomaterial being assessed.

### 6.2.1 Fundamental Concerns and Considerations

The process progressing from the laboratory bench to *in vitro* methodologies yielding biocompatibility data outcomes neither ensures fidelity of those biocompatibility measures to *in vivo* measures, nor may the *in vitro* to *in vivo* observations enable a seamless transition. Is this a concern?

It is not a concern that *in vitro* outcome data may not be equivalent to *in vivo* outcome data. For example, a biomaterial may be cytotoxic to a cell line *in vitro*, however, in a subcutaneous implantation site, the tissue fluid will buffer the biomaterial affects and the implant may in fact be biocompatible.

In yet another example, the pharmacokinetics of a growth factor released from a biomaterial tested with an *in vitro* system may yield an outcome that is distinctly different than if the biomaterial was implanted in an animal femur model. Again, these differences between *in vitro* and *in vivo* outcome measures are not concerns. It is important to the process of biomaterials evaluation, therefore, that the experimental scientist is aware there may not be fidelity between the *in vitro* and *in vivo* test systems.

A significant area of focus at this stage of biological characterization is the chemical and physical characterization of the device or material used in the biological testing. Biomaterials come in any number of physical and chemical types and as a result, there exists a large number of means to characterize them. The fundamental consideration is that the results from any biological test must be representative of the material that is destined for the clinic, for example, a biomaterial (i.e., the product) that will be sterilized by radiation. Radiation sterilization can alter either the chemical or physical characteristics

**TABLE 6.1**

Material Characterization. A Representative Design Characterization for a Medical Device That Could Be Used in Orthopedic Applications as a Bone Void Filler

| Design Criteria | Characterization |
| --- | --- |
| Physical characteristics | Examples of these tests include mass, volume and density, porosity and surface area. Shape and dimensional specifications are also considered important. For bioresorbable materials, the pH and dissolution rate *in vitro* is also assessed. Setting and reaction times are assessed for devices that are mixtures and may be exothermic. For devices meant to be injected, the injectability of the final device examining pressures needed to place the material into the defect site are defined |
| Chemical make-up | Examples of these tests include the identification of the crystalline and noncrystalline phases, phase purity and weight percentage of phases by x-ray diffraction (XRD), Identity testing by FT-IR, elemental analysis and heavy metals by ICP are performed Elemental analyses and assessments for all impurities are assessed |
| Biological properties | Most devices are expected to be sterile and nonpyrogenic. As a result, sterility testing using standard United States Pharmacopoeia (USP) methods and endotoxin testing using LAL are employed. Bioresorbable devices are often characterized by their dissolution rate *in vivo*. Further, for devices containing an active or biological component to the *in vitro* and *in vivo* tests are used to determine the biological properties, and can include cell proliferation assays, viability and functional screenings |

of the product and therefore the biological characteristics of the product may be affected. Consequently, the material undergoing testing also must be sterilized. A standard means to characterize a biomaterial is by defining its principle physical, chemical and biological properties (summarized in Table 6.1). These chemical, physical, and biological criteria are further used to describe the device design.

Moreover, at each stage during the series of the biomaterial product development, prior test results and the conclusions must be validated to enable progress to the subsequent testing. This strategy exploits a fundamental underpinning of the biomaterial product development process — risk assessment.

Risk assessment generally follows the outline described in the ISO 14971 standard entitled Medical Devices — Application of Risk Management to Medical Devices. This standard has defined measures that must be addressed for each device. Importantly, a checklist included in Appendix 3 is often employed prior to initiating each human clinical trial.

Paramount during the risk assessment process is awareness that appearance of animal model testing success does not necessarily predict success in the human clinical indication. There may be, for example dosing issues, pharmacokinetic and pharmacodynamic differences between the animal model and the human patient. Is this a fundamental concern for biomaterials testing?

The answer is: No. The FDA routinely requires a platform of outcome data derived from standard testing protocols that exploit *in vitro* and *in vivo* tests. Moreover, the transition from a successful series of outcomes in the preclinical *in vivo* model system to the clinical *in vivo* system is generally understood and expected to require modification in the clinical *in vivo* system. *In vitro* and animal model testing can provide reasonable assurance of human safety but are not by themselves a prognosticator of human outcome application which requires a separate developmental programme. The antecedent *in vitro* and preclinical testing paradigms do not unequivocally predict how a biomaterial will perform in humans. Therefore, the staging to evaluate biomaterials using clinical *in vivo* system testing is accomplished in steps (i.e., phases). The recognized drug developmental definitions of Phase I, II, and III clinical trials in patients are not recognized in the device development. The prominent definition used in device development is a pilot programme to show safety and assess the study design which is equivalent to Phases I and II drug studies. The next stage of device development is the pivotal trial. The pivotal trial is the device equivalent of a Phase III drug programme. However, as in the drug analogy, the Phase I/II clinical trial (pilot) neither ensures a biomaterial will be successful in the pivotal or Phase III trial nor obtain FDA approval for the intended clinical target. (Clinical trials will be discussed briefly later in this chapter.)

### 6.2.2 The Clinical Target and Preclinical Correlate

We learned in Chapter 2 that *in vivo* assessments of biocompatibility are expressly selected to simulate end use applications. The end use application is identified as a clinical target. The dilemma often encountered with animal models is there may not be an adequate preclinical target correlate for the human clinical indication.

The end use application must be adequately identified for a biomaterial. However, in terms of a suitable preclinical application correlate, sometime there is a correlate and sometimes there is not.

An important question that needs to be addressed for biomaterials design and development is: Are the targeted clinical properties of the biomaterial consistent with the end use application? The answer to this question is sometimes yes and sometimes no.

The reason for this duality is that very often the biology of the target site for which the biomaterial is intended, may not be satisfactorily characterized. We emphasize that biology of the clinical target is key to the rational, instructive guidance for the design and development of the biomaterial(s) and their end stage use. Furthermore, understanding and appreciating the liabilities and virtues of the most suitable, representative preclinical correlate for the end use application of the biomaterial further strengthen the outcome observations.

It is therefore prudent at this time to look at some *in vivo* animal models that can be used for biomaterials testing for targeted clinical indications.

## 6.3　Animal Models: Preliminary Steps to *In Vivo* Testing

It is already clear that prior to reaching the tier of testing that involves animal models, a comprehensive platform of *in vitro* tests will have been executed to validate biocompatibility (i.e., safety) for the biomaterial intended for human clinical application. Chapter 2 provides a broad overview of these *in vitro* testing approaches. In Chapter 3 a focused emphasis on the *in vitro* tests is provided that is based on the Medical Device Bill passed by the U.S. Congress, 1976; the National Heart, Lung and Blood Institute publications, 1980 and 1985; the ISO 10993 standards of 1992; and the U.S. Pharmacopeia: Biological tests *in vitro*, 2004). These neatly defined testing paradigms included agar diffusion, direct contact, extract dilution (elution), specific endpoint assessments as well as assays for cell function (e.g., MTT, BrdU), mutagenesis and blood–materials interactions (BMIs).

In distinction to the specifics available for *in vitro* testing, preclinical animal models are neither as comprehensively described nor are outcome measures as neatly and unambiguously defined for *in vivo* paradigms as they are for *in vitro* tests.

As we learned in Chapter 2, extensive efforts and progress have been made to provide procedures, protocols, guidelines and standards, predominantly for tissue compatibility of medical devices (AAMI Standards, 1997; the FDA Blue Book Memorandum, 1995; ISO 10993 Biological Evaluation of Medical Devices, with emphasis on 10993-1: Evaluation and testing, ISO 10993-2: Animal Welfare requirements, ISO 10993-6: Test for local effects after implantation; and the American Society for Testing Materials (ASTM), Annual Book of ASTM standards, specifically ASTM F-981-93: Practice for Assessment of Compatibility of Biomaterials (Nonporous) for Surgical Implants with Respect to Effects of Materials on Muscle and Bone and ASTM F-763-93: Practice for Short Term Screening of Implant Materials, 1999). Chapter 2 offered several brief perspectives on the general types of *in vivo* tests (Chapter 2, Table 1 to Table 4).

Important ASTM standards for *in vivo* animal models for biomaterial testing are ASTM standard F 981-04, the assessment of compatibility of biomaterials for surgical implants with respect to the effects of materials on muscle and bone and ASTM F 749-98 standard practice for evaluating material extracts by intracutaneous injection in the rabbit (to determine biocompatibility of materials used in medical devices).

It is highly noteworthy that biomaterials intended for an end use as a device have to employ a preclinical *in vivo* model that complies with defined standards promulgated by the Department of Health and Human Services in the Good Laboratory Practice (GLP) for Nonclinical Laboratory Studies (1992).

The preclinical pathway selected for *in vivo* materials testing will be determined by the material's end use application. As a result, there is the potential that the preclinical programme is flawed if the reader of the ISO 10993 standard with the regulatory framework documents misunderstands the overall developmental programme. The guidance is not simply several checklists of required studies that need to be performed prior to initiation of a human trial. A close reading of the ISO 10993 standard reveals that each device developer should examine the end use and design the preclinical safety programme around the associated risks of the clinical application. Routinely, a preclinical plan will be drawn up in concert with an expert in toxicology for each material and its application. The predetermined studies will be executed under GLP and individual reports generated. The individual study reports are critiqued by the toxicology expert and the rationale for initiating a clinical study can be prepared.

For example, a biomaterial designed for a device such as an implantable stent will proceed through a testing pathway that is different than a device such as a bone void filler. Moreover, combination materials that include a biological agent, for example the growth factor platelet derived growth factor (abbreviated as PDGF), will proceed through yet another pathway. Each pathway has unique as well as overlapping regulatory ramifications and outcome measures intended to validate safety and efficacy.

Initially, some combination materials plus biologicals were labelled by the FDA as devices and designated as an Investigational Device Exemption (IDE), even though a biological component was included. These combination products were under the auspices of either the Center of Device Evaluation and Research (CDER) or the Center for Biologics Evaluation and Research (CBER). Moreover, the FDA requires that all clinical evaluations of IDEs (unless they are exempt) have an approved IDE prior to commencing the study. Further, the IDE regulations define two types of device studies: Significant Risk (SR) and Nonsignificant Risk (NSR). The SR and NSR study requirements are essentially identical with the exception that NSR studies do not require a formal FDA filing and approval prior to study initiation.

In the same manner that *in vitro* and *in vivo* safety studies are performed in conformance with rigorous GLP standards, clinical studies, whether SR or NSR, must conform to rigorous good clinical practice (GCP) requirements which are described later.

## 6.4 Opportunities by an IDE Pathway

Assuming the required *in vitro* assays and *in vivo* animal model testing data have demonstrated safety and efficacy, a medical device (under the IDE) may follow five possible routes to market (Kahan, 2000). The most frequently taken pathway is either a 510(k) or Premarket Approval (PMA).

### 6.4.1   510(k) Notification Process

The FDA will need to determine whether the biomaterial device (e.g., a calcium phosphate bone void filler) is equivalent to an already marketed product (device) or predicate device that is either a Class I or Class II device of a pre-amendment Class III (The Federal Food Drug and Commerce Act, FDC, Medical Device Amendment, 1976).

*Class I.*   These are devices where there are general controls sufficient enough to ensure safety and effectiveness. Examples include elastic bandages, examination gloves and hand held surgical instruments.

*Class II.*   These are devices where general controls are determined as being insufficient to provide reasonable assurance that safety and effectiveness will be assured. However, there is adequate information to establish performance standards that can provide safety and effectiveness assurance. Examples of this class of devices include powered wheelchairs and infusion pumps.

*Class III.*   These are devices that cannot be classified as either Class I or Class II due to insufficient information to determine the general controls and performance standards assuring for safety and efficacy. Class III devices are usually dedicated to life-sustaining and life-supporting application, or are implanted in the patient. Typical Class III examples can include replacement heart valves, breast implants, TMJ implants.

### 6.4.2   Premarket Approval Application (PMA)

The PMA pathway is followed when the approval for higher-risk devices does not exist. For example, when either Class III devices or devices where a substantial equivalent predicate does not exist or the device has been classified as a Class III due to its potential risk to health.

## 6.5   The Investigational New Drug (IND) Option

In order for a new drug to reach the clinical market, a tremendous amount of focused data must be acquired from *in vitro* and *in vivo* tests. Moreover, the definition of a drug may be perceived as being broad and there is susceptibility to become bogged down by a commensurately broad base of tests.

Furthermore, conceptually the notion of the definition of a drug can be less than obvious. For example, a COX2 inhibitor such as Celebrex is a drug and the growth factor known as bone morphogenetic protein (BMP) is also a drug. Both the COX2 inhibitor and BMP operate through different physiological pathways and elicit different biological and pharmacological processes. However, they are drugs and fall under the FDA's category IND.

Different types of categories of drugs follow a different *in vivo* testing pathway. There are both overlaps in required outcome information as well as uniquely different information that will be necessary to validate safety and efficacy.

In addition, screening a therapeutic molecule that will follow an IND pathway is more daunting than the IDE regulatory pathway. Therefore, as emphasized earlier, the academic is very strongly encouraged to engage with a corporate entity having expertise in the regulatory process and establish a dialog with the FDA to lay out the most logical roadmap to follow for regulatory approval.

## 6.6   Considerations and Pathway to the Clinic

Prior to entry into the clinic, a decision must be made whether the intended biomaterial product has substantial equivalence to a currently approved product or whether the new product is distinctly different than currently existing products. The differences may be as a consequence of unique formulation (e.g., composition), biological mechanism of action or, of equal importance, the clinical application. In this last case, an existing biomaterial may be used for a different clinical purpose where it has a different means of anatomical implantation or it is implanted at a different anatomical site. These similarities and differences are all part of the risk assessment prior to human (clinical) use.

*Substantial equivalence.*   A substantially equivalent device must have the same intended end use as a currently approved (by the FDA) predicate device. Moreover, the fundamental characteristics of the as yet unapproved device must be substantially equivalent.

*Filing.*   PMAs take longer and are more expensive than 510(k) filings. Data collection and preparation for the PMA usually occurs over several years and runs into millions of dollars, whereas a 510(k) may take 3 to 6 months and cost less than six figures. There are legal or statutory differences that make the 510(k) process different than a PMA process as well. Three of the most critical differences are:

1. Clinical study requirements for the PMA
2. Detailed manufacturing information provided in a PMA
3. Quality systems requirements that are needed in the process development or product development life cycle

*Device Design and Product Life-Cycle.* The product life-cycle and associated documentation requirements are a relatively recent concept. The Medical Device Quality System regulations were established in 1996 and have been amended several times since that date. The original concept was to better harmonize the global manufacturing requirements for medical devices, particularly between the U.S. legal requirements and the ISO 13485 standards for medical device quality systems. The U.S. regulations were meant to take the place of the historical Good Manufacturing Practice (GMP) requirements and to expand the GMPs into the device development process.

Early in the history of medical device regulation in the United States, the longest lead-time to gain market approval was the clinical trial which was generally only used for Class III, PMA-type devices. The length of the clinical study requirement has recently been supplanted by the length of time required to address the commercial manufacturing standards and ensure that the commercial device is representative of the device from which the data in the preclinical and clinical stages were derived.

One of the most important differences between the 510(k) and PMA filing is the role of the manufacturing standards or quality systems used in the production of a device and the role of the manufacturing validation documentation requirements in the PMA filing. In the case of a 510(k) device, the sponsor commits to a validation programme in association with a published FDA guidance or recognized standard. The validations are not specifically filed with the 510(k) but are referenced for future inspection. These validations for 510(k) devices are later assessed by the FDA's field operations group as part of their routine inspectional requirements.

In the PMA filing, the sponsor must provide the FDA detailed manufacturing information showing the validity of the manufacturing process. The validation requirements for combination products involving a device plus a drug or biologic is complicated by the differences in the regulation of the different manufacturing processes. The United States and other countries will use different standards from the traditional device standards in assessing the validity of the manufacturing processes for the drug or biological component. In other words, the regulatory manufacturing standards are complicated by the combination nature of the device and the fact that there is no single manufacturing covering drugs or biologicals and devices.

Finally, as described earlier, the regulatory system for gaining market approval for devices includes a series of design assessments at discrete points in the developmental process. Each sponsor of a Class III medical device submission is required to have a device design system that includes specified elements under the heading design control.

*Design Control.* Design control is a system to examine the safety, performance and dependability of a specified design of a medical device. The design is often defined by the previously mention chemical, physical and biological properties. For any specific design, the purpose of the device including its performance is documented by a series of characteristics that the device must achieve and these are defined as the "design inputs." The testing results showing that the device meets its performance requirements are termed the "design outputs." This information is formally termed the device's "design review," which is filed in a "design history file."

Two additional critical documents are noteworthy in the regulatory development program:

1. *Quality Plan.*  Quality planning is a requirement for manufacturing of Class III devices and it becomes particularly important in the manufacture of devices containing biologically active components. As there are a number of regulations and standards defining the requirements of an active or biological material. Prior to the manufacture of device containing a combination of a biomaterial or device and an active material, a quality plan describing the standards that are to be met should be prepared. For example, the drug component may follow the regulatory framework specific to drugs and the biomaterial may follow the device regulations, but the combination will often have a mix of standards used in production and testing. As a result, a "quality plan" laying out the regulatory standards is prepared which is also termed the "quality map."

2. *Failure Mode Effects Analysis (FMEA).*   The use of FMEA is common in the device field and is a growing concept within the drug and biologics arena. A failure by definition, is the inability of the device to meet any of its design intents. These can include improper processing, assembly, packaging, storage, or labelling. A failure can occur through wear, improper storage, fatigue, material failures or poor workmanship.

The FMEA is a system to identify, analyze and rank each potential failure mode according to its severity and likelihood of occurrence. Other factors taken into consideration include consequences or severity of the failure and its probability of detection. A risk priority is assigned to each failure mode based on these criteria and the controls are assessed to control or eliminate the potential defect. Most importantly, the effect of the failure on the end user or patient is assessed, particularly potential failures that can cause injury or death.

## 6.7  Comments on Clinical Testing

Most clinical trials for drugs and biologics are executed in steps, referred to as phases (summarized in Table 6.2). Each phase is set up to determine different information. The patient inclusion criteria for each phase must be precisely documented and is a rigorously controlled process.

The drug and biological process is referred to as the Phase I, II, and III approach. For medical devices, the nomenclature is somewhat different in that devices generally fall under pilot and pivotal studies. Devices can undergo more than one pilot study depending on the clinical application and generally each additional clinical use will require a separate pivotal trial (i.e., study).

The standard nomenclature for drug and biologicals is as follows:

*Phase I.*  In this phase, the best way to administer a new treatment of a determination of dosage for safety is determined. A small number of healthy patients are included and the pharmacology of the drug is determined at this stage to establish the lowest possible therapeutic administration of that drug. Side effects are very closely scrutinized.

**TABLE 6.2**

Clinical Development Paradigm

| Phase | | | |
|---|---|---|---|
| Drug and Biologic | Device | Definition | Comment |
| I | Pilot | Small-scale study examining safety. For drugs, in healthy patients. For devices, in the patient population intended to receive the treatment | IDE for Device; IND for drugs and biologics |
| II | — | For drugs, initial assessment of the drug in the patient population for whom the treatment is intended | Overlapping pilot stage with pivotal |
| III | Pivotal | Large-scale study examining the effectiveness of the therapy in the patient population expected to receive the treatment | Generally randomized controlled trial (RCT); masked. Large numbers of patients to address statistical considerations |

*Phase II.* This phase includes the controlled clinical studies conducted to evaluate the effectiveness of the drug for a particular indication or indications in patients with the disease or condition under study. Moreover, a Phase II study will determine the common short-term side effects and risks associated with the drug. Phase II studies are typically well controlled, closely monitored and conducted in a relatively small number of patients, usually involving no more than several hundred subjects. Phase I and Phase II studies are generally considered part of the pilot stage for device developmental purposes.

*Phase III.* A Phase III study for drug trials are large, multicentred, randomized, controlled studies (RCT) examining safety and effectiveness. The regulatory standard for approval of a drug or biological requires "two well-controlled" studies. For devices, the requirement for approval is that scientific information derived from the studies must show safety and effectiveness to the "preponderance of scientific evidence." This difference between drugs and devices allows devices to utilize a number of supplemental data supporting its market approval to include foreign clinical results and bench or animal testing. Further, a device pivotal trial is generally a single trial subject to the results (Table 6.2)

The patient pool being administered the therapy, e.g., biomaterial such as calcium phosphate and a biological such as PDGF may involve several hundred patients at different medical (treatment) centres and patients receive placebo therapies or the current standard of care for a comparison to determine efficacy outcome with the new treatment.

The FDA regulatory function and product development through clinical testing is far beyond the scope and intent of this chapter. However, we do offer a number of key references in the bibliography section for the inquisitive reader.

## 6.8 Biomaterial or Biological or Combination?

Whether candidate therapeutics fall into the biomaterial category or biological category will often not be determined by what may seem to be apparent and distinguishing features.

It is not unusual in the medical field to encounter a biological that has been classified by the FDA as a device. An example is a craniofacial therapeutic/dental therapeutic that promotes the regeneration of alveolar bone, tooth cementum and periodontal ligament. The product is called Emdogain (produced and manufactured by BIORA). The Emdogain product is a biologically derived partially purified mixture of protein and extracellular matrix derived from porcine tooth germ to treat human patients. Yet, the FDA has approved Emdogain as a device, not as a biologic.

The academic investigator focused on applied research with a clinical target should include corporate engagement where the corporate entity has seasoned regulatory personnel experienced in dealing with the FDA and where FDA guidance can be obtained to assist in the selection of the most appropriate and effective preclinical models. Those preclinical models must be guided by the most likely regulatory approval pathway (i.e., either 510(k) or PMA and defined by either the IDE or IND).

An exciting new therapeutic has been developed by Professor Stephen Feinberg and his team at the University of Michigan (Izumi et al., 2004). The product involves a tissue engineered mucosal equivalent, known as *ex vivo* produced oral mucosa equivalent (EVPOME) that has been categorized by the FDA as a drug. Therefore, the Feinberg team will apply for an Investigational New Drug (IND) through the CBER and the group will engage in a highly regulated testing hierarchy of *in vitro* test and a focused *in vivo* animal model prior to entering into human clinical trails (beginning with a Phase I clinical trial).

With the *in vivo* test system (animal model), vertebrate use must comply with the epochal Animal Welfare Act (1985 and subsequent amendments) and the National Institutes of Health policy (e.g., The Public Health Service Policy on Humane Care and Use of Laboratory Animals, 1986). Moreover, all animal research protocols must be reviewed and approved by an IACUC. Relevant to biomaterials testing, the IACUC will insist on quantifiable outcome measures from the *in vivo* experiment.

There are many new combination products in development consisting of biomaterials plus biologics, which can include human cells, referred to as human somatic cell therapy and the Center of Biologic Evaluation and Research (CBER) is the organization arm overseeing control. The FDA also has different centers that regulate materials/biologics.

The Medical Device User Fee and Modernization Act (2002) established the Office of Combination Products to develop guidelines for combination products.

---

## 6.9   The "Bench to Bedside" Process: An Approach to Design and Develop a Bone Regeneration Therapy

The clinical target for an example bone therapy is identified and the biology and biomechanics of the clinical target (also known as the clinical indication) are defined. The pathway and skill set (i.e., personnel resources) are set in place and a process is executed to design and develop a therapy with targeted properties that will address a defined clinical need (Figure 6.1).

The bench to bedside process can be summarized in three stages.

*Stage 1: Integration of the disciplines basic biology, biomechanics and biomaterials.*   Personnel with expertise in these disciplines will engage with clinicians and identify a clinical target. Candidate therapeutics will be designed and developed that will progress through the process to Stage 2. For example, if the clinical target is a nonloadbearing bone void, the therapeutic composition could include a particulate calcium phosphate such as tricalcium phosphate (TCP) that will deliver PDGF.

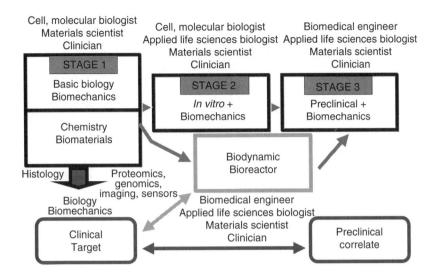

**FIGURE 6.1**
Bench to bedside: process. Regulatory standards, testing protocols, FDA guidelines. ASTM, IDE, IND, Class I-III, ISO 1099. IP.

*Stage 2: Testing.* The *in vitro* and biomechanical testing (e.g., defined ISO or ASTM tests) will determine a hierarchy of performance standards that must be fine tuned and calibrated to fulfil the biological and biomechanical standards of the clinical target. This stage will determine properties that include biocompatibility, the impact of the therapy on cell viability, function (e.g., expression of key functional markers that for osteoblasts could include alkaline phosphatase, osteocalcin and/or osteonectin), biofunctional performance (e.g., compression, torsion and tensile properties) and release kinetics of, for example, the PDGF from the TCP. Those candidate therapeutics that appeared to promote the optimal biological responses will be transitioned to the preclinical correlate: The *in vivo* animal model that most closely represents the clinical target.

An exciting alternative opportunity illustrated in Figure 6.1 is the anticipated strategy to use a biodynamic bioreactor that will be programmed to fulfil the biological milieu encountered with an animal model.

*Stage 3: Animal model.* The preclinical correlate to the clinical indication will become the test bed for the therapeutic. For example, a targeted clinical need is bone regeneration in a gap defect in the skull. A preclinical correlate is the rat calvaria bone gap model that exploits a critical-sized defect (CSD) (Figure 6.2a). A CSD will not spontaneously heal with bone unless it is treated with a bone regeneration therapy. The top series of animal model views (Figure 6.2a) indicate preparation of the CSD (far left) and no bone healing either radiographically (middle view) or histologically (far right). When demineralized bone matrix, a bone regenerating biomaterial derived from bone, is implanted into the preclinical rat calvaria bone gap model (i.e., CSD), new bone formation occurs (Figure 6.2a: lower panels, middle: radiographic and far right: histologic).

Quantitative outcome measures are required by IACUCs as we emphasized earlier in the chapter. Consequently, techniques that include radiomorphometry (Figure 6.2b) and histomorphometry (Figure 6.2c) are used in preclinical tests to quantitate radiographic and histologic responses of the animal model to biomaterials destined for targeted human clinical therapies.

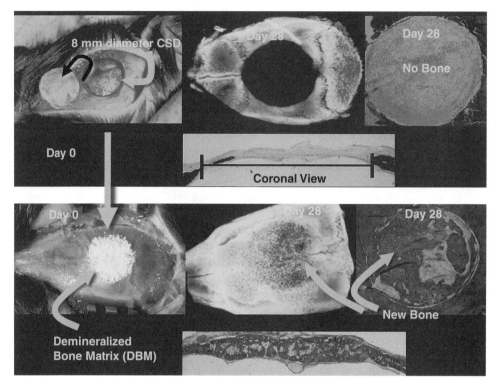

**FIGURE 6.2**
(**See color insert following page 498.**) Rat Calvaria: bone gap model.

Challenging clinical conditions include bony clefts in the maxilla (i.e., the upper jaw) and gap defects in long bones (radius and ulna, for example) of the forearm, which may occur from trauma or surgical resection due to cancer. A preclinical correlate used for the maxillary cleft is a dog model to test poly(lactide-co-glycolide): PLGA and recombinant human bone morphogenetic protein-2: rhBMP-2 (Figure 6.3). In Figure 6.3 the upper photo includes the radiograph where new bone (left side) formed in the treated side of the cleft

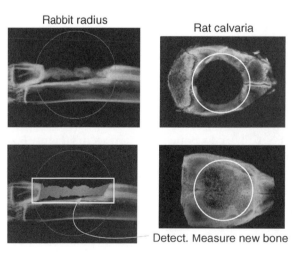

Detect. Measure new bone

**FIGURE 6.3**
Radiomorphometry.

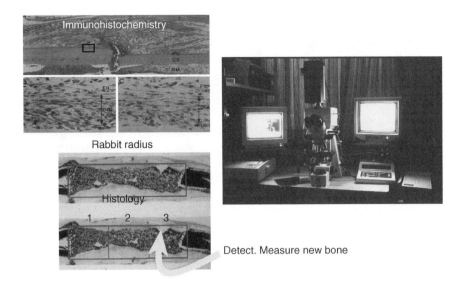

**FIGURE 6.4**
Histomorphometry.

and no bone formed on the right side. The histological outcome is shown in the panel directly below the radiograph.

The rabbit radius gap model (Figure 6.4a) is used to test combination therapies (i.e., delivery system biomaterial plus biologic) for bone regeneration. The outcome from treatments using the rabbit long bone gap model (Figure 6.4a) is shown in Figure 6.4b. The histological and radiographical results are seen across test conditions (Figure 6.5–6.7).

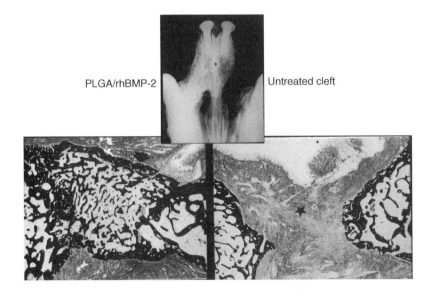

**FIGURE 6.5**
Preclinical correlate: surgically prepared cleft.

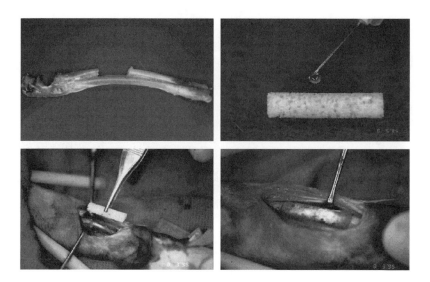

**FIGURE 6.6**
Rabbit long bone gap model. RhBMP-2 and Poly(D,L-lactide).

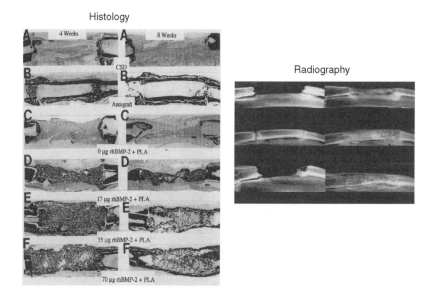

**FIGURE 6.7**
Histology and radiography.

## 6.10   Conclusion

There is considerable diversity in biological responses when a biomaterial and biomaterial–biological are implanted into a living system (e.g., a patient). Consequently, a standardized, rigorous and reproducible paradigm that as accurately as possible will predict the clinical outcome for a targeted clinical indication is a fundamental requirement for therapeutic development. This chapter stresses the importance of testing standards and identified key organizations involved with standards for *in vivo* biomaterials testing.

There are many potential clinical indications for biomaterials. Consequently, there must be a rational, effective approach in animal model selection to ensure unambiguous efficacy validation of the biomaterial and biomaterial–biological combination.

The animal models to test biomaterials must follow standards and permit unambiguous outcome measures that must be quantifiable. Moreover, animal models must be repeatable among laboratories and yield reproducible outcome data among laboratories. It has therefore been the emphasis of this chapter to underscore the importance of standards, especially those standards based on consensus organizations within the American Society for Testing Materials Committee F-4 (ASTM F-4). The standards are available in the public domain on an annual basis from the ASTM.

---

## Ten Questions

**Question 1.** Describe the considerations and cite the organizations integral to humane care and use of experimental animals for materials testing.

**Answer 1.** Anyone using an *in vivo* system is responsible for humane use of that test system (i.e., the animal model). When vertebrates are used, there must be compliance with the Animal Welfare Act (1985) and the National Institutes of Health Policy on Humane Care and Use of Laboratory Animals (1986). Moreover, *all in vivo* research protocols must be reviewed and approved by an IACUC that will insist on measurable, quantifiable outcome measures from the experiment.

Specific standards and stringent criteria must be fulfilled by vivaria administering animal husbandry that includes veterinary care, record keeping, dedicated space per animal, human interaction, feeding and fluid management, waste disposal, environmental policy and regulations, temperature, air circulation, personnel training, credentialing, the operating theatre, methods of restraint and transport to and from the holding facilities to the operating theatre, as well as anaesthesia, euthanasia and disposal.

**Question 2.** Does the process from the laboratory bench to *in vitro* methodologies ensure fidelity of those biocompatibility measures to *in vivo* measures? Provide support for the answer you choose.

**Answer 2.** It is not a concern that *in vitro* outcome data may not be equivalent to *in vivo* outcome data. For example, a biomaterial may be cytotoxic to a cell line *in vitro*, however, in a subcutaneous implantation site, the tissue fluid will buffer the biomaterial affects and the implant may in fact be biocompatible. Moreover, the pharmacokinetics of a growth factor released from a biomaterial tested with an *in vitro* system may yield an outcome that is distinctly different than if the biomaterial was implanted in an animal femur model.

**Question 3.** Does animal model testing success predict success in the human clinical indication? Provide support for the answer you choose.

**Answer 3.** Animal model testing success does not necessarily predict success in the human clinical indication. There may be dosing issues, pharmacokinetic and pharmacodynamic differences between the animal model and the human patient.

The FDA routinely requires phases of outcome data derived from standard testing protocols that exploit *in vitro* and *in vivo* tests. The transition from a successful series of outcomes in the preclinical *in vivo* model system to the clinical *in vivo* system is generally understood and expected to require modification in the clinical *in vivo* system. *In vitro* and animal model testing can provide reasonable assurance of human safety but are not by themselves a prognosticator of human outcome application which requires a separate developmental programme. The antecedent *in vitro* and preclinical testing paradigms do not unequivocally predict how a biomaterial will perform in humans. Therefore, the staging to evaluate biomaterials using clinical *in vivo* system testing is accomplished in either stages or phases.

**Question 4.** What are the stages and phases associated with drugs and devices, respectively?

**Answer 4.** The recognized drug developmental definitions of Phase I, II, and III clinical trials in patients are not recognized in the device development, which proceeds first through a pilot and second through a pivotal trial.

For a biological, the three phases are as follows:

In Phase I, the best way to administer a new treatment of a determination of dosage of the biological for safety is determined. A small number of patients are included. When a drug is the focus, the lowest possible therapeutic administration of that drug is emphasized. Side effects are very closely scrutinized.

In Phase II, usually less than 100 patients are involved and the expectation is that with a larger patient pool than in the Phase I study, a broader range of responses will be elicited from the biological.

In Phase III, the patient pool being administered the biological therapy may involve several hundred patients at different medical (treatment) centres and patients receive placebo therapies or the current standard of care for a comparison to determine efficacy outcome with the new treatment.

The prominent definition used in device development is a pilot programme to show safety and assess the study design which is in general, equivalent to Phases I and II drug (biological) studies. The next stage of device development is the pivotal trial. The pivotal trial is the device equivalent of a Phase III drug programme.

**Question 5.** Are the targeted clinical properties of the biomaterial consistent with the end use application? Provide support for the answer you choose.

**Answer 5.** Sometimes yes and sometimes no. The biology of the target site for which the biomaterial is intended may not be satisfactorily characterized and biology of the clinical target is key to the rational, instructive guidance for the design and development of the biomaterial(s) and their end stage use.

**Question 6.** How is the preclinical pathway selected for *in vivo* materials testing? And, is there a concern in the selection approach?

**Answer 6.** The preclinical pathway selected for *in vivo* materials testing will be determined by the material's end use application. As a result, there is the potential that the preclinical programme may be flawed. For example, a close reading of the ISO 10993 standard reveals that each device developer should examine the end use and design the preclinical safety programme around the associated risks of the clinical application.

**Question 7.** Describe the IDE pathway a biomedical device make take, including the classification levels, and describe and provide examples of those classes.

**Answer 7.** A biomaterial device such as a calcium phosphate bone void filler may be considered by the FDA to be equivalent to an already marketed product (device) or predicate device. This pathway is the 510(k) pathway. In this pathway, the device may then be classified according to one of three levels of classification.

Class I devices are those where general controls sufficient enough to ensure safety and effectiveness. Examples include elastic bandages, examination gloves and hand-held surgical instruments.

Class II devices are those where general controls are determined as being insufficient to provide reasonable assurance that safety and effectiveness will be assured. However, there is adequate information to establish performance standards that can provide safety and effectiveness assurance. Examples of this class of devices include powered wheelchairs and infusion pumps

Class III devices cannot be classified as either Class I or Class II due to insufficient information to determine the general controls and performance standards assuring for safety and efficacy. Class III devices are usually dedicated to life-sustaining and life-supporting application, or are implanted in the patient. Typical class III examples can include replacement heart valves, breast implants, and TMJ implants.

The PMA pathway is followed when the approval for higher-risk devices does not exist. For example, when either Class III devices or devices where a substantial equivalent predicate does not exist or the device has been classified as a Class III due to its potential risk to health.

**Question 8.** Contrast and compare the clinical development paradigm of a drug and biologic versus a device.

**Answer 8.** Most clinical trials for drugs and biologics are executed in phases. Each phase is set up to determine different information

*Phase I.* In this phase, the best way to administer a new treatment of a determination of dosage for safety is determined. A small number of patients are included. When a drug is the focus, the lowest possible therapeutic administration of that drug is emphasized. Side effects are closely scrutinized.

*Phase II.* This phase usually involves less than 100 patients and the expectation is that with a larger patient pool than in the Phase I study, a broader range of responses will be elicited.

*Phase III.* In this phase, the patient pool being administered the therapy may involve several hundred patients at different medical (treatment) centres and patients receive placebo therapies or the current standard of care for a comparison to determine efficacy outcome with the new treatment.

In contrast to the biologic and drug, a device pathway will involve a pilot study first and then a pivotal trial study as the final stage.

**Question 9.** Describe a strategy that can be used to design and develop a therapeutic.

**Answer 9.** The clinical target for a therapy is identified and the biology and biomechanics of the clinical target (also known as the clinical indication) are defined.

The *first stage* in the design and development strategy will integrate clinicians and individuals with expertise in the disciplines basic biology, biomechanics and biomaterials. This group will define the clinical indication in terms of biology and if necessary, biomechanical properties. Possible combinations of biologicals will be considered for the clinical indication.

The *second stage* in the strategy will involve *in vitro* and biomechanical testing that will determine a hierarchy of performance standards that will be fine tuned and calibrated to fulfil the biological and biomechanical standards of the clinical target. These standards may include those defined according to ISO or ASTM tests. This stage will answer questions about biocompatibility, the impact of the therapy on cell viability, function, biofunctional performance (e.g., compression, torsion and tensile properties) and release kinetics. Those candidate therapeutics that promote the optimal biological response (and when relevant, biomechanical performance) will be transitioned to the preclinical correlate.

The *in vivo* animal model that most closely represents the clinical target (i.e., most appropriate preclinical correlate) will be selected.

The *third and final stage* in the strategy will be the preclinical correlate to the clinical indication. This stage will involve the animal model testing. The animal models to test biomaterials will follow standards and permit unambiguous outcome measures that will be quantifiable and repeatable among laboratories.

**Question 10.** Why are standards necessary in the design and development of therapeutics to treat clinical problems?

**Answer 10.** Standards are necessary to unify the biological and biomechanical functional performance of biologics (drugs) and devices and to ensure they perform according to a consensus, and an acceptable level of criteria. The established standards for performance criteria are the best way to ensure the highest level of predictability that the biologic or device will be safe and efficacious in the clinical environment.

Therefore, consensus standards, such as the American Society for Testing and Materials Committee F-4 (ASTM F-4) have been established for most implant devices.

Moreover, the establishment of a standardized testing paradigm for biologics and devices will ensure that among laboratories, there is a common protocol for testing and that results from the knowledge that common protocols can be compared, contrasted and reproduced. Repeatability among laboratories strengthens the validation of outcome and further underscores the safety and efficacy of the biological or device that will be used for a targeted clinical indication.

## Appendix 6.1:  American Society for Testing and Materials (ASTM)

(Some example ASTM documents with sample subject standards. Please refer to the ASTM website, http://www.astm.com for a comprehensive listing as well as the ASTM Annual Book of Standards that is published each year.)

| ASTM Document | Subject Standard |
|---|---|
| ASTM F-619-97 | Practice for extraction of medical plastics |
| ASTM F-720-96 | Practice for testing guinea pigs for contact allergens |
| ASTM F-748-95 | Practice for selection generic biological test methods for materials and devices |
| ASTM F-749-98 | Practice for evaluating material extracts by intracutaneous injection in the rabbit |
| ASTM F-981-93 | Practice for assessment of compatibility of nonporous biomaterials for surgical implants: Effects of materials on muscle and bone |
| ASTM F-1439-96 | Guide for the performance of lifetime bioassay for the tumorgenic potential of implant materials |
| ASTM F-763-93 | Practice for the short-term screening of implant materials |

## Appendix 6.2:  ISO 10,993, Biological Evaluation of Medical Devices International Standards Organization (ISO)

(Please refer to the ISO website, http://www.iso.org for a comprehensive overview as well the details on the subject standards.)

| ISO Document | Subject Standard |
|---|---|
| ISO 10,993-1 | Evaluation and testing |
| ISO 10,993-2 | Animal welfare requirements |
| ISO 10,993-3 | Tests for genotoxocity, carcinogenicity, reproductive toxicity |
| ISO 10,993-4 | Selection of tests for interactions with blood |
| ISO 10,993-5 | Tests for cytotoxicity: *In vitro* methods |
| ISO 10,993-6 | Tests for local effects after implantation |
| ISO 10,993-7 | Ethylene oxide sterilization residuals |
| ISO 10,993-8 | Being redone. No topic |
| ISO 10,993-9 | Framework for the identification and quantification of potential degradation products |
| ISO 10,993-10 | Tests for irritation and sensitization |
| ISO 10,993-11 | Test for systemic toxicity |
| ISO 10,993-12 | Sample preparation and reference material |
| ISO 10,993-13 | Identification and quantification of degradation products from polymers |
| ISO 10,993-14 | Identification and quantification of degradation products from ceramics |
| ISO 10,993-15 | Identification and quantification of degradation products from metals and alloys |
| ISO 10,993-16 | Toxicokinetic study design for degradation products and leachables |

## Appendix 6.3:  Risk Analysis Form

Device Name/Code: _____ Dated:

| Question | Response |
|---|---|
| a) What is the intended use? | |
| b) Is the device intended to contact the patient or other persons? | |
| c) What materials and/or components  are used? | |
| d) Is energy delivered to and/or extracted from the patient? | |
| e) Are substances delivered to and/or extracted from the patient? | |
| f) Are biological materials processed by the device for subsequent reuse? | |
| g) Is the service supplied sterile or intended to be sterilized by the user? | |
| h) Is the device intended to modify the patient environment? | |
| i) Are measurements made? | |
| j) Is the device interpretive? | |
| k) Is the device intended to control or to interact with other devices or drugs? | |
| l) Are there unwanted outputs of energy or substances? | |
| m) Is the device susceptible to environmental influences? | |
| n) Are there essential consumables or accessories associated with the device? | |
| o) Is routine maintenance and/or calibration necessary? | |
| p) Does the device contain software? | |
| q) Does the device have a restricted shelf-life? | |
| r) Possible delayed and/or long-term use effects? | |
| s) To what mechanical forces will the device be subjected? | |
| t) What determines the lifetime of the device? | |
| u) Is the device intended for single use or reuse? | |

## Appendix 6.4:   Possible Hazards Associated with Medical Devices

Device Name/Code: _____ Dated:

| | Estimation of Risk | | | |
| Possible Hazard | Normal Condition | Fault Condition | Is Risk Acceptable? | Rationale |
| --- | --- | --- | --- | --- |
| I) Energy Hazards | | | | |
| a)  Electricity | | | | |
| b)  Heat | | | | |
| c)  Mechanical force | | | | |
| d)  Ionizing radiation | | | | |
| e)  Nonionizing radiation | | | | |
| f)  Electromagnetic fields | | | | |
| g)  Moving parts | | | | |
| h)  Suspended masses | | | | |
| i)  Patient support device failure | | | | |
| j)  Pressure (vessel rupture) | | | | |
| k)  Acoustic pressure | | | | |
| l)  Vibration | | | | |
| m) Magnetic fields, e.g., MRI | | | | |
| II) Biological Hazards | | | | |
| a)  Bioburden/biocontamination | | | | |
| b)  Bioincompatibility | | | | |
| c)  Incorrect output (substance/energy) | | | | |
| d)  Incorrect formulation (chemical composition) | | | | |
| e)  Toxicity | | | | |
| f)  (Cross-)infection | | | | |
| g)  Pyrogenicity | | | | |
| h)  Inability to maintain hygienic safety | | | | |
| i)  Degradation | | | | |
| III) Environmental Hazards | | | | |
| a)  Electromagnetic interference | | | | |
| b)  Inadequate supply of power or coolant | | | | |
| c)  Restriction of cooling | | | | |
| d)  Likelihood of operation outside prescribed environmental conditions | | | | |
| e)  Incompatibility with other devices | | | | |
| f)  Accidental mechanical damage | | | | |
| g)  Contamination due to waste products and/or device disposal | | | | |
| IV) Hazard Related to Use of the Device | | | | |
| a)  Inadequate labelling | | | | |
| b)  Inadequate operating instructions | | | | |
| c)  Inadequate specification of accessories | | | | |
| d)  Inadequate specification of preuse checks | | | | |

**Appendix 6.4** (Continued)

| | Estimation of Risk | | | |
| | Normal Condition | Fault Condition | Is Risk Acceptable? | Rationale |
| Possible Hazard | | | | |
|---|---|---|---|---|
| e) Over-complicated operating instructions | | | | |
| f) Unavailable or separated operating instructions | | | | |
| g) Use by unskilled personnel | | | | |
| h) Use by untrained/unskilled personnel | | | | |
| i) Reasonably forseeable misuse | | | | |
| j) Insufficient warning of side effects | | | | |
| k) Inadequate warning of hazards likely with reuse of single use device | | | | |
| l) Incorrect measurement and other metrological aspects | | | | |
| m) Incorrect diagnosis | | | | |
| n) Erroneous data transfer | | | | |
| o) Misrepresentation of results | | | | |
| p) Incompatibility with consumables/ accessories/other devices | | | | |
| V) Hazards Arising from Function Failure, Maintenance and Aging | | | | |
| a) Inadequacy of performance characteristics for the intended use | | | | |
| b) Lack of or inadequate specification of maintenance, including specification of postmaintenance functional checks | | | | |
| c) Inadequate maintenance | | | | |
| d) Lack of adequate determination of end of device life | | | | |
| e) Loss of mechanical integrity | | | | |
| f) Inadequate packaging (contamination and/or deterioration of device) | | | | |
| g) Improper reuse | | | | |

## Appendix 6.5: Risk Analysis Instructions

The purpose of this procedure is to provide a risk analysis of a medical device that meets the intent of EN 1441. The analysis will include the investigation of available information to identify hazards and estimate risks. The risk analysis form (attached) details the required elements for a risk analysis.

*Note*: "Step" numbers shown refer to the procedural steps outlined in EN 1441.

Step 1 — Product definition and description

Step 2 — Identification of qualitative and quantitative characteristics

Consistent with the intent of EN 1441, the risk analysis procedure includes the consideration of a series of questions related to the purpose and use of the device under analysis. These questions and responses are to be tabulated in Form No. 046.

Step 3 — Identification of possible hazards

Step 4 — Estimation of the risk of each hazard

Step 5 — Acceptability of risk

Consistent with the intent of EN 1441, the risk analysis procedure includes the consideration of a list of possible hazards associated with medical devices, an estimation of risk associated with these hazards, and the acceptability of these risks. This association is to be tabulated in the risk analysis form.

Step 6 — Risk reduction

The hazards identified by a means of the interrogatory analysis above are of sufficiently low risk and low probability that a risk reduction initiate is deemed unnecessary.

Step 7 — Generation of other hazards

There were no additional hazards created by a risk reduction initiative.

Step 8 — Evaluation of all identified hazards

It is believed that all hazards have been identified through the process shown above.

Step 9 — Adequacy of device safety

Approval of the risk analysis signifies that with regard to the intended application and use of the device, it is the position of the reviewer(s) that the risks associated with the identified hazards are acceptable.

## References

Izumi, K., Song, J., and Feinberg, S., Development of a tissue-engineered human oral mucosa: from the bench to the bedside cells, *Tissues Organs*, **176**, 134–152 (2004).

Black, J., *Biological Performance of Materials. Fundamentals and Biocompatibility*, 2nd ed., Marcel Dekker, New York (1992).

Dee, K., Puleo, D., and Bizios, R., Eds., *Tissue–Biomaterials Interactions*, Wiley-Liss, New York (2003).

An, Y. and Friedman, R., Eds., *Animal Models in Orthopaedic Research*, CRC Press, Boca Raton (1999).

Ratner, B., Hoffman, A., Schoen, F., and Lemons, J., Eds., *Biomaterials Sciences. An Introduction to Materials in Medicine*, 2nd ed., (2004).

Kahan, J., *Medical Device Development*, Paraexel Press, Alexandria, VA (2000).

Witikin, K., *Clinical Evaluation of Medical Devices*, Humana Press, Clifton, UK (1998).

## Recommended Websites

ASTM International Standards Worldwide. http://www.astm.com/cgi-bin/SoftCart.exe/ABOUT/aboutASTM.html..

FDA: IDE, IND, Clinical trials. http://www.fda.gov.

ISO Standards. http://www.iso.org/iso/en/ISOOnline.frontpage.

# 7

## Fibrin and Its Applications

**Bill Tawil**

## CONTENTS

Tissue engineering products have been generated by nature since the beginning of life at no cost and introducing no inflammation or rejection side effects. While these natural tissue-engineering products are formed during the healing process of most defects in healthy individuals, they fail to overcome similar defects in compromised patients. Examples of these untreated diseases include chronic wounds in diabetic or obese patients, bone defects in osteoporosis patients, functional deterioration in Parkinson and Alzheimer patients, muscle weakening in muscular dystrophy, etc. Thus, there are unmet needs requiring the generation of tissue engineering products. A successful man-made tissue-engineering product should have the same components as a natural tissue-engineering product, i.e., a scaffold, cells, and signaling molecules.

In this chapter, the use of fibrin as a scaffold in generating tissue-engineering products is discussed. Examples are presented on the use of fibrin in delivering bioactive substances or skin cells such as fibroblasts and keratinocytes for the treatment of chronic wounds, mesenchymal stem cells to treat bone defects, or neural stem cells to overcome neuronal diseases. Other uses of fibrin in tissue engineering that is not covered here are the use of fibrin to make blood vessels and fibrin tubes to be used as axonal bridges.

By the end of the chapter, one should have an appreciation of why so many scientists and companies have been using fibrin in generating tissue-engineering products over the last three decades.

## 7.1  Fibrin as a Natural Scaffold during Wound Healing

While the main purpose of fibrin formation during the wound healing process is hemostasis, its subsequent function as a scaffold for migrating cells into the wound bed is very critical for the onset of a proper and complete wound healing process. Within seconds of an injury, activated thrombin, an enzyme, assembles fibrinogen molecules into fibrils that are crossed-linked by factor XIII to form an insoluble fibrin clot (Figure 7.1(a),(b);

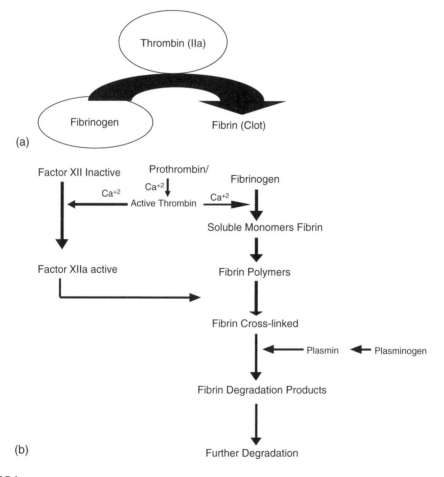

**FIGURE 7.1**
(a) The formation of fibrin from fibrinogen. Thrombin acts as an enzyme in this transformation. (b) More detailed scheme of the formation of fibrin from fibrinogen. Various players are involved in the formation and degradation of fibrin.

reviewed in Amrani, 2001; Ariens et al., 2002). There are many factors that modulate the formation of fibrin clots from three chains ($\alpha$, $\beta$, and $\gamma$) and affect the fibrin degradation (Figure 7.1b). Mutations in these chains could lead to various diseases; for example, dysfibrinogemias results from the mutation in the $\gamma$ fibrinogen chain leading to either no effect, bleeding, or thrombosis (reviewed in Cote et al., 1998). Fibronectin and many growth factors such as TGFb1, EGF, FGF, and VEGF are trapped within the formed fibrin clot (Werner and Grose, 2003) forming a biomatrix rather than an inert scaffold. This biomatrix fibrin presents an excellent natural scaffold allowing various cells such as fibroblasts to migrate into the wound bed. The wound healing process from this point on has been reviewed many times over the years (Clark, 1998; Figure 7.2). Briefly, neutrophils and monocytes are recruited to the injury site as a response to inductive proteins originating from the cell debris and bacterial contamination caused by the injury. As the first stage of wound healing, the cleaning stage, is completed by the removal of any bacteria or cell debris by neutrophils and the macrophages (activated monocytes), the construction process begins with fibroblasts, keratinocytes, and endothelial cells migrating into the fibrin-filled wound. As the fibrin clot starts to degrade, the invading cells deposit matrix molecules such as collagen, laminin, and other extracellular matrix molecules (ECM) rebuilding the dermis, epidermis, and the vasculature network. The proliferation of these various cells, their coordinated invasion, their deposition of matrix molecules, and the degradation of the fibrin clot are all orchestrated by various growth factors secreted initially by platelets and then activated macrophages (Werner and Grose, 2003). As the growth factor-packed fibrin biomatrix starts to receive cells, a naturally formed tissue-engineering product is created. The role of fibrin in the various stages of wound healing is illustrated in Table 7.1.

These natural characteristics of fibrin contribute to the vast literature, over the last 30 years, on the use of fibrin in delivering cells or bioactive substances to treat various diseases. Below are some examples of how fibrin is used in making tissue-engineering products, presenting in the process its intrinsic bioactive characteristics.

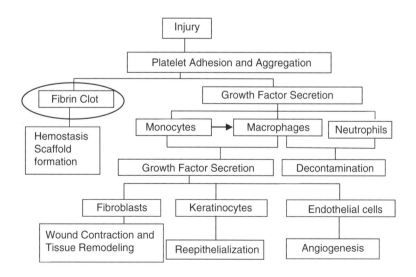

**FIGURE 7.2**
A schematic of the wound healing process.

**TABLE 7.1**

The Role of Various Proteins in Wound Healing

| | Phases of Wound Healing | | |
|---|---|---|---|
| | **Inflammation** | **Proliferation** | **Maturation** |
| Fibrin(ogen) | Attracts and activates leukocytes. Promotes platelet adhesion | Stimulates angiogenesis. Promotes cell migration and adhesion | |
| Thrombin | Cleaves fibrinogen leading to clot formation and hemostasis. Activates factor XIII | Activates would healing related receptors on epithelial cells, fibroblasts, endothelial cells, and other cell types | |
| Fibronectin | Provides binding sites for migrating fibroblasts. Acts as bridge for cells migrating into clot | | |
| Factor XIII | Cross-links fibronectin with fibrin and collagen | Stimulates fibroblasts. Stimulates collagen synthesis | |
| EGF | | Stimulates cell proliferation of keratinocytes and fibroblasts | Regulates MMP expression in keratinocytes |
| bFGF | | Stimulates angiogenesis and is also a mitogen for fibroblasts. Chemotactic factor for both fibroblasts and keratinocytes | |
| TGFβ | | Stimulates fibroblast growth and differentiation. Stimulates matrix deposition, re-epithelialization, and angiogenesis | Regulates MMP production in keratinocytes |
| VEGF | | Stimulates angiogenesis and induces endothelial cell proliferation | |

## 7.2   Fibrin in Hemostasis and Tissue Sealing

The use of fibrin product in hemostasis is based on the concept of promoting a quicker hemostasis by increasing the concentration of fibrinogen to more than 3 to 4 mg/ml, which is the concentration detected in the plasma of most healthy individuals. Fibrin sealant products are the most advanced in this concept/technology. Fibrin products are approved in the United States for hemostasis and tissue sealing indications in various surgical procedures including cardio-pulmonary bypass surgery, trauma to the spleen, and sealing of colostomy closure (see Table 7.2 for some examples). Historically, fibrin products originated 30 years ago from a much primitive state. Initially, hemostasis was achieved by concentrating fibrinogen from plasma taken from the patient. This fibrinogen was then reintroduced into the patient's wound along with thrombin. While this process is still in use, it has been declining sharply over the last few years because of the realization that

**TABLE 7.2**

Examples of the Use of Fibrin in Surgery

| Indication | References |
|---|---|
| Cardiovascular — antibiotics | Surgical treatment of active infective endocarditis with paravalvular involvement. Watanabe G. et al. *The Journal of Thoracic and Cardiovascular Surgery*, 1994 |
| Cardiovascular — growth factors | The use of biologic glue for better adhesions between the skeletal muscle flap and the myocardium and for increasing capillary ingrowth. Chekanov V et al. *The Journal of Thoracic and Cardiovascular Surgery*, 1996 |
| Growth factors | Experimental use of a modified fibrin glue to induce site-directed angiogenesis from the aorta to the heart. Fasol R et al. *The Journal of Thoracic and Cardiovascular Surgery*, 1994 |
| Orthopedics — antibiotics | Treatment of experimental osteomyelitis with a fibrin sealant antibiotic implant. Mader J.T. et al. *Clinical Orthopaedics*, 2002 |
| Plastics — skin grafting/burns | The effect of fibrin glue on skin grafts in infected sites. Jabs A.D. et al. *Plastic and Reconstructive Surgery*, 1992 |
| | Fibrin glue in the treatment of dorsal hand burns. Boeckx W. et al. *Burns*, 1992 |
| | Fibrin glue: its use for skin grafting of contaminated burn wounds in areas difficult to immobilize. Vedung S. and Hedlund A. *Journal of Burn Care and Rehabilitation*, 1993 |
| | Cologne burn center experiences with glycerol-preserved allogenic skin: part 1: clinical experiences and histological findings (overgraft and sandwich technique). Horch R. et al. *Burns*, 1994 |
| | Cologne burn center experiences with glycerol-preserved allogenic skin: part 2: combination with autologous cultured keratinocytes. Stark G.B. and Kairser H.W. *Burns*, 1994 |
| | Role and innocuity of Tisseel, a tissue glue, in the grafting process and in vivo evolution of human cultured epidermis. Auger F.A. et al. *British Journal of Plastic Surgery*, 1993 |

there are various issues with this approach. First, blood is withdrawn from a patient; this could be a problematic if the patient is already bleeding or very ill. Second, the amount of fibrinogen that is concentrated by this process is not consistent among various individuals; it maximally concentrates fibrinogen to 10 mg/ml vs. 100 mg/ml in some available fibrin products. Third, and a major issue in this process, is the lack of a heat-inactivation step exposing the nurses and doctors to viral or bacterial contamination originating from the patient's own plasma as it is processed. The fourth point is the lack of fibrinolysis inhibitor leading to fibrin clot degradation in 4 to 5 days. Existing fibrin products overcome these problems; there is a consistent high concentration of fibrinogen in the range of 100 mg/ml, 30-fold higher than the fibrinogen concentration in a healthy individual. The fibrin is heat-inactivated to eliminate any viral transmission. Most importantly, a fibrinolysis inhibitor is added increasing the life of the formed fibrin clot to 10 to 14 days depending on the location of fibrin in the body. An example of existing fibrin products is shown in Figure 7.3.

An important point to make here is that while various fibrin sealant products consist of the same two components, fibrinogen-rich and thrombin, there are a lot of variations between them regarding how quick they adhere, how long they last before dissolving,

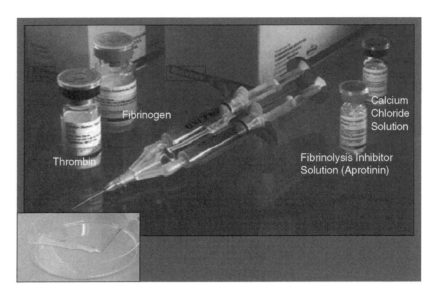

**FIGURE 7.3**
An example of fibrin products available in the United States.

and, most importantly, their toxicity issue. For example, one of these fibrin sealant products has a warning box on it indicating its neurotoxicity characteristic due to the presence of tranexamic acid; the toxic effect of tranexamic acid was supported by many studies (Schlag et al., 2000, 2002; Cox et al., 2003). The toxicity aspect of this specific fibrin product will prevent it from being used in making tissue-engineering products. So in conclusion, one should not make the assumption that all fibrin sealants are equivalent.

## 7.3   The Use of Fibrin in Tissue Engineering

As indicated above, to compose a fibrin clot during wound healing, two components are needed; a fibrinogen enriched sealer protein complex and thrombin. It is also indicated that the existing fibrin products use the same approach, i.e., they consist of two human-derived components, fibrinogen-rich and thrombin, that when mixed form a fibrin clot. While the approved use of these products is in hemostasis and tissue sealing, the future of fibrin sealant is in the field of tissue engineering. Some fibrin products consist of a fibrinogen concentration of about 100 mg/ml, which is about 30-fold more than it is normally in the plasma and thrombin concentration of 500 units/ml. Recent work (Cox et al., 2004; Mooney et al., 2004) clearly indicates that changing the fibrinogen or thrombin concentration in the formed fibrin clot leads to major changes in the biochemical and mechanical characteristics of the fibrin clot. These changes could explain the difference in cell growth and differentiation by various cells in these formulations. There have been hundreds of papers published over the last three decades showing the use of fibrin in tissue engineering including its use in delivering cells and bioactive substances to treat soft and hard tissue defects.

As described above, the fibrin clot eventually degrades within 1 to 2 weeks depending on its environment. Within this time frame, the fibrin clot could retain many bioactive substances and invaded cells in active and viable form localizing them, as a consequence, to the injury site. Various studies have supported the use of fibrin in tissue engineering both *in vitro* as well as *in vivo* (Albes et al., 1994; Arnaud et al., 1994; Perka et al., 2000; Horch et al., 2001).

### 7.3.1 Fibrin Sealant as a Delivery Vehicle for Bioactive Substances

There are many studies that show fibrin as an ideal delivery vehicle for delivering growth factors and peptides in an active form. Some of these proteins bind weakly within the fibrin clot and diffuse from the fibrin clot at various diffusion rates (MacPhee et al., 1996; Wong et al., 2003). Other growth factors such as basic fibroblast growth factor (bFGF) and vascular endothelial growth factor (VEGF) bind specifically and strongly to fibrin (ogen) (Hasimoto et al., 1992; Albes et al., 1994; Sahni and Francis, 2000; Wong et al., 2003) and diffuse slowly from the fibrin clot. Recent studies used a cross-linking approach to bind growth factors to the fibronectin or factor XIII within the fibrin clot (Schense et al., 2000; Andree et al., 2001). These modifications support the slow release of these growth factors over an extended period of time. This cross-linking approach allows the binding of any growth factor which is naturally does not bind to fibrin. This powerful technology combines the hemostatic effect of fibrin with a wound healing effect generated by the added growth factors. This technology could also be expand to link antibiotics or painkillers to fibrin in such way that when the surgeon uses fibrin in hemostasis and tissue sealing, he will also be able to control infection and pain locally over a period of 1 to 2 weeks, the life of the fibrin clot.

An example of how added bioactive substances to the fibrin clot influence the cell behavior is the use of fibrin to deliver mycoplasma lipopeptide-2 (MALP-2; Cole et al., 2002). MALP-2, which is secreted by mycoplasma, plays an essential role in the early influx of leukocytes and monocytes to the injury site. MALP-2 is mixed with fibrin and the secretion of various cytokines and chemoattractants is measured from monocytic cells seeded on the fibrin clots. Monocytes seeded on 3D fibrin clots containing MALP-2 secrete more cytokines such as IL-6, TNF-alpha, and chemoattractants such as MIP-1 alpha and MCP-1 when compared to monocytes seeded on fibrin clots without MALP-2. Two factors affected the amount of proteins secreted by monocytes: MALP-2 concentration and the fibrinogen and thrombin concentration in the final formed fibrin clot (Figure 7.4a). Furthermore, the above study shows that the secreted cytokines and chemoattractants enhanced fibroblast migration using *in vitro* migration assay (Figure 7.4b). Additionally, using RT-PCR approaches, the gene expression of about 1200 genes in various cell types is measured at different time points in the presence and absence of MALP-2 incorporated in the fibrin clot. The results show that MALP-2 affects the gene expression of many genes including its own receptors (TLR2 and TLR4). In conclusion, this study supports the use of fibrin sealant in delivering MALP-2, and possibly other peptides, in an active form that might enhance skin-wound healing. The most important point of the above study is that the interaction between the delivered bioactive substances and the fibrin clot could be manipulated and controlled to achieve a desirable environment that supports cell proliferation, cell differentiation, cell migration, etc. Other studies show the effect of glial cell-line-derived neurotrophic factor incorporated in fibrin glue on developing dopamine neurons (Cheng et al., 1995).

### 7.3.2 Fibrin Sealant as a Delivery Vehicle for Cells

Fibrin sealant has been used for years to deliver autologous cells to various skin defects. For example, BioSeed® is a product produced by a German company, BioTissue; the product is manufactured by mixing keratinocytes from the patient, after isolation and propagation in culture, with fibrin to successfully treat chronic wounds (Horch et al., 2001).

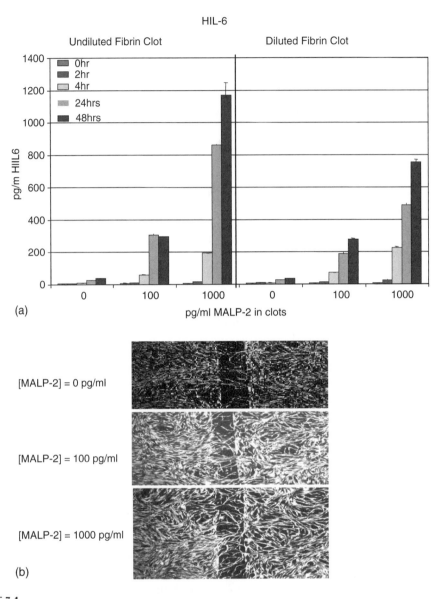

(a)

(b)

**FIGURE 7.4**
(a) The fibrinogen and thrombin concentration as well as the peptide MALP-2 concentration in the final clot affect cytokine secretion from monocyte seeded on MALP-2-fibrin construct. (b) Cytokines secreted from monocots seeded in MAL-2-fibrin construct enhance fibroblast cell migration in a wound culture assay.

The fibrin sealant becomes a much more acceptable delivery vehicle as new studies showed that by simply changing the concentration of fibrinogen and thrombin in the final fibrin clot, one could optimize the ideal environment for delivering various cell types. This fibrin-driven cell-delivery platform was tested on human-derived fibroblasts, keratinocytes and mesenchymal stem cells using *in vitro* and *in vivo* studies (Cole et al., 2002; Ferguson et al., 2003; Catelas et al., 2004, 2005; Cox et al., 2004; Ho et al., 2005; Mana et al., 2005; Mogford et al., 2005). Other studies have shown the successful delivery of autologous urothelial cells onto a prefabricated pouch (Wechselberger et al., 1998), or the use of osteoblasts in fibrin to improve bone cellular outgrowth (Van Griensven et al., 2000). This optimized cell-delivery platform could be used for generating more successful cell-based therapy to overcome various diseases. Below are some examples on using fibrin for cell delivery.

### 7.3.2.1 The Use of Fibrin Sealant for Delivering Human Mesenchymal Stem Cells (hMSCs)

MSCs are easy to isolate, easy to expand in culture, and easy to transfect. They also differentiate into different cell types such as osteoblasts, chondrocytes, and muscle cells. Moreover, there are no ethical issues for their use when compared to fetal stem cells. Thus, MSCs could be used for both cell and gene therapies in various tissue-engineering applications. Human-derived mesenchymal stem cells proliferate well on top (Wiedemann et al., 2002) as well as inside the 3D fibrin clots (Figure 7.5; Ho et al., 2005). Their rate of proliferation depends on the final concentration of fibrinogen and thrombin in the formed fibrin clot. Moreover, some fibrin formulations seem to induce the differentiation of mesenchymal stem cells into the osteogenic lineage in the absence of any osteogenic differentiation factors (Catelas et al., 2004, 2005). The ability of MSCs to grow robustly within fibrin clot and its potential ability to induce these cells into different lineages in the absence or perhaps with a minimum addition of other bioactive substances transforms fibrin sealant from an excellent hemostatic agent to also an excellent inexpensive platform to be used for treating bone, cartilage, and muscle defects.

### 7.3.2.2 The Use of Fibrin Sealant for Delivering Human Neuronal Stem Cells (hNSCs)

Similar work was also preformed on hNSCs with similar results (Ferguson et al., 2003). hNSCs are viable within the 3D fibrin sealant matrix and they proliferate within the 3D fibrin sealant matrix (Figure 7.6). The rate of proliferation, again, varies depending on the fibrinogen and thrombin concentration in the 3D fibrin clot. The NSCs morphology within

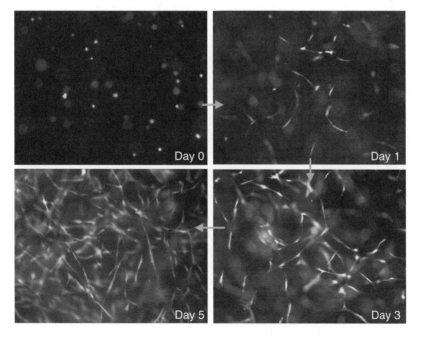

**FIGURE 7.5**
Human mesenchymal stem cell proliferation within 3D fibrin construct.

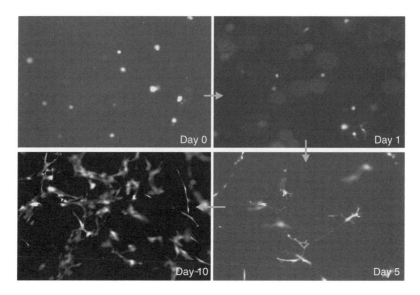

**FIGURE 7.6**
Human neural stem cell proliferation and possible differentiation within 3D fibrin construct.

the 3D fibrin clot is also different depending on the fibrin formulation and it correlates with the period of time in which the hNSCs are inside the fibrin clot. In some formulations, hNSCs extend what looks like axons. Future studies are needed to determine the differentiation of these stem cells using various neuronal markers. In conclusion, fibrin presents an excellent milieu for neuronal stem cells to grow and potentially differentiate.

### 7.3.2.3  The Use of Fibrin Sealant for Delivering Normal Human-Derived Keratinocytes (NHK)

Similar to the studies preformed on human-derived mesenchymal stem and neuronal stem cells, fibrin formulations support keratinocytes proliferation (Sese et al., 2003). More specifically, low fibrinogen and thrombin concentrations in the final fibrin clot provide for optimal keratinocyte adhesion and proliferation on the top of the fibrin clots allowing in some fibrin formulations for significant cell–cell interactions. On the other hand, it was determined that a high concentration of fibrinogen and thrombin in the final fibrin clots provide for an optimal NHK proliferation within the 3D fibrin clots. Cell morphology is also different depending on the fibrinogen and thrombin concentration, for example, low fibrinogen concentration in the final fibrin clot leads to a linear/spread keratinocytes morphology in contrast to that seen in fibrin clots containing a high fibrinogen concentration (Figure 7.7). These conclusions are different from the findings obtained for fibroblasts and mesenchymal stem cells. Thus, different modified formulations of fibrin sealant may be chosen when delivering various cell types.

### 7.3.2.4  The Use of Fibrin Sealant for Delivering Human-Derived Fibroblasts

Most of the work on cell delivery using fibrin was preformed on the human-derived fibroblasts (Cox et al., 2004). Fibroblasts, similar to keratinocytes and mesenchymal stem cells, adhere and proliferate well on various fibrin sealant formulations. They also proliferate well within all tested formulations of 3D fibrin clots (Figure 7.8). Furthermore,

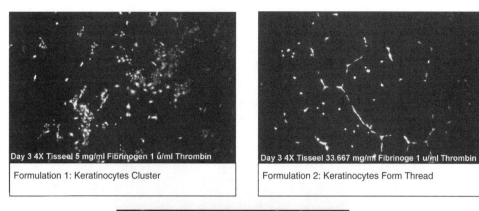

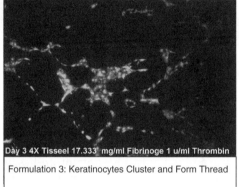

**FIGURE 7.7**
Human keratinocyte cell morphology on various fibrin constructs.

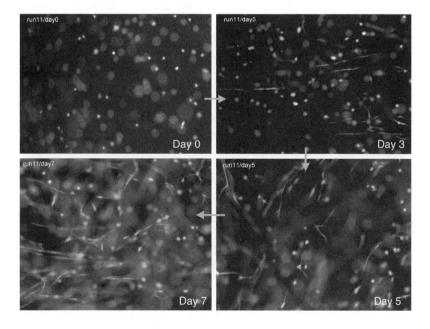

**FIGURE 7.8**
Human dermal fibroblasts proliferation in 3D fibrin constructs.

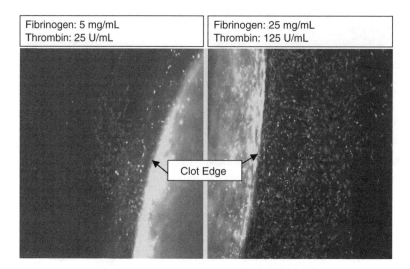

**FIGURE 7.9**
Human dermal fibroblasts migrate out of fibrin constructs after a few days.

the study shows how and when fibroblasts migrate out of the 3D fibrin clots in a viable form (Figure 7.9). Moreover, fibrin clots modulate the gene and protein expression in fibroblasts seeded on and within the fibrin clot (Cox et al., 2004). The delivery of fibroblasts using fibrin sealant was also examined in various animal studies. In the first animal model, green fluorescent protein (GFP)-tagged mouse dermal fibroblasts were transplanted into full-thickness open wounds created on the mouse's head. After 5 to 7 days, tissue sections from the wounds showed the GFP-labeled fibroblasts to be localized to the wounded area. In the second animal model, an increasing number of LacZ-transfected dermal rat fibroblasts mixed with fibrin sealant were added to full-thickness wounds created on the backs of rats. The blood supply to the wounded area was reduced to create a hypoxic environment. The rat fibroblasts, detected with anti-LacZ, enhanced the wound closure as well as increased reepithelization of the wounded area; this increase positively correlated with an increase in the cell numbers in the fibrin clots. Finally, rabbit dermal fibroblasts mixed in fibrin sealant were added to hypoxic full-thickness cutaneous wounds in the rabbit ear ulcer model and were found to enhance wound healing as measured by the increase of the wound closure, granulation and reepithelization. Thus, some modified formulations of fibrin sealant present an excellent delivery vehicle for fibroblast delivery leading to an enhancement in wound healing.

In conclusion, fibrin sealant is a moldable 3D matrix that can be adapted to any shape and seeded with cells or bioactive molecules for tissue regeneration and promotion of wound healing in soft and hard tissue defects.

## 7.4   What Is Next in Fibrin Technology

### 7.4.1   Understanding the Physical Characteristics of Fibrin

The structure of a fibrin clot as seen by scanning electron microscopy (SEM) is shown in Figure 7.10a (Amrani and DiOrio, unpublished data). A higher magnification view of an individual fiber bundle as seen by transmission electron microscopy (TEM) is shown in Figure 7.10b. The thrombin concentration affects the porosity of the fibrin clot; a higher

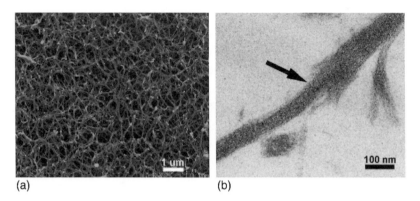

(a) (b)

**FIGURE 7.10**
(a) Scanning electron microscopy (SEM) of a fibrin construct. (b) Transmission electron microscopy (TEM) of a fibrin construct.

thrombin concentration usually leads to a less porosity than a low thrombin concentration. Salt concentration also plays a role in the porosity within the 3D fibrin clots. Furthermore, the fibrinogen concentration influences the mechanical structure of the fibrin clot as measured in breaking strength and adhesiveness (Sierra, 1993; Khare et al., 1998;). Factor XIII is also shown to influence the elastic characteristics of fibrin clots (Roberts et al., 1973; Mosesson et al., 2001). Recently, some labs have started looking into the correlation between cell proliferation, differentiation, and fibrin microstructure, including pore size and fibril thickness. A recent work by Dr. Shaw's lab at CLU is an example of such essential studies to understand the relationship between fibrin structure and cell behavior (Mooney et al., 2004, 2005). He measured specific mechanical characteristics over a period of 10 days on fibrin–fibroblast constructs prepared in a culture dish using a newly-established indentation protocol to determine the nominal elastic modulus of fibrin or cell–fibrin constructs at specified time points. The study shows that unpopulated fibrin has a linear ($R = 0.983$) relationship between the indentation stiffness and fibrinogen concentration. Their preliminary data also show that the indentation stiffness of cell-populated fibrin steadily decreases with an increasing incubation time (1 to 10 days), suggesting that the cells exert a significant effect on the construct structure and hence mechanical function (Figure 7.11). Furthermore, the studies on collagen production by fibroblasts incorporated in fibrin gels (Tuan et al., 1996) are now followed up with studies on the effect of mixing collagen and fibrin on the mechanical characteristics of the fibrin/collagen construct (Mooney et al., 2004, 2005).

### 7.4.2 Understanding the Bioactive Characteristics of Fibrin

Recent works have shown that plasma fractions, which are used to produce some fibrin products, contain fibronectin and various growth factors (Colin Newton, unpublished data). The activity of these proteins is now under investigation. Many studies point to the conclusion that fibrin is a biomatrix and not inert material such as synthetic polymers. That should not be surprising based on the information presented above on the use of fibrin for cell delivery.

### 7.4.3 The Use of Fibrin to Deliver Synthetic Materials

The new focus of fibrin is on its use in delivering synthetic materials (Daculsi et al., 2004). Dalcusi uses fibrin to deliver macroporous biphasic calcium phosphate (MBCP), showing

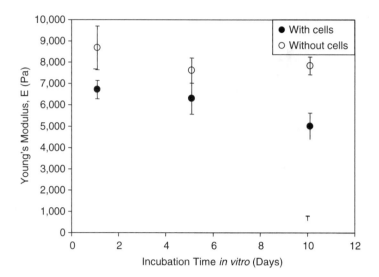

**FIGURE 7.11**
Mechanical characteristics — stiffness of fibrin constructs in the presence and absence of fibroblasts.

excellent handling characteristics and enhanced bone ingrowth. Further studies including clinical studies will support the above strategy, since synthetic materials will provide the mechanical strength needed for hard tissue repair, while fibrin provides the ideal environment for cell growth and differentiation.

## 7.5   Conclusions

While fibrin has been used for 25 years globally and successfully in hemostasis and tissue sealing, it has been established, over the last 5 years, as a platform for bioactive substance and cell delivery. A possible contributing factor to successful fibrin use in such a platform is the intrinsic presence of many extracellular matrix proteins such as fibronectin and growth factors that are known to play a role in cell adhesion, proliferation, and differentiation. While most of the studies so far on fibrin use for bioactive substance and cell delivery are at the preclinical level, some products that use fibrin to deliver cells are available, such as BioSeed® in Germany. The interest in using fibrin in various indications and applications is clearly demonstrated by the hundreds of published papers every year.

## References

Due to the vast publications on fibrin, the author apologizes for not including all important references.

Albes, J.M., Klenzner, T., Kotzerke, J., Thiedemann, K.U., Schafers, H.-J., and Borst, H.-G., Improvement of tracheal autograft revascularization by means of fibroblast growth factor, *Ann. Thorac. Surg.*, **57**, 444 (1994).

Amrani, D., Wound healing: role of commercial fibrin sealants, *Ann. NY Acad. Sci.*, **936**, 566 (2001).

Andree, C., Voigt, M., Wenger, A., Erichsen, T., Bittner, K., Schaefer, D., Walgenbach, K.J., Borges, J., Horch, R.E., Eriksson, E., and Stark, G.B., Plasmid gene delivery to human keratinocytes through a fibrin-mediated transfection system, *Tissue Eng.*, **7**, 757 (2001).

Ariens, R.A., Lai, T.-S., Weisel, J.W., Greenberg, C.S., and Grant, P.J., Role of factor XIII in fibrin clot formation and effects of genetic polymorphisms, *Blood,* **100** (3), 743 (2002).

Arnaud, E., Morieux, C., Wybier, M., and de Vernejoul, M.C., Potentiation of transforming growth factor (TGF-beta 1) by natural coral and fibrin in a rabbit cranioplasty model, *Calcif. Tissue Int.,* **54** (6), 493 (1994).

Catelas, I., Sese, N., Helgerson, S., and Tawil, B., *Effects of fibrin gel formulation on mesenchymal stem cell proliferation and differentiation.* 8th World Biomaterials Congress, Sydney, Australia (2004).

Catelas, I., Sese, N., Wu, B., Dunn, J., Helgerson, S., and Tawil, N.J., Human mesenchymal stem cells proliferation and osteogenic differentiation in fibrin gels *in vitro*, submitted for publication.

Cheng, H., Hoffer, B., Stromberg, I., Russell, D., and Olson, L., The effect of glial cell line-derived neurotrophic factor in fibrin glue on developing dopamine neurons, *Exp. Brain Res.,* **104** (2), 199 (1995).

Clark, R.A.F., *The Molecular and Cellular Biology of Wound Repair*, Plenum Press, New York (1998).

Cole, M., Cox, S., Inman, E., Chan, C., and Tawil, N., *Fibrin sealant tisseel® as a vehicle for peptide delivery:* in vitro *studies*. The Wound Healing Society 12th Annual Conference, Baltimore (2002).

Cote, H.C.F., Lord, S.T. and Pratt, K.P., γ-chain dysfibriongenemias: molecular structure–function relationships of naturally occurring mutations in the γ chain of human fibrinogen, *Blood,* **92** (7), 2195 (1998).

Cox, S., Cole, M., Mankarious, S., and Tawil, B., The effect of tranexamic acid incorporated in fibrin sealant clots on cell behavior of neuronal and non-neuronal cells, *J. Neuronal Res.,* **72**, 734 (2003).

Cox, S., Cole, M., and Tawil, N., The behavior of human dermal fibroblasts in 3 dimensional fibrin clots: dependence on the fibrinogen and thrombin concentration, *Tissue Eng.,* **10** (5/6), 942 (2004).

Daculsi, G., Goyenvalle, E., Aguado, E., Bilban, M., Bittner, K., Gobin, C., and Spaethe, R. *Osteopromoting properties of new injectable fibrin–bioceramic composite for bone regeneration*, 8th World Biomaterials Congress, Sydney, Australia (2004).

Ferguson, R., Cox, S., Sese, N., Cole, M., and Tawil, B., *The use of fibrin sealant to deliver neuronal stem cell:* in vitro *studies*. Society for Biomaterials 29th Annual Meeting, Reno, Nevada (2003).

Hasimoto, J., Kurosaka, M., Yoshiya, S., and Hirohata, K., Meniscal repair using fibrin sealant and endothelial cell growth factor, *Am. J. Sports Med.,* **20**, 537 (1992).

Ho, W., Tawil, N.J., Dunn, J.C.Y., Wu, B.M., The behavior of human mesenchymal stem cells in 3D fibrin clots: dependence on fibrinogen concentration and clot structure, *Tissue Eng.,* accepted (2006).

Horch, R.E., Bannasch, H., and Stark, G.B., Transplantation of cultured autologous keratinocytes in fibrin sealant biomatrix to resurface chronic wounds, *Transplant. Proc.,* **33** (1–2), 642 (2001).

Khare, A., Woo, L., Mclean, A., and Helgerson, S., Mechanical characterization of fibrin gels, *Blood Coagul. Fibrin.,* **9** (7), 105 (1998).

MacPhee, M.J., Singh, M.P., Brady, R. Jr., Akhyani, N., Liau, G., Lasa, C. Jr., Hue, C., Best, A., and Drohan, W., Fibrin sealant: a versatile delivery vehicle for drugs and biologics, In: *Surgical Adhesives and Sealants Current Technology and Applications*, Sierra, D.H. and Saltz, R., Eds., Techomic Publishing Co., Lancaster, PA (1996).

Mana, M., Cole, M., Cox, S., and Tawil, B., The effect of fibrinogen and thrombin on human monocytes behavior and protein expression on various formulations of fibrin clot, *Wound Repair and Regeneration.,* accepted (2006).

Mogford, J., Tawil B., and. Mustoe, T., Fibrin sealant combined with fibroblasts and PDGF enhance wound healing in excisional wounds, submitted for publication.

Mooney, R.G., Costales, C., Doerfler, A., Toland, G., Tawil, B., and Shaw, M.C., *Indentation Micromechanics of Fibroblast–Fibrin and Keratinocyte–Fibrin Constructs*, Society for Biomaterials, Philadelphia, PA (2004).

Mooney, R.G., Costales, C., Shaw, M.C., Tuan, T.-L., Wu, B., and Tawil, B., *Mechanical characteristics of fibroblast–fibrin constructs: effect of fibrinogen and thrombin concentration*, The Wound Healing Society 15th Annual Conference, Chicago, Illinois (2005).

Mosesson, M.W., Siebenlist, K.R., and Meh, D.A., The structure and biological features of fibrinogen and fibrin, *Ann. NY Acad. Sci.,* **936**, 11 (2001).

Perka, C., Schultz, O., Spitzer, R.S., Lindenhayn, K., Burmester, G.R., and Sittinger, M., Segmental bone repair by tissue-engineered periosteal cell transplants with bioresorbable fleece and fibrin scaffolds in rabbits, *Biomaterials*, **21**, 1145 (2000).

Roberts, W.W., Lorand, L., and Mockros, L.F., Viscoelastic properties of fibrin clots, *Biorheology*, **10**, 29 (1973).

Sahni, A. and Francis, C.W., Vascular endothelial growth factor binds to fibrinogen and fibrin and stimulates endothelial cell proliferation, *Blood*, **96**, 3772 (2000).

Schense, J.C., Bloch, J., Aebischer, P., and Hubbell, J.A., Enzymatic incorporation of bioactive peptides into fibrin matrices enhances neurite extension, *Nat. Biotechnol.*, **18**, 415 (2000).

Schlag, M.G., Hopf, R., and Redl, H., Convulsive seizures following subdural application of fibrin sealant containing tranexamic acid in a rat model, *Neurosurgery*, **47**, 1463 (2000).

Schlag, M.G., Hopf, R., Zifko, U., and Redl, H., Epileptic seizures following cortical application of fibrin sealants containing tranexamic acid in rats, *Acta Neurochir.*, **144**, 63 (2002).

Sese, N., Cole, M., Cox, S., and Tawil, B., *Delivering human keratinocytes using fibrin sealant:* in vitro *studies.* The Wound Healing Society 13th Annual Conference, Seattle, Washington (2003).

Sierra, D.H., Fibrin sealant adhesive systems: A review of their chemistry, material properties, and clinical applications, *J. Biomater. Appl.*, **7**, 309 (1993).

Tuan, T.L., Song, A., Chang, S., Younai, S., and Nimni, M.E., *In vitro* fibroplasia: matrix contraction, cell growth, and collagen production of fibroblasts cultured in fibrin gels, *Exp. Cell Res.*, **223**, 127 (1996).

Van Griensven, M., Zeichen, J., Pape, H.C., Lehmann, U., Bosch, U., and Seekamp, A.A., Modified method to culture human osteoblasts using Tissuecol® to improve bone sample adhesion and cellular outgrowth, *Cells Tissues Organs*, **166**, A501 (2000).

Wechselberger, G., Schoeller, T., Stenzl, A., Ninkovic, M., Lille, S., and Russell, R.C., Fibrin glue as a delivery vehicle for autologous urothelial cell transplantation onto a prefabricated pouch, *J. Urol.*, **160**, 583 (1998).

Werner, S. and Grose, R., Regulation of wound healing by growth factors and cytokines, *Physiol. Rev.*, **83**, 835 (2003).

Wiedemann, U., Cox, S., Cole, M., and Tawil, B., *The use of fibrin sealant for the delivery of human mesenchymal stem cells:* in vitro *studies*, The Wound Healing Society 12th Annual Conference, Baltimore, MD (2002).

Wong, C., Inman, E., Spaethe, R., and Helgerson, S., Fibrin-based biomaterials to deliver human growth factors, *Thromb. Haemostasis*, **89**, 573 (2003).

# 8

# *Proteins and Amino Acid-Derived Polymers*

**Joshua C. Haarer and Kay C. Dee**

**CONTENTS**

## 8.1   Introduction

### 8.1.1   Why Use Proteins as Biomaterials?

Proteins are essentially polymers of amino acids, folded into three-dimensional shapes. Proteins are a major structural or mechanical component of many tissues, and are also biochemically important as directive substrates for cell adhesion and migration, as signaling molecules, as enzymes, as active regulators of cellular differentiation and function, and more. Because the structure and properties of natural tissues depend so strongly on component proteins, proteins and industrially-created polymers containing amino acids have been developed as biomaterials for tissue repair and replacement. Because the amino acids that comprise proteins are produced by the human body, one would expect protein-based biomaterials to undergo naturally-controlled degradation processes (Lu et al., 2004) into products less toxic than those produced by some synthetic polymers, and to perhaps elicit lower immune responses than some synthetic polymeric biomaterials like poly(lactic acid) (Meinel et al., 2005). The chemical and mechanical properties of protein-based biomaterials can be tailored for specific applications, depending on the amino-acid composition and on any further chemical modifications added by a biomaterials scientist or engineer. This chapter will focus on a select set of proteins and amino-acid derived matrices that are broadly studied and/or commonly used as bio-materials, presenting fundamental and overview information that should be helpful in understanding the general field of research and the specialized chapters on different types of protein/amino acid-based polymeric biomaterials presented elsewhere in this book.

### 8.1.2   Protein Structure and Synthesis

When proteins are synthesized in the body, the precursor molecules pass through four stages on the way to becoming a functional protein (Figure 8.1). The general structure of an amino acid can be represented as a central α-carbon atom surrounded by a hydrogen atom, a carboxyl group, a side chain group, and an amino group. Individual amino acids are held together with peptide bonds. These are rigid, planar bonds that join the carboxyl group of one amino acid with the amino group of another. The primary structure of a protein is simply the linear sequence of the constituent amino acids held together with peptide bonds. The secondary structure is achieved when hydrogen bonds are formed between the amino acids of the primary structure. The once-linear primary structure folds to form a more complicated structure, typically α-helices or β-pleated sheets, as these two forms are the most stable of all secondary structure forms. Secondary structures are joined together to form three-dimensional tertiary structures. These tertiary structure subunits may then interact with each other to form the three-dimensional quaternary structure of a multi-unit protein.

## 8.2   Collagen

### 8.2.1   Sources and Refinement

A variety of cells, perhaps most notably fibroblasts, within the human body produce collagen. For the purposes of engineering tissues and implants, collagen is often harvested from bovine, equine, and porcine tissues, and can be processed into various forms

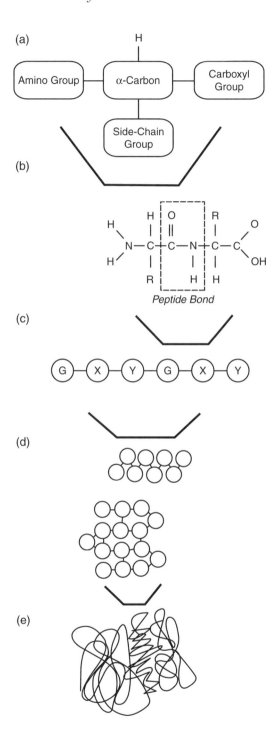

**FIGURE 8.1**
Amino acid structure and the fundamental stages of protein synthesis. The general amino acid structure is shown in (a). Amino acids are joined together with peptide bonds (b), a rigid planar unit between the carboxyl and amino groups of adjacent amino acids. The primary structure of a protein is a simple sequence of amino acids held together by peptide bonds (c). For collagen, this sequence is primarily glycine alternated with various other amino acids, as shown. The secondary structure of proteins is generally in the form of α-helices or β-pleated sheets (d). Tertiary structures are combinations of secondary structures and quaternary structures (e) are further combinations of tertiary structures or further refined tertiary structures.

including films, mats, fibers, and gels. In order to avoid rapid degradation *in vivo* and to increase mechanical strength the collagen must be fixed, or cross-linked, either chemically or physically. Photooxidation, dehydrothermal treatments, and ultraviolet irradiation are examples of physical cross-linking methods. Although one advantage of physical cross-linking methods is that no potentially toxic chemical residues could be left in the collagen, chemical fixatives are more commonly used because physical methods tend to result in weaker cross-linking (Ma et al., 2004). Chemical cross-linking methods include treatment with carbodiimides, glutaraldehydes, and polyglycidyl ether. Varying the chemical treatment parameters (time, temperature, fixative strength) allows varying levels of fixation and, thus, varying mechanical properties and resistance to degradation.

The amino acid composition of a collagen species may also affect cross-linking and, thereby, mechanical properties. Lysine and hydroxylysine are necessary for natural intra- and inter-molecular cross-linking of collagen (Angele et al., 2004). The more lysine and hydroxylysine present in a type of collagen, the more resistant it will be to enzymatic and thermal degradation. Because of its higher lysine content, equine collagen resists the enzymatic actions of collagenases — enzymes that specifically degrade collagen — better than bovine or porcine collagen. Lysine can also be used as an additive to chemical fixatives to enhance their actions (Angele et al., 2004).

Given that collagen is found in nearly every tissue in the human body, and is relatively inexpensive and easy to manufacture/process in the laboratory, it is not surprising that collagen has been tested or used as a biomaterial for a wide variety of tissue-engineered implants. Collagen has been used in biomaterial applications involving the regeneration of blood vessels, heart valves, tendon and ligament, skin, peripheral nervous system, and cartilage and meniscal tissue, as well as in drug delivery and plastic surgery applications (Yannas, 1996).

### 8.2.2  Molecular Structure

Ten different polypeptide chains form the primary structure, or α-chains, of the collagen protein. Generally, these are composed of repeating triplets of amino acids in the form [Gly-X-Y]$_n$, where X and Y are varying amino acids, but quite often proline (Ottani et al., 2002). This repetitive sequence helps give collagen repeatable and predictable mechanical properties (Altman et al., 2003). In the secondary collagen structure, α-chains fold into a right-handed helix. At this point, the glycine residues are arranged linearly along the helix. As the secondary structure winds together with two other secondary structures, a left-handed triple helix is formed (the tertiary collagen structure). One period of the helix measures approximately 300 nm (Gelse et al., 2003). The glycine residues are the smallest residues of the collagen molecule, and these end up packed together on the inside of the triple helix (Gelse et al., 2003). The amount of glycine has been shown to correlate with the mechanical flexibility of polypeptide chains. Elastin and spider silk, for example, have high glycine content (Debelle and Tamburro, 1999) and are relatively flexible proteins. After formation of the tertiary structure, the precollagen molecule is excreted from the fibroblast to the extracellular space. As the molecules are completed, the nonhelical portion of the molecule is added in the form of various carbohydrates, finalizing a molecule massing approximately 285 kDa (Yannas, 1996).

As collagen forms the multi-molecule structure known as a microfibril, the individual molecules do not contact each other axially but instead are separated by a gap of approximately 40 nm (Figure 8.2) (Ottani et al., 2002). It is this separation that gives collagen its characteristic banding pattern, the "D-period," when viewed using a microscope.

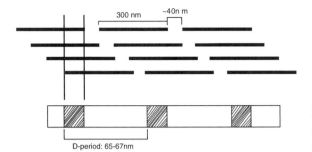

300 nm  ~40n m

D-period: 65-67nm

**FIGURE 8.2**
Demonstration of the fiber alignment resulting in the D-period and banding pattern of collagen.

### 8.2.3 Types and Distributions

Over 20 types of collagen have been identified. A summary of collagen types and distributions within the human body is presented in Table 8.1. Type I collagen is ubiquitously distributed and comprises the largest proportion of the total collagen within the human body (Fung, 1993).

### 8.2.4 Mechanical Properties

With over 20 species of collagen, all possessing varying chemical and mechanical properties, the biomedical community has only begun to take advantage of the possible opportunities associated with this material. Some of the fundamental mechanical

**TABLE 8.1**

Collagen Types, Constituent $\alpha$-Chains (the Three Individual Fibrils That Make up the Collagen Triple Helix), and Distribution within the Body

| Type | $\alpha$-Chains | Distribution |
|------|-----------------|--------------|
| I | $\alpha 1, \alpha 2$ | Bone, tendon, ligament, cornea, dermis |
| II | $\alpha 1$ | Hyaline cartilage |
| III | $\alpha 1$ | Skin, vessel wall, distensible tissues |
| IV | $\alpha 1 - \alpha 6$ | Basement membrane |
| V | $\alpha 1 - \alpha 3$ | Same as Type I, but with smaller contribution |
| VI | $\alpha 1 - \alpha 3$ | Dermis, cartilage, placenta, lungs, intervertebral disc |
| VII | $\alpha 1$ | Dermal–epidermal junctions, cervix, oral mucosa |
| VIII | $\alpha 1, \alpha 2$ | Endothelial cells, Descemet's membrane |
| IX | $\alpha 1 - \alpha 3$ | Cartilage, cornea |
| X | $\alpha 3$ | Fetal or juvenile cartilage |
| XI | $\alpha 1 - \alpha 3$ | Cartilage |
| XII | $\alpha 1$ | Ligament, tendon, perichondrium |
| XIII | $\alpha 1$ | Epidermis, hair follicle, intestine, liver, lung |
| XIV | $\alpha 1$ | Dermis, tendon, vessel wall, placenta, lung |
| XV | $\alpha 1$ | Fibroblasts, smooth muscle cells, kidney, pancreas |
| XVI | $\alpha 1$ | Fibroblasts, keratinocytes, amnion |
| XVII | $\alpha 1$ | Dermal–epidermal junctions |
| XVIII | $\alpha 1$ | Lung, liver |
| XIX | $\alpha 1$ | Rhabdomyosarcoma |
| XX | $\alpha 1$ | Embryonic skin, sternal cartilage, tendon |
| XXI | $\alpha 1$ | Vessel wall |

*Note*: There are numerous subtypes of each $\alpha$-chain. (*Source:* Adapted from Table 1 in Gelse, K., Poschl, E., and Aigner, T., *Adv. Drug Deliv. Rev.* **55**, 1531–1546 (2003). With permission.)

properties (and structure–property relationships) of collagen have yet to be fully explored. However, because collagen is the most prevalent structural protein in the body and can be found in every tissue, it is a logical biomaterial choice for many types of tissue and implant engineering.

Temperature and pH are known to affect protein stability, and biomaterial scientists often alter these variables in order to digest natural materials and extract a desired portion. For example, the material behavior of collagen is relatively unaffected over the range of temperature from 0 to 37°C (Rigby et al., 1958). At or above 37°C, the triple-helix structure denatures (Yannas, 1996; Mirnajafi et al., 2005). The same effect is achieved by exposing collagen to a low pH solvent.

When mechanically tested, collagen fibers and soft collagenous tissues display a characteristically shaped, nonlinear stress–strain curve (Figure 8.3). This nonlinearity is caused by the natural "crimp" in relaxed collagen. Under low strains, the crimp is expanding, and the collagen molecule becomes more linear. As strain increases beyond what is allowed by expansion of the crimp, the cross-links supporting the molecule become stressed. This extension beyond the crimp is what produces the linear region of the stress–strain curve. During everyday activities, collagen in tissues will generally operate in the lower stress–strain area, known as the "toe region." While materials scientists often investigate and report peak stress or strain values for materials, it is within the lower boundaries of stress–strain behavior that collagenous biomaterials will experience the vast proportion of use. After the toe region, the stress–strain curve for collagen reaches a generally linear region similar to that which would be demonstrated by a linear elastic material.

The tangent modulus (obtained from the linear portion of the stress–strain curve) for collagen fibers has a reported range between 350 and 1000 MPa (Fung, 1993; Gentleman et al., 2003); reported tensile strengths for collagen fibers range between 50 and 100 MPa (Fung, 1993). Collagen fibers have exhibited two behaviors that appear at first to be counterintuitive. First, when compared to large-diameter fibers, smaller-diameter collagen fibers tend to display larger values of tangent modulus and peak stress. It has been suggested that larger-diameter fibers are more likely to possess defects and thus break more easily; smaller fibers have a larger surface-to-volume ratio, allowing a greater number of surface cross-links per fiber unit length, which would effectively "stiffen" the

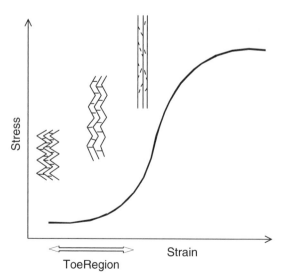

**FIGURE 8.3**
Characteristic stress–strain curve of collagen and location of the "Toe Region." Above the stress–strain curve are the stages of collagen uncrimping that generate this stress–strain plot.

fiber (Gentleman et al., 2003). Large diameter fibers do show greater resistance to low-level strain (Christiansen et al., 2000). Second, the tangent modulus obtained from a stress–strain curve is a material property, and therefore should not be dependent upon the size of a specimen (as opposed to stiffness, the slope of a load–elongation curve, which is a structural property). However, different lengths of collagen fibers, either fabricated in the same ways or dissected from the same tissues, have been determined to have significantly different moduli (Haut, 1986; Gentleman et al., 2003).

Finally, it should be noted that it is possible to combine multiple forms of collagen into one biomaterial construct — for example, embedding collagen fibers of various lengths in collagen gels — creating a construct that derives major biomechanical properties (e.g., tensile or compressive modulus) from one form of collagen while deriving another type of property (e.g., hospitable to cell culture and possibly vascular ingrowth) from the other form. Such constructs mimic the natural tissue environment in which collagen fibers function as part of a matrix composed of a host of proteins, cells and other components.

### 8.2.5 Physiological Responses

One benefit of naturally-derived biomaterials, such as collagen, is that the materials are normally experienced by the body. Collagenases and metalloproteinases are produced by cells degrading/digesting collagen in tissues. The products of this degradation will be amino acids that the body copes with in the course of its normal metabolic processes. That said, collagen used for implants often comes from a nonautologous source and can provoke an immune response if not treated properly.

The quaternary structure of collagen regulates many interactions with the surrounding environment. In particular, platelet aggregation has been shown to be a property of the quaternary structure (Yannas, 1996). Collagen is also chemotactic to leukocytes and fibrogenic cells (Gentleman et al., 2003) and binds growth factors and cytokines (Gelse et al., 2003). Different collagen types may even be semi-specific with regard to what biomolecules are bound or attracted to the collagen. For example, Type II collagen preferentially binds TGF-β and BMP-2 (Gelse et al., 2003).

The triple helix structure of collagen is evolutionarily conserved, meaning that this structure is present in many species and has been maintained from an evolutionary ancestor. Type I collagen in particular is an evolutionarily conservative molecule, and therefore tends to be better tolerated across species and elicits a lower immune response than other collagen types (Yannas, 1996). The composition of the terminal regions of the collagen molecule varies between species, and for biomaterial applications, the terminal regions are often removed or chemically modified with the intent of reducing any immune response to the material. However, the central helix of collagen contains sites that can be antigenic (can bind to circulating antibodies), and because the immune response to collagen can depend on the donor and recipient species as well as the implantation site, treatments that in theory should reduce immunogenicity may not, in fact, remove all antigenic sites (Lynn et al., 2004). It is important, therefore, when developing a collagenous biomaterial, to experimentally confirm any theoretically-probable hypotheses regarding the potential immune response. Patients awaiting an implant can be tested to determine whether they have a pre-existing allergy to collagen; it has been reported that only between 2.5 and 4% of the population has a preexisting allergy to bovine collagen (Cukier et al., 1993; Soo et al., 1993; Cretel et al., 2001), and that adverse reactions to implanted collagen in patients without preexisting allergies are similarly rare (<3%) (Lynn et al., 2004). The remarkably low incidence of severe immune reactions to the collagen biomaterials commonly clinically used for skin substitutes, tissue augmentation, heart valves, etc., provides motivation to continue developing new applications for this promising biomaterial.

---

## 8.3 Elastin

### 8.3.1 Sources and Refinement

Human elastin is found predominantly within blood vessel walls and lung tissue. The ligamentum nuchae (the well-developed ligament that connects the base of the skull to and along the spinous processes of cervical vertebrae) of ungulates (hoofed herbivorous quadrupeds) is almost pure elastin, with a small amount of collagen (Fung, 1993). Other elastic proteins similar to elastin are resilin, retrieved from the flexible joints of arthropods (spiders, crustaceans, centipedes, insects), and abductin, harvested from the hinges of scallops (Fung, 1993). Due to the difficulty of purifying elastin, the protein has not been widely used as a biomaterial, nor its mechanical properties studied extensively (Debelle and Tamburro, 1999; Daamen et al., 2001).

Elastin, unlike collagen, cannot be fixed with aldehydes (Fung, 1993). Tannic acid has been shown to be a more effective cross-linker for elastin. This acid binds to hydrophobic regions of proline-dense proteins, like elastin and collagen, and forms hydrogen bonds (Isenburg et al., 2004). As an added benefit, tannic acid exhibits an antibacterial effect.

For biomaterial applications, elastin is most often formed into gels or fibers. Gels are achieved by chemical hydrolysis, using oxalic acid or potassium hydroxide. Temperature and molecule concentration are then raised to form the gel (Debelle and Tamburro, 1999). Elastin will denature above 66°C, but repeated heating and cooling below 66°C will not change the mechanical properties (Fung, 1993).

### 8.3.2 Molecular Structure

Elastin is an insoluble, tightly cross-linked polymer (Mithieux et al., 2004) composed of a number of tropoelastin molecules covalently bonded together. Tropoelastin is produced intracellularly and cross-linked extracellularly (Fung, 1993). The cross-links occur at hydrophilic regions, while hydrophobic regions separate the cross-links. Despite being mostly hydrophobic, elastin is highly hydrated (Debelle and Tamburro, 1999).

The secondary structure of elastin is a β-turn, but this β-turn is dynamic. The aforementioned cross-links continually change conformation, resulting in the high-entropy nonstressed state of elastin. The amino acid composition of elastin includes glycine, alanine, valine and proline, in order of respective proportions from greatest to least (Debelle and Tamburro, 1999). Again, glycine can be correlated to high levels of elasticity.

### 8.3.3 Mechanical Properties

Elastin is the most linearly elastic natural protein material. A consistent tensile tangent modulus of approximately 0.6 MPa (Fung, 1993) makes elastin a simple and predictable material with which to work in engineering applications. The elasticity of elastin is entropically driven (Fung, 1993). When in a relaxed state, elastin is more hydrated and less structured, with higher entropy. When extended, elastin is less hydrated and more structured, with lower entropy (Debelle and Tamburro, 1999).

### 8.3.4  Physiological Responses

It has been suggested that elastin elicits an immune response similar to that provoked by collagen implants (Mithieux et al., 2004). Fibroblasts and monocytes are chemotactically attracted to elastin, and the most common outcomes to implantation of elastic materials *in vivo* are fibrous encapsulation and a foreign body response (Debelle and Tamburro, 1999; Mithieux et al., 2004). Elastin does not activate platelets as readily as collagen does, so less coagulation occurs at an elastin/blood interface than at a collagen–blood interface. For this reason, elastin coatings have been applied to synthetic vascular implants with some success (Woodhouse et al., 2004).

## 8.4  Silk

### 8.4.1  Sources and Refinement

Both spiders and silkworms (the larvae of *Bombyx mori*, the domestic silk moth) produce natural fibers of silk. Silkworm-derived fibers are generally used for biomaterial research and applications due to the fact that spiders have a low production rate when compared to silkworms. Spiders are also predatory and territorial, and thus cannot be bred domestically in close quarters (Winkler and Kaplan, 2000). Silk moths are fully domesticated, and one *B. mori* cocoon can yield 300 to 1200 m of usable silk fiber (Winkler and Kaplan, 2000).

Before use as a biomaterial, a protein (sericin) that coats silk fibers must be removed to reduce the chance of an undesirable immune response. To accomplish this, often the silk is washed with a sodium carbonate solution (Sofia et al., 2001; Fini et al., in press; Altman et al., 2002) or with urea (Saitoh et al., 2004). After the sericin is removed, a wax or silicone is applied to keep the underlying fibers (fibroin) from fraying (Sofia et al., 2001). When sericin is removed during silk refinement, the fibers experience an approximately 15% decrease in ultimate tensile strength and an approximately 28% decrease in linear stiffness (Altman et al., 2002). If the silk is to be solubilized, after sericin removal the fibers are decomposed in a concentrated salt solution such as calcium chloride, lithium bromide, or lithium thiocyanate (Winkler and Kaplan, 2000).

Silk scaffolds can be prepared without the use of chemical cross-linking agents (Kim et al., in press), and may be processed as foams, fibers, films, or meshes (Altman et al., 2003). This flexibility in processing allows silks to be woven to match desired mechanical properties and spatial structures (Altman et al., 2002). For example, Altman et al. (2002) designed a silk fiber matrix that closely matched the mechanical properties of human anterior cruciate ligament (ACL).

### 8.4.2  Molecular Structure

Unmodified *B. mori* silk fibers consist of two or more core fibers, fibroin, held together by sericin, a glue-like protein (Altman et al., 2003). The fibroin is composed of two polypeptide chains, a 25-kDa and a 350-kDa variant, held together with disulfide bonds. Glycine, alanine, and serine make up the majority of these core fibers (Kim et al., in press). The secondary structure of the silk protein from *B. mori* is a β-sheet with a repeating dipeptide sequence of the pattern [Gly-X-Gly-Y-Gly-Z]$_n$, where X, Y, and Z variably represent the amino acids alanine and serine (Saitoh et al., 2004).

Because spider silk is used in many different functions, including prey capture, sensory function, safety lines, and more, spider silks are much more variable in composition than

*B. mori* silk fibers. The amino acid content may even vary on a day-to-day basis for fibers spun by a single spider (Winkler and Kaplan, 2000). This variability makes spider silk difficult to work with as a biomaterial. But, the many different types of spider silk offer opportunities to study changing mechanical properties caused by changing amino acid compositions.

### 8.4.3   Mechanical Properties

Silk is a very stable protein with a high density of hydrogen bonds. This stability leads to slow degradation times *in vivo* (Altman et al., 2003), although the actual degradation rate of an implant formed from silk depends upon the constructed form of the implant as well as the location of the implant within the body (Postlethwait, 1970; Salthouse et al., 1977; Bucknall, 1983; Greenwald et al., 1994; Lam et al., 1995). Therefore while it has been estimated that a silk yarn will lose 100% of its tensile strength in a period of 5 months (Horan et al., in press), it should be understood that statistics like this should not be universally applied and actual figures for silk degradation will vary depending on implant form and location. It is currently hypothesized that slow degradation times are desirable to allow the gradual transfer of a load-bearing burden from the implanted biomaterial to the natural tissue remodeling around the biomaterial (Horan et al., in press).

Fibroin is a predominantly hydrophobic molecule, possessing smaller hydrophilic regions alternated with hydrophobic regions (Bini et al., 2004). The overall hydrophobicity allows tight packing of the molecule within fibers, which in turn results in solid mechanical properties. Silk is highly resistant to thermal decomposition: neither spider nor silkworm silks denature until reaching a temperature of 210°C (Winkler and Kaplan, 2000). Select mechanical properties of silk are compared to other commonly-used biomaterials in Table 8.3.

### 8.4.4   Physiological Responses

The most important aspect of processing silk for use as a biomaterial is the removal of the protein sericin. Type I allergic reactions (an abnormally strong immune reaction to naturally occurring proteins) have resulted from the surgical use of unmodified silk fibers, possibly due to sensitization from previous exposure to unmodified silk. The glue-like protein sericin has been implicated as the causative agent for immune responses to silk, but only when in conjunction with fibroin—sericin by itself does not elicit an immune response (Panilaitis et al., 2003). With the removal of sericin, silk elicits a mild immune response with the possibility of provoking a foreign body reaction (Bucknall, 1983; Altman et al., 2003). The strongest immune responses may be directed at the gaps and inconsistencies in manufactured silk films (Meinel et al., 2005). Improved manufacturing methods may therefore enhance the functionality of silk as a biomaterial.

The effectiveness of silk as a tissue culture scaffold has yet to be resolved. Bone marrow stromal cells have been demonstrated to grow more proficiently on silk than on biomaterials like collagen and poly(lactic acid) (Meinel et al., 2005). Other studies have shown that keratinocytes and endothelial cells prefer a silk matrix only when the silk is coated with Type I collagen or fibronectin (Sung et al., 1999; Meinel et al., 2005). Fortunately, even if chemical modifications to silk are required to create a successful cell culture substrate, possibilities for bonding growth factors and/or adhesive proteins to silk have already been identified (Altman et al., 2003). Some difficulties have been reported in achieving good cell perfusion to the innermost portions of a silk matrix, but this issue may prove solvable with better cell seeding methods (Altman et al., 2002).

Fibroin strongly binds to components of the coagulation cascades. Silk sutures are highly thrombogenic immediately after implantation, but show a lower level of thrombus than synthetic sutures (e.g., poly(lactic acid)) at later points in time (Altman et al., 2003). One benefit of silk over other naturally-derived biomaterials is that silk avoids any bioburdens or possible xenozoonoses (novel cross-species infections) associated with using animal-derived materials (Altman et al., 2002).

## 8.5 Fibrin and Fibrinogen

### 8.5.1 Sources and Refinement

Fibrin is a naturally-occurring polymer, threads of which form at the conclusion of coagulation cascades to consolidate and trap cells/proteins at the site of newly-formed clots. Because of fibrin's role in the clotting cascade as a "glue" that holds clots together, the most popular biomaterial applications for fibrin have been sealants and glues. These glues are used to repair wounds incurred during surgical procedures, to adhere skin grafts, to promote nerve tissue repair, and more. Fibrin glue is generally a combination of thrombin, fibrinogen, Factor XIII, a fibrinolytic inhibitor such as aprotinin, and tranexamic acid or aminocaproic acid (Webster and West, 2002). The glue may be delivered by syringe, spray, or endoscopically.

Thrombin, the catalytic enzyme that generates fibrin monomers, can be derived in human or bovine forms. Given current apprehensions concerning xenozoonoses (particularly Bovine Spongiform Encephalopathy), the human form is preferably used (Webster and West, 2002). Human plasma fibrinogen is also used in fibrin glues (Weisel, 2004). Like thrombin, animal forms of fibrinogen are available; fibrinogen has even been harvested from salmon (Manseth et al., 2004).

The superior adhesive strength of mussels in their underwater environment has directed much attention toward studying the success of this function, with the intent of creating alternative tissue sealants or bioglues. Mussel adhesive proteins can be purified from native tissue, but synthetic production of these proteins will be much more efficient since 1 kg of adhesive would require the harvesting of 5 to 10 million mussels (Webster and West, 2002). Recombinant technology has been used to produce mussel protein analogues, and this work will surely continue.

### 8.5.2 Molecular Structure

Fibrinogen, the polymeric precursor to fibrin, is a 45-nm elongated dimer (Weisel, 2004) composed of two identical halves, each with three polypeptide chains: A$\alpha$, B$\beta$, and $\gamma$. When fibrin molecules assemble, thrombin cleaves the A fibrinopeptides and B fibrinopeptides to form fibrin monomers. Factor XIII, activated by thrombin and $Ca^{2+}$, strengthens the fibrin network by creating covalent disulfide bonds between the glutamyl and lysyl residues of two adjacent fibrin molecules, thereby hardening the clot and reducing its susceptibility to proteolytic degradation (Hanson and Harker, 1996; Kohn and Langer, 1996; Webster and West, 2002).

The stiffness and density of a fibrin matrix depends upon the diameter and number of fibrin monomers formed when thrombin cleaves fibrinogen (Urech et al., 2005). However, fibrin fiber size is limited. Fibrin has a natural periodicity of 22.5 nm that is maintained irrespective of fiber size. Therefore, the molecules on the outside of a larger diameter fiber will be stretched axially to maintain that periodicity. A fibrin fiber has reached its maximum diameter when the energy to stretch a molecule exceeds the energy of the bond that adheres the new molecule to the aggregate fiber (Weisel, 2004).

### 8.5.3    Mechanical Properties

The relative concentrations of the components of fibrin glues control the mechanical properties of the final product. Increased concentration of fibrinogen will upregulate the density and strength of fibrin glue. The absence of $Ca^{2+}$ reduces the yield strength of glue clots (Webster and West, 2002). The addition of Factor XIII correlates with an increase in elastic modulus (Urech et al., 2005).

Because of this inherent variability, mechanical properties of fibrin matrices can be best presented in ranges. The elastic modulus, for example, ranges over multiple orders of magnitude (Cummings et al., 2004; Urech et al., 2005). It is possible, however, for fibrin glues to exhibit a higher tensile strength than staples after 3 to 4 days (Webster and West, 2002). In its pure form, fibrin is less stiff and more elastic than collagen, experiencing a very sudden failure (Cummings et al., 2004). However, a fibrin–collagen composite matrix exceeds both pure fibrin and pure collagen ultimate tensile strengths, and demonstrates a more gradual failure beyond the yield point (Cummings et al., 2004).

### 8.5.4    Physiological Responses

It has been suggested that fibrin is relatively nonthrombogenic compared to other biomaterials, due to the fact that it does not activate platelets as readily (Cummings et al., 2004). Fibrin matrices are not only the last step of coagulation cascades, they are the first structural step toward angiogenesis and the formation of new tissue. Fibrin has been shown to be a natural ingrowth matrix for endothelial cells (Cummings et al., 2004). Fibrin matrices also promote extracellular matrix (ECM) synthesis by smooth muscle cells and fibroblasts (Grassl et al., 2002).

---

## 8.6    Extracellular Matrix

### 8.6.1    Sources and Refinement

ECM scaffolds may be derived from numerous sources, including: porcine small intestine submucosa (SIS), porcine urinary bladder submucosa (UBS), porcine urinary bladder matrix (basement membrane derived) (UBM), bovine pericardium, canine stomach submucosa, dermis and basement membrane of the skin, Achilles tendon, and liver stroma. In all cases, the natural tissue is washed with a detergent to remove cells and leave only the structural and functional proteins of the ECM. A natural matrix remains, without cells and the associated antigens that cause xenografts to elicit such a strong immune response.

Prior to use as a biomaterial, ECM is commonly cross-linked to reduce its *in vivo* degradation time. Glutaraldehyde or epoxies bond the lysine, hydroxylysine, or arginine amino groups (Sung et al., 1999) and increase the stiffness and bond density of the ECM (Mirnajafi et al., 2005). Cross-linking retards degradation and cellular infiltration (Courtman et al., 2001) by reducing the number of available bonding sites. Other modifications to ECM include layering the decellularized tissue to attain desired mechanical properties and altering the structure of the matrix. For example, Wei et al. (2005) modified the porosity of ECM to suit tissue engineering needs, using acetic acid and collagenase.

### 8.6.2    Molecular Structure

ECM is a combination of structural and functional proteins that provide structural support for tissues, is an attachment site for host cells, and acts as chemoattractants that induce and control tissue remodeling, as well as other functions (Badylak, 2002). Growth factors commonly found in ECM include: vascular endothelial growth factor, fibroblast growth factor, endothelial growth factor, transforming growth factor beta, keratinocyte growth factor, hepatocyte growth factor, and platelet-derived growth factor. All of these can be present in ECM biomaterials in naturally occurring quantities and distributions (Badylak, 2002).

### 8.6.3   Material Properties

The material properties of ECM biomaterials vary greatly due to different methods of preparation and the physiological source of the material; in this case, "source" refers to both harvesting regions (bladder, stomach, intestine, etc.) and species (porcine, bovine, canine, etc.). Canine SIS has a reported elastic modulus of 85 MPa, while the modulus of bovine SIS has been estimated to be 7 MPa (Freytes et al., 2004). Mechanical properties of ECM biomaterials are directly related to the original site of harvest. Intestinal wall experiences large axial hoop stresses *in vivo*, and harvested SIS demonstrates anisotropic properties. Stomach and bladder walls experience more multi-directional stresses, and exhibit more directionally uniform mechanical properties (Freytes et al., 2004). The alignment of structural protein fibers (collagen, for example) will correspond to the primary direction of stresses in the native tissue (Mirnajafi et al., 2005).

For general reference, ball-burst strength tests were performed on a number of two-ply ECM materials. The observed burst strengths, from greatest to least, were canine SIS, UBS/UBM combination, and porcine UBS, ranging from 260 to 20 N (Freytes et al., 2004).

The mechanical properties of ECM biomaterials can be customized through layering, but general guidelines for manufacturing have not yet been discovered. Noncross-linked UBS has a multidirectional ultimate tensile strength of approximately 40 N as a single sheet (Badylak, 2002). If UBS is doubled to create a two-ply material, the ultimate tensile strength increases to approximately 60 N. As a four-ply material, UBS again increases its ultimate tensile strength to around 175 N. In contrast, stomach submucosa demonstrates a lower ultimate tensile strength as a four-ply material than as a two-ply material (262 vs. 175 N) (Freytes et al., 2004).

### 8.6.4   Physiological Responses

A small number of xenogenic cells can remain after the ECM refinement process, so ECM will generally elicit at least a slight immune response. The effect of cross-linking ECM on any subsequent immune response is currently unclear. It may be argued that the reduced number of bonding sites that exist in this biomaterial after cross-linking will reduce opportunities for interactions with the host environment; alternatively it may be argued that residues from the fixing agents themselves can increase immune response to the implanted biomaterial (Sung et al., 1999; Courtman et al., 2001). As with any biomaterial, it will be important to continue experimentally investigating potential immune responses to implants derived from ECM.

## 8.7   Synthetic Amino Acid Polymers

Artificially-designed polymers of amino acids (i.e., sequences created by humans, rather than as naturally occurring proteins) are not widely used as biomaterials at present, but are an area of active research. Synthetic amino acid polymers tend to be formed using one of five general strategies (Bourke and Kohn, 2003; Link et al., 2003): amino acid side chains can be grafted to a synthetic polymer backbone; copolymers can be created by combining nonamino acid monomers with amino acids; peptides or poly(amino acid) blocks can be incorporated in alternating, repetitive sequence block copolymers; naturally-occurring amino acids may be linked by nonamide bonds (for example, ester or carbonate bonds); or, naturally occurring amino acids may be individually modified and arranged as desired.

The development of tyrosine-derived polycarbonates is one example of current research on synthetic amino acid polymers. Tyrosine-derived polymers have a relatively long degradation time (much longer than poly(lactic acid)) (Bourke and Kohn, 2003), which makes these polymers biomaterial candidates for prolonged drug release applications, or for orthopedic implants. Tyrosine-derived polycarbonates do not form a locally acidic environment upon degradation as does poly(lactic acid), a common synthetic polymer that has been used for bone tissue engineering (Tangpasuthadol et al., 2000) and that is reviewed elsewhere in this volume. While biocompatibility aspects (including potentially induced immune responses) of tyrosine-derived polymers are still under investigation, initial results have indicated a positive future for these biomaterials (Hooper et al., 1998; James et al., 1999). A second example of continuing research in the area of synthetic amino acid polymers is the effort to modify the structures of individual amino acids, and to incorporate these nonstandard amino acids into peptide structures. Rather than relying on the mechanical and chemical properties of available amino acids, this technology attempts to engineer new amino acids with customized properties (Di Zio and Tirrel, 2002; Heilshorn et al., 2003; Link et al., 2003; Nowatzki and Tirrell, 2004).

Combining selected, naturally-occurring proteins into biomaterials allows some degree of material property customization: the resulting material can be designed to possess specifically-desired characteristics due to the selected components. The field of synthetic amino acid polymers takes this principle one step further and could theoretically provide near-complete control of material and chemical characteristics. Unfortunately, synthetic amino acid polymers are not, at present, widely used as biomaterials due to difficulties in processing, in predicting swelling kinetics and release rates of incorporated biological agents or drugs, and concern over potential immune reactions (Kohn et al., 2004). Continued research on how individual amino acids and bonding methods affect overall resultant polymer properties will help these biomaterials reach their full potential.

## 8.8  Conclusion

Selected chemical and mechanical properties of the biomaterials that were discussed in this chapter are presented in Table 8.2 and Table 8.3, along with properties of a few comparison materials. To maintain the brevity of this chapter, discussion of

**TABLE 8.2**

Selected Properties of Proteins Discussed in This Chapter

| Protein | Function | Size | Thermal Stability |
|---------|----------|------|-------------------|
| Collagen | ECM Protein | 285 kDa | Denatures at 39°C (Stryer, 1981) |
| Fibrinogen | Clotting | 340 kDa | Denatures at 56°C (Loeb and Mackey, 1972) |
| Elastin | ECM protein | — | Denatures at 66°C (Fung, 1993) |
| Silk (*B. bombi*) | Reproductive | Variable | Denatures at 210°C (Winkler and Kaplan, 2000) |

**TABLE 8.3**

Selected Mechanical Properties of Protein-Based Biomaterials and Other Materials for Comparison

| Material | UTS (MPa) | Elastic Modulus (GPa) | Percent Strain at Failure |
|---|---|---|---|
| Silk with sericin | 500 | 5–12 | 19 (Perez-Rigueiro et al., 2000) |
| Silk without sericin | 610–690 | 15–17 | 4–16 (Perez-Rigueiro et al., 2000) |
| Collagen | 50–100 (Fung, 1993) | 0.35–1 (Fung, 1993) | |
| Tendon | 28–47 (Gentleman et al., 2004) | 0.085–0.137 (Gentleman et al., 2004) | |
| PLA | 28–50 (Kohn and Langer, 1996) | | 2–6 (Kohn and Langer, 1996) |
| Bone | 100 (Fung, 1993) | 10 (Fung, 1993) | |
| Elastin | | 0.6 (Fung, 1993) | |
| Fibrin | ~0.015 (Cummings et al., 2004) | 19–37 (Cummings et al., 2004) | |

multi-component protein-based biomaterials was limited to only a short section on ECM, but it should be noted that a great number of successful biomaterials are derived by combining multiple protein components. This approach can synergistically enhance both mechanical and biochemical properties of the resulting biomaterial.

Although all of the protein/amino acid polymer-based biomaterials discussed in this chapter are subject to at least some concern about the potential for undesirable immune responses, biomaterials that undergo naturally-controlled degradation processes into nontoxic products and that can be fabricated to possess the chemical and mechanical properties needed for specific applications have clear benefits over other alternatives. Proteins and amino-acid derived polymers should continue to be a fruitful and clinically useful area of biomaterials development.

# References

Altman, G.H., Diaz, F., Jakuba, C., Calabro, T., and Horan, R.L. et al., Silk-based biomaterials, *Biomaterials*, **24**, 401–416 (2003).

Altman, G.H., Horan, R.L., Lu, H.H., Moreau, J., and Martin, I. et al., Silk matrix for tissue engineered anterior cruciate ligaments, *Biomaterials*, **23**, 4131–4141 (2002).

Angele, P., Abke, J., Kujat, R., Faltermeier, H., and Schumann, D. et al., Influence of different collagen species on physico-chemical properties of crosslinked collagen matrices, *Biomaterials*, **25**, 2831–2841 (2004).

Badylak, S.F., The extracellular matrix as a scaffold for tissue reconstruction, *Semin. Cell Dev. Biol.*, **13**, 377–383 (2002).

Bini, E., Knight, D.P., and Kaplan, D.L., Mapping domain structures in silks from insects and spiders related to protein assembly, *J. Mol. Biol.*, **335**, 27–40 (2004).

Bourke, S.L. and Kohn, J., Polymers derived from the amino acid L-tyrosine: polycarbonates, polyarylates and copolymers with poly(ethylene glycol), *Adv. Drug Deliv. Rev.*, **55**, 447–466 (2003).

Bucknall, T.E., Teare, L., and Ellis, H., The choice of suture to close abdominal incisions, *Eur. Surg. Res.*, **15**, 59–66 (1983).

Christiansen, D., Huang, E.K., and Silver, F.H., Assembly of type I collagen: fusion of fibril subunits and the influence of fiber diameter on mechanical properties, *Matrix Biol.*, **19**, 409–420 (2000).

Courtman, D.W., Errett, B.F., and Wilson, G.J., The role of crosslinking in modification of the immune response elicited against xenogenic vascular acellular matrices, *J. Biomed. Mater. Res.*, **55**, 576–586 (2001).

Cretel, E., Richard, M.A., Jean, R., and Durand, J.M., Still's-like disease, breast prosthesis, and collagen implants, *Rheumatol. Int.*, **20**, 129–131 (2001).

Cukier, J., Beauchamp, R.S., Spindler, J.S., Spindler, S., Lorenzo, C., and Trentham, D.E., Association between bovine collagen dermal implants and a dermatomyositis of a polymyositis-like syndrome, *Ann. Intern. Med.*, **188**, 920–928 (1993).

Cummings, C.L., Gawlitta, D., Nerem, R.M., and Stegemann, J.P., Properties of engineered vascular constructs made from collagen, fibrin, and collagen–fibrin mixtures, *Biomaterials*, **25**, 3699–3706 (2004).

Daamen, W.F., Hafmans, T., Veerkamp, J.H., and van Kuppevelt, T.H., Comparison of five procedures for the purification of insoluble elastin, *Biomaterials*, **22**, 1997–2005 (2001).

Debelle, L. and Tamburro, A.M., Elastin: molecular description and function, *Int. J. Biochem. Cell Biol.*, **31**, 261–272 (1999).

Di Zio, K. and Tirrel, D.A., Mechanical properties of artificial protein matrices engineered for control of cell and tissue behavior, *Macromolecules*, **36**, 1553–1558 (2002).

Fini, M., Motta, A., Torricelli, P., Giavaresi, G., and Nicoli Aldini, N. et al., The healing of confined critical size cancellous defects in the presence of silk fibroin hydrogel, *Biomaterials*, **26**, 3527–3536 (2005).

Freytes, D.O., Badylak, S.F., Webster, T.J., Geddes, L.A., and Rundell, A.E., Biaxial strength of multilaminated extracellular matrix scaffolds, *Biomaterials*, **25**, 2353–2361 (2004).

Fung, Y.C., *Biomechanics: Mechanical Properties of Living Tissues*, Springer, Berlin (1993).

Gelse, K., Poschl, E., and Aigner, T., Collagens — structure, function, and biosynthesis, *Adv. Drug Deliv. Rev.*, **55**, 1531–1546 (2003).

Gentleman, E., Lay, A.N., Dickerson, D.A., Nauman, E.A., Livesay, G.A., and Dee, K.C., Mechanical characterization of collagen fibers and scaffolds for tissue engineering, *Biomaterials*, **24**, 3805–3813 (2003).

Gentleman, E., Livesay, G.A., Dee, K.C., and Nauman, E.A., Tissue engineering of ligament, *Encyclopedia of Biomaterials and Biomedical Engineering*, Vol. 69, Marcel Dekker, New York pp. 1559–1569 (2004).

Grassl, E.D., Oegema, T.R., and Tranquillo, R.T., Fibrin as an alternative biopolymer to type-I collagen for the fabrication of a media equivalent, *J. Biomed. Mater. Res.*, **60**, 607–612 (2002).

Greenwald, D., Shumway, S., Albear, P., and Gottlieb, L., Mechanical comparison of 10 suture materials before and after *in vivo* incubation, *J. Surg. Res.*, **56**, 372–377 (1994).

Hanson, S. and Harker, L., Blood coagulation and blood–materials interactions, In: *Biomaterials Science*, Ratner, B., Hoffman, A., Schoen, F., and Lemons, J., Eds., Academic Press, New York, pp. 193–199 (1996).

Haut, R.C., The influence of specimen length on the tensile failure properties of tendon collagen, *J.Biomech.*, **19**, 951–955 (1986).

Heilshorn, S.C., DiZio, K.A., Welsh, E.R., and Tirrell, D.A., Endothelial cell adhesion to the fibronectin CS5 domain in artificial extracellular matrix proteins, *Biomaterials*, **24**, 4245–4252 (2003).

Hooper, K.A., Macon, N.D., and Kohn, J., Comparative histological evaluation of new tyrosine-derived polymers and poly(L-lactic acid) as a function of polymer degradation, *J. Biomed. Mater. Res.*, **41**, 443–454 (1998).

Horan, R.L., Antle, K., Collette, A.L., Wang, Y., and Huang, J. et al., *In vitro* degradation of silk fibroin, *Biomaterials*, in press, **26**, 3385–3393 (2005).

Isenburg, J.C., Simionescu, D.T., and Vyavahare, N.R., Elastin stabilization in cardiovascular implants: improved resistance to enzymatic degradation by treatment with tannic acid, *Biomaterials*, **25**, 3293–3302 (2004).

James, K., Levene, H., Parsons, J.R., and Kohn, J., Small changes in polymer chemistry have a large effect on the bone–implant interface: evaluation of a series of degradable tyrosine-derived polycarbonates in bone defects, *Biomaterials*, **20**, 2203–2212 (1999).

Kim, U.-J., Park, J., Kim, H.J., Wada, M., and Kaplan, D.L., Three-dimensional aqueous-derived biomaterial scaffolds from silk fibroin, *Biomaterials*, **26**, 2775–2785 (2005).

Kohn, J., Abramson, S., and Langer, R., Bioresorbable and bioerodible materials, In: *Biomaterials Science*, Ratner, B., Hoffman, A., Schoen, F., and Lemons, J., Eds., Elsevier/Academic Press, Amsterdam/New York, pp. 115–127 (2004).

Kohn, J. and Langer, R., Bioresorbable and bioerodible materials, In: *Biomaterials Science*, Ratner, B., Hoffman, A., Schoen, F., and Lemons, J., Eds., Academic Press, New York, pp. 64–72 (1996).

Lam, K.H., Nijenhuis, A.J., Bartels, H., Postema, A.R., Jonkman, M.F., Pennings, A.J., and Nieuwenhuis, P., Reinforced poly(L-lactic acid) fibers as suture material, *J. Appl. Biomater.*, **6**, 191–197 (1995).

Link, A.J., Mock, M.L., and Tirrell, D.A., Non-canonical amino acids in protein engineering, *Curr. Opin. Biotechnol.*, **14**, 603–609 (2003).

Loeb, W.F. and Mackey, W.F., A "Cuvette Method" for the determination of plasma fibrinogen, *Bull. Am. Soc. Vet. Clin. Pathol.*, **1**, 5–8 (1972).

Lu, Q., Ganesan, K., Simionescu, D.T., and Vyavahare, N.R., Novel porous aortic elastin and collagen scaffolds for tissue engineering, *Biomaterials*, **25**, 5227–5237 (2004).

Lynn, A.K., Yannas, I.V., and Bonfield, W., Antigenicity and immunogenicity of collagen, *J. Biomed. Mater. Res. Part B: Appl. Biomater.*, **71B**, 343–354 (2004).

Ma, L., Gao, C., Mao, Z., Zhou, J., and Shen, J., Enhanced biological stability of collagen porous scaffolds by using amino acids as novel cross-linking bridges, *Biomaterials*, **25**, 2997–3004 (2004).

Manseth, E., Skjervold, P.O., Fjaera, S.O., Brosstad, F.R., Bjornson, S., and Flengsrud, R., Purification and characterization of Atlantic salmon (*Salmo salar*) fibrinogen, *Comp. Biochem. Physiol. Part B: Biochem. Mol. Biol.*, **138**, 169–174 (2004).

Meinel, L., Hofmann, S., Karageorgiou, V., Kirker-Head, C., and McCool, J. et al., The inflammatory responses to silk films *in vitro* and *in vivo*, *Biomaterials*, **26**, 147–155 (2005).

Mirnajafi, A., Raymer, J., Scott, M.J., and Sacks, M.S., The effects of collagen fiber orientation on the flexural properties of pericardial heterograft biomaterials, *Biomaterials*, **26**, 795–804 (2005).

Mithieux, S.M., Rasko, J.E.J., and Weiss, A.S., Synthetic elastin hydrogels derived from massive elastic assemblies of self-organized human protein monomers, *Biomaterials*, **25**, 4921–4927 (2004).

Nowatzki, P.J. and Tirrell, D.A., Physical properties of artificial extracellular matrix protein films prepared by isocyanate crosslinking, *Biomaterials*, **25**, 1261–1267 (2004).

Ottani, V., Martini, D., Franchi, M., Ruggeri, A., and Raspanti, M., Hierarchical structures in fibrillar collagens, *Micron*, **33**, 587–596 (2002).

Panilaitis, B., Altman, G.H., Chen, J., Jin, H.-J., Karageorgiou, V., and Kaplan, D.L., Macrophage responses to silk, *Biomaterials*, **24**, 3079–3085 (2003).

Perez-Rigueiro, J., Viney, C., Llorca, J., and Elices, M., Mechanical properties of a single-brin silkworm silk, *J. Appl. Polym. Sci.*, **75**, 1270–1277 (2000).

Postlethwait, R.W., Long-term comparative study of nonabsorbable sutures, *Ann. Surg.*, **171**, 892–898 (1970).

Rigby, B.J., Hirai, N., Spikes, J.D., and Eyring, H., The mechanical properties of rat tail tendon, *J. Gen. Physiol.*, **43**, 265–283 (1958).

Saitoh, H., Ohshima, K.-I., Tsubouchi, K., Takasu, Y., and Yamada, H., X-ray structural study of noncrystalline regenerated *Bombyx mori* silk fibroin, *Int. J. Biol. Macromol.*, **34**, 259–265 (2004).

Salthouse, T.N., Matlaga, B.F., and Wykoff, M.H., Comparative tissue response to six suture materials in rabbit cornea, sclera, and ocular muscle, *Am. J. Ophthalmol.*, **84**, 224–233 (1977).

Sofia, S., McCarthy, M.B., Gronowicz, G., and Kaplan, D.L., Functionalized silk-based biomaterials for bone formation, *J. Biomed. Mater. Res.*, **54**, 139–148 (2001).

Soo, C., Rahbar, G., and Moy, R.L., The immunogenicity of collagen implants, *J. Dermatol. Surg. Oncol.*, **19**, 431–434 (1993).

Stryer, L., *Biochemistry*, W.H. Freeman, San Francisco (1981).

Sung, H.-W., Chang, Y., Chiu, C., Chen, C., and Liang, H., Crosslinking characteristics and mechanical properties of a bovine pericardium fixed with a naturally occurring crosslinking agent, *J. Biomed. Mater. Res.*, **47**, 116–126 (1999).

Tangpasuthadol, V., Pendharkar, S.M., and Kohn, J., Hydrolytic degradation of tyrosine-derived polycarbonates, a class of new biomaterials. Part I: study of model compounds, *Biomaterials*, **21**, 2371–2378 (2000).

Urech, L., Bittermann, A.G., Hubbell, J.A., and Hall, H., Mechanical properties, proteolytic degradability and biological modifications affect angiogenic process extension into native and modified fibrin matrices in vitro, *Biomaterials*, **26**, 1369–1379 (2005).

Webster, I. and West, P., Adhesives for medical applications, In: *Polymeric Biomaterials*, Dimitriu, S., Ed., Marcel Dekker, New York, pp. 703–738 (2002).

Wei, H.-J., Liang, H.-C., Lee, M.-H., Huang, Y.-C., Chang, Y., and Sung, H.-W., Construction of varying porous structures in acellular bovine pericardia as a tissue-engineering extracellular matrix, *Biomaterials*, **26**, 1905–1913 (2005).

Weisel, J.W., The mechanical properties of fibrin for basic scientists and clinicians, *Biophys. Chem.*, **112**, 267–276 (2004).

Winkler, S. and Kaplan, D.L., Molecular biology of spider silk, *Rev. Mol. Biotechnol.*, **74**, 85–93 (2000).

Woodhouse, K.A., Klement, P., Chen, V., Gorbet, M.B., Keeley, F.W. et al., Investigation of recombinant human elastin polypeptides as non-thrombogenic coatings, *Biomaterials*, **25**, 4543–4553 (2004).

Yannas, I.V., Natural materials, In: *Biomaterials Science*, Ratner, B., Hoffman, A., Schoen, F., and Lemons, J., Eds., Academic Press, New York, pp. 84–93 (1996).

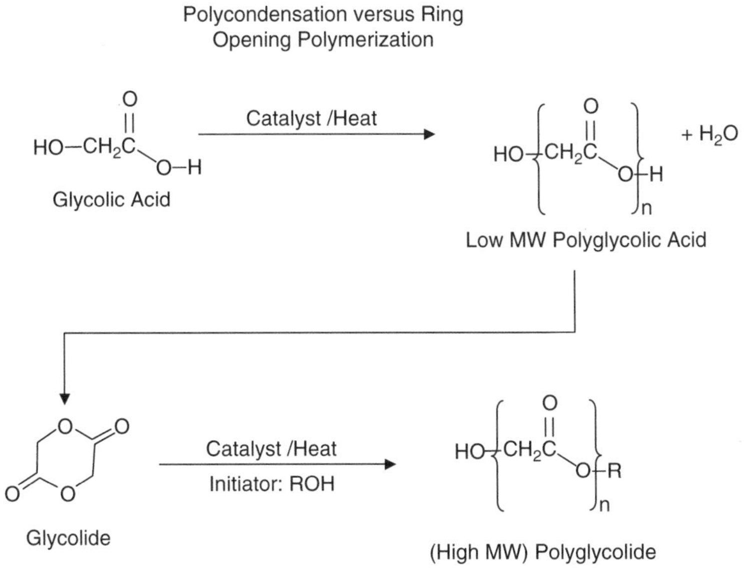

Polycondensation versus Ring
Opening Polymerization

**FIGURE 9.1**
The preparation of low molecular weight polyglycolic acid by a polycondensation process followed by "back-biting" depolymerization to form the six-member lactone, glycolide. The lactone can then be made to undergo ring-open polymerization to produce polyglycolide. Molecular weight can be controlled by the amount of initiator, typically an alcohol.

and D(+)-lactide, *not* a single compound. The polymer formed from racemic lactide is usually a random copolymer of the two stereoisomers and does not readily crystallize. The racemic mixture has found particular utility in the area of controlled drug delivery. Another monomer having an oxygen adjacent to an α-carbon that has found commercial use is the lactone *p*-dioxanone. Additionally, two other lactones have been used quite successfully via copolymerization, trimethylene carbonate, and ε-caprolactone, although they do not possess oxygens adjacent to α-carbons (see Figure 9.2).

Besides glycolide and lactide, three other cyclic monomers are used in the production of synthetic absorbable polyesters; these are *p*-dioxanone, ε-caprolactone, and trimethylene carbonate. The first of these, *p*-dioxanone (CA index name: 1,4-dioxan-2-one), can be homopolymerized to an absorbable material, and has found practical utility as a

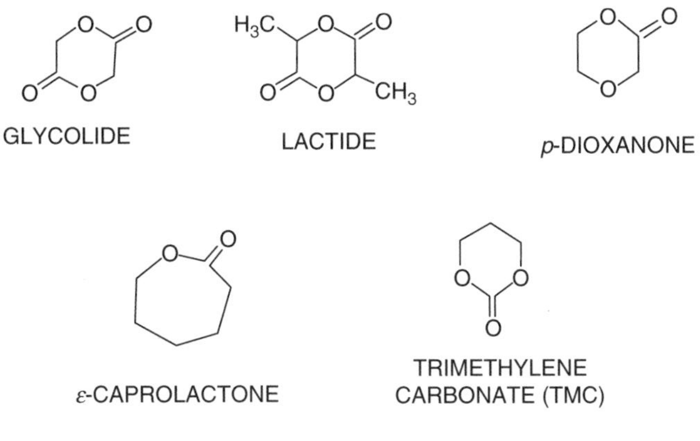

**FIGURE 9.2**
Five monomers that have been used extensively in the preparation of synthetic absorbable polyesters.

homopolymer. This monomer can also be readily copolymerized. The second, ε-capro-lactone (2-oxepanone or 6-hydroxyhexanoic acid lactone), can be polymerized to result in a commercially useful semicrystalline polymer, but the homopolymer poly(ε-caprolactone) exhibits limited susceptibility to hydrolysis in the body, and hence has limited utility as an implantable biomaterial. It, along with the last monomer, trimethylene carbonate or TMC (CA index name: 1,3-dioxan-2-one but also known as 1,3-propylene carbonate) finds use through copolymerization where it serves to modify polymer properties to make them better suited to particular applications. With their ability to lower glass transition temperatures in copolymers, these monomers provide an especially valuable approach to produce softer, more pliable materials. It is interesting to note that the monomeric trimethylene carbonate can still be viewed as a lactone; it is a cyclic ester of carbonic acid.

## 9.3   Synthetic Routes/Polymerization

### 9.3.1   Ring-Opening Polymerization

Ring-opening polymerization (ROP) is a very important synthetic route, utilizing not only the lactones themselves but also involving catalysts and initiators to facilitate the desired polymerization outcome. Key points that need to be understood include thermodynamics (especially the driving force to ring-open and its effect on the equilibrium level of monomer) and reaction kinetics (which affect the rate at which the equilibrium level is reached). Catalyst type and amount are tied to kinetics, while polymerization initiators are largely responsible for controlling molecular weight. Polymerization time and tempera-ture also play roles as will be outlined below (see Figure 9.1)

First a few words on the thermodynamic aspects of lactone monomers, focusing initially on the six-member ring, glycolide. This lactone possesses high ring strain; this means that the open chain species is greatly preferred over the closed six-member ring. The ring strain that this compound possesses is high enough to drive the ring-opening polymerization reaction with efficiency. Thus under the right conditions, the reaction can be driven to near completion. The monomer–polymer equilibrium, however, is temperature dependent. As temperatures increase, although the rate of reaction increases, the equilibrium is shifted more and more to disfavor the polymeric species.

If one considers the lactone lactide as glycolide with two methyl groups attached, conformational arguments can help envision that the methyl groups "push" the ring in a bit. This effect serves to stabilize lactide when compared to glycolide, resulting in less ring strain and a corresponding decrease in the driving force to ring-open. Thus the equilibrium monomer level of lactide at high temperatures is much greater than that of glycolide. Residual monomer level is of practical concern for the application of these polymers since it will influence their melt processing behavior, storage stability, and biological interactions upon implantation.

Let us now discuss the control of the final molecular weight, as it is an important consideration in producing a polymer with the right balance of melt processability and physical properties for practical utility. The molecular weight of polylactones can be controlled by the inclusion of a specified level of polymerization initiator. Each initiator molecule will form a new polymer chain. Thus for a fixed amount of monomer, an increase in the initiator level will increase the number of chains and result in a lower overall molecular weight. Important initiators for the reaction are hydroxyl-containing compounds. They may be monofunctional such as the 12-carbon alcohol, dodecanol, or multifunctional, such as diethylene glycol. Interestingly, it is not the total number of initiating chemical groups (e.g., hydroxyl groups) that determines the number average molecular weight, but rather the amount of initiating molecules. Although it is easy to see that for each initiator possessing a single functional group, a new chain is formed, notice that a diol initiator having two hydroxyl groups still results in the formation of a single linear chain. Initiators with a higher number of hydroxyl groups will, however, result in branched materials. It is possible to produce "star molecules" when highly functional initiators are utilized.

Catalysts are required to allow the polymerization to be conducted in a reasonable time frame, and therefore the efficiency of the catalyst is very important. If the polymerization proceeds too rapidly, the heat of polymerization (due to the release of ring strain) cannot be efficiently dissipated, leading to overheating and the formation of undesirable species within the polymer. As the catalysts are generally difficult to remove from the formed polymer, there are other considerations in their selection as well. Medical applications of these materials require that the catalysts be highly biocompatible and not pose any concern for implantation inside the body. Although numerous catalysts can be used from purely a chemistry standpoint, specific tin catalysts have found the most favor since in addition to their functional effectiveness, they have been shown to be biologically safe at the levels they are employed. Stannous octoate, based on one of the octanoic acids, 2-ethylhexanoic acid, and stannous chloride dihydrate are among the most commercially relevant polymerization catalysts.

Polymerization may be conducted in solution or in solventless melt processes. Solution polymerization has found little commercial utility because of the difficulty of reducing the residual solvent level to an acceptable point. The method however can be very useful in synthesizing special polymers with very narrow molecular weight distributions or very specific monomer sequence distributions. Solution polymerization also allows for efficient heat removal.

A number of bulk (solventless) polymerization approaches may be utilized in which reaction temperature plays a role. Again let us illustrate using glycolide as the example. Reaction temperatures for the ROP of glycolide can range from below 150°C to as high as about 260°C. Temperatures between approximately 190 and 230°C have found the greatest utility in practice. The product, polyglycolide, melts at about 224°C, making it possible for the forming polymer to begin to crystallize during the polymerization if the reaction temperature is sufficiently low. This behavior is used to advantage, and the approach is referred to as solid-state polymerization. If instead the polymerization is conducted entirely in the melt state, it is referred to as a melt polymerization. Finally, although glycolide can be ring-opened in solution, homopolymerization in solution is generally not conducted because the forming chains quickly crystallize and precipitate. This leads to problems in achieving high molecular weight. Among these potential methods, the most popular commercial approach of preparation is bulk-melt polymerization.

### 9.3.2  Macroinitiators

One of the consequences of the reaction of hydroxyl groups with lactones is the ability to produce copolymers with nonrandom sequence distributions. Polymers that are designed to be blocky in nature have been made, and have lead to some very successful products because they can provide an unusual combination of properties. These copolymers will generally be made in a sequential addition polymerization in which the monomer feed is added in steps; by adjusting the composition of the monomer, the composition along the forming polymer chains can be adjusted. An example is as follows.

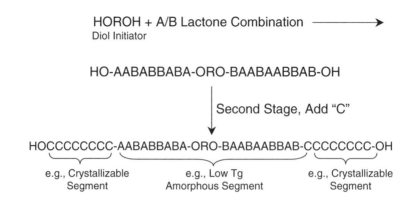

**FIGURE 9.3**
Illustration of a synthetic scheme utilizing a two-step polymerization process. It can be used, for instance, to produce a segmented copolymer of soft and hard blocks.

An initial bulk polymerization is conducted using a mixture of monomers, a diol as the initiator, and an appropriate level of a suitable catalyst. The reaction mass is brought up to the polymerization temperature along with suitable agitation provided by a stirrer. In due time a random copolymer is formed; it happens to be noncrystallizable because there is not enough symmetry in the resulting chain segments to support crystal formation (see Figure 9.3). Note that this formed polymer still has hydroxyl groups attached at each end of the chain and that these can still act as an initiating species. It can be viewed as an $\alpha,\omega$-dihydroxy macroinitiator. Instead of discharging the random copolymer as a finished product, a third monomer (or perhaps one of the pure monomers used in the initial polymerization step) is introduced into the reactor and the polymerization is continued. The random copolymer, as an $\alpha,\omega$-dihydroxy macroinitiator, begins ring-opening the new lactone monomer of the second stage of the polymerization incorporating new sequences. If the newly incorporated sequences are crystallizable, the new copolymer has the potential to crystallize. As will be discussed later, crystallizing a polymeric article provides one means of achieving dimensional stability, especially if the level of molecular orientation is very high, as might be seen in a fiber. Multiple-step polymerizations have been employed commercially to produce copolymers with soft, noncrystallizable, low glass transition temperature segments and hard, crystallizable segments that provide dimensional stability.

### 9.3.3 Polycondensation

As useful as the lactones are, they still cannot completely fulfill all of the property requirements that might be sought from synthetic absorbable polymers. For instance, the polylactones tend to be limited in their intrinsic hydrophilicity. One approach to overcome this attribute is to use an $\alpha,\omega$-dihydroxy polyethylene glycol (PEG) as a macroinitiator to render the resulting copolymer more hydrophilic. As there is a limit to the molecular weight of the PEG that can be used in an implantable device, this approach is a bit restricting. (Very high molecular weight PEG cannot be easily eliminated from the body.) Another approach that is being explored is based on aliphatic diacids possessing oxygen atoms adjacent to their $\alpha$-carbons. These diacids are then polymerized in conjunction with a diol by means of a polycondensation reaction. Because organic chemists have used the term "oxa" to designate the replacement of an ethylene group by an oxygen, these diacids have been called oxa-diacids and the resulting polymers polyoxaesters (POEs) (Bezwada and Jamiolkowski, 2000).

It is interesting to note that polycondensation polymerizations can also be combined with ring-opening polymerizations in certain circumstances. If one prepares a polyester by polycondensation using a large excess of the diol, one can insure hydroxyl termination of the formed polymer. This resulting polymer can be used in a copolymerization in which a lactone is feed into the reactor at the end of the polycondensation. A polylactone sequence is then added to the ends of each of the chains. This approach has been used to make POE/lactone copolymers with controlled hydrophilicity and a broad array of other attributes.

## 9.4   The Polymers

The monomers described in this chapter can be used to make a wide variety of polyesters. A number are useful as homopolymers, that is, polymers made from a single monomer species. The monomers are frequently used to make copolymers, both with random sequence distributions, as well as with more ordered structures. A number of very successful commercial products based on these polymers are shown in Figure 9.4. The following section will provide a bit more detail on the polymers.

### 9.4.1   Homopolymers

There are presently three lactone monomers that are homopolymerized to produce absorbable polymers used in commercial medical/surgical products. These are glycolide, L(−)-lactide, and *p*-dioxanone. Polyglycolide has found use as suture material (Dexon™), poly(L(−)-lactide) as an injection molding resin for absorbable surgical devices, and poly(*p*-dioxanone) as both a suture material as well as an injection molding resin. These materials will be described later in this chapter.

### 9.4.2   Copolymers

There are a number of very successful absorbable products based on copolymers. One such product is Coated Vicryl Suture™ of Ethicon, Inc. This product is based on a 90/10 random copolymer of glycolide and lactide (Craig et al., 1975). This polymer possesses a glass transition temperature above room temperature, such that its Young's modulus is rather high. This feature would result in a very stiff monofilament fiber, not suitable for application as a suture. To circumvent this behavior, very fine filaments are manufactured, and the resulting multifilament yarns are braided to provide sutures that are adequately pliable. In some surgical procedures, monofilament sutures are preferred over multi-filament braids. This requires the polymer to have a low glass transition temperature, as alluded to earlier, yet be crystallizable enough so as to be dimensionally stable when high molecular orientation is imparted to achieve the high strength demanded by this application.

Monocryl Monofilament Suture™ of Ethicon, Inc. is made from a polymer based on a sequential addition polymerization (Bezwada et al., 1995). First a mixture of ε-caprolactone and glycolide is polymerized using a diol as an initiator. Additional glycolide is added to the resultant "prepolymer" in a second stage polymerization step.

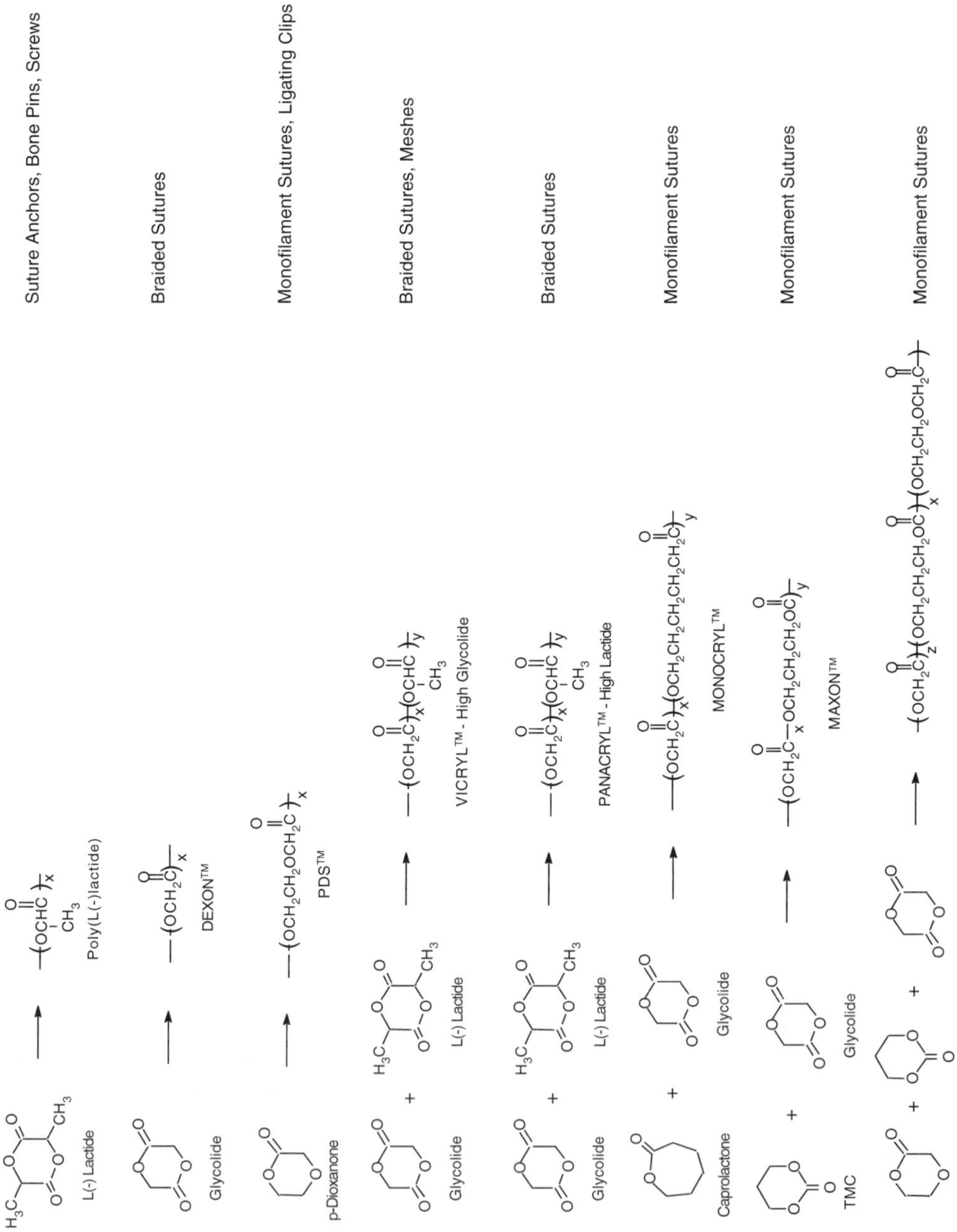

Suture Anchors, Bone Pins, Screws

Braided Sutures

Monofilament Sutures, Ligating Clips

Braided Sutures, Meshes

Braided Sutures

Monofilament Sutures

Monofilament Sutures

Monofilament Sutures

L(-) Lactide → Poly(L(-)lactide)

Glycolide → DEXON™

p-Dioxanone → PDS™

L(-) Lactide + Glycolide → VICRYL™ - High Glycolide

L(-) Lactide + Glycolide → PANACRYL™ - High Lactide

Caprolactone + Glycolide → MONOCRYL™

TMC + Glycolide → MAXON™

p-Dioxanone + TMC + Glycolide → BIOSYN™

**FIGURE 9.4**

## MOLECULAR WEIGHT DISTRIBUTION

The molecular weight distribution of the polymer systems is an important characteristic, as it influences the physical properties, flow behavior, and morphology development. One needs to understand the difference between weight average molecular weight and number average molecular weight to fully appreciate their importance and relevance. Consider for a moment trying to get a measure of the average body length of a collection of snakes in a large tub. One of your friends looks into the tub, spots the head of one of the snakes, and then carefully reaches in and grabs it just behind its neck; he measures it and then returns it to the tub. After doing this a fair number of times, he arrives at an average value that changes little with additional measurements — he declares an average. A second friend is not as careful, and he does not even look in the tub; each time he reaches into the tub and grabs at the first snake he touches. He also arrives at a value, but it is much larger than the value determined by your first friend.

How can this be? The explanation is quite simple and is at the heart of number vs. weight average molecular weight. In the first case, every snake had an equal chance of being picked, as each snake had only one head. The average that resulted is known as the number average. In the second case, snakes that were longer had a greater chance of being selected. In fact, the chance of being selected was proportional to its body length. Because longer snakes were being selected in the measurement process, it is not surprising that the resulting average was larger. Although the details will not be shown here, this second average is a "weight" average. If the population being measured is "normally" distributed, the weight average will be twice the value of the number average. An important characteristic of polyesters is their ability to undergo a process called transesterification when heated. The net result of the transesterification process is to drive the chain lengths toward a normal molecular weight distribution.

## 9.4.3  Blends

Resin blending has been used for years to achieve performance advantages or to lower overall costs. The blending of the synthetic absorbable polyesters of the present chapter has been explored as well.

In an unexpected discovery, it has been found that when the homopolymers, poly (L(−)-lactide) and poly(D(+)-lactide), are blended together, they form a higher melting stereocomplex (Loomis et al., 1989; Murdock and Loomis, 1988). The stereocomplex polylactide formed is found to exhibit very high strength. In another example, consider the case of a need for an injection molding resin, which exhibits a failure mechanism of softening with time rather than catastrophic brittle failure. In an effort to achieve these particular performance characteristics, unattainable by copolymerization means, polyglycolide has been (melt)-blended with a lactide-rich lactide/glycolide copolymer. These two materials are immiscible on a molecular level. When the relative amount favors polyglycolide, the result is a material in which polyglycolide is the matrix phase and the copolymer is the dispersed phase. The polyglycolide is normally readily crystallizable, and it is found that the matrix phase of the blend is as well. Thus parts molded from this blend will be able to retain their shapes, however complex, due to the dimensional stability imparted by the crystallinity developed in the matrix. What then is the role of the dispersed phase in this system? When this resin blend is injection molded, the lactide rich copolymeric phase is transformed by the shear forces generated — from dispersed spheres within the polyglycolide matrix into elongated fiber-like domains. These elongated domains act as crack arrestors. Once the molded part is implanted, the two polymers begin to degrade, but at quite different rates; the polyglycolide degrades faster. Normally, an initiated crack would propagate completely through causing catastrophic failure. Here, however, initial cracks are "arrested" allowing the part to remain relatively intact. With time, additional cracks form and are arrested. On a macroscopic level, the part appears to soften with time until all of the polyglycolide matrix breaks down leaving the copolymer "fibers", which will ultimately absorb as well. The aforementioned example is one in which a fundamental knowledge of the performance of not only the polymeric material, but as well consideration of the final morphology of the finished article is utilized to great advantage.

### 9.4.4   Some Specific Important Polymers

#### 9.4.4.1   *Polyglycolic Acid/Polyglycolide*

With a repeat unit of $[C_2H_2O_2]_n$, the simplest aliphatic polyester is polyglycolic acid (PGA). Low molecular weight polymer can be prepared directly from the polycondensation of glycolic acid. Due to the high temperatures involved in this synthetic route, the resulting side reactions limit the molecular weight that can be reached. For example, to achieve a number average molecular weight of 35,000, the extent of reaction must be 0.998, which is very difficult to achieve. The high reaction temperature is needed in order to form the ester linkage directly from the acid and the alcohol. Polymer chemists refer to glycolic acid as an AB system in which both chemical groups are on the same molecule; the reaction of terephthalic acid with ethylene glycol to form the commercially important poly(ethylene terephthalate) (PET) is an AA–BB system in which the acid groups are on one molecule and the alcohol groups are on another. PET can be formed by polycondensation methods because it is inherently more stable.

   To achieve molecular weights of commercial relevance, the preferred approach is to start with glycolide. Although glycolide can be prepared through the elimination of sodium chloride from sodium chloroacetate (Chujo et al., 1967), it is usually prepared in a two-step process in which glycolic acid is first made to undergo polycondensation under moderate conditions, removing water and forming low molecular weight PGA. This is followed by a second step, during which the low molecular weight chains undergo a backbiting reaction that forms the six-member lactone and causes the end of the chain to "unzip." This second step is conducted under reduced pressure and relatively high temperatures. The crude glycolide monomer that is distilled off must be further purified before polymerization. Recrystallization from ethyl acetate is often used for this purification step. The polymerization of glycolide can result in a high molecular weight product. It should be noted that the polymer resulting from this scheme should be called polyglycolide (PG) as opposed to polyglycolic acid, PGA, but many authors do not make this distinction. The heat of polymerization is reported by Chujo et al. (Chujo et al., 1967) to be 6.3 kcal/mole. Polyglycolide crystallizes with an orthorhombic unit cell with dimensions: $a = 5.22$ Å, $b = 6.19$ Å, $c = 7.02$ Å (Chatani et al., 1968). The planar zigzag chains form a sheet structure parallel to the *ac* plane. The chains however crystallize in what is described as an antiparallel fashion. That is, chains between two adjacent sheets orient in opposite directions, resulting in a tightly packed material, and hence a high density. Chujo et al. report a specific gravity of the perfect crystal of 1.707, with the completely amorphous state giving a value of 1.50. For an aliphatic organic molecule containing only carbon, hydrogen, and oxygen, these are indeed high values.

The heat of polymerization reported by Chujo et al. as 6.3 kcal/mole refers to the energy released when the ring is opened. The heat of fusion extrapolated to the fully crystallized polymer has been reported to be 12 kJ/mol or 45.7 cal/g; this refers to energy needed to melt the polymer. The Tm of PG is regarded by many to be 224°C, but values as high as 253°C have been observed in carefully prepared samples. The glass transition temperature is about 36 to 40°C, and depends in part on the amount of residual monomer present.

### 9.4.4.2  The Polylactides

Although polyglycolide is the simplest of the poly(alpha esters), polylactide received much of the initial research attention. It must be understood that the polylactides (PL) are a family of materials, possessing a very wide range of properties depending on the details of the material. At the heart of the matter is stereochemistry (see also insert). As mentioned earlier, there are three lactide monomers (L(−)-lactide, D(+)-lactide, and *meso*-lactide).

---

**LACTIDE NOMENCLATURE AND STEREOCHEMISTRY**

The moiety upon which this polyester is based, lactic acid, contains a chiral carbon. There exists two optically active stereoisomers, or enantiomers, of lactic acid, the D-form and the L-form. The assignments of capital D and capital L are based on the special arrangements of the atoms about the chiral carbon. Optically active enantiomers can rotate polarized light either to the right or to the left. The symbols + and − are often used to denote rotation to the right and left, respectively. Additionally, lower case d (dextrorotatory, from the Latin *dexter*) is often used to indicate optical rotation to the right, while lower case l (levorotatory, from the Latin *laevus*) indicates rotations to the left. This convention has often lead to pervasive nomenclature problems in the literature with the lactic acids, their lactones, and the corresponding polyesters. One of the two lactic acids having a three-dimensional structure corresponding to the L configuration happens to rotate polarized light to the right; it is correctly designated L(+)-lactic acid. The corresponding enantiomer has the D structural configuration and rotates polarized light to the left. It is D(−)-lactic acid. So far, so good. Problems arise, however, when these acids are made into their lactide derivatives, the cyclic dimer lactones. L(+)-lactic acid can be converted to L-lactide, but the optical rotation of this molecule is in the minus (−) or levorotatory direction. The monomer should then be known as L(−)-lactide; although it is not recommended, it can also be designated l-lactide because the lower case l would indicate a rotation of polarized light to the left. Employing the *R* and *S* designations, L(−)-lactide is also known as 3*S*,6*S*-3,6-dimethyl-1,4-dioxane-2,5-dione while the D(+) isomer is known as 3*R*,6*R*-3,6-dimethyl-1,4-dioxane-2,5-dione. The *meso*-isomer is 3*R*,6*S*-rel-3,6-dimethyl-1,4-dioxane-2,5-dione.

Polymerizing L(−)-lactide monomer leads to the polyester, poly(L(−)-lactide). Researchers have often used the acid-based nomenclature to designate the polymer even though it was formed by reaction of the lactone, not directly from the acid. Many have used poly(L-lactic acid). The confusion arises when the lower case l is used to designate this polymer, poly(l-lactic acid), as this refers to the polymer made from the *monomer* rotating light to the left and this was *not* the case in our example.

Remember, poly(L(−)-lactide) is made from polymerizing L(−)-lactide, which in turn is made from L(+)-lactic acid, which is also known as d-lactic acid because it rotates light to the right. Although it should not be done in the eyes of a polymer chemist, referring to poly(L(−)-lactide) as poly(L-lactic acid) would not be a sin. Referring to it as poly(l-lactic acid) would be however, as it is based on d-lactic acid.

The presence of the methyl groups in the various PLs alters their physical characteristics, mechanical performance, ability to retain their mechanical strength postimplantation, as well as their chemical hydrolysis profiles. From a thermodynamic standpoint, the methyl group stabilizes the six-member ring lactone monomer over glycolide. The effects of this stabilization are seen at many levels. Lactide is easier to prepare from lactic acid than glycolide is to prepare from glycolic acid. Secondly, the monomer–polymer equilibrium in the lactide family is slightly shifted toward the monomer when compared to that of glycolide–polyglycolide, generally resulting in more residual (unreacted) monomer during polymerization. In the course of melt processing, because the lactide monomer is slightly favored when compared to glycolide, polylactide polymer is less stable than polyglycolide; the polymer can readily unzip to regenerate more monomer. This behavior creates a challenge for melt processing of lactide polymers. This mode of polymer degradation results not so much in a rapid loss of molecular weight, but in the production of a species, the monomer, that is more susceptible to chemical hydrolysis than is the polymer itself. Finally, from a thermodynamic standpoint, the methyl groups alter the thermal properties of the polymer. Poly(L($-$)-lactide) and poly(D($+$)-lactide) homopolymers are crystallizable; when crystalline they exhibit melting transitions between about 170 and 182°C, although melting points as high as 200°C have been observed. The higher values have been observed with well-annealed higher molecular weight samples; therefore, preparation of the polymer through solid-state polymerization results in very high crystallinity and high melting. Glass transition temperatures have been reported between about 56 and 65°C. Keep in mind that residual monomer or regenerated monomer will lower the measured $T_g$.

Besides making polylactide more hydrophobic than polyglycolide, from a chemistry standpoint, the methyl group alters the reactivity of the ester group through an electronic influence and from a steric hindrance aspect. Sterically, the water molecule has a more difficult time physically approaching the ester group to form the transition state leading to hydrolysis. Overall, this results in a material that reacts much more slowly with water than polyglycolide. In medical device applications, this slower reactivity has made the polylactides very well suited for orthopedic surgery applications where healing times are longer than that required for soft tissue repair.

### 9.4.4.3  Poly(p-Dioxanone)

As the name implies, this homopolymer is based on the monomer *p*-dioxanone, a six-member lactone structurally not unlike glycolide. If one substitutes a methylene group for one of glycolide's carbonyl groups, the result is *p*-dioxanone. Poly(*p*-dioxanone) is a low-melting (approximately 115 to 120°C) aliphatic polyester with a low glass transition temperature (approximately $-10$°C). The low $T_g$ allows for a low Young's modulus, and because the polymer can be crystallized to impart dimensional stability, this polymer has found use as a monofilament suture (Ray et al., 1981). Again, dimensional stability is a particular issue in fibers because of the high molecular orientation that needs to be imparted; this orientation is a thermodynamic driving force for shrinkage as the chains look to resume a random coil configuration. Dimensional stability is perhaps even more important in injection-molded parts. One way of achieving dimensional stability in a molded part made from a polymer with a low $T_g$, is to crystallize the part in the mold. The crystallization rate of poly(*p*-dioxanone) is fast enough to be injection molded into absorbable medical devices that will not warp or distort by allowing it to crystallize within the mold cavity. Because of its low $T_g$, parts can be made that can be flexed without breaking. This has led to the use of poly(*p*-dioxanone) for devices such as clips that require hinges to function.

Poly(*p*-dioxanone) is also known as poly(1,4-dioxan-2-one), while the hydroxyl-acid that is generated upon hydrolysis of this polymer is 2-hydroxyethoxy-acetic acid. Again this polymer is generally made by the ring-opening polymerization of the corresponding lactone monomer. The monomer–polymer equilibrium is not as favorable to the polymer, however, as what is seen with glycolide; hence the homopolymer is not as thermally stable as polyglycolide. This has a number of implications. During polymerization, the reaction temperature must be much lower than what would be used for glycolide. The patent literature describes a solid-state polymerization in which the reaction temperature is lower than the melting point of the forming polymer. The resulting polymer must then be ground for use. Because of the unfavorable equilibrium, a higher level of unreacted monomer remains in the polymer. This residual monomer is removed by a volatilization process in which the ground resin is heated under vacuum at temperatures lower than the resin's melting point. Bezwada et al. details the copolymerization of *p*-dioxanone with other lactones (Bezwada et al., 1997), further covering the utility of this monomer beyond its homopolymer use.

## 9.5 Applications

### 9.5.1 Satisfying Product Requirements: The Interconnection of Chemistry, Processing, Polymer Morphology, and Design

Many factors are interconnected in achieving and controlling product performance. Depending on the product category, important performance criteria may be based on mechanical properties and the rates at which they are lost after implantation, biological performance (including the rate of absorption and tissue reaction profile), or possibly on diffusion characteristics (e.g., in controlled drug delivery devices). This section will briefly review some of these interconnections (see also Figure 9.5).

### 9.5.2 Mechanical Devices

Absorbable mechanical devices can range from sutures to orthopedic screws to ligating clips. Inherent is these devices are the mechanical property requirements that must be met. For suture materials, the tensile strength is of course very important, but elongation-to-break and other characteristics play a vital role in the articles performance. Readers of this chapter will know at this point that mechanical properties depend greatly on the amount of molecular orientation imparted during processing (Weiler and Gogolewski, 1996). The greater the orientation, the greater is the driving force to distort as the polymer chains try to restore a random coil shape. This can result in fiber shrinkage or distortion of molded parts. The development of some crystallinity helps to insure dimensional stability. The level of crystallinity required to maintain part integrity will depend on the maximum temperature that the product will be exposed to in shipping, storage, and use. At a given maximum exposure temperature, the lower the glass transition temperature of the polymer and the higher the molecular orientation, the greater the crystallinity level needs to be to insure dimensional stability. When the polymers described in this chapter are made into fibrous products (suture materials, meshes, etc.), the crystallinity level in these products is typically 35 to 45%. If the products are formed by an injection molding process,

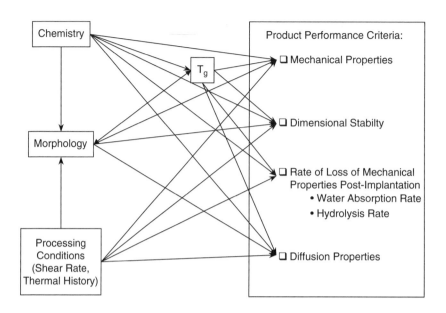

**FIGURE 9.5**
Interconnection of chemistry, processing, and polymer morphology.

crystallinity levels can be reduced because the driving force for distortion, the degree of orientation, is lower.

Processing history is a phrase that is used to reflect the time–temperature–shear profile that a polymer is exposed to during melt processing and/or subsequent storage. It is of particular importance for this class of polymers due to their high susceptibility to chemical changes when heated, especially in the presence of moisture. Processing history is also important for these materials in that it influences the final part morphology — which then plays a key role in the stability and biological performance of the part upon implantation. Successful fabrication of useful articles requires one to take deliberate actions to control aspects such as exposure of the raw materials to the ambient environment, residence times and shear rates in the melt state when in a constrained environment (e.g., inside of an extruder or injection molding machine), and thermal and environmental conditions in the melt state when in a nonconstrained flow configuration (e.g., fiber formation through spinning or drawing, etc). In addition, the manner in which these polymers are crystallized plays an important role in determining the performance characteristics of the finished article. Considerations include aspects such as cooling rates, quiescent vs. flow, and subsequent thermal/stress treatments such as annealing, controlled relaxation or stretching (Abuzaina et al., 2002). Particular care must be paid to these processing aspects to insure that the characteristics of the finished article match the required performance attributes.

Consideration of several aspects in a bit more detail will be useful in understanding how control of the processing history can be utilized to advantage, and must be considered to avoid disaster. During melt processing, the higher the melt temperature and longer the residence time at high temperature, the greater the potential for a drop in molecular weight due to degradation. This loss of molecular weight can be accompanied by undesirable changes to the polymer resulting in discoloration or a propensity for accelerated hydrolysis when in use.

This behavior requires very careful selection of both processing equipment and processing conditions when utilizing these polymers. As a second example, fibers or molded parts are often subjected to a heat treatment to increase crystallinity. This annealing is done for a number of reasons, not the least of which is to provide dimensional stability — avoiding shrinkage in the case of fibers and warping in the case of molded parts. The annealing cycles must be carefully selected not only because mechanical properties will be affected, but biological performance, such as tissue reaction and absorption profiles will also depend on the polymer morphology (Migliaresi et al., 1991; Gogolewski and Mainil-Varlet, 1996; Park and Cima, 1996; Andjelić and Jamiolkowski, 2001; Fitz et al., 2002). An additional consideration is the use environment for the part. For example, if a part is to be flexed in its use, one may desire a smaller crystal size to minimize part failure upon flexure. Such a morphology is more easily achieved by crystallization under conditions which favor nucleation over crystal growth rate — e.g., annealing at lower temperatures. Although fibers can be annealed "in-line" through heated chambers while being further oriented or allowed to relaxed, they can as well be wound on racks to be annealed in an off-line operation. While it is relatively easy to constrain the "shape" of a fiber through such "rack annealing," this is not necessarily the case for small molded parts. Annealing conditions must be identified that will not warp the part while it is undergoing the very treatment that is meant to preserve its shape.

As seen in the above, the processing history of parts fabricated from this class of polymers is of great importance. Even small changes in processing history, introduced either intentionally or accidentally, can influence polymer performance so significantly that product attributes can vary wildly. Measures must be put in place to insure that processing results in robust products.

### 9.5.3 Controlled Drug Delivery Devices

Many of the controlled drug delivery products that use the polymers of this chapter are based on microsphere technology. The common microsphere fabrication methods involve solutions of polymer. Solubility in appropriate solvents is not a universal quality of the polyesters described in this chapter. Of particular utility is the incorporation of polymerized lactide sequences. Because the amount of molecular orientation is very low, materials can be amorphous provided their glass transition temperatures are high enough.

### 9.5.4 Sterilization

Requirements of implantable surgical devices or controlled drug delivery products usually include being sterile. Although heat treatment has been used to sterilize for a very long time, synthetic absorbable poly(α-esters) do not readily lend themselves to this methodology because of rapid hydrolysis at elevated temperatures, and limited dimensional stability. The most popular sterilization method is based on exposure to ethylene oxide (EO). The design of an EO sterilization process is not without careful considerations. The article to be sterilized must be exposed to the EO gas only after it has been humidified to a suitable level. The time–temperature profile must be selected to be both efficacious as well as efficient. EO can act as a plasticizer during the sterilization process and reduced the $T_g$. The part behaves at any given temperature as if it is being exposed to a higher temperature. In some cases, under poorly selected conditions, the article can shrink or warp, or unexpectedly crystallize. Besides achieving sterility, a key consideration for the process engineer is to insure that the amount of residual EO is below acceptable levels. Gamma irradiation is a convenient sterilization method. It can however produce a drop in molecular weight resulting in a reduction of mechanical properties. The possibility of the formation of undesirable species must be carefully examined; this is particularly important for drug delivery vehicles.

## 9.6    Characterization and Methods of Analysis

Typical analytical techniques to characterize the described polyesters are gel permeation chromatography (GPC) and solution viscosity for molecular weight; nuclear magnetic resonance (NMR) for composition and sequence distribution; differential scanning calorimetry (DSC) for crystallinity level; x-ray diffraction for crystallinity level and morphological information; and hot stage optical microscopy (HSOM) for visualization of developing supramolecular structures. Many others techniques supplement these. Proper analytical characterization can make the seemingly impossible possible. Likewise, improper analytical characterization can make the possible, impossible.

## 9.7    Closing Remarks

As described in this chapter, poly($\alpha$-esters) are an important class of biomaterials, especially well suited for use in implantable medical device and drug delivery applications. Their complex chemistry and certain unique aspects of their behavior during polymerization and processing have presented significant hurdles to their successful application. Nonetheless, these materials find numerous applications in critical medical and surgical applications. This chapter has sought to provide a technical foundation, and to describe successful examples where the challenges were overcome to great commercial and scientific advantage. Finally, it has sought to provide the tools and basis to allow the reader to appreciate the complexities and interdependencies of chemistry, processing, and design.

## Problems

### Problem 1
You are working with a lactide/glycolide copolymer reported to have a composition of 65/35. (a) If this is on a mole basis, what does this correspond to on a weight basis? (b) If it is 65/35 on a weight basis, what does this correspond to on a mole basis?
### Answers to Problem 1
1. 69.75/30.25
2. 59.93/40.07

The easiest way to attack part (a) of this problem is to assume the existence of a hypothetical copolymer in which a total of 1 mole of monomer was used to make it. Because 65 mol% of the copolymer is based on lactide, the polymerized lactide must correspond to 0.65 mol; a similar argument provides that this copolymer sample is based on 0.35 mol of polymerized glycolide. The molecular weights of lactide and glycolide are 144.13 and 116.07 g/mol, respectively. Because 0.65 mol of lactide correspond to 93.38 g (0.65 mol × 144.13 g/mol) and 0.35 mole of glycolide correspond to 40.62 g (0.35 mol × 116.07 g/mol), our hypothetical copolymer must have weighed 134.30 g (93.38 + 40.62).

Dividing the individual lactide and glycolide weights by the total copolymer's weight provides the composition on a weight basis. Thus 93.38 g/134.30 g gives rise to a value of 69.75 wt% lactide and 40.62 g/134.30 g gives rise to 30.25 wt% glycolide.

An insight to easily solve part (b) of this problem is to imagine a hypothetical copolymer of this composition which weight 100.00 g. Because 65 wt% of the copolymer is based on lactide, the polymerized lactide must correspond to 65 g; again, a similar argument provides that this copolymer sample is made of 35 g of polymerized glycolide. The molecular weights of lactide and glycolide are 144.13 and 116.07 g/mol, respectively. Because 65 g of lactide correspond to 0.4510 mole (65 g/144.13 g/mol) and 35 g of glycolide correspond to 0.3015 mole (35 g/116.07 g/mol), our hypothetical copolymer must have been based on 0.7525 mole of total monomer.

Dividing the individual lactide and glycolide moles by the total number of moles provides the composition on a mole basis. Thus 0.4510 mol/0.7525 mol gives rise to a value of 59.93 mol% lactide and 0.3015 mol/0.7525 mol gives rise to 40.07 mol% glycolide.

## Problem 2

You are starting with a polyethylene glycol resin (PEG) having a molecular weight of 1200 g/mol. Its molecular weight is very narrowly distributed and it is difunctional, possessing an alcohol group on each chain end. You want to use this material as a macroinitiator to incorporate PEG sequences in a lactide polymer. You use (a) 10 wt% PEG in one polymerization and (b) 20 wt% in another. Estimate the molecular weight of each of the resulting resins, assuming a normal molecular weight distribution.

**Answer to Problem 2**
1. $M_w$ is 24,000 g/mol while $M_n$ is 12,000 g/mol
2. $M_w$ is 12,000 g/mol while $M_n$ is 6000 g/mol

As before, it is easiest to solve these kinds of problems by envisioning a hypothetical case of a convenient weight or mole size. Because this particular problem starts off in weight, we will assume a certain initial weight, say 100 g. Because 10 wt% of the resin is made of the PEG, this corresponds to 10 g of incorporated PEG. At 1200 g/mol, this is 0.008333 mole (10 g/1200 g/mol). Because one polymeric chain is produced for every molecule of PEG, we can assume that there are 0.008333 mole of polymeric chains present. The weight of the resin was 100 g. We can now estimate the number average molecular weight by dividing the weight (100 g) by the number of moles (0.008333 mole). The $M_n$ is 12,000 g/mol. If we assume a normal molecular weight distribution, the estimated $M_w$ will be two times the $M_n$.

Let us now consider the case in which the PEG is present at 20 wt%. Using a hypothetical case of total 100 g of resin, the number of moles of incorporated PEG is 0.01667 mole (20 g/1200 g/mol). The estimated $M_n$ is 6000 g/mol (100 g/0.01667 mole) and the estimated $M_w$ is twice that value.

In doing these kinds of estimations, greater error is introduced as the molecular weight and the weight fraction of the PEG increases.

## Problem 3

A sample of L(−)-lactide is homopolymerized. The resulting homopolymer exhibits a melting point of 180°C when measured by DSC, differential scanning calorimetry. A sample of D(+)-lactide is then polymerized. What is the expected melting point of this second homopolymer?

## Answer to Problem 3

180°C.

The melting point of the corresponding stereoisomer, poly(D + )-lactide, should be identical. Note the situation is very different if one mixed the corresponding polymers; a sterocomplex of the two types of chains forms with a higher melting point.

## Problem 4

An experiment is conducted in which equal amounts of L(−)-lactide and D(+)-lactide are mixed and the mixture polymerized. What is the melting point of the resulting copolymer?

## Answer to Problem 4

No melting point; this is a trick question.

The resulting copolymer does not crystallize so, by definition, it cannot have crystals that melt and thus, does not have a melting point.

## Problem 5

Many researchers report a glass transition temperature for polyglycolide of approximately 40°C, while providing a value for poly(L(−)-lactide) of 65°C. You have synthesized a copolymer based on a 50/50 weight mixture of the two monomers, glycolide and lactide.

Two means of approximating the glass transition temperature are the Gordon–Fox Equation:

$$T_g = T_{ga}\,\varnothing_a + T_{gb}\varnothing_b$$

and the Fox Equation:

$$1/T_g = W_a/T_{ga} + W_b/T_{gb}$$

where

$T_{ga}$ and $T_{gb}$ = the glass transition temperatures of polymers "a" and "b"

$\varnothing_a$ and $\varnothing_b$ = volume fraction of polymers "a" and "b"

$W_a$ and $W_b$ = the weight fraction of polymers "a" and "b."

Both predict that the glass transition of your copolymer will be above room temperature. (In fact, it should never fall below the glass transition temperature of the homopolymer having the lowest $T_g$.) In spite of this, you find that films and dogbones of your copolymer are quite soft and pliable indicating a $T_g$ below RT. What explanation can you provide?

## Answer to Problem 5

The conversion of monomer to polymer may not be complete leaving residual monomer to plasticize the resin. This residual monomer will lower the $T_g$ substantially, making the polymer soft and pliable at room temperature. Were this material to be used for a device that was implanted in the body, an unusually high tissue reaction may result. This is because a burst of acid groups is created due to the high reactivity of the monomer to water.

## Problem 6

You blend two synthetic absorbable polyesters together using appropriate melt processing equipment. The characteristics of the resulting blend are a function of the blending conditions. At first the blend is crystallizable, but as the blending process continues, the rate of crystallization decreases and eventually the material is rendered noncrystallizable. What is going on?

### Answer to Problem 6

Initially, because of thermodynamic considerations, the blend is a mixture of two separate phases that are not miscible. As blending continues there is a small amount of transesterification that takes place at the phase interface. The small number of resulting block-copolymeric chains then act as emulsifying agents further increasing the amount of intimate mixing. More chains transesterify leading eventually to a single phase. As transesterification continues, the sequence distribution is more and more randomized driving the blend to a random copolymer.

The described phenomena can be observed by following glass transition temperatures: two $T_g$s indicate a biphasic system, while a single glass transition is indicative of a miscible system. Further support for a single miscible phase could come from microscopy and scattering (neutron, x-ray, and light can all be used to characterize miscibility). The rate of crystallization, as well as the ultimate attainable level, decreases as the sequence distribution of the monomer repeat units of the chains randomize.

## Problem 7

You have a small supply of melt-prepared polyglycolide, which was made using dodecanol as the initiator. This resin has a weight average molecular weight of 80,000 g/mol. A sample of the resin is partially dried and then injection molded into test pieces. This requires heating the resin to 240°C, at which point all the water present reacts with the polyester. You find that the molecular weight drops down to 52,000 g/mol. Assume (1) that the drop in molecular weight is entirely due to reaction with the water still present in the only partially dry resin, and (2) a normal molecular weight distribution. (a) What is the relative amount of water originally present? (b) What would the water content have been if the $M_w$ dropped the same percentage, but from 160,000 to 104,000?

### Answer to Problem 7

1. 243 ppm
2. 121 ppm

The $M_w$ is initially 80,000 g/mol; since we are asked to assume a normal molecular weight distribution, the $M_n$ must have been 40,000 g/mol. The "final" $M_w$ is 52,000 g/mol so the "final" $M_n$ must be 26,000 g/mol.

For purposes of problem solving, we can consider the hypothetical case in which the resin has an initial weight of 100 g. (This assumption will have no bearing on the final answer; proof is left to the reader.) If you started with 100 g of polymer and the (number average) molecular weight is 40,000 g/mol, we can calculate that the number of moles of chains present had to be 0.0025 mole (100 g/40,000 g/mol). Once the water reacted with the resin and its $M_n$ dropped to 26,000 g/mol, the number of chains increased to 0.00384615 mole (100 g/26,000 g/mol). Because the reaction of one molecule of water is required to cleave a chain to result in two, shorter chains, we can now calculate the moles of water to be 0.00134615 mole (0.00384615 − 0.0025 mole). Knowing the MW of water, we can calculate the weight of water required to be 0.02425 g (0.00134615 mole × 18.015 g/mol). Because we assume a polymer weight of

100 g, this weight of water and weight of polymer corresponds to a water content of 243 ppm ($0.02425 \text{ g}/100 \text{ g} \times 10^6$). It should be noted that even a small amount of water causes a great drop in molecular weight, which then affects many important properties. It serves to point out the importance of limiting the exposure of these polymers to moisture, even that present in the air, prior to melt processing.

With regards to (b), one uses the same methodology. Note however that at higher molecular weight, the amount of water needed to get the same percent decrease in molecular weight is smaller.

## Problem 8

One encounters difficulty dissolving a particular drug in a DL-lactide/glycolide resin, when it was possible to do so with a previous batch of the "same" material. What could be some of the issues with the new copolymer batch?

### Answer to Problem 8

Overall resin composition/monomer sequence distribution in the copolymer/molecular weight of the resin

There may be a slight variation in the overall composition of the resin; e.g., increasing the incorporated glycolide level slightly could shift solubility. For a given overall composition, monomer sequence distribution may vary from copolymer lot to copolymer lot. If the resin has polymerized glycolide sequences long enough, they may crystallize. Such a material will often not fully dissolve.

Molecular weight may have an impact. If the new resin is higher in molecular weight it may take longer to dissolve; if it is a lot higher, the amount that can be dissolved may be reduced as well.

## Problem 9

I made a sample of a random copolymer based on 13/87 lactide/glycolide. It degrades a bit too fast for the application I have in mind. My colleague suggested making a second material a little richer in lactide because polylactide is known to absorb slower than polyglycolide. I do not follow this advice. Why not?

### Answer to Problem 9

Although homopolymeric polylactide does indeed absorb slower than homopolymeric polyglycolide, copolymerization is a bit more complex. Assume the lactide was doubled to give a composition of 26/74. The relatively larger amount of polymerized lactide interferes with crystallization of the resulting resin. Besides affecting mechanical properties, the amorphous nature of this second resin more readily allows water to enter and react with the ester groups. In the first resin, the esters groups present in the crystals have a reduced rate of reaction because of the close packing that crystallization provides.

## Problem 10

You and your associates have designed a medical implant that you envision to be made of an alpha polyester. You secure resin, and make the device by injection molding. The parts look great. You send them to a contract sterilizer to have them sterilized by ethylene oxide, and the parts come back warped. This is surprising because your contractor assured you that the parts would not be exposed to temperatures higher than 55°C, which is lower than the glass transition of the resin you used to mold the parts. What is the source of your problem and how might you minimize the distortion?

### Answer to Problem 10

Just as residual monomer can lower the $T_g$ of a polylactone, ethylene oxide can plasticize the polymer as well. Although the amount of molecular orientation that is imparted by injection molding is much lower than that imparted by extrusion, it can still be a driving force to cause distortion upon relaxation. A molding engineer might refer to this as "built-in stress". To minimize distortion, employ molding cycles that will lower the initial "stress" in the part, and then employ sterilization cycles that will expose your parts to the lowest possible temperatures when they still have absorbed EO present. In some cases annealing the part to induce crystallization prior to EO exposure may also help, but the biological performance may then shift in an undesirable way.

---

# References

Abuzaina, F.M., Fitz, B.D., Andjelić, S., and Jamiolkowski, D.D., Time resolved study of shear-induced crystallization of poly(*p*-dioxanone) polymers under low-shear, nucleation-enhancing shear conditions by small angle light scattering and optical microscopy, *Polymer*, **43**, 4699 (2002).

Andjelić, S. and Jamiolkowski, D., Tensile property examinations of isothermally grown semi-crystalline films made from absorbable poly(*p*-dioxanone), *J. Appl. Med. Polym.*, **5**, 16 (2001).

Andjelić, S., Fitz, B.D., and Jamiolkowski, D.D., Crystallization in synthetic absorbable polymers, In: *Recent Research Developments in Biomaterials*, Ikada, Y., Ed., Research Signpost, Kerala, India, pp. 153–177 (2002), Chap. 8.

Andjelić, S., Fitz, B.D., and Jamiolkowski, D.D., Advances in morphological development to tailor the performance of absorbable medical devices, In: *Absorbable and Biodegradable Polymers*, Shalaby, S.W. and Burg, K.J.L., Eds., CRC Press, Boca Raton, FL, pp. 113–141 (2003), Chap. 9.

Bezwada, R.S. and Jamiolkowski, D.D., Hydrophilic synthetic absorbable polyoxaesters, *Trans. Sixth World Biomater. Congr.*, **2**, 430 (2000).

Bezwada, R.S., Jamiolkowski, D.D., and Cooper, K., Poly(*p*-dioxanone) and its copolymers, In: *Handbook of Biodegradable Polymers*, Domb, A.J., Kost, J., and Wiseman, D.M., Eds., Harwood Academic Publishers, Australia, pp. 29–61 (1997), Chap. 2.

Bezwada, R.S., Jamiolkowski, D.D., Lee, I.-Y., Agarwal, V., Persivale, J., Trenka-Benthin, S., Erneta, M., Suryadevara, J., Yang, A., and Liu, S., MONOCRYL™ Suture, a new ultra-pliable absorbable monofilament suture, *Biomaterials*, **16**, 1141 (1995).

Chatani, Y., Suehiro, K., Okita, Y., Tadokoro, H., and Chujo, K., Structural studies of polyesters. I. Crystal structure of polyglycolide, *Makromol. Chem.*, **113**, 215 (1968).

Chujo, K., Kobayashi, H., Suzuki, J., Tokuhara, S., and Tanabe, M., Ring-opening polymerization of glycolide, *Makromol. Chem.*, **100**, 262 (1967).

Craig, P.H., Williams, J.A., Davis, K.W., Magoun, A.D., Levy, A.J., Bogdansky, S., and Jones, J.P., A biological comparison of polyglactin 910 and polyglycolic acid synthetic absorbable sutures, *Surg. Gynecol. Obstet.*, **141**, 1 (1975).

Fitz, B.D., Jamiolkowski, D.D., and Andjelić, S., Tg depression in poly(L(−)-lactide) crystallized under partially constrained conditions, *Macromolecules*, **35**, 5869 (2002).

Gogolewski, S. and Mainil-Varlet, P., The effect of thermal treatment on sterility, molecular and mechanical properties of various polylactides; I. Poly(L-lactide), *Biomaterials*, **17**, 523 (1996).

Hollinger, J.O., Jamiolkowski, D.D., and Shalaby, S.W., Poly(alpha esters) and bone repair, In: *Biomedical Applications of Synthetic Biodegradable Polymers*, Hollinger, J.O., Ed., CRC Press, New York, pp. 197–222 (1995), Chap. 9.

Loomis, G.L., Murdock, J.R., and Gardner, K., New materials from the organization of enantiomeric polylactides, *Trans. 15th Annu. Mtg. Soc. Biomater.*, **12**, 73 (1989).

Migliaresi, C., De Lollis, A., Fambri, L., and Cohn, D., The effect of thermal history on the crystallinity of different molecular weight PLLA biodegradable polymers, *Clin. Mater.*, **8**, 111 (1991).

Murdock, J.R. and Loomis, G.L., U.S. Patents 4,719,246 and 4,766,182, (1988).

Park, A. and Cima, L.G., *In Vitro* cell response to differences in poly-L-lactide crystallinity, *J. Biomed. Mater. Res.*, **31**, 117 (1996).

Ray, J.A., Doddi, N., Regula, D., Williams, J.A., and Melveger, A., Polydioxanone (PDS™), a novel monofilament synthetic absorbable suture, *Surg. Gynecol. Obstet.*, **153**, 497 (1981).

Weiler, W. and Gogolewski, S., Enhancement of the mechanical properties of polylactides by solid-state extrusion; I. Poly(D-lactide), *Biomaterials*, **17**, 529 (1996).

## Further Information

Chu, C.C., von Fraunhofer, J.A., and Greisler, H.P., *Wound Closure Biomaterials and Devices*, CRC Press, Boca Raton, FL (1996).

Shalaby, S.W., *Biomedical Polymers: Designed-to-Degrade Systems*, Hanser Publishers, New York (1994).

# 10

## *Polyurethanes*

Scott A. Guelcher

**CONTENTS**

Polyurethanes comprise a diverse family of materials, including thermoplastic and cast elastomers, flexible and rigid foams, fibers, coatings, and sealants. First commercialized in the 1930s, polyurethane products are sold into a number of industrial markets, including automotive, seating, apparel, and insulation. They were initially developed for biomedical applications in the 1960s (Lelah and Cooper, 1986) with the introduction of the segmented polyurethane elastomer Biomer® into the cardiovascular market. Applications of polyurethanes in medicine have been reviewed (Wilkes, 1975; Woodhouse and Skarja, 2001). Through the careful selection of raw materials and processing conditions, materials having a wide range of mechanical, biological, and physical properties can be prepared. For example, tissue engineered scaffolds are designed to support significant attachment and proliferation of cells, while blood-contact materials (such as heart valves and catheters) are designed to promote minimal protein adhesion. Another important design consideration is the biostability of polyurethane implants. Specifically, tissue engineered scaffolds for bone are designed to degrade at a rate in register with tissue healing and remodeling, while pacemaker lead insulation is designed to resist degradation for many years.

   This chapter comprises three sections. In Section 10.1, the fundamentals of polyurethane chemistry, including synthesis, processing, and structure-property relationships, are presented. Nondegradable biomedical polyurethane implants are discussed in Section 10.2 and degradable tissue engineered polyurethane scaffolds are reviewed in Section 10.3.

## 10.1   Fundamentals of Polyurethane Chemistry

### 10.1.1   Isocyanates

Isocyanates, characterized by $-N=C=O$ functionality, react with nucleophiles (e.g., alcohols and amines) by addition to the carbon-nitrogen double bond as shown in Figure 10.1. Their chemistry has been extensively reviewed (Oertel, 1994; Szycher, 1999). Isocyanates react with alcohols to form urethane linkages (Figure 10.1a) and with amines to form urea linkages (Figure 10.1b). Isocyanates also react with water to

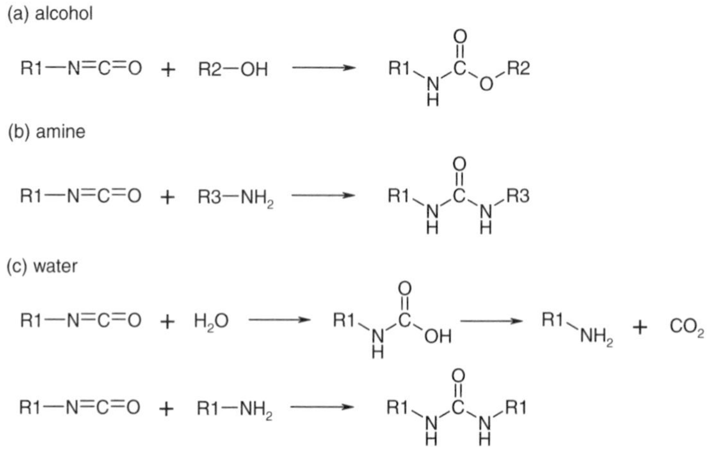

**FIGURE 10.1**
Reactions of isocyanates with molecules containing an active hydrogen.

form carbamic acid, an unstable compound that decomposes to an amine and carbon dioxide gas (Figure 10.1c). The water reaction is important in the synthesis of polyurethane foams, where the carbon dioxide gas functions as a biocompatible blowing agent. Other compounds with active hydrogens, such as carboxylic acids, ureas, urethanes, and amides also react with isocyanates; these reactions have been reviewed elsewhere (Oertel, 1994; Szycher, 1999).

Polyurethanes are synthesized from both aromatic and aliphatic isocyanates. The structures of commercially significant polyisocyanates are shown in Table 10.1. Aromatic polyisocyanates include 4,4′-methylenebis (phenyl isocyanate) and toluene diisocyanate (TDI), while aliphatic isocyanates include 4,4′-methylenebis (cyclohexyl isocyanate), hexamethylene diisocyanate (HDI), isophorone diisocyanate (IPDI), 1,4-diisocyanato-butane (BDI), and lysine methyl ester diisocyanate (LDI). Aromatic isocyanates are approximately 5 to 10 times more reactive (Szycher, 1999) and typically yield polyurethanes with superior mechanical properties (Frisch et al., 1971) relative to aliphatic isocyanates; however, they are generally more toxic. The free NCO content of a

**TABLE 10.1**

Commercially Significant Polyisocyanates

| Chemical Name | Structure |
| --- | --- |
| 4,4′-methylenebis (phenyl isocyanate) | |
| 2,4- and 2,6-toluene diisocyanate (TDI) | |
| 1,6-diisocyanatohexane (HDI) | |
| 1,4-diisocyanatobutane (BDI) | |
| Isophorone diisocyanate (IPDI) | |
| 4,4′-methylenebis (cyclohexyl isocyanate) | |
| Lysine methyl ester diisocyanate (LDI) | |

polyisocyanate, typically measured by titration, is an important quantity in formulating polyurethanes

$$\% \text{ free NCO} = \frac{42}{w} = \frac{42f}{M} \tag{10.1}$$

where $w$ $\langle \text{Da eq}^{-1} \rangle$ is the equivalent weight, $f$ is the functionality, and $M$ is the molecular weight of the polyisocyanate.

### 10.1.2 Polyols

Polyols are compounds comprising a polyether, polycarbonate, polyester, polydimethyl-siloxane, or polybutadiene backbone and hydroxyl end groups. They are typically viscous liquids with molecular weights ranging from 400 to 5000 g/mol. Synthesis of polyols has been reviewed elsewhere (Oertel, 1994; Szycher, 1999). Examples of commercially significant polyols are listed in Table 10.2.

Polyols are typically prepared by reacting a small starter molecule with a monomer(s) to increase molecular weight. The functionality $f$ is defined as the number of reactive terminal hydroxyl or amine groups and is controlled by the choice of starter, which typically is a small molecule such as butanediol ($f = 2$), glycerol ($f = 3$), pentaerythritol ($f = 4$), or sucrose ($f = 8$). The molecular weight of the polyol is controlled by varying the ratio of monomers to starter. The polyol component of the polyurethane significantly affects the *in vivo* stability of the material. Typically, the hydrolytic stability of polyols observes the order polycarbonate > polyether > polyester.

The hydroxyl number (OH number) of a polyol is typically measured by titration and is an important quantity in formulating polyurethanes

$$\text{Hydroxyl number} = \frac{56.1 \times 10^3}{w} = 56.1 \times 10^3 \frac{f}{m} \tag{10.2}$$

### 10.1.3 Prepolymers and Chain Extension

NCO-terminated prepolymers are oligomeric intermediates with isocyanate functionality synthesized by reacting a polyol with an excess of diisocyanate as shown in Figure 10.2.

**TABLE 10.2**

Commonly Used Polyols

| Chemical Name | Structure |
|---|---|
| Poly(propylene oxide) (PPO) | 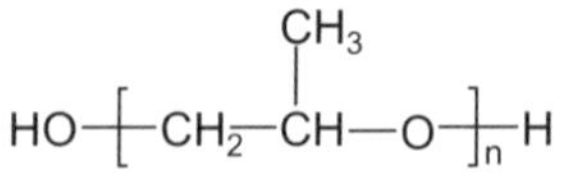 HO-[CH₂-CH(CH₃)-O]ₙ-H |
| Poly(ethylene oxide) (PEO) | 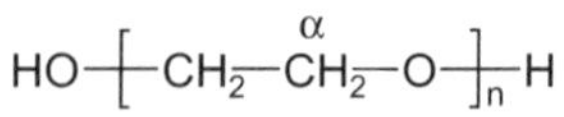 HO-[CH₂-CH₂-O]ₙ-H |
| Poly(tetramethylene oxide) (PTMO) | 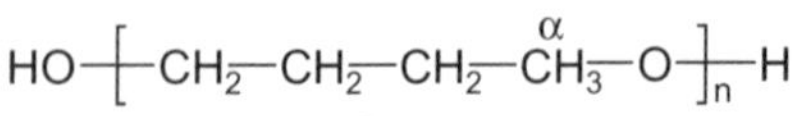 HO-[CH₂-CH₂-CH₂-CH₃-O]ₙ-H |
| Polycaprolactone diol (PCL) | 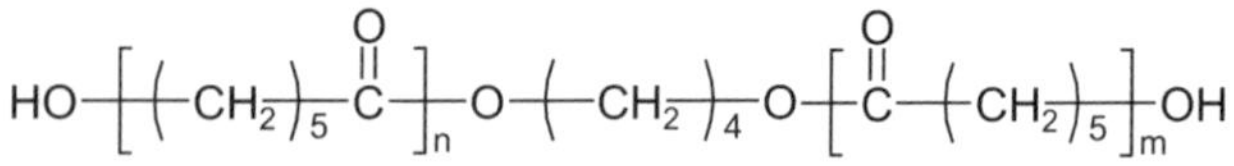 HO-[(CH₂)₅-C(=O)]ₙ-O-(CH₂)₄-O-[C(=O)-(CH₂)₅]ₘ-OH |
| Poly(di(ethylene glycol)adipate) (PDEA) (structure of repeat unit) | 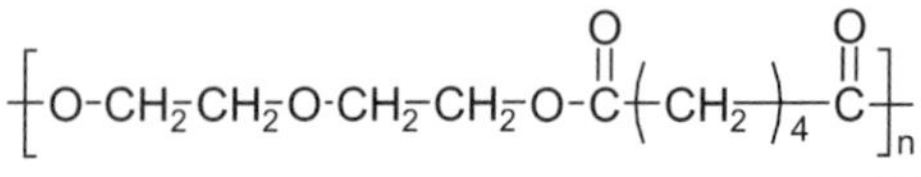 [O-CH₂CH₂O·CH₂CH₂O-C(=O)-(CH₂)₄-C(=O)]ₙ |

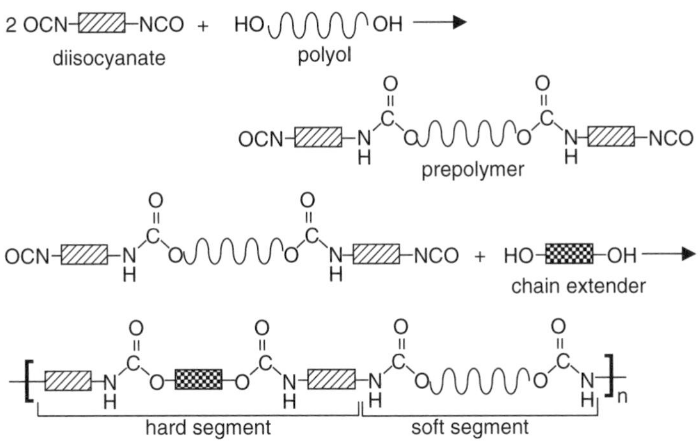

**FIGURE 10.2**
Schematic of polyurethane synthesis via the prepolymer process.

Prepolymers are typically prepared at 60–90°C in the presence of a urethane catalyst, such as dibutyltin dilaurate. The NCO:OH ratio of the prepolymer is defined as

$$\text{NCO : OH ratio} = \frac{q_{\text{NCO,I}}}{q_{\text{OH,P}}} = \frac{m_{\text{I}}/w_{\text{I}}}{m_{\text{P}}/w_{\text{P}}} \tag{10.3}$$

where $q_i = m_i/w_i$ is the number of equivalents and $m_i$ is the mass of component i (subscript I denotes the isocyanate, C the chain extender, and P the polyol). By varying the NCO:OH equivalent ratio it is possible to prepare prepolymers with targeted free NCO content and average molecular weight; this ability to tailor-make intermediates differentiates polyurethanes from other polymers, such as polyolefins. The free NCO content (see Equation 10.1) of prepolymers typically ranges from 1 to 15 wt%; materials with free NCO contents ranging from 16 to 32 wt% have a significant amount of free isocyanate monomer and are referred to as quasi-prepolymers (Szycher, 1999). A large excess of isocyanate (e.g., NCO:OH equivalent ratio > 3) is required to prepare quasi-prepolymers.

In the chain extension step (Figure 10.2), a short-chain (e.g., <500 g/mol) diamine or diol chain extender is added to the prepolymer to yield a high molecular weight polyurethane. Typical chain extenders are listed in Table 10.3. Chain extenders with functionality equal to two yield linear segmented polyurethanes, while chain extenders with functionality greater than two yield chemically cross-linked materials. Using the prepolymer process, greater control can be gained over the structure and properties of the polyurethane than can be achieved using the one-shot process where all the reactants are mixed at once (Oertel, 1994). For example, a more uniform hard segment size distribution resulting in enhanced microphase separation (Spaans et al., 1998) can typically be achieved via the prepolymer process compared to the one-shot process.

The index is defined as the ratio of NCO equivalents in the isocyanate to the total number of OH and NH$_2$ equivalents in the polyol and chain extender:

$$\text{INDEX} = 100 \times \frac{q_{\text{NCO,I}}}{q_{\text{OH,C}} + q_{\text{OH,P}}} = 100 \times \frac{m_{\text{I}}/w_{\text{I}}}{m_{\text{C}}/w_{\text{C}} + m_{\text{P}}/w_{\text{P}}} \tag{10.4}$$

**TABLE 10.3**

Chain Extenders

| Chemical Name | Structure |
| --- | --- |
| 1,4-Butanediol (BDO) | 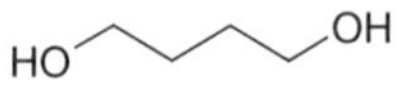 |
| Ethylenediamine (EDA) | 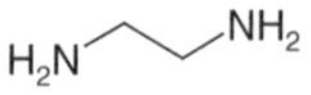 |
| Putrescine | 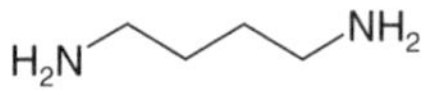 |
| 1,3-Diamino-2-hydroxypropane | 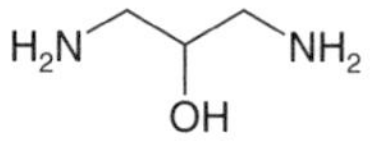 |
| BDO.BDI.BDO (Spaans et al., 1998a) | 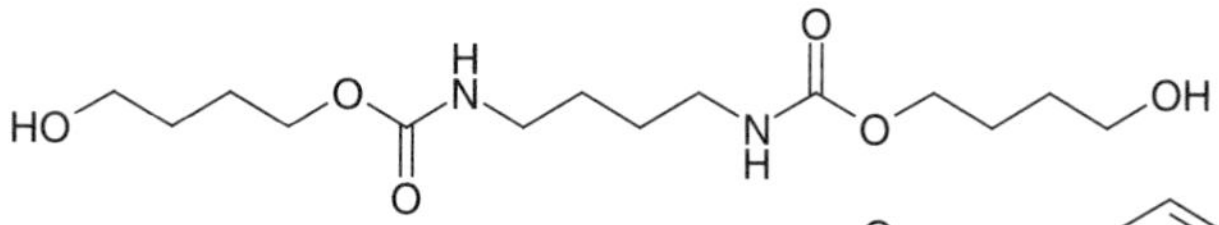 |
| TyA.BDI.TyA (Guelcher et al., 2005a) | 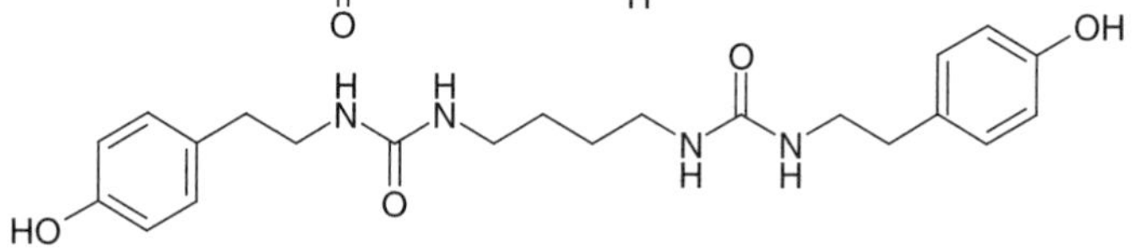 |
| Phe.CHDM.Phe (Skarja and Woodhouse 1998, 2000) | 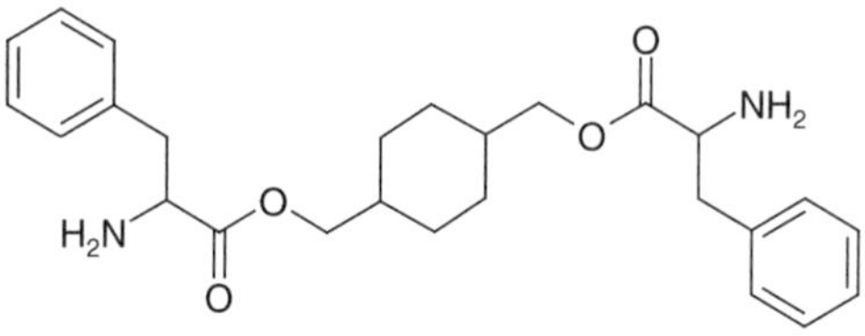 |

The index typically varies between 100 and 125 to ensure complete conversion to high molecular weight polymer. It is important to note that although the sum of hydroxyl and amine equivalents is specified by the index, the ratio of chain extender to polyol in the polyurethane can be varied over a wide range by modulating the free NCO content of the prepolymer.

### 10.1.4 Segmented Polyurethane Elastomers

#### 10.1.4.1 *Microphase Separation and Hydrogen Bonding*

Segmented polyurethane elastomers are linear block copolymers composed of alternating hard and soft segments. As shown in Figure 10.2, the isocyanate and chain extender comprise the hard segment while the polyol comprises the soft segment. The high-melting (typically > 100°C), polar hard segments are generally incompatible with the low-melting or amorphous, nonpolar soft segments, thereby promoting microphase-separation of the segmented polyurethane as shown in Figure 10.3. Urethane and urea groups in the hard segments of adjacent polymer chains can form hydrogen bonds (Figure 10.4) that induce the formation of ordered hard segments. Hard segments have been suggested to aggregate to form ordered cylinders 25 Å in diameter by 55 Å long as illustrated in Figure 10.3b (Eisenbach et al., 1994). These microphase-separated, ordered hard domains function as physical cross-links that resist flow when stress is applied to the material. The physical cross-links can be disrupted by heating the material above the hard segment melting

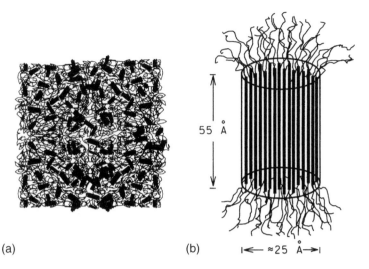

**FIGURE 10.3**
(a) Microphase separation and (b) formation of domain structure in segmented polyurethanes (*Source*: Eisenbach, C.D., Ribbe, A., and Gunter, C., *Macromolecular Rapid Communications*, **15**, 395, (1994). With permission.)

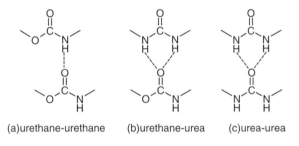

**FIGURE 10.4**
Examples of hydrogen bonding that commonly occur in polyurethanes (*Source*: Gisselfält K. *Structure Dependent Chemical and Biological Interactions of Poly (urethane urea)s*, Chalmers University of Technology, Göteborg, Sweden (2002). With permission.)

transition or by dissolving the material in an aprotic solvent (e.g., dimethylformamide (DMF) or dimethylacetamide (DMAc)). The soft segment typically has a glass transition temperature less than 0°C and is therefore rubbery and amorphous at the use temperature.

### 10.1.4.2 Structure–Property Relationships

The structure of the hard segment has a profound effect on hard segment ordering and material properties. Diamine chain extenders yield poly(urethane urea)s, which typically have higher hard segment melting temperatures, and therefore harder mechanical properties, compared to polyurethanes prepared from diol chain extenders (Oertel, 1994). Furthermore, chain extenders with an even number of carbon atoms in the backbone promote enhanced hard segment ordering relative to those having an odd number of carbon atoms (Oertel, 1994). The relative fractions of the hard and soft segments also affect the mechanical properties of segmented polyurethanes. Hard segment content increases with decreasing polyol molecular weight, thereby yielding harder and stiffer polymers with higher tear strength but lower elongation at break. The data in Table 10.4 illustrate the effect of hard segment content on polymer stiffness and elongation at break. As the poly(ε-caprolactone) (PCL) diol soft segment molecular weight decreases from 2000 to

**TABLE 10.4**

Mechanical Properties of Poly(Urethane Urea) Fibers Prepared From MDI-Polyester Diol Prepolymers and an Ethylenediamine (EDA) Chain Extender

| Polyester diol Soft Segment | Hard Segment Content (%) | Stiffness (kN mm$^{-1}$) | Elongation at Break (%) |
|---|---|---|---|
| PDEA500 | 52.8 | 17 ± 1 | 50 ± 5 |
| PDEA1000 | 35.9 | 6 ± 0.4 | 120 ± 10 |
| PDEA2000 | 21.9 | 6 ± 0.5 | 130 ± 13 |
| PCL530 | 51.4 | 45 ± 2 | 32 ± 8 |
| PCL1250 | 30.9 | 6 ± 0.4 | 74 ± 14 |
| PCL2000 | 21.9 | 6 ± 0.3 | 77 ± 12 |

Data reproduced from Gisselfält K. *Structure Dependent Chemical and Biological Interactions of Poly (urethane urea)s*, Chalmers University of Technology, Göteborg, Sweden (2002). With permission. Two different polyester diols were evaluated: polycaprolactone diol (PCL) and poly(di(ethylene glycol) adipate) (PDEA).

530 g mol$^{-1}$, the hard segment content increases from 21.9 to 51.4 wt%, the stiffness increases from 6 to 45 N mm$^{-1}$, and the elongation at break decreases from 77 to 32%. As expected, the polymer becomes harder and less elastic with increasing hard segment content. The poly(di(ethylene glycol)adipate) (PDEA) diol soft segments yield poly-urethane fibers that are somewhat softer and weaker than those prepared from PCL diols, possibly due to the lesser degree of microphase-separation in the PDEA polyurethanes.

### 10.1.4.3  Processing

Segmented polyurethane elastomers are processed by a variety of techniques depending on the composition of the material. They are often synthesized by solution polymerization in DMF or DMAc. Polyurethanes with hard segment melting temperatures below the decomposition temperature are thermoplastic and can therefore be processed by extrusion, melt spinning, or injection molding. Poly(urethane urea)s prepared from diamine chain extenders typically have hard segment melting transitions greater than the decomposition temperature ($\sim 250°C$) and therefore must be processed in aprotic solvents (DMF, DMAc) by techniques such as solvent casting of films, wet-spinning of fibers, or electro-spinning of fibers (Stankus et al., 2004). Segmented polyurethanes can also be cast by reactive liquid molding (Section 10.1.5) if the intermediates are liquids at the process temperature.

### 10.1.5  Cast Polyurethanes

As shown in Figure 10.5, two-component polyurethanes are prepared via a reactive liquid molding process wherein an NCO-functional resin is mixed with an OH-functional hardener and cast into a mold. The reactive liquid mixture cures in the mold where it hardens to form a solid. The NCO-functional resin can either be a polyisocyanate or an NCO-terminated prepolymer. The OH-functional hardener comprises all components with an active hydrogen (e.g., polyols, chain extenders, cross-linkers, and water) and optional additives, such as catalyst, stabilizer, fillers, and pore opener. Segmented polyurethane elastomers, cross-linked thermosets, and porous foams can all be processed by reactive liquid molding.

Chemically cross-linked polyurethanes are cast from components with functionality greater than two. If the extent of chemical cross-linking is sufficiently high, then the material is an insoluble thermoset. Polyols, such as triols and hexols, and low molecular

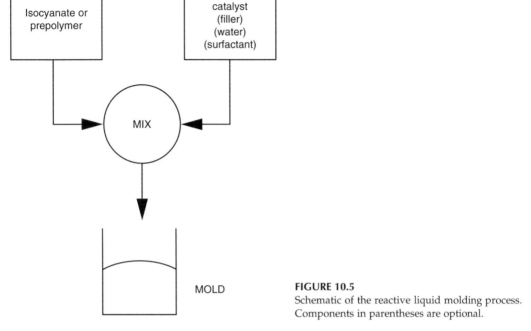

**FIGURE 10.5**
Schematic of the reactive liquid molding process. Components in parentheses are optional.

weight triol and triamine cross-linkers are commonly used to prepare chemically cross-linked polyurethanes (Oertel, 1994).

## 10.2 Biomedical Implants

Due to their toughness, versatility, durability, biocompatibility, and biostability, polyurethanes have been used in a wide variety of implantable biomedical devices (Lelah and Cooper, 1986; Stokes and McVenes, 1995). Examples of commercial applications are presented in Section 10.2.1 and Section 10.2.2. As with other implanted devices, monocytes are recruited to the surface of the material *in vivo*, where they can differentiate into macrophages and foreign body giant cells (FBGC) (Matheson et al., 2004). When activated, macrophages can release components which facilitate the chemical degradation of polyurethane implants. The mechanisms of degradation, as well as efforts to stabilize polyurethane implants, are reviewed in Section 10.2.3.

### 10.2.1 Historical Background

Segmented polyurethane elastomers are widely used in the manufacture of biomedical implants intended for long-term service. Due to their excellent mechanical properties and adequate biocompatibility (Lelah and Cooper, 1986), biomedical-grade polyurethane elastomers have been used in a number of applications, such as ligament reconstructions (Spaans et al., 2000), blood-contact materials (Thomas et al., 2001), infusion pumps (Szycher, 1999), heart valves (Hoffman et al., 1993), insulators for pacemaker electrical leads (Capone, 1992), bandages (Oertel, 1994), blood dialyzers (Oertel, 1994), and cardiovascular catheters (Oertel, 1994; Szycher, 1999).

**TABLE 10.5**

Commercial Biomedical-Grade Polyurethanes

| Trade Name | Manufacturer | Isocyanate | Chain Extender | Polyol |
|---|---|---|---|---|
| Duraflex™ | VASCOR, Inc. (Capone, 1992) | H12MDI | 1,4-butanediol | Non-polyether |
| Tecoflex® EG-85A | Thermedics, Inc. (Capone, 1992) | H12MDI | 1,4-butanediol | Polyether |
| Tecothane TT1074A | Termedics, Inc. (Alferiev, 2002) | MDI | 1,4-butanediol | PTMEG |
| Biomer® | Ethicon (Reed et al., 1994) | MDI | Ethylene diamine/1,3-diaminocyclohexane | PTMEG |
| ChronoFlex® AR | PolyMedica (Reed et al., 1994) | MDI | Ethylene diamine/1,3-diaminocyclohexane | Polycarbonate |
| PurSil™ | Polymer Technology Group | MDI | Low molecular weight glycol | Polydimethylsiloxane/PTMEG |
| CarboSil™ | Polymer Technology Group | MDI | Low molecular weight glycol | Polydimethylsiloxane/polycarbonate |
| Elasthane™ | Polymer Technology Group | MDI | Butanediol | PTMEG |
| Bionate® | Polymer Technology Group | MDI | Diamine | Polycarbonate |
| BioSpan® | Polymer Technology Group | MDI | Diamine | Polyether |
| Pellethane® 2363-55D | Dow Chemical (Martin et al., 1999) | MDI | 2,4-butanediol | PTMEG |

Biomer was withdrawn from the market in 1991.

One of the first biomedical polyurethanes, Biomer® (Table 10.5), was commercialized in the 1960s by Ethicon, Inc., which had licensed the technology from DuPont (Reed et al., 1994). Biomer® was first investigated as a biomaterial in 1967 (Pierce and Turner, 1967) and has been used in cardiovascular applications, such as heart-assist pumps, catheters, and artificial hearts. However, in 1991 Ethicon withdrew Biomer® from the market due to surface microcracking of the polyether soft segment.

Commercial biomedical-grade polyurethane elastomers are manufactured from a variety of intermediates, as shown in Table 10.5. Biomedical polyurethane implants are typically prepared from either MDI or $H_{12}MDI$, a short-chain glycol chain extender, and either a polyether or polycarbonate polyol.

## 10.2.2 Commercial Applications

### 10.2.2.1 Cardiac Pacemakers

When the natural electrical system of a patient's heart is impaired, cardiac pacemakers are used to electrically stimulate the heart to restore its regular muscular contractions necessary for the adequate flow of blood through the body. Connectors, insulators, tines, and adhesives composed of poly(ether urethanes) commonly used in cardiac pacemakers have performed reliably in clinical applications for almost 30 years (Szycher, 1999; Coury, 2004). Thermoplastic polyurethanes are useful for pacemaker lead insulation because of a favorable combination of properties, such as high tensile strength ($>35$ MPa), high elasticity, and adequate blood compatibility (Szycher, 1999). Furthermore, the polyurethane softens significantly 1 h after insertion into the body, which enables the clinician to insert a rigid lead that softens *in vivo* to avoid damage to the heart. In some cases, poly(ether urethane) lead insulation has exhibited surface cracks after months to years post implantation, which has been attributed to degradation by metal ion-induced oxidation (Coury, 2004).

### 10.2.2.2 Cardiovascular Disease

Segmented polyurethane elastomers are also used in a number of treatments for cardiovascular disease, such as angiography catheters and transluminal angioplasty catheters (Szycher, 1999). In the coronary angiography procedure, a thin and flexible catheter is inserted into the aorta of a patient. A radiopaque dye is then injected which enables the visualization of the coronary arteries, as well as the source of the blockage, under radiography.

For patients whose coronary arteries are partially blocked by fatty deposits, angioplasty offers a lower-cost and lower-risk alternative to bypass surgery. In the angioplasty procedure illustrated in Figure 10.6, a catheter with a balloon at the tip is inserted into a clogged artery where the balloon is then repeatedly inflated to flatten the deposits. Balloons are frequently prepared from fabric-reinforced polyurethane elastomers due to their favorable biological and mechanical properties, such as low permanent deformation, high elongation at break, and adequate blood compatibility that results in a minimal risk of forming blood clots during the procedure.

### 10.2.2.3 Infusion Pumps

In recent years, there has been an increased interest in controlled drug delivery techniques. Compared to more conventional treatments, infusion pumps that intravenously deliver a constant dosage of a drug offer significant advantages, such as increased patient compliance and reduced drug side effects (Szycher, 1999). The pump is connected to a vein

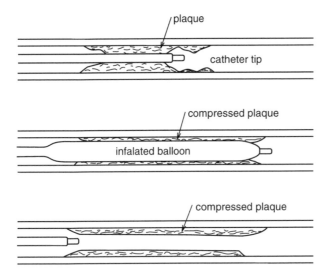

**FIGURE 10.6**
Schematic of the angioplasty procedure. (a) A balloon-tipped catheter is inserted into a blocked artery. (b) The balloon is repeatedly inflated, thereby compressing the atherosclerotic plaque against the artery wall. (c) The catheter is withdrawn from the artery, which now has an increased cross-sectional area. (*Source*: Adapted from Szycher, M., *Szycher's Handbook of Polyurethanes*, CRC Press, Boca Raton, FL (1999). With permission.)

via a needle and catheter. Infusion pump systems incorporating Tecoflex® poly(ether urethane) catheters with an outer diameter of only 0.38 mm have been utilized for cancer treatment and control of diabetes. Because they can deliver medication directly to the diseased organ (e.g., the liver), infusion pumps have the potential to significantly reduce side effects associated with conventional chemotherapy.

### 10.2.2.4   *Peritoneal Dialysis*

In patients afflicted with end-stage kidney disease (ESKD), the kidneys no longer execute their important task of cleansing the patient's blood. Peritoneal dialysis is a treatment wherein sterile fluids are periodically injected into the patient's abdomen through a catheter. The peritoneum, a membrane that surrounds the abdomen, is used as a pathway for the removal of waste products from the blood. Tecoflex® poly(ether urethane) has been approved by the FDA for use as peritoneal dialysis catheters (Szycher, 1999).

### 10.2.3   Biostability of Polyurethane Implants

The soft segment of polyurethane elastomers is subject to chemical degradation *in vivo*. Recent work has focused on identifying the mechanisms of degradation *in vivo* (Zhao et al., 1991, 1995; Anderson et al., 1992). *In vitro* treatments have been developed that simulate the *in vivo* degradation (Anderson et al., 1998). Based on improved understanding of the degradation mechanisms, new soft segment compositions have been developed to improve the biostability of polyurethane elastomers.

### 10.2.3.1   *Polyester Soft Segments*

In the 1950s, polyurethane foams prepared from aromatic polyisocyanates and polyester polyols were commercialized for orthopedic reconstructive surgery and plastic surgery applications (Bloch and Hastings, 1972). Although acute inflammation was minimal, there were undesirable long-term effects resulting from hydrolytic degradation of the adipate ester soft segment (Bloch and Hastings, 1972). However, despite the known hydrolytic degradation of poly(ester urethanes), clinicians have continued to use poly(ester urethane) foam-coated silicone mammary implants for many years (Blais, 1990).

### 10.2.3.2 Polyether Soft Segments

Due to their improved resistance to hydrolysis, polyether polyols have replaced polyester polyols for many biomedical implant applications. However, although hydrolytically stable, polyethers undergo environmental stress cracking through a combination of both chemical degradation and mechanical stress (Zhao et al., 1995; Schubert et al., 1995; Szycher, 1988). The mechanism of chemical degradation appears to be oxidative attack on the $\alpha$-methylene carbon of the polyether (Stokes et al., 1990; Zhao et al., 1993; Wu et al., 1992; Schubert et al., 1997) (see Table 10.2 for the location of the $\alpha$-methylene carbon). The oxidative attack results in chain scission of the polyether to form an ester (Anderson et al., 1998). Coury has presented a detailed review of the process of oxidative biodegradation (Coury, 2004).

Cells are an important component of the degradation process. Recognizing the polyurethane implant as a foreign body, monocytes are recruited to the surface of the implant where they may differentiate into macrophages that fuse to form foreign body giant cells (FBGC)s (Matheson et al., 2004). These cells then release hydroxyl and/or hydroperoxide radicals (Zhao et al., 1991), which promote oxidation and chain scission of the polyether soft segment (Anderson et al., 1998). Diffusion of oxygen into the polyurethane provides a source of radicals for the autooxidation process. If the polymer is not stressed, the depth of the degraded layer (which is controlled by oxygen diffusion) is about 10 μm (Schubert et al., 1997).

Chemical degradation and mechanical deformation contribute synergistically to environmental stress cracking of polyurethane implants. The effects of both stress and strain on oxidative degradation have been investigated but are not completely understood. Some evidence indicates that stress or strain can accelerate failure of polyurethane implants through propagation of cracks in the degraded surface layer into the bulk (Wu et al., 1994). Initially, chemical degradation resulting in chain scission creates small flaws which can grow into small pits under the influence of an applied deformation. The small pits coalesce to form large pits which can eventually result in tearing and failure of the implant (Anderson et al., 1998). Other evidence (e.g., creep (Wu et al., 1994) and constant strain studies (Schubert et al., 1995, 1997)) indicates that the primary effect of deformation is a reduction in the degradation rate due to stress-induced crystallization of the polyether soft segment (Wu et al., 1994). Under conditions of uniaxial stress, orientation and crystallization of the soft segment is more easily attained than under conditions of biaxial stress (Anderson et al., 1998).

### 10.2.3.3 Stabilization of Biomedical Implants

The stability of polyurethane implants can be increased by decreasing the susceptibility of the polyether soft segment to oxidative degradation. Antioxidants, such as vitamin E ($\alpha$-tocopherol), have been added to poly(ether urethane urea)s to slow degradation (Anderson et al., 1998). An alternative approach to improving soft segment stability is incorporating ether- and ester-free soft segments, such as polycarbonates, polydimethyl-siloxane (PDMS), dimerized fatty acid derivatives, and hydrogenated polybutadiene polyols (Coury et al., 1990; Pinchuk et al., 1991; Takahara et al., 1991, 1994; Kato et al., 1995; Mathur et al., 1997; Anderson et al., 1998; Coury, 2004). Polyurethanes with PDMS soft segments have been reported to be stable *in vitro* to both hydrolysis and oxidation (Takahara et al., 1991). Polyurethanes with polycarbonate soft segments have improved resistance to oxidative degradation relative to polyethers (Capone, 1992; Anderson et al., 1998). However, hydrolytic degradation of poly(carbonate urethanes) is possible due to the acidic environment (pH 3.5 to 3.7) at the macrophage/FBGC-material interface which catalyzes the hydrolysis of the carbonate linkage (Ward et al., 1996; Anderson et al., 1998).

In short-term studies, poly(carbonate urethanes) implanted in an *in vivo* cage for time intervals of 1, 2, 3, 5, and 10 weeks demonstrated no indications of degradation in SEM analysis. However, after 5 weeks there was a decrease in the amount of carbonate bonds, which was attributed to hydrolysis (Mathur et al., 1997). Hydrolysis was also detected in longer term (i.e., up to 3 years) *in vivo* studies (Seifalian et al., 2003). Long-term studies of 5 years or longer are necessary to determine the feasibility of poly(carbonate urethane) implants (Coury, 2004).

More recently, surface-modifying end groups (SMEs) (Ward et al., 1995, 1998; Ward and White, 1996) and surface-modifying macromolecules (SMMs) (Santerre et al., 2000) have been developed to improve the oxidative stability of polyurethane implants. SMMs are typically fluorocarbon polymers that are mechanically blended with a polyurethane prior to fabrication of the implant. The fluorocarbon component migrates to the surface of the implant where it protects the polyurethane from oxidative degradation. SMEs are moieties (e.g., 2000 Da polydimethylsiloxaneamine) that are covalently bound to the polymer backbone during synthesis via terminal isocyanate groups. The surface-active endgroups migrate to the surface of the polymer but leave the original polymer backbone intact. The advantage of the technology is that it enables the preparation of polyurethane implants with surfaces that are more resistant to oxidative attack. *In vivo* studies have demonstrated that both SMMs and SMEs enhance the stability of polyurethane implants.

## 10.3   Degradable Tissue Engineered Scaffolds

The design criteria for tissue engineered scaffolds differ considerably from those for nondegradable implants. For bone and cartilage regeneration, scaffolds are designed to degrade *in vivo* over a specified time period to nontoxic degradation products. Excessively rapid degradation can result in accumulation of decomposition products that damage neighboring tissue (Aurell et al., 2002). However, if the degradation rate is too slow, then stress-shielding can occur, resulting in degradation of neighboring tissue (Silvaggio and Fu, 1990; Aurell et al., 2002; Gisselfält et al., 2002). Scaffolds must also support the in-growth of tissue and meet mechanical and physical properties targets.

An important design consideration is the toxicity of the degradation products associated with the diisocyanates. Biomedical implants fabricated from segmented polyurethane elastomers (e.g., catheters and pacemaker leads) frequently incorporate the aromatic diisocyanate MDI in order to obtain favorable mechanical properties such as low permanent deformation and high elongation. However, these materials are typically prepared from polyether, polycarbonate, and polydimethlysiloxane soft segments that are more hydrolytically stable than polyesters. Poly(ester urethanes) prepared from aromatic diisocyanates have been reported to degrade to acutely toxic, carcinogenic, and mutagenic aromatic diamines (Szycher and Siciliano, 1991), although the question of whether the concentrations of these harmful degradation products attain physiologically relevant levels is currently unresolved and strongly debated (Blais, 1990; Szycher and Siciliano, 1991; Coury, 2004). Therefore, research has been undertaken to synthesize degradable polyurethanes that mitigate the potential risk associated with toxic aromatic diamine degradation products. In one approach, aliphatic diisocyanates, particularly lysine methyl ester diisocyanate (LDI) and 1,4-diisocyanatobutane (BDI), have been used to synthesize biodegradable polyurethane scaffolds. Potential degradation products associated with these aliphatic diisocyanates include the biological diamines lysine and putrescine, respectively.

Degradable scaffolds have been prepared from segmented polyurethane elastomers and from two-component polyurethanes cast via reactive liquid molding processes. These materials have been reported to support the attachment, proliferation, and differentiation of cells *in vitro*, to support tissue in-growth with minimal immunogenic response *in vivo*, and to degrade *in vitro* and *in vivo* to nontoxic components.

## 10.3.1   Segmented Polyurethane Elastomers

### 10.3.1.1   *Musculoskeletal*

In order to prepare biodegradable tissue engineered scaffolds from MDI, the potential risk associated with toxic aromatic diamine degradation products must be mitigated (Szycher and Siciliano, 1991). By controlling the frequency of ester linkages in the backbone, aromatic segmented poly(ester urethanes) have been synthesized that degrade to noncytotoxic fragments smaller than 2000 Da that are eliminated from the body. (Aurell et al., 2002; Gisselfält, 2002; Gisselfält et al., 2002). The hard segment of the poly(ester urethane) comprises MDI and a diamine (e.g., ethylenediamine or 1,3-diaminopropane) chain extender while the soft segment comprises either poly(di(ethylene glycol)adipate) (PDEA) or poly(ε-caprolactone) (PCL) diol. These degradable poly(urethane urea)s have been processed by wet-spinning to yield fibers trademarked by Artimplant (Sweden) as Artelon®. *In vivo* studies in rabbits and minipigs were performed to evaluate the biocompatibility of Artelon® fibers and their efficacy for ACL reconstruction by suturing the fibers to the synovial membrane of the knee (Liljensten et al., 2002). The implants demonstrated no evidence of mutagenicity and no evidence of severe fatigue after repeated cyclic loading. No adverse joint reaction or macroscopic inflammation was observed; however, macrophages and foreign body multinuclear giant cells were observed near the surface of the implant. Ingrowth of connective tissue (shown in Figure 10.7) was observed at observation times longer than 6 months post-implantation and degradation of the polymer was observed after 24 months post implantation.

Degradable scaffolds designed to promote healing of the knee-joint meniscus have been fabricated from segmented poly(ester urethane) elastomers. Healing of meniscal lesions has been observed in dogs after implantation of porous polymer scaffolds fabricated from MDI-based poly(ester urethane)s (Klompmaker et al., 1992, 1993, 1996; De Groot et al., 1996). Due to concern about the potential toxicity of degradation products associated

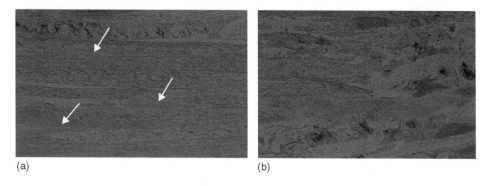

(a)                                                                (b)

**FIGURE 10.7**
**(See color insert following page 498.)** Photomicrographs of rabbit knee joints implanted with poly(urethane urea) (PUUR) band. (a) 6 months post implantation. Arrows denote tissue in-growth between the PUUR fibers. (b) 18 months post implantation. Note the disruption of the fibers relative to 6-months post implantation. (*Source*: Adapted from Gisselfält, K. *Structure Dependent Chemical and Biological Interactions of Poly(urethane urea)s*, Ph.D. thesis, Chalmers University of Technology, Göteborg, Sweden (2002). With permission.)

with MDI, degradable segmented polyurethane elastomers were prepared from BDI and a 50/50 poly(ε-caprolactone-co-L-lactide) diol via the prepolymer process. NCO-terminated prepolymers were first synthesized from BDI and poly(L-lactide-*co*-ε-caprolactone) and poly(ε-caprolactone) (PCL) diols followed by chain-extension with short-chain diols and diamines (Spaans et al., 1998a, 1998b, 1999, 2000, 2001, 2003; De Groot et al., 1996, 1997a, 1997b). Butanediamine (BDA) and butanediol (BDO) chain extenders were evaluated, as well as a novel chain extender (BDO.BDI.BDO, see Table 10.3) prepared by reacting an excess of BDO with BDI followed by precipitation of the chain extender in a nonsolvent. Microphase-separation of the BDO.BDI.BDO-based polyurethane into semi-crystalline hard and soft segments has been reported (Spaans et al., 1998). The polyurethane prepared from the BDO.BDI.BDO chain extender had a higher modulus (70.0 MPa) relative to that prepared from the BDO chain extender (23.3 MPa), presumably due to the larger hard segment (Spaans et al., 1998, 2003). Porous scaffolds have been prepared from the BDO.BDI.BDO-based polyurethane using the salt leaching/freeze drying technique (Spaans et al., 1998a, 1998b). Salt crystals (150 to 300 μm) were dispersed in a solution of the polymer in DMF. The solvent was then freeze-dried and the salt extracted with water, resulting in a combination of interconnected macropores (150 to 300 μm) and micropores (<50 μm). The scaffolds had a compression modulus of 200 kPa, which is suitable for the regeneration of fibrocartilage (De Groot et al., 1997).

Biocompatible polyurethanes with hard segments similar in structure to that of MDI-based polyurethanes have been synthesized from aliphatic diisocyanates (BDI and LDI), diurea diol chain extenders based on tyrosine and tyramine (see Table 10.3), and a poly (ethylene glycol) (PEG) soft segment (Guelcher et al., 2005). The tyramine and tyrosine moieties in the backbone contain phenyl groups which reportedly impart rigidity to the hard segment (Oertel, 1994). The nonbranched, symmetric polyurethane with a hard segment comprising BDI and a tyramine-based chain extender had the highest modulus at 37°C. Short-chain branches (SCBs) introduced into the hard segment by incorporating LDI and tyrosine-based chain extenders reduced the modulus by one to two orders of magnitude. All of the tyrosine- and tyramine-based polyurethanes supported the attachment, proliferation, and viability of MG-63 human osteoblast-like cells *in vitro*.

### 10.3.1.2  *Cardiovascular*

Biodegradable segmented polyurethane elastomers have been investigated for cardio-vascular applications. Segmented elastomers have been prepared from BDI, putrescine and lysine ethyl ester chain extenders, and polyether and polyester diols (Guan et al., 2002, 2003; Stankus et al., 2004). Materials with elongations at break ranging from 325 to 895% and tensile strengths ranging from 8 to 29 MPa have been synthesized. The materials also supported adhesion of endothelial cells *in vitro* and the degradation products exhibited no signs of cytotoxicity. Blends of poly(ester urethane urea)s (PEUU) and Type I collagen were electro-spun to construct strong elastic matrices designed to support cell adhesion and enzymatic matrix remodeling. The resulting materials mimicked elastic extracellular matrices by incorporating both a biological molecule (e.g., collagen) to improve cell adhesion and a synthetic molecule (e.g., PEUU) to provide acceptable mechanical properties.

To facilitate enzymatic hard segment degradation, diester diamine chain extenders have been synthesized from cyclohexanedimethanol (CHDM) and L-phenylalanine (see Table 10.3) (Skarja and Woodhouse, 1998, 2000; Woodhouse and Skarja, 2001; Elliott et al., 2002). The enzyme chymotrypsin has been demonstrated to cleave ester bonds adjacent to phenylalanine residues in the polymer backbone, thereby promoting hard segment degradation. However, the phenyl short-chain branches present in the phenylalanine chain extender disrupt hard segment ordering, resulting in an amorphous hard segment.

### 10.3.1.3 Nerve

In addition to cardiovascular and musculoskeletal applications, poly(ester urethane) elastomers have used to fabricate biodegradable nerve guidance channels (NGCs). Poly(ester urethane)s with tunable degradation rates and mechanical properties have been prepared from alternating blocks of crystalline poly[(R)-3-hydroxybutyric acid-co-(R)-3-hydroxyvaleric acid]-diol (PHB) and amorphous poly[glycolide-co-(ε-caprolactone)]-diol linked by aliphatic polyisocyanates (LDI and 2,2,4-trimethyl-hexamethylene diisocyanate) (Saad et al., 1997, 1999; Borkenhagen et al., 1998). *In vitro* and *in vivo* studies have demonstrated that the materials are biodegradable and are cell- and tissue-compatible. Nerve regeneration in rats was investigated in a 10 mm long NGC using a transected sciatic nerve model with an 8 mm gap. Twenty-three of the 26 NGC implants exhibited regenerated tissue cables within the channel lumen that were composed of Schwann cells and myelinated axons. The inflammatory response resulting from the degradation of the polymer did not hinder the process of nerve regeneration.

## 10.3.2 Cast Polyurethane Scaffolds

Biocompatible and biodegradable polyurethane foams have been prepared by mixing an NCO-functional resin with an OH-functional hardener (both liquid components) and casting the resulting reactive liquid mixture in a mold (see Figure 10.5). Porosity is introduced by incorporating water (a blowing agent) and/or a leachable porogen in the hardener component. The scaffold can be cast before implanting into the body or cast directly into a wound where it cures *in situ*. By selecting appropriate intermediates, polyurethanes that degrade to nontoxic degradation products have been prepared. Degradable scaffolds and implants have been fabricated for bone and cartilage tissue engineering applications.

### 10.3.2.1 Salt Leaching Process

Biocompatible and biodegradable polyurethane scaffolds have been prepared via reactive liquid molding processes from LDI, polyester polyols, and a porogen (such as salt (Bruin et al., 1988; Adhikari and Gunatillake, 2004) or gelatin (Adhikari and Gunatillake, 2004; Adhikari et al., 2004)). After the polymer has cured, the porogen is leached from the material to yield a porous scaffold. Relatively high (e.g., 85%) concentrations of porogen are required to prepare scaffolds with interconnected pores. Both one-shot (Bruin et al., 1988) and prepolymer (Adhikari and Gunatillake, 2004; Adhikari et al., 2004a, 2004b; Gunatillake et al., 2004) processes have been utilized. Polyurethanes prepared from LDI and poly(D,L-lactide) (750 g eq$^{-1}$) and poly(ε-caprolactone) (600 g eq$^{-1}$) triols demonstrate the effects of polyol composition on mechanical properties (Wiggins and Storey, 1992). The D,L-lactide-based material was a rigid plastic with a modulus of 752 MPa, tensile strength of 15.2 MPa, and elongation at break of 10% due to its relatively high glass transition temperature ($T_g = 48°C$). The ε-caprolactone-based material was a soft elastomer with a modulus of 1.7 MPa, tensile strength of 2.29 MPa, and elongation at break of 118% due to its relatively low glass transition temperature ($T_g = -63°C$). The equivalent weight of the polyol also affects the mechanical properties of crosslinked polyurethanes. Generally, higher crosslink density (e.g., lower polyol equivalent weight) increases the hardness and brittleness of the material.

*In vitro* (Gunatillake et al., 2004) and *in vivo* studies in guinea pigs (Bruin et al., 1988) and rats (Adhikari and Gunatillake, 2004) have demonstrated that cast porous polyurethane scaffolds prepared from LDI and polyester polyols degrade to nontoxic by-products and support the migration of cells and in-growth of new tissue. A 4-month subcutaneous implant study in rats exhibited fibroblast infiltration near the surface pores of the implant after 2 months (Adhikari and Gunatillake, 2004). After 4 months a soft capsule had formed around the implants and fibroblast infiltration had progressed into the core of the implant. No adverse tissue response to the implants was observed.

### 10.3.2.2  Foaming Process

Porous scaffolds have been prepared from BDI and poly(L-lactide-*co*-ε-caprolactone) diol via a combination of the porogen and foaming processes (Spaans et al., 2000). A prepolymer prepared from BDI and the polyester diol was chain-extended with a mixture comprising water, salt, dodecyl sulfate (surfactant), and polyester diol. The salt was leached from the scaffold by contacting it with water after the polymer had cured. Dodecyl sulfate was added as a surfactant to regulate the pore size. Scaffolds having a porosity of ~75% and suitable mechanical properties for the knee-joint meniscus (e.g., modulus > 150 kPa) were prepared by this process. Further improvements in mechanical properties were achieved by the addition of adipic acid to the chain extender mixture.

Biocompatible and biodegradable porous polyurethane foams for bone tissue engineering have been prepared from aliphatic diisocyanates (Zhang et al., 2000, 2002, 2003a, 2003b; Beckman et al., 2004). LDI-glycerol and LDI-glucose prepolymers were reacted with water to yield porous polyurethane foams having pores ranging from 125 to 500 μm. The foams supported the attachment, proliferation, and differentiation of bone marrow stromal cells *in vitro*, degraded to nontoxic degradation products *in vitro*, and did not induce antibody responses *in vivo*. Degradable foams designed for use as bone graft substitutes have been prepared from prepolymers comprising hexamethylene diiso-cyanate (HDI) and polyether and polyester polyols, organometallic catalysts, surfactants, and inorganic fillers (Gorna and Gogolewski, 2003). The compressive moduli of the scaffolds ranged from 9 to 1960 kPa. All the materials induced the deposition of calcium phosphate crystals and underwent controlled degradation *in vitro*.

Injectable polyurethane porous scaffolds have been synthesized via a one-shot process from LDI, poly(ε-caprolactone-co-glycolide) triols, water, and triethylenediamine (catalyst) (Guelcher et al., 2004, 2004). Stabilizers (sulfated castor oil and polyethersiloxanes) and a pore opener (calcium stearate) were added to control the surface chemistry and promote the generation of stable, interconnected pores. The foams were characterized by rise times less than 20 min, porosities greater than 95%, and interconnected pores ranging from 100 to 1000 μm. An SEM image of a typical polyurethane foam is shown in Figure 10.8. The foams supported the attachment of viable MG-63 cells *in vitro* and demonstrated about 5 to 10% mass loss after 8 weeks in phosphate-buffered saline at 37°C.

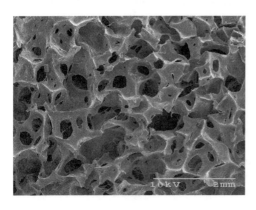

**FIGURE 10.8**
SEM image of an injectable polyurethane foam.

An injectable bone void filler has been prepared by mixing an LDI-polyester polyol prepolymer with calcium phosphate and water in the presence of diethanolamine, a urethane blowing catalyst which catalyzes the reaction of isocyanates with water (Bennett et al., 1996). The material is mixed prior to implantation and cures *in situ* to form a porous implant. The initial transient inflammatory reaction, characterized by a minimal number of foreign body giant cells, subsided on day 3 post implantation. The implants were characterized by good integration with host tissue, in-growth of vascular buds, and fibrovascular penetration.

### 10.3.3 Bioactive Polyurethane Sensors

Biologically active molecules can be covalently bound to polyurethanes through isocyanate chemistry. Because diisocyanates react vigorously with primary amines and alcohols, any biologically active molecule with amine and/or hydroxyl groups can in principle react with free NCO and covalently bind to the polyurethane. A number of enzymes, such as phosphotriesterase (LeJeune et al., 1997), organophosphorus hydrolase (OPH), organophosphorus acid anhydrolase (OPAA), urease, butyrylcholinesterase, and acetylcholinesterase, have been incorporated into polyurethane foams (LeJeune et al., 2001). An enzyme that catalyzes the reaction of a toxic analyte is incorporated in the polyurethane foam to convert the analyte to a marker compound. The concentration of the marker compound is measured by an indicator also present in the foam. Sensors have been developed for a number of analytes, including toxic nerve agents and pesticides. The technology has been commercialized by Agentase, LLC (Pittsburgh, PA) in the manufacture of polymeric sensors.

## 10.4 Summary

Polyurethanes are versatile materials that can be prepared with a wide variety of mechanical and biological properties through the judicious selection of raw materials and processing conditions. Segmented polyurethane elastomers are incorporated in numerous commercial cardiovascular devices, such as catheters and pacemaker leads, due to their adequate biocompatibility and excellent mechanical properties. In recent years, considerable research has been directed toward enhancing the biostability of polyurethane implants by identifying the mechanisms of degradation and improving their resistance to oxidative degradation. In contrast to polyurethane implants designed to be biostable, degradable tissue engineered polyurethane scaffolds for tissue regeneration are designed to degrade *in vivo* at a controlled rate, preferably in register with tissue healing. Poly(ester urethane) scaffolds have been reported to degrade to nontoxic by-products and support the migration of cells and ingrowth of new tissue *in vivo*.

## References

Adhikari, R. and Gunatillake, P.A., Commonwealth Scientific and Industrial Research Organization, assignee, *Biodegradable Polyurethane/urea Compositions*, Australia patent WO 2004/009227 A2 (2004).

Adhikari, R., Gunatillake, T., Le, T.P., Danon, S.J., Seymour, K., Thissen, H., Werkmeister, J., Ramshaw, J.A., and Jacinta, W., *Injectable Biodegradable Polyurethanes for Tissue Engineering: Effect of Phosphorylcholine*, Abstract Presented at the Seventhth World Biomaterials Congress, Sydney, Australia (2004).

Adhikari, R., Gunatillake, P.A., Le, T.P., Mayadunne, R., Danon, S.J., Seymour, K., Bean, P., Thissen, H., Werkmeister, J., and Ramshaw, J.A., *Injectable Biodegradable Polyurethanes for Cartilage Repair: Evaluation of Biocompatibility and Biodegradability*, Abstract presented at the Seventh World Biomaterials Congress, Sydney, Australia (2004).

Alferiev, I.S., Novel elastomeric polyurethanes with pendant epoxy groups as highly reactive auxiliary groups for further derivatizations, *J. Polym. Sci. A: Polym. Chem.*, **40**, 4378 (2002).

Anderson, J.M., Hiltner, A., Wiggins, M.J., Schubert, M.A., Collier, T.O., Kao, W.J., and Mathur, A.B., Recent advances in biomedical polyurethane biostability and biodegradation, *Polym. Int.*, **46**, 163 (1998).

Anderson, J.M., Hiltner, A., Zhao, Q., Wu, Y., Renier, M., Schubert, M.A., Brunstedt, M., Lodoen, G., and Payet, C.R., Cell/polymer interactions in the biodegradation of polyurethanes, In: *Biodegradable Polymers and Plastics*, Vert, M., Feijen, J., Albertsson, A., Scott, G., and Chiellini, E., Eds., Royal Society of Chemistry, Cambridge, pp. 122 (1992).

Aurell, C.-J., Flodin, P., and Artimplant AB, assignee, *New Linear Block Polymer*, PCT (2002).

Bennett, S., Connolly, K., Lee, D.R., Jiang, Y., Buck, D., Hollinger, J.O., and Gruskin, E.A., Initial biocompatibility studies of a novel degradable polymeric bone substitute that hardens in situ, *Bone*, **19**, 101S (1996).

Beckman, E., Doll, B., Guelcher, S., Hollinger, J., and Zhang, J., Carnegie Mellon University and University of Pittsburgh, assignee, Biodegradable polyurethanes and use thereof patent WO2004065450 (2004).

Blais, P., Letter to the editor, *J. Appl. Biomater.*, **1**, 197 (1990).

Bloch, B. and Hastings, G., *Plastics Materials in Surgery*, Charles C. Thomas, Springfield, IL (1972).

Borkenhagen, M., Stoll, R.C., Neuenschwander, P., Suter, U.W., and Aebischer, P., *In vivo* performance of a new biodegradable polyester urethane system used a nerve guidance channel, *Biomaterials*, **19**, 2155 (1998).

Bruin, P., Veenstra, G.J., Nijenhuis, A.J., and Pennings, A.J., Design and synthesis of biodegradable poly(ester-urethane) elastomer networks composed of non-toxic building blocks, *Makromol. Chem. Rapid Commun.*, **9**, 589 (1988).

Capone, C.D., Biostability of a non-ether polyurethane, *J. Biomater. Appl.*, **7**, 108 (1992).

Coury, A., Chemical and biochemical degradation of polymers. In: Ratner, B., Hoffman, A., Schoen, F., and Lemons. J., Eds., *Biomaterials Science: An Introduction to Materials in Medicine*, Ratner, B., Hoffman, A., Schoen, F., and Lemons, J., Eds., Elsevier Academic Press, Boston, pp. 411 (2004).

Coury, A., Hobot, C., Slaikeu, P., Stokes, K., and Cahalan, P., *A New Family of Implantable Biostable Polyurethanes*, Abstract Presented at the Transactions of the 16th Annual Meeting Society for Biomaterials, 1990. p. 158.

De Groot, J.H., de Vrijer, R., Pennings, A.J., Klompmaker, J., Veth, R.P.H., and Jansen, H.W.B., Use of porous polyurethanes for meniscal reconstruction and meniscal prosthesis, *Biomaterials*, **17**, 163 (1996).

De Groot, J.H., de Vrijer, R., Wildeboer, B.S., Spaans, C.J., and Pennings, A.J., New biomedical polyurethane ureas with high tear strengths, *Polym. Bull.*, **38**, 211 (1997a).

De Groot, J.H., Kuijper, H.W., and Pennings, A.J., A novel method for fabrication of biodegradable scaffolds with high compression moduli, *J. Mater. Sci. Mater. Med.*, **8**, 707 (1997b).

Eisenbach, C.D., Ribbe, A., and Günter, C.,. Morphological studies of model ployurethane elastomers by element-specific electron microcopy. *Macromol. Rapid Commun.*, **15**, 395 (1994).

Elliott, S.L., Fromstein, J.D., Santerre, J.P., and Woodhouse, K.A., Identification of biodegradation products formed by L-phenylalanine based segmented polyurethaneureas, *J. Biomater. Sci. Polym. Ed.*, **13**, 691 (2002).

Frisch, K., Reegen, S., and Rumano, L., *Advances in Urethane Science and Technology*, Frisch, K. and Reegen, S., Eds., Technomic Publishing, Lancaster, pp. 49 (1971).

Gisselfält, K., Edberg, B., and Flodin, P., Synthesis and properties of degradable poly(urethane urea)s to be used for ligament reconstructions, *Biomacromolecules*, **3**, 951 (2002).

Gorna, K. and Gogolewski, S., Preparation, degradation, and calcification of biode-gradable polyurethane foams for bone graft substitutes, *J. Biomed. Mater. Res.*, **67A**, 813 (2003).

Guan, J., Sacks, M., Beckman, E., and Wagner, W., Synthesis, characterization, and cytocompatibility of elastomeric, biodegradable poly(ester-urethane)ureas based on poly(caprolactone) and putrescine, *J. Biomed. Mater. Res.*, **61**, 493 (2002).

Guan, J., Sacks, M., Beckman, E., and Wagner, W., Biodegradable poly(ether ester urethane)urea elastomers based on poly(ether ester) triblock copolymers and putrescine: synthesis, characterization and cytocompatibility, *Biomaterials*, **25**, 85 (2003).

Guelcher, S.A., Gallagher, K., Didier, J.E., Klinedinst, D., Doctor, J.S., Goldstein, A., Wilkes, G., Beckman, E., and Hollinger, J.O., Synthesis of biocompatible segmented polyurethanes from aliphatic diisocyanates and diurea diol chain extenders, *Acta Biomater.*, **1**, 471 (2005).

Guelcher, S., Patel, V., Gallagher, K., Connolly, S., Didier, J., Doctor, J., and Hollinger, J., *Injectable Polyurethane Scaffolds for Bone Tissue Engineering*. Abstract Presented at the American Institute of Chemical Engineering Annual Meeting, Austin, TX, p. 63a (2004).

Guelcher, S., Patel, V., Gallagher, K., Connolly, S., Didier, J., Doctor, J., and Hollinger, J., Synthesis and biocompatibility of polyurethane foam scaffolds from lysine diisocyanate and polyester polyols, *Tissue Eng.* (2005) in press.

Gunatillake, P.A., Adhikari, R., Le, T.P., Danon, S.J., Seymour, K., McFarland, C., Bean, P., Mitchell, S., Dalton, A., Werkmeister, J., Ramshaw, J.A., White, J.F., Glattaner, V., and Tebb, T.A., *Injectable Biodegradable Polyurethanes for Tissue Engineering*, Abstract Presented at the 7th World Biomaterials Congress, Sydney, Australia (2004).

Hoffman, D., Gong, G., Pinchuk, L., and Sisto, D., Safety and intracardiac function of a silicone-polyurethane elastomer designed for vascular use, *Clin. Mater.*, **13**, 95 (1993).

Kato, Y., Dereume, J., Kontges, H., Frid, N., Martin, J., MacGregor, D., and Pinchuk, L., *Preliminary Mechanical Evaluation of a Novel Endoluminal Graft*, Abstract Presented at the Transactions of the 21st Annual Meeting Society for Biomaterials, p. 81 (1995).

Klompmaker, J., Jansen, H.W.B., Veth, R.P.H., Nielsen, H.K.L., De Groot, J.H., and Pennings, A.J., Porous polymer implants for repair of full-thickness defects of articular cartilage. An experimental study in the dog, *Biomaterials*, **13**, 625 (1992).

Klompmaker, J., Jansen, H.W.B., Veth, R.P.H., Nielsen, H.K.L., De Groot, J.H., and Pennings, A.J., Porous implants for the knee joint meniscus reconstruction: a preliminary study on the role of pore sizes in ingrowth and differentiation of fibrocartilage, *Clin. Mater.*, **14**, 1 (1993).

Klompmaker, J., Jansen, H.W.B., Veth, R.P.H., Nielsen, H.K.L., De Groot, J.H., and Pennings, A.J., Meniscal replacement using a porous polymer prosthesis: a preliminary study in the dog, *Biomaterials*, **17**, 1169 (1996).

LeJeune, K.E., Mesiano, A.J., Bower, S.B., Grimsley, J.K., Wild, J.R., and Russell, A.J., Dramatically stabilized phophotriesterase-polymers for nerve agent degradation, *Biotechnol. Bioeng.*, **54**, 105 (1997).

LeJeune, K.E., Russell, A.J., and Agentase, L.L.C., assignee, Enzyme-containing polymeric sensors, United States patent 6,291,200 (2001).

Lelah, M.D. and Cooper, J.L., *Polyurethanes in Medicine*, CRC Press, Boca Raton, FL (1986).

Liljensten, E., Gisselfaelt, K., Edberg, B., Bertilsson, H., Flodin, P., Nilsson, A., Lindahl, A., and Peterson, L., Studies of polyurethane urea bands for ACL reconstruction, *J. Mater. Sci. Mater. Med.*, **13**, 351 (2002).

Martin, D.J., Meijs, G.F., Gunatillake, P.A., Yozghatlian, S.P., and Renwick, G.M., The influence of composition ratio on the morphology of biomedical polyurethanes, *J. Appl. Polym. Sci.*, **71**, 937 (1999).

Matheson, L.A., Santerre, J.P., and Labow, R.S., Changes in macrophage function and morphology due to biomedical polyurethane surfaces undergoing biodegradation, *J. Cell Physiol.*, **199**, 8 (2004).

Mathur, A.B., Collier, T.O., Kao, W.J., Wiggins, M.J., Schubert, M.A., Hiltner, A., and Anderson, J.M., *In vivo* biocompatibility and biostability of modified polyurethanes, *J. Biomed. Mater. Res.*, **36**, 246 (1997).

Oertel, G., *Polyurethane Handbook*, Hanser Gardner Publications, Berlin (1994).

Pierce, W.S. and Turner, M.C., Mechanical left ventricular assistance: experimental studies using an implantable roller pump, *Trans. Am. Soc. Artif. Int. Org.*, **13**, 299 (1967).

Pinchuk, L., Esquivel, M., Martin, J., and Wilson, G., *Corethane: A New Replacement for Polyether Urethanes for Long-Term Implant Applications*, Abstract presented at the Transactions of the 17th Annual Meeting of the Society for Biomaterials, p. 1 (1991).

Reed, A.M., Potter, J., and Szycher, M., A solution grade biostable polyurethane elastomer: ChronoFlex AR, *J. Biomater. Appl.*, **8**, 210 (1994).

Saad, B., Hirt, T.D., Welti, M., Uhlschmid, G.K., Neuenschwander, P., and Suter, U.W., Development of degradable polyesterurethanes for medical applications: in vitro and in vivo evaluations, *J. Biomed. Mater. Res.*, **36**, 65 (1997).

Saad, B., Neuenschwander, P., Uhlschmid, G.K., and Suter, U.W., New versatile, elastomeric, degradable polymeric materials for medicine, *Int. J. Biol. Macromol.*, **25**, 292 (1999).

Santerre, J.P., Meek, E., Tang, Y., and Labow, R.S., Use of fluorinated surface modifying macromolecules to inhibit the degradation of polycarbonate-urethanes by human macrophages, *Trans. Sixth World Biomater. Congr.*, 77 (2000).

Schubert, M.A., Wiggins, M.J., Anderson, J.M., and Hiltner, A., The effect of strain state on the biostability of a poly(etherurethane urea) elastomer, *J. Biomed. Mater. Res.*, **35**, 319 (1997a).

Schubert, M.A., Wiggins, M.J., Anderson, J.M., and Hiltner, A., The role of oxygen on poly(etherurethane urea) degradation, *J. Biomed. Mater. Res.*, **34**, 519 (1997b).

Schubert, M.A., Wiggins, M.J., Schaefer, M.P., Hiltner, A., and Anderson, J.M., Oxidative biodegradation mechanisms of biaxially strained poly(etherurethane urea) elastomers, *J. Biomed. Mater. Res.*, **29**, 337 (1995a).

Schubert, M.A., Wiggins, M.J., Schaefer, M.P., Hiltner, A., and Anderson, J.M., *J. Biomed. Mater. Res.*, **29**, 337 (1995b).

Seifalian, A., Salacinski, H., Tiwari, A., Edwards, E., Bowald, S., and Hamilton, G., In vivo biostability of a poly(carbonate-urea)urethane graft, *Biomaterials*, **24**, 2549 (2003).

Silvaggio, V. and Fu, F., *Articular Cartilage and Knee Joint Function: Basic Science and Arthroscopy*, Ewing, J., Ed., Raven Press, New York, pp. 273 (1990).

Skarja, G.A. and Woodhouse, K.A., Synthesis and characterization of degradable polyurethane elastomers containing an amino-acid based chain extender, *J. Biomater. Sci. Polym. Ed.*, **9**, 271 (1998).

Skarja, G.A. and Woodhouse, K.A., Structure-property relationships of degradable polyurethane elastomers containing an amino acid-based chain extender, *J. Appl. Polym. Sci.*, **75**, 1522 (2000).

Spaans, C.J., Belgraver, V.W., Rienstra, O., De Groot, J.H., Veth, R.P.H., and Pennings, A.J., Solvent-free fabrication of micro-porous polyurethane-amide and polyurethane-urea scaffolds for repair and replacement of the knee-joint meniscus, *Biomaterials*, **21**, 2453 (2000).

Spaans, C.J., De Groot, J.H., Belgraver, V.W., and Pennings, A.J., A new biomedical polyurethane with a high modulus based on 1,4-butanediisocyanate and ε-caprolactone, *J. Mater. Sci. Mater. Med.*, **9**, 675 (1998).

Spaans, C.J., De Groot, J.H., Dekens, F.G., and Pennings, A.J., High molecular weight polyurethanes and a polyurethane urea based on 1,4-butanediisocyanate, *Polym. Bull.*, **41**, 131 (1998).

Spaans, C.J., De Groot, J.H., Dekens, F.G., Veth, R.P.H., and Pennings, A.J., Development of new polyurethanes for repair and replacement of the knee joint meniscus, *Polym. Prepr.*, **40**, 589 (1999).

Spaans, C.J., De Groot, J.H., Van der Molen, L.M., and Pennings, A.J., New biodegradable polyurethane-ureas, polyurethane and polyurethane-amide for *in-vivo* tissue engineering: structure-properties relationships, *Polym. Mater. Sci. Eng.*, **85**, 61 (2001).

Spaans, C.J., Dekens, F.G., De Groot, J.H., Pennings, A.J., and Polyganics B.V., Assignee, Biomedical polyurethane, its preparation and use, EP patent EP 1 308 473 A1 (2003).

Stankus, J., Guan, J., and Wagner, W., Fabrication of biodegradable elastomeric scaffolds with sub-micron morphologies, *J. Biomed. Mater. Res.*, **70A**, 603 (2004).

Stokes, K. and McVenes, R., Polyurethane elastomer biostability, *J. Biomater. Appl.*, **9**, 321 (1995).

Stokes, K., Urbanski, P., and Upton, J., The in vivo auto-oxidation of polyether polyurethane by metal ions, *J. Biomater. Sci. Polym. Ed.*, **1**, 207 (1990).

Szycher, M., *Szycher's Handbook of Polyurethanes*, CRC Press, Boca Raton, FL (1999).

Szycher, M., Biostability of polyurethane elastomers: a critical review, *J. Biomater. Appl.*, **3**, 297 (1988).

Szycher, M. and Siciliano, A., An assessment of 2,4-TDA formation from Surgitek polyurethane foam under stimulated physiological conditions, *J. Biomater. Appl.*, **5**, 323 (1991).

Takahara, A., Coury, A., and Cooper, S.L., *Molecular Design of Biologically Stable Polyurethanes*, Abstract Presented at the Transactions of the 20th Annual Meeting Society for Biomaterials, p. 44 (1994).

Takahara, A., Coury, A., Hergenrother, R., and Cooper, S.L., Effect of soft segment chemistry on the biostability of segmented polyurethanes. I. *In vitro* oxidation, *J. Biomed. Mater. Res.*, **25**, 341 (1991).

Thomas, V., Kumari, T.V., and Jayabalan, M., In vitro studies on the effect of physical cross-linking on the biological performance of aliphatic poly(urethane urea) for blood contact applications, *Biomacromolecules*, **2**, 588 (2001).

Ward, R.S. and White, K.A., The Polymer Technology Group, Assignee, Surface-modifying endgroups for biomedical polymers, U.S. patent **5**, 589, 563 (1996).

Ward, R.S., White, K., Gill, R., and Lim, F., *The Effects of Phase Separation and Endgroup Chemistry on in vivo Biostability*, Abstract Presented at the Transactions of the ASAIO Meeting, Washington, DC, p. 17 (1996).

Ward, R.S., White, K.A., Gill, R., and Wolcott, C., *Development of Biostable Thermoplastic Polyurethanes with Oligomeric Polydimethylsiloxane End Groups*, Abstract Presented at the Transactions of the 21st Annual Meeting Society for Biomaterials, p. 268 (1995).

Ward, R.S., Tian, Y., and White, K.A., Improve polymer biostability via oligomeric end groups incorporated during synthesis, *Polym. Mater. Sci. Eng.*, **79**, 526 (1998).

Wiggins, J. and Storey, R., *Synthesis and Characterization of L-lysine Based Poly(ester-urethane) Networks*, Abstract Presented at the American Chemical Society, Division of Polymer Chemistry, Washington, DC, p. 516 (1992).

Wilkes, G., Ed., *Necessary Considerations for Selecting a Polymeric Material for Implantation with Emphasis on Polyurethanes*, Vol. 8. Plenum Press, New York, pp. 45 (1975).

Woodhouse, K.A. and Skarja, G.A., Biodegradable polyurethanes, U.S. patent **6**, 221, 997 (2001).

Wu, Y., Lodoen, G., Anderson, J.M., Baer, E., and Hiltner, A., *J. Biomed. Mater. Res.*, **28**, 515 (1994).

Wu, Y., Sellitti, C., Anderson, J.M., Hiltner, A., Lodoen, G., and Payet, C.R., An FTIR-ATR investigation of in vivo poly(ether urethane) degradation, *J. Appl. Polym. Sci.*, **46**, 201 (1992).

Wu, Y., Sletten, K.R., Topolkaraev, V., Lodoen, G., Anderson, J.M., Baer, E., and Hiltner, A., *J. Appl. Polym. Sci.*, **53**, 1037 (1994).

Zhang, J.-Y., Beckman, E.J., Hu, J., Yuang, G.-G., Agarwal, S., and Hollinger, J.O., Synthesis, biodegradability, and biocompatibility of lysine diisocyanate-glucose polymers, *Tissue Eng.*, **8**, 771 (2002).

Zhang, J.-Y., Beckman, E.J., Piesco, N.J., and Agarwal, S., A new peptide-based urethane polymer: synthesis, biodegradation, and potential to support cell growth *in vitro*, *Biomaterials*, **21**, 1247 (2000).

Zhang, J., Doll, B., Beckman, J., and Hollinger, J.O., Three-dimensional biocompatible ascorbic acid-containing scaffold for bone tissue engineering, *Tissue Eng.*, **9**, 1143 (2003a).

Zhang, J., Doll, B., Beckman, E., and Hollinger, J.O., A biodegradable polyurethane-ascorbic acid scaffold for bone tissue engineering, *J. Biomed. Mater. Res.*, **67A**, 389 (2003b).

Zhao, Q., Casas-Bejar, J., Urbanski, P., and Stokes, K., Glass wool-H2O/CoCl2 test system for in vitro evaluation of biodegradative stress cracking in polyurethane elastomers, *J. Biomed. Mater. Res.*, **29** (1995).

Zhao, Q., McNally, A.K., Rubin, K.R., Reiner, M., Wu, Y., Rose-Caprara, V., Anderson, J.M., Hiltner, A., Urbanski, P., and Stokes, K., Human plasma $\alpha_2$-macroglobulin promotes in vitro oxidative stress cracking of Pellethane 2363-80A: in vivo and in vitro correlations, *J. Biomed. Mater. Res.*, **27**, 379 (1993).

Zhao, Q., Topham, N., Anderson, J.M., Hiltner, A., Lodoen, G., and Payet, C.R., Foreign-body giant cells and polyurethane biostability: in vivo correlation of cell adhesion and surface cracking, *J. Biomed. Mater. Res.*, **25**, 177 (1991).

# 11

## Polymers Derived from L-Tyrosine

**Joachim Kohn and Jaap Schut**

## CONTENTS

## 11.1 Introduction

This chapter describes polymeric biomaterials based on the natural amino acid L-tyrosine. We will discuss the synthesis of tyrosine-derived monomers and polymers, the processing and physicomechanical properties of these polymers, their hydrolytic degradation mechanism, their *in vitro* and *in vivo* behavior, and will conclude with a description of the utility of these polymers in drug delivery applications.

Naturally occurring metabolites have often been employed as monomers in the design of biodegradable polymers in an attempt to create materials that degrade *in vivo* to nontoxic degradation products. Examples of such polymers are found throughout this book; poly(L-lactic acid) (PLLA) and poly(glycolic acid) (PGA) and their copolymers (PLGA), polycaprolactone (PCL), polydioxanone, and polyanhydrides. However, these materials are almost exclusively based on aliphatic structural units, while most high strength engineering plastics contain one or more aromatic ring structures in their polymer backbone. Some examples are: poly(phenylene terephthalamide) (also known as Kevlar®), poly(ethylene terephthalate) (PET), poly(bisphenol-A carbonate), and poly-etherimide (also known as Kapton®) (Crawford, 1998).

Aliphatic polyesters are widely used in biomedical engineering research and in the manufacture of the majority of clinically used, biodegradable implants (such as, for example, sutures, drug delivery systems, and bone pins). However, the lack of structural variation limits the range of physicomechanical properties available among the aliphatic polyesters. Since a biomaterial should match the mechanical properties of the surrounding tissue as closely as possible, there is a need for a diverse range of biodegradable polymers that can be adapted to interact optimally with such mechanically diverse tissues as bone, cartilage, muscles, or blood vessels.

Based on their similarity to natural proteins, synthetic poly(amino acids) have been investigated as possible biocompatible and biodegradable polymers. The conventional polymerization of amino acids forms polymers with a polypeptide backbone that may have a variety of reactive and nonreactive side groups. Despite the low systemic toxicity of these materials and their degradation products (i.e., naturally occurring amino acids), they have not been widely employed as practical biomaterials (Kohn et al., 2004). This is largely due to the extensive intrachain hydrogen bonding present in these materials that causes high crystallinity, low solubility, poor processability, and extensive water uptake and swelling upon exposure to the physiological environment. Furthermore, poly(amino acid)s rely on enzymatic degradation of the amide bond as the predominant mechanism of degradation. Because enzymatic activity can vary strongly among different patients it is difficult to reproduce and control the degradation of these polymers in vivo. Additional issues are the cost of preparing poly(amino acids) of high molecular weight and the inherent antigenicity of poly(amino acids) containing more than three different amino acids in their backbone (Pachence and Kohn, 2000).

The development of pseudo-poly(amino acids) (Kohn and Langer, 1987; Kohn, 1990; Kohn, 1991; Pulapura and Kohn, 1992; Kohn, 1993; James and Kohn, 1997; Pachence and Kohn, 2000) represents an attempt to utilize naturally occurring amino acids as monomeric building blocks without creating conventional poly(amino acids). Pseudo-poly(amino acids) are characterized by the presence of nonamide bonds-such as ether, ester, urethane, or carbonate-in their backbone structure. Usually this is accomplished by polymerization of the reactive side chain groups of the amino acids, as opposed to polymerization via the α-amino and α-carboxylic acid groups. This approach reduces the number of interchain hydrogen bonds by at least a factor of two, leading to an increased solubility in common organic solvents, reduced water uptake and swelling, and often a loss of crystallinity, which in turn results in a large improvement of the processing behavior.

## 11.2  Synthesis of Tyrosine-Derived Monomers and Polymers

Aromatic rings are a common structural element in high strength engineering plastics. When comparing aromatic monomers in the diphenol class, even the least toxic monomer that is most likely to be biocompatible, bisphenol-A, proved to be cytotoxic to chick embryo fibroblasts (Kohn and Langer, 1986; Kohn, 1991), leading to the conclusion that there are no diphenolic monomers commercially available for the synthesis of biocompatible and biodegradable polymers. To impart to polymeric biomaterials properties resembling engineering plastics, a monomer family was developed based on the naturally occurring amino acid L-tyrosine that combines a diphenolic monomer structure with excellent biocompatibility. The structures of L-tyrosine, its alkyl ester derivatives as well as 4-hydroxyphenyl propionic acid (also known as desaminotyrosine, e.g., tyrosine without an amino group) are shown in Figure 11.1. The carbodiimide-mediated reaction between L-tyrosine alkyl ester and desaminotyrosine creates a diphenolic monomer, *Desaminotyrosyl-L-Tyrosine Alkyl* ester, abbreviated as DTR where R stands for alkyl). For comparison, Figure 11.1 also shows the structure of bisphenol A.

Figure 11.2a illustrates the versatility of the DTR as a monomer; it can be polymerized by reaction with a wide variety of reagents to form a family of different polymers with diverse physical and biological properties. In analogy to the synthesis of

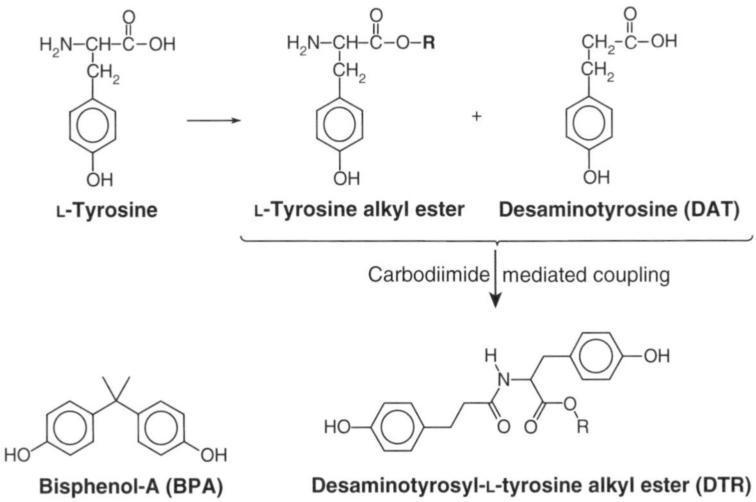

**FIGURE 11.1**
The structure of bisphenol-A compared to desaminotyrosyl-L-tyrosine alkyl ester (DTR), and the tyrosine derivatives used to prepare this diphenolic, biodegradable monomer (for the structure of group R see Figure 11.2).

poly(bisphenol-A carbonate), reaction of DTR with phosgene forms poly(DTR carbonate)s (Pulapura and Kohn, 1992). However, in contrast to poly(bisphenol-A carbonate), poly(DTR carbonate)s are slowly biodegradable. The reaction of DTR with dicarboxylic acids results in poly(DTR arylate)s (Fiordeliso et al., 1994; Brocchini et al., 1997, 1998), while reaction with alkyl- or aryl dichlorophosphates leads to poly(DTR phosphate ester)s (Gupta and Lopina, 2002, 2004). The DTR monomer can also be copolymerized with poly(ethylene glycol) (PEG) of varying molecular weight to form either alternating polyethers (d'Acunzo and Kohn, 2002; d'Acunzo et al., 2002), or random poly(DTR-co-PEG carbonate)s (Yu and Kohn, 1999). End capping of poly(DTR carbonate)s or poly(DTR arylate)s with PEG results in triblock copolymers (Sheihet et al., 2003).

Figure 11.2b and c provides examples of the ester and diacid groups that have been employed in the synthesis of these polymers. This illustrates that polymers derived from DTR monomers provide a versatile source of biomedical materials.

Polymers bearing a chemically reactive pendent chain have the significant advantage that biologically active ligands or drugs can be covalently attached to the polymer backbone. The lack of such a reactive pendent chain is one of the major limitations of poly(lactic acid) and most other polymers used currently as degradable implant materials. Using DTR as a monomer, polymers having a chemically reactive carboxylic acid pendent chain can be obtained by an indirect synthetic route: If a selectively removable protecting group, such as a benzyl ester, is used in place of the alkyl ester group (R), the corresponding polymers can be subjected to a deprotection reaction that removes the benzyl ester protecting group without significant reduction in the polymer molecular weight. This reaction sequence results in the formation of polymers containing free carboxylic acid groups. By mixing regular DTR (R is a nonselectively removable alkyl ester group) with DTBz (Bz is the selectively removable protecting group), copolymers can be prepared having any desirable ratio free carboxylic acid groups. These polymers can be regarded as having been derived from desaminotyrosyl-tyrosine (DT). For example, the corresponding polycarbonates are designated as poly(DTR-co-x% DT carbonate)

(a)

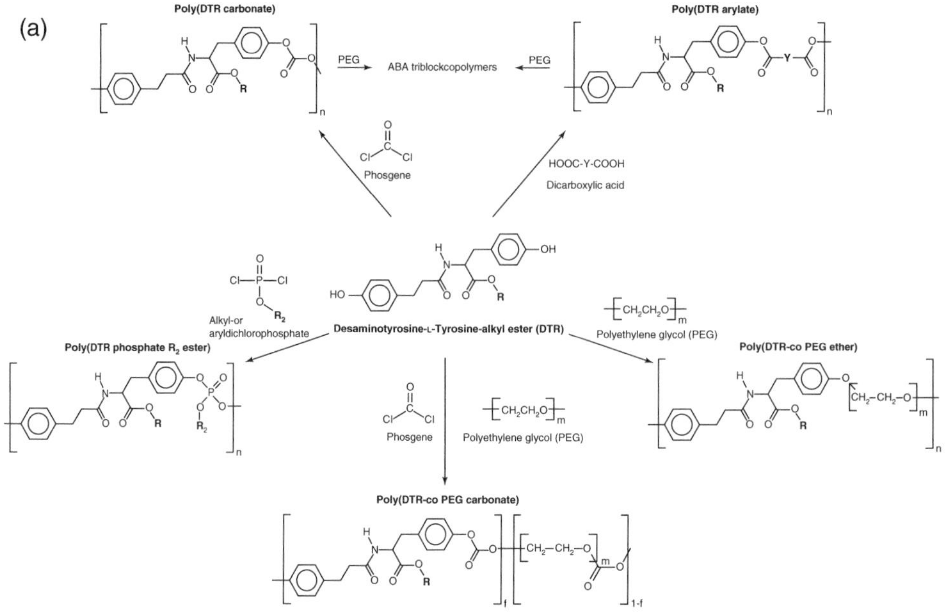


(b)

| Alkyl group | Abbreviation* | Structure (R) |
|---|---|---|
| None, free acid | XT | -H |
| Methyl | XTM | |
| Ethyl | XTE | |
| i-Propyl | XTiP | |
| n-Butyl | XTB | |
| i-Butyl | XTiB | |
| s-Butyl | XTsB | |
| Hexyl | XTH | |
| Octyl | XTO | |
| 2-(2-Ethoxyethoxy)ethanol | XTG | |
| Dodecyl | XTD | |
| Benzyl | XTBz | |

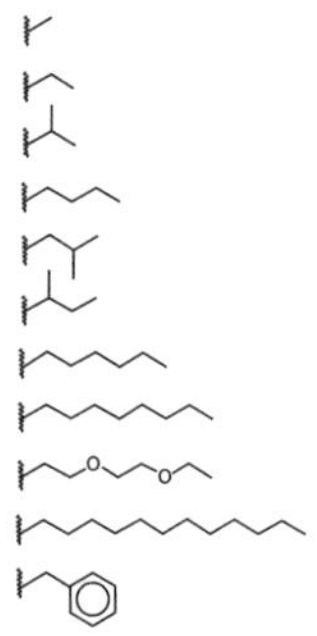

*Where X = D, H or C:
D = Desaminotyrosine-L-tyrosine alkyl ester
H = 4-Hydroxyphenyl acetic acid L-tyrosine alkyl ester
C = 4-Hydroxycinnamic acid L-tyrosine alkyl ester

(c)

| Diacid | Structure (Y) |
|---|---|
| Succinic | |
| Glutaric | |
| Diglycolic | |
| Adipic | |
| 3-Methyl adipic | |
| Suberic | |
| Dioxaoctanoic | |
| Sebacic | |
| Dodecanedioic | |

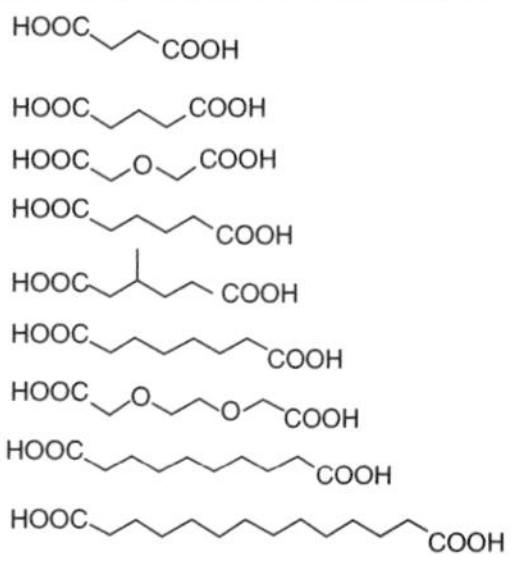


**FIGURE 11.2**
(a) The synthesis of a wide variety of biodegradable polymers from desaminotyrosyl-L-tyrosine alkyl ester monomer (DTR); (b) structure of the alkyl ester group; (c) structure of the diacid group.

where x represents the molar fraction of repeat units having a free carboxylic acid group (Hoven et al., 2004). The presence of DT in the polymer backbone results in an increased hydrolysis rate, making it possible to tune the polymer lifetime from years to weeks (Tschopp et al., 2000; Kohn, unpublished results).

By varying the molecular composition of DTR derived polymers, one can generate polymers whose physicomechanical and biological properties fit most biomedical applications. For example, the introduction of iodine atoms into the phenolic ring (Pendharkar et al., 1998) introduces radiopacity to the bulk polymer, a property that is imperative when x-ray imaging of implanted devices is to be performed. Replacement of the DTR structural unit by other naturally occurring substances has been investigated: replacement of the ethyl unit ($-CH_2CH_2-$) in tyrosine by methyl ($-CH_2-$) or ethenyl ($-CH=CH-$), has led to *HTR* (4-*Hydroxyphenylacety-L-Tyrosine Alkyl* ester) and *CTR* (4-hydroxycinnamyl-L-Tyrosine *Alkyl* ester) derived polymers, respectively (Brocchini et al., 1997; Kohn). Because these monomers have a more rigid structure, the resulting polymers exhibit an increased glass transition temperature ($T_g$) and stiffness.

An interesting recent development has been the use of phosphate esters as the linking group by reacting the diphenol monomer with alkyl- or arylphosphates resulting in polyphosphate esters (Mao and Leong, 1999; Gupta and Lopina, 2002, 2004). The phosphate group is ubiquitous in nature, and fully biocompatible and resorbable. Although these polymers are still in an experimental stage, they have shown promise in a number of biomedical studies such as peptide and growth factor release, gene delivery, nerve guides, contact lenses, and stent coating (Chaubal et al., 2003).

## 11.3 Physicomechanical Properties and Processing

Most of the important engineering properties of polymers are dependent on both the molecular weight and the polymer's processing history. It is therefore difficult to describe the properties of a polymer in absolute terms and it is impossible to compare the properties of two different polymers without specifying their molecular weight and the way in which the polymer specimens were fabricated and tested. It is therefore not surprising that the values reported in the literature for specific polymer properties are not always consistent. This point must be kept in mind when interpreting the information provided in this section.

A library of 112 tyrosine containing polyarylates has been synthesized through reaction of 14 different DTR and HTR diphenolic monomers with 8 different dicarboxylic acids (Brocchini et al., 1997). The polymers in this library exhibit a spectrum of physical properties, as illustrated in Figure 11.3a and b. From Figure 11.3a one sees that the glass transition temperature ($T_g$)—the temperature at which the polymer makes a transition from hard to soft—ranges from 2 to 91°C, depending on polymer structure. The polymers with short ester side chains and short diacid backbone groups generally have a higher $T_g$, while the opposite is true for polymers having longer ester side chains and longer diacid backbone groups. The materials in this library range from fairly strong and tough (for example: poly(DTE succinate)) to soft and flexible (for example: poly(DTO sebacate)). A correlation between polymer structure and the hydrophobicity of the polymer surface was established by measuring the air–water contact angle of solvent cast polymer surfaces by goniometry. The measured air–water contact angles, used as a rough estimate of surface hydrophobicity, range from 64 to 101° and increase with increasing lengths of side chain and diacid (Figure 11.3b).

Copolymerization of DTR monomers with short chains of PEG provides another means to alter the physical properties of a polymer significantly (Yu and Kohn, 1999). Poly(DTE carbonate) is a strong, tough, and stiff polymer that shows around 1 to 2% of equilibrium water uptake. In contrast, poly(DTE-co-PEG carbonate) that contains 5, 15, and 30 mol% PEG shows 10, 25, and 92% of equilibrium water uptake, respectively. When these copolymers contain more than 15 mol% PEG, they start to behave like hydrogels, while copolymers containing 70% PEG or more are water soluble.

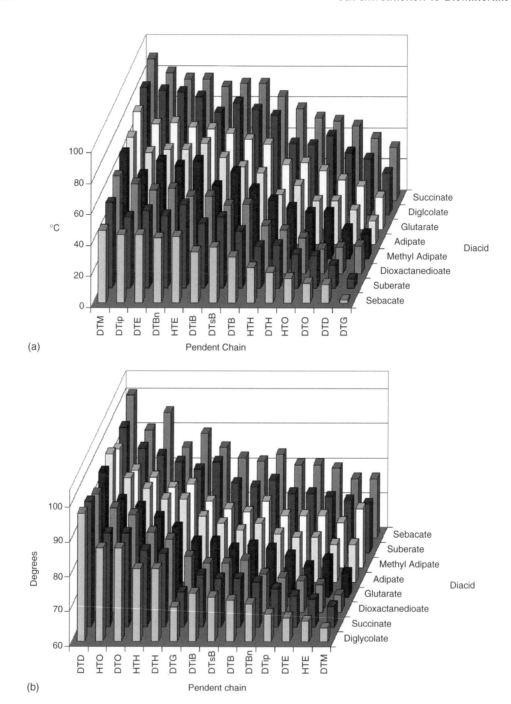

**FIGURE 11.3**
Physical properties in a library of L-tyrosine derived polyarylates. (a) Glass transition temperature (°C); (b) air–
water contact angle (degrees).

Most DTR derived polymers are soluble in organic solvents, opening the possibility
to fabricate films and fibers by solution processing techniques such as solvent casting,
electro-spinning, and wet-spinning. In addition, there is a large enough gap between
the glass transition ($\sim 0$ to 100°C) and decomposition ($\sim 250$ to 300°C) temperatures

in these materials to allow for an adequate temperature window for thermal processing methods. Thus, most DTR derived polymers can be processed by extrusion, compression and injection molding, allowing the fabrication of disks, rods, and devices with intricate shapes. Thus, polymer properties have been reported using many different types of specimens. The ease with which tyrosine-derived polymers can be processed makes it possible to consider these materials for a wide range of biomedical applications.

The ability to prepare polymer fibers is important for biomedical applications, such as the preparation of fiber meshes for use as tissue engineering scaffolds, sutures, implants for tendon reconstruction, or fiber mats for the prevention of tissue adhesions after surgery. In view of this, a number of publications describe the preparation and use of fibers prepared from various tyrosine-derived polymers. For example, fibers that were melt spun from poly(DTE carbonate) had a tensile modulus of 3.1 GPa and a tensile strength of 230 MPa. These fibers retained about 87% of their initial tensile strength after 30 weeks of incubation in phosphate buffered saline. For comparison, similar fibers made of PLLA retained only about 7% of their initial strength under identical experimental conditions. Based on these observations, it was suggest that poly(DTE carbonate) fibers may be used in the design of implants for the reconstruction of the anterior cruciate ligament (ACL) (Bourke et al., 2004). In contrast, fibers made from poly(DTD dodecanedioate) showed a comparable strength (200 MPa) but were less stiff (tensile modulus: 1 to 2 GPa). These fibers may be useful when soft tissue compliance is needed.

It was recently discovered that the poly(DTR arylate)s containing large side groups as well as large diacid groups showed orientation upon processing, up to the point of exhibiting liquid crystalline behavior (Jaffe et al., 2002, 2003a,b). Interchain hydrogen bonding as well as hydrophobic interactions between the ester group and diacid alkyl chain may be involved in the formation of a superstructure that leads to this interesting behavior. This discovery might open up the way for high strength polymeric biomaterials. Currently, additional studies are needed to define how the supramolecular structure can be fine-tuned through small variations in polymer processing.

The preparation of highly porous, sponge-like devices is of particular interest to tissue engineers. Such devices can serve as scaffolds for tissue regeneration. Tyrosine-derived polycarbonates and polyarylates have been used to prepare such scaffolds by a salt-leaching, solvent phase separation technique (James and Kohn, 1996; Lhommeau et al., 1998; Bouevich et al., 2000). These scaffolds exhibit a bimodal pore size distribution, where the macro pores have sizes in the order of 200 to 400 $\mu$m, and the micropores have sizes in the order of 1 to 10 $\mu$m. Figure 11.4 shows an illustrative example of a tissue engineering scaffold prepared from poly(DTE carbonate).

After being shaped into the desired structure, biomaterials need to be sterilized prior to implantation. Two standard techniques are treatment by ethylene oxide or gamma radiation. Gamma radiation sterilization is often preferred as this does not demand extensive degassing of the material after treatment. While sterilization by ethylene oxide has comparable effects on both PLA and poly(DTR carbonate)s, treatment with gamma radiation caused less loss of molecular weight in poly(DTR carbonate)s than in PLA (Bourke and Kohn, 2003). This fact, a result of the presence aromatic ring structures in the polymer, makes poly(DTR carbonate)s more suited for preimplant sterilization by gamma radiation than PLA.

Table 11.1 illustrates the variety of mechanically different materials that can be made by altering the chemical structure of tyrosine-derived polymers. It lists the glass transition and melting temperatures, as well as tensile strength data for a selected number of tyrosine-derived polymers. A selection of engineering plastics and established polymeric biomaterials is shown for comparison.

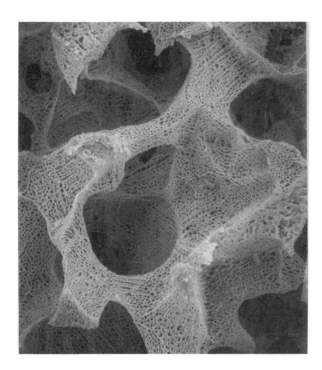

**FIGURE 11.4**
A porous tissue scaffold with bimodal pore size distribution made from poly(DTE carbonate).

## 11.4   Degradation Mechanism of DTR Polymers

The poly(hydroxy acid)s (such as PLA) degrade with the concomitant release of acid. The acidic degradation products have been shown to cause aberrant tissue responses, in particular when large devices (such as pins, screws, and plates) are implanted in bones (Böstman and Pihlajamaki, 2000). An inherent advantage of tyrosine-based polymers is that their degradation does not lead to a high local concentration of acidic degradation products. When comparing the amount of acid degradation products that are released upon hydrolysis, the following values are found for PGA, PLLA, poly(DTE adipate), and poly(DTE carbonate): 15.5, 11.4, 6.4, and 2.6 meq acid per gram of polymer (Bourke and Kohn, 2003), respectively.

DTR derived polymers exhibit *in vitro* and *in vivo* lifetimes that are tunable from several hours to several years depending on the backbone and pendent chain structure (Ertel and Kohn, 1994; Ertel et al., 1995), Incorporation of PEG into these polymer reduces its glass transition temperature and hydrophobicity, while incorporation of desaminotyrosine (DT), which has a free carboxylic acid group, increases its degradation rate (Tschopp et al., 2000).

The hypothesis that these polymers would degrade to naturally occurring substances under physiological conditions was confirmed by experiments. Studies on the hydrolysis kinetics of model compounds of poly(DTR carbonate) showed that under physiological conditions (a) the backbone carbonate group hydrolyzes at a higher rate than the ester side group, (b) increasing the length of the pendent ester group lowers the hydrolysis rate of both ester and carbonate group, and (c) the amide group showed no cleavage *in vitro* under physiologically relevant conditions (Tangpasuthadol et al., 2000a,b; Bourke and Kohn, 2003).

**TABLE 11.1**

Comparison of Some Physical Properties of Selected Engineering Plastics, Biodegradable Polymers, and L-Tyrosine Derived Polymers

| Material | $T_g^*$ (°C) | $T_m^{**}$ (°C) | Tensile Modulus (GPa) | Tensile Strength (MPa) | Elongation at Break (%) |
|---|---|---|---|---|---|
| Poly(butylenes terephthalate) (PBT) | 50 | 223 | 2.6 | 55 | 200–300 |
| Poly(ethylene terephthalate) (PET) | 70 | 265 | 1.7 | 50 | 180 |
| Poly(phenylene sulphide) (PPS) | 85 | a | 2.6–4.7 | 65–480 | 2–40 |
| Poly(bisphenol-A carbonate) (PC) | 150 | a | 2–2.4 | 45–66 | 100–110 |
| Nylon 6,6 | 162 | 265 | 1.7–3.3 | 62–82 | 30–60 |
| Polyethersulfone (PES) | 204 | a | 2.4 | 83 | 40–80 |
| Polyetherimide (PEI) | 215 | a | 3 | 105 | 60 |
| Kevlar®[b] | 425 | 554 | 76–165 | 2000–3000 | 1–2.5 |
| UHMWPE[c] | 90 | 140 | | | |
| Teflon®[e] | 126 | 335 | 0.34 | 7–270 | 100–600 |
| Polyorthoesters | 55–95 | | 0.82–1.2 | 19–27 | 7–220 |
| Polycaprolactone (PCL) | 62 | 57 | 0.4 | 16 | 80–700 |
| Poly(L-lactic acid) (PLLA) | 50–59 | 159–190 | 1.2–12 | 28–2300 | 2–26 |
| Poly(glycolic acid) (PGA) | 35 | 210–230 | 1.2–6.5 | 0.34–0.40 | 15–35 |
| Poly(hydroxy butyrate) (PHB) | 1 | 170–190 | 3.5–4 | 40 | 3 |
| Poly(DTE carbonate) (Ertel and Kohn, 1994; Kohn, 1998) | 93 | a | 1.5 | 67 | |
| Poly(DTB carbonate) (Ertel and Kohn, 1994; Kohn, 1998) | 90 | a | 1.6 | 60 | |
| Poly(DTH carbonate) (Ertel and Kohn, 1994; Kohn, 1998) | 63 | a | 1.4 | 32–220 | 120 |
| Poly(DTO carbonate) (Ertel and Kohn, 1994; Kohn, 1998) | 52 | a | 1.2 | 198 | |
| Poly(DTH succinate) | 53 | a | 1.20 | 31 | 9 |
| Poly(DTO succinate) | 48 | a | | | |
| Poly(DTE adipate) | 61 | a | 1.52 | 34 | 157 |
| Poly(DTH adipate) | 38 | a | 0.43 | 30 | 418 |
| Poly(DTO adipate) | 28 | a | 0.01 | 28 | 424 |

*(continued)*

**TABLE 11.1**　(Continued)

| Material | $T_g^*$ (°C) | $T_m^{**}$ (°C) | Tensile Modulus (GPa) | Tensile Strength (MPa) | Elongation at Break (%) |
|---|---|---|---|---|---|
| Poly(DTE sebacate) | 44 | LC | | | |
| Poly(DTH sebacate) | 20 | | 0.0026 | 23 | 449 |
| Poly(DTD sebacate) | 12 | LC | | | |
| Poly(DTE-co-x% PEG2k carbonate) | | a | 1.8[w]/0.97[d] | 36[w]/29[d] | 460[w]/820[d] |
| Poly(DTE-co-2% DT-co-PEG2k carbonate) | | a | 0.35[w]/0.023[d] | 21[w]/2.8[d] | 980[w]/230[d] |
| Poly(DTE-co-5% PEG1k carbonate) | | a | 1.2[w]/0.58[d] | 37[w]/19[d] | 590[w]/500[d] |

[a] Amorphous polymer; [LC] liquid crystalline behavior has been observed; [b] Kevlar® = poly(p-phenylene terephthalamide) from Dupont; [c] UHMWPE = ultra-high molecular weight polyethylene; [e] Teflon® = polytetrafluorethylene from Dupont; [w] in wet state; [d] in dry state.

*$T_g$ = glass transition temperature.

**$T_m$ = melting temperature.

## 11.5   *In Vitro* and *In Vivo* Biological Interactions

Protein adsorption on to biomaterial surfaces is recognized as the crucial first step to cell adhesion that in turn determines the ultimate *in vivo* performance of the biomedical construct. Figure 11.5 shows the amount of fibrinogen adsorbed onto polyarylate surfaces as measured by an immunofluorescence assay, and compares it to adsorption onto PLLA and PGA surfaces (Weber et al., 2004).

The amount of adsorbed fibrinogen varies from 55 to 220% of the control surface value (polypropylene) depending on the specific polymer structure. PLLA and PGA are among the more strongly binding surfaces, as are the polyarylates with shorter pendent ester and diacid groups. Longer ester and diacid groups are generally correlated with a decrease in fibrinogen adsorption. Since fibrinogen plays a key role in platelet activation and thrombosis, these measurements may indicate that polyarylates with long alkyl ester pendent chains and long diacids may be more hemocompatible than the commonly used PLLA and PGA. Of special interest is the comparison between poly(DTR glutarate)s and poly(DTR diglycolate)s (See Figure 11.2 for their structures). In spite of their structural

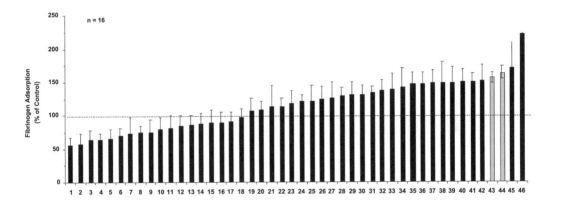

| 1  | p(DTiB sebacate)          | 16 | p(DTsB suberate)          | 31 | p(DTE adipate)            |
|----|---------------------------|----|---------------------------|----|---------------------------|
| 2  | p(HTH sebacate)           | 17 | p(DTBn suberate)          | 32 | p(DTM adipate)            |
| 3  | p(DTO glutarate)          | 18 | p(HTE suberate)           | 33 | p(DTsB glutarate)         |
| 4  | p(DTH adipate)            | 19 | p(DTsB adipate)           | 34 | p(DTO diglycolate)        |
| 5  | p(DTO sebacate)           | 20 | p(HTE adiapte)            | 35 | p(DTsB 3-methyl adipate)  |
| 6  | p(HTH suberate)           | 21 | p(DTM 3-methyl adipate)   | 36 | p(DTBn 3-methyl adipate)  |
| 7  | p(DTO adipate)            | 22 | p(DTH succinate)          | 37 | p(DTiP 3-methyl adipate)  |
| 8  | p(DTO suberate)           | 23 | p(DTB suberate)           | 38 | p(DTB adipate)            |
| 9  | p(HTH adipate)            | 24 | p(DTiP adipate)           | 39 | p(DTB 3-methyl adipate)   |
| 10 | p(DTBn sebacate)          | 25 | p(DTO succinate)          | 40 | p(DTH diglycolate)        |
| 11 | p(DTH 3-methyl adipate)   | 26 | p(DTB succinate)          | 41 | p(DTE 3-methyl adipate)   |
| 12 | p(DTH suberate)           | 27 | p(DTB glutarate)          | 42 | p(DTE glutarate)          |
| 13 | p(DTH glutarate)          | 28 | p(DTM suberate)           | 43 | *p(lactic glycolic acid)* |
| 14 | p(DTiB adipate)           | 29 | p(DTBn adipate)           | 44 | *p(lactic acid)*          |
| 15 | p(DTM sebacate)           | 30 | p(HTE 3-methyl adipate)   | 45 | p(HTE succinate)          |
|    |                           |    |                           | 46 | p(DTB diglycolate)        |

**FIGURE 11.5**

Human fibrinogen adsorption on flat and smooth polymer surfaces made of polymers from library of polyarylates, compared to PLLA and PLGA (gray bars). Values are normalized against noncoated polypropylene as a reference.

similarity and overall closely matched physicomechanical properties, the poly(DTR diglycolate)s show much higher fibrinogen adsorption than the poly(DTR glutarate)s. This fact demonstrates that even small structural variations within the same polymer family can have a significant effect on protein adsorption. This polymer structure dependant response can also be seen on a more complex, biological level. Table 11.2 summarizes results from several cell and animal studies using different polycarbonates and polyarylates.

**TABLE 11.2**

Overview of Selected Cell and Animal Studies on Different Polycarbonates and Polyarylates

| *In vitro* studies | |
|---|---|
| **Cell type** | **Polymer** |
| *Rat lung fibroblasts* | *Poly(DTR carbonate)s* |
| *Chick embryonal dorsal root ganglion cells* (James and Kohn, 1996) | |

Fibroblasts preferred hydrophilic surfaces, while nerve cells preferred hydrophobic surfaces, as judged by their relative proliferation rates.

| | |
|---|---|
| *Rat lung fibroblasts and osteoblasts* (Yu and Kohn, 1999) | *Poly(DTR-co-PEG1000 carbonate)s* |

Cell attachment and proliferation decreased significantly going from the ethyl via butyl to the hexyl ester. Incorporation of 1, 5, or 10% of PEG decreased cell attachment and proliferation even more.

| | |
|---|---|
| *Human keratinocytes* (Sharma et al., 2004) | *Poly(DTR-co-PEG1000 carbonate)s* |

Keratinocytes were shown to migrate at increasing speed with PEG contents increasing from 0, 4, to 8%.

| *In vivo* studies | |
|---|---|
| **Animal (implantation site)** | **Polymer** |
| *Rat (subcutaneous)* (Hooper et al., 1998) | *Poly(DTE carbonate), poly(DTE adipate)* |

Poly(DTE adipate) showed milder tissue response than than poly(DTE carbonate) and significant tissue in-growth. Estimated lifetime in nonloadbearing, soft tissue devices: poly(DTE carbonate) 3 years, poly(DTE adipate) 200 days. Poly(DTE carbonate) and poly(DTE adipate) are more hydrophobic than PLLA: less swelling of the implant during degradation, onset of mass loss in later stage of degradation in tyrosine polymers than PLLA.

| | |
|---|---|
| *Rats (subcutaneous)* (Silver et al., 1992) | *Poly(DTH carbonate)* |

Poly(DTH carbonate) exhibited good tissue compatibility and milder inflammation response than HDPE and PLLA controls. Polycarbonate had thinner fibrous capsule around implant than HDPE.

| | |
|---|---|
| *Rabbit (distal femur)* (Ertel et al., 1995) | *Poly(DTH carbonate)* |

Poly(DTH carbonate) demonstrated bone apposition (i.e., direct contact between bone and implant without intervening scar tissue), while polydioxanone showed a fibrous layer surrounding the implant during whole 6-month study.

| | |
|---|---|
| *Rabbits (transcortically)* (James et al., 1999a,b) | *Poly(DTR carbonate) R = Et, Bu, Hex, Oct* |

Poly(DTE carbonate) showed highest degree of bone apposition, least encapsulation and strength loss in study of this series in 1280 day study. Neither mechanical strength nor stiffness is source of osteocompatibility, but changing polymer chemistry upon degradation: easily hydrolyzable ethyl ester group liberates carboxylate groups that complex calcium ions.

| | |
|---|---|
| *Dog (femur)* (Choueka et al., 1996) | *Poly(DTR carbonate) R = Et, Hex* |

Bone in-growth increased continuously in DTE and DTH over 48 weeks, while PLLA control peaked at 24, then decreased. Fibrous capsule around PLLA implant, while bone apposition on to DTE and DTH. 50% weight loss after 48 weeks in all samples.

| | |
|---|---|
| *Pig (coronary artery)* (Zeltinger et al., 2004) | *Polycarbonates* |

Interarterial stent was well apposed to vessel wall with little damage to internal elastic lamina. Negligible inflammation and thrombosis in 28-day study. Antiproliferative drugs blended into polymer can regulate formation of neointima.

It is clear from this table that these polymers induce a biological response that depends both on their specific structure, as well as on the cell or tissue that they are brought in contact with. An illustration of a tissue dependent response is found for poly(DTE carbonate): in contact with soft tissue it forms a fibrous capsule identical to the response seen for PLA and other clinically used biomaterials, while in hard tissue an exceptional degree of bone apposition is observed, leading to the conclusion that poly(DTE carbonate) is superior to most other polymers in terms of bone tissue compatibility (Hooper et al., 1998). Thus, under certain conditions, it is possible to optimize the cell-material or tissue–material interactions of a medical implant by carefully fine-tuning the chemical structure of the biomaterial used in the fabrication of the implant.

## 11.6   Drug Delivery and Device Coatings

The versatile chemistry of L-tyrosine derived polymers makes it possible to independently vary the glass transition temperature ($T_g$) of the polymer and its hydrophobic/hydrophilic nature. This makes them promising candidates for use as drug delivery vehicles or coatings since changes in polymer structure can be used to tune the drug release properties over a wide range.

In most drug delivery applications, a drug and polymer are mixed, forming either a homogeneous or phase-separated blend. The rate of drug release is usually controlled by the rate of diffusion of the drug through the polymeric matrix, and the rate of diffusion, in turn, is critically affected by $T_g$ and the hydrophobicity/hydrophilicity of the polymer matrix: In most cases, there is a sharp increase in the rate of drug diffusion, when an amorphous polymer is warmed from below its $T_g$ (glassy state) to above its $T_g$ (rubbery state). Obviously, for practical applications, the temperature of drug release is fixed at body temperature (37°C). Therefore, it is important to be able to vary the polymer's $T_g$ through small structural changes. In the case of polyarylates, this can be achieved by varying side chain length: Poly(DTE adipate) is glassy at 37°C, while poly(DTH adipate) is rubbery. The simple change from an *ethyl* ester pendent chain in DTE to a *hexyl* ester pendent chain in DTH resulted in a tenfold higher release rate of p-nitro aniline, a model compound for low molecular weight, hydrophobic drugs (Fiordeliso, 1993; Fiordeliso et al., 1994).

Another way to dramatically affect drug release is through a change in the hydrophobicity of the polymer matrix. In the case of tyrosine-derived polymers, where the monomer (DTR) is hydrophobic, drug release rates can be accelerated by copolymerization with a hydrophilic component such as PEG. This was shown by the incorporation of p-nitro aniline in microspheres made of copolymers of DTB (B stands for butyl) and PEG. In a series of copolymers, designated as poly(DTB-co-x% PEG carbonate), the diffusion controlled release of p-nitro aniline increased with increasing PEG content in the polymer (Yu and Kohn, 1999).

Using the principles described above, tyrosine-derived polymers have been studied in a wide range of drug delivery applications. For example, poly(DTH carbonate) was used in an intercranial, long-term, controlled release device for dopamine (Coffey et al., 1992; Dong, 1993). This hydrophilic drug molecule is usually rapidly degraded under physiological conditions. After formulation of the release device, the polymeric matrix provided protection against degradation. About 15% of the total dopamine loading was released over 180 days, which translated into a therapeutically relevant release rate of 1 to 2 μg/day.

In some drug delivery applications it is desirable to obtain a time delayed, pulsatile release profile. Integrilin® is a clinically used, antithrombotic heptapeptide.

When this water soluble peptide was blended into different poly(DTR arylates), no release of the peptide was observed when the peptide-loaded polymer was kept in phosphate buffer solution for more than 40 days. This surprising finding was explained by a strong, hydrogen bond mediated interaction between the peptide and the polymer matrix. As hydrogen bonding is weakened when the pH drops, it was hypothesized that peptide release should occur upon acidification of the polymer matrix. Based on this idea, small quantities of fast degrading lactide–glycolide copolymers (PLGA) were added to the poly(DTR arylate)–peptide blends. As the PLGA degraded, releasing acidic degradation products within the interior of the poly(DTR arylate) matrix, the peptide–polymer interaction was weakened and the release of peptide commenced. The time lag of peptide release was dependent on the molecular weight of the PLGA: Lag times of 5, 18, and 27 days were observed when the PLGA had molecular weights of 12,000, 18,000, and 62,000, respectively (Schachter et al., 1996; Schachter and Kohn, 2002).

Tyrosine-derived polymers have also been explored for the effective delivery of water insoluble drugs. Such drugs pose a significant delivery problem since a minimum level of solubility in body fluids is required for bioavailability. Using a different molecular architecture, a triblock copolymer, designated as PEG5000–*block*-oligo(DTO suberate)–*block*-PEG5000, was synthesized. This amphiphilic triblock copolymer self-assembles when dispersed in an aqueous medium to form nanospheres with a diameter of about 45 to 70 nm. While the exterior of the nanospheres is hydrophilic, the interior is hydrophobic and allows for the solubilization of drugs that would otherwise be insoluble in water. For example, the clinical use of the hydrophobic antitumor drug Paclitaxel is limited by its low solubility in aqueous media. However, Paclitaxel-nanosphere complexes could be dispersed in aqueous media readily and had the same strong antiproliferative activity as the drug itself when tested against KB cervical carcinoma cells (Sheihet et al., 2003, submitted for publication).

## 11.7   Conclusions

In this chapter we discussed polymeric biomaterials derived from L-tyrosine. In the past decade the biomedical and biomaterials communities have come to realize that using non-optimized, off-the-shelf polymers for a wide variety of biomedical applications often does not allow meeting the very goal-specific material demands. The use of L-tyrosine derived polymers opens up versatile ways to adjust the material properties to match the requirements of specific individual applications.

The DTR (desaminotyrosyl-L-tyrosine alkyl ester) diphenolic monomers that are presented in this chapter can be modified at their pendant ester group, and they can be polymerized in a variety of ways to form polycarbonates, polyarylates, or poly(phosphate ester)s, that may additionally contain DT (desaminotyrosyl-L-tyrosine) and PEG (poly(ethylene glycol)) as comonomers. All of these polymers are biocompatible, their degradation products are natural metabolites or biologically benign substances. They offer a range of tunable chemical, physical, and mechanical properties, are solvent soluble, and have convenient thermal processing windows. Although they are generally amorphous, some of these polymers exhibit liquid crystalline-like behavior that might be used to fabricate high strength biomaterials.

Prehydrolyzation of a controlled amount of the pendant ester groups to generate free carboxylic acid groups increases the hydrolytic degradation rate of the polymers, allowing for *in vivo* lifetimes of implanted devices that can range from years to days. Protein adsorption and cell interaction behavior of these materials can be tuned through the introduction of hydrophobic or hydrophilic groups. These polymers can also be made inherently x-ray visible by covalent iodination of the phenyl ring in the backbone. Another noteworthy property is the fact that L-tyrosine derived polymers do not generate a high flux of acidic components upon *in vivo* degradation.

Research undertaken over the past 15 years has shown that the family of L-tyrosine derived monomers are promising biomaterials candidates. They may find a wide range of practical applications in the near future.

## Problems

### Problem 1
How much more acid does PLLA release per gram material upon hydrolytic degradation than does poly(DTE carbonate)?
**Answer to Problem 1**
PLLA produces $11.4/2.6 = 4 \times$ more acid per gram material than poly(DTE carbonate).

### Problem 2
What method was used to create tyrosine-derived biomaterials that are x-ray visible? Can that method be used for other polymer systems?
**Answer to Problem 2**
The phenolic rings present in the tyrosine-derived monomers (DTR) were permanently iodinated. Iodine, like all heavy elements, scatters x-rays effectively, resulting in visibility of the material by x-ray imaging. This approach is limited to those polymers that contain aromatic rings (benzyl or phenyl), which can be readily iodinated. Aliphatic iodine derivatives tend to be toxic and are therefore less useful for the creation of x-ray visible biomaterials.

### Problem 3
Arrange the following chemical bonds in order of increasing rate of degradation under physiological conditions and comment on the principle mechanism of degradation: ester, ether, carbonate, anhydride, and amide (peptide).
**Answer to Problem 3**
Ether (usually stable, slow oxidative cleavage possible) < amide (enzymatic degradation only, stable to hydrolysis) < ester (hydrolysis) ~ carbonate (hydrolysis) ≪ anhydride (fast hydrolysis).

### Problem 4
How could the level of cell adhesion and polymer degradation be optimized for different applications and which L-tyrosine derived polymer compositions could one use for:
  (A) An application that requires a strong, stiff, but fast degrading polymer with a high level of cell adhesion?

  (B) An application that requires a flexible polymer with little cell adhesion?
**Answer to Problem 4**
Poly(DTE carbonate) is a very good choice for a strong, stiff polymer with a high level of cell adhesion, but it degrades too slowly. The rate of degradation can be increased by the

incorporation of "DT" units into the polymer backbone. Thus, poly(DTE-co-x% DT carbonate) fulfills the stated requirements of (A). The value of "x" would have to be optimized depending on the rate of degradation required. Tyrosine-derived polyarylates are more flexible than polycarbonates. Among the polyarylates, those with longer diacid backbone structures tend to be more flexible than those with shorter diacids. Therefore, poly(DTR suberate) or poly(DTR sebacate) would be good starting points. However, these polymers are good substrates for cell adhesion. To reduce the cell adhesion and increase polymer flexibility further, copolymerization with PEG is a good approach. Therefore, poly(DTR-co-x% PEG suberate) or poly(DTR-co-x% PEG sebacate) would be good choices. The nature of "R" and the value of "x" depend on the specific application and could be used to further fine-tune the polymer properties.

## Problem 5
Poly(DTR diglycolate)s and poly(DTR glutarate)s have only slightly different chemical structures, and almost the same surface hydrophobicity (the R group being the same). However, the adsorption of fibrinogen is markedly different on both surfaces. How would you explain the large difference in the fibrinogen adsorption onto these materials?

**Answer to Problem 5**
The ether oxygen atom in the diglycolate monomer provides a selective adsorption site for the fibrinogen molecule. This unique site is not present in the glutarate monomer.

## Problem 6
Write the structural formula for the following tyrosine-derived polymers:
poly(DTE carbonate), poly(DTH-co-10 mol%PEG$_{2000}$ carbonate), poly(DTO suberate), poly (DTB-co-5 mol%DT-co-10mol%PEG$_{1000}$ adipate).

**Answer to Problem 6**
See Figure 11.6.

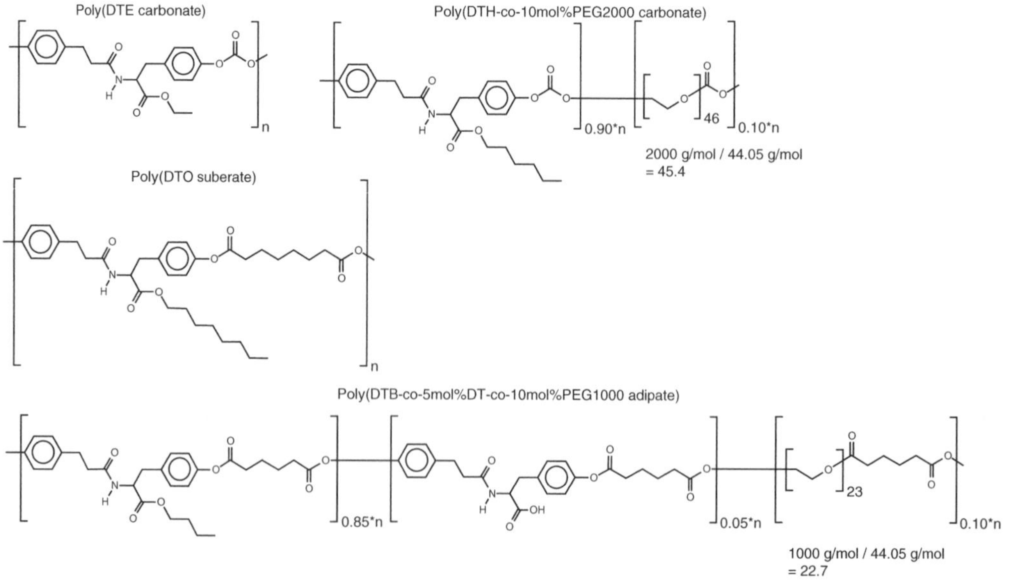

**FIGURE 11.6**
Answer to problem 6.

## Problem 7
What changes in the structure of poly(DTE carbonate) would you suggest to:
   (A) Increase the rate of degradation without affecting the polymer's stiffness?
   (B) Increase the rate of degradation slightly while also making the polymer more flexible? What other property would be affected by that structural modification?

### Answer to Problem 7
   (A) Incorporate "DT" units into the polymer backbone. This will significantly increase degradation rate without affecting mechanical properties. The other alternative is to incorporate PEG into the polymer backbone. While this, too, increases the degradation rate, it significantly reduces stiffness and strength as well.
   (B) As outlined in (A), incorporation of PEG would achieve the stated goals, but this approach would also reduce the hydrophobicity of the polymer matrix and would result in a polymer with higher equilibrium water uptake than poly(DTE carbonate).

## Problem 8
Which of the tyrosine-derived polymers are good candidates for use as a load-bearing orthopedic implant such as a small bone fixation pin or screw? First, state the requirements of the polymer for this specific application, then the material of your choice.

### Answer to Problem 8
Good osteoconductivity, $T_g$ significantly above body temperature, high stiffness, high strength, high toughness, and medium- to long-range degradation time with strength retention for at least 6 months. One of the best candidate materials among the tyrosine-derived polymers with this property profile is poly(DTE carbonate).

## Problem 9
Why are polymers derived from desaminotyrosyl-tyrosine alkyl esters (DTR) more processible than conventional poly(L-tyrosine)?

### Answer to Problem 9
Poly(L-tyrosine) is nonprocessable since it is virtually insoluble in most organic solvents and since it thermally decomposes before it melts, eliminating any of the thermal processing techniques such as compression or injection molding. The nonprocessability of poly(L-tyrosine) is a consequence of strong interchain hydrogen bonding mediated by the amide bonds in the polymer backbone. In DTR-derived polymers, 50% of all amide bonds are replaced by other bonds such as ester or carbonate bonds, which are not hydrogen-bond donors. This reduces interchain hydrogen bonding leading to (a) increased solubility and (b) reduced melt viscosity so that the polymer can be extruded or molded at temperatures that are below its thermal decomposition temperature.

## References

Böstman, O.M. and Pihlajamaki, H., Clinical biocompatibility of biodegradable orthopedic implants for internal fixation: a review, *Biomaterials*, **21**, 2615 (2000).
Bouevich, F. et al., Microscopic analysis of porous biodegradable scaffolds for tissue engineering, *Microscopy and Microanalysis*, (2000), Philadelphia (2000).

Bourke, S.L. et al., Preliminary development of a novel resorbable synthetic polymer fiber scaffold for anterior cruciate ligament reconstruction, *Tissue Engineering*, **10**, 43 (2004).

Bourke, S.L. and Kohn, J., Polymers derived from the amino acid L-tyrosine: polycarbonates, polyarylates and copolymers with poly(ethylene glycol), *Adv. Drug Del. Rev.*, **55**, 447 (2003).

Brocchini, S. et al., A combinatorial approach for polymer design, *J. Am. Chem. Soc.*, **119**, 4553 (1997).

Brocchini, S. et al., Structure–property correlations in a combinatorial library of degradable biomaterials, *J. Biomed. Mater. Res.*, **42**, 66 (1998).

Chaubal, M.V. et al., Polyphosphates and other phosphorus-containing polymers for drug delivery, *Critical Reviews in Therapeutic Drug Carrier Systems*, **20**, 295 (2003).

Choueka, J. et al., Canine bone response to tyrosine-derived polycarbonates and poly(L-lactic acid), *J. Biomed. Mater. Res.*, **31**, 35 (1996).

Coffey, D. et al. Evaluation of a tyrosine derived polycarbonate device for the intracranial release of dopamine, in *Symposium on Polymer Delivery Systems presented at the 203rd Meeting of American Chemical Society*, San Francisco, CA (1992), CELL 0058.

Crawford, R.J., *Plastics Engineering*, 3rd ed., Butterworth-Heinemann, Oxford (1998).

d'Acunzo, F. et al., Alternating multiblock amphiphilic copolymers of peg and tyrosine-derived diphenols. Ii. Self-assembly in aqueous solution and at hydrophobic surfaces, *Macromolecules*, **35**, 9366 (2002a).

d'Acunzo, F. and Kohn, J., Alternating multiblock amphiphilic copolymers of peg and tyrosine-derived diphenols. I. Synthesis and characterization, *Macromolecules*, **35**, 9360 (2002b).

Dong, Z., Synthesis of four structurally related tyrosine-derived polycarbonates and in vitro study of dopamine release from poly(desaminotyrosyl-tyrosine hexyl ester carbonate), M.Sc. thesis, Rutgers University (1993).

Ertel, S.I. et al., Evaluation of poly(DTH carbonate), a tyrosine-derived degradable polymer, for orthopaedic applications, *J. Biomed. Mater. Res.*, **29**, 1337 (1995).

Ertel, S.I. and Kohn, J., Evaluation of a series of tyrosine-derived polycarbonates for biomaterial applications, *J. Biomed. Mater. Res.*, **28**, 919 (1994).

Fiordeliso, J., Aliphatic polyarylates derived from L-tyrosine: *A New Class of Biomaterials for Biomedical Applications*, M.S. thesis, Rutgers University (1993).

Fiordeliso, J. et al., Design, synthesis, and preliminary characterization of tyrosine-containing polyarylates: New biomaterials for medical applications, *J. Biomater. Sci (Polym. Ed.)*, **5**, 497 (1994).

Gupta, A.S. and Lopina, S.T., L-Tyrosine-based backbone-modified poly(amino acids), *J. Biomater. Sci. Polym. Ed.*, **13**, 1093 (2002).

Gupta, A.S. and Lopina, S.T., Synthesis and characterization of L-tyrosine based novel polyphosphates for potential biomaterial applications, *Polymer*, **45**, 4653 (2004).

Hooper, K.A. et al., Comparative histological evaluation of new tyrosine-derived polymers and poly(L-lactic acid) as a function of polymer degradation, *J. Biomed. Mater. Res.*, **41**, 443 (1998).

Hoven, V.P. et al., Acid-containing tyrosine-derived polycarbonates: Wettability and surface reactivity, *Macromol. Symp.*, **216**, 87 (2004).

Jaffe, M. et al., Process–structure–property relationships of erodable polymeric biomaterials, i: poly (desaminotyrosyl arylates), *Pol. Adv. Tech.*, **13**, 926 (2002).

Jaffe, M. et al., Process–structure–property relationships of erodable polymeric biomaterials, ii: long range order in poly (desaminotyrosyl arylates), *Polymer*, **44**, 6033 (2003a).

Jaffe, M. et al., Biorelevant characterization of biopolymers, *Thermochim. Acta*, **396**, 141 (2003b).

James, K. et al. Small animal surgical and histological procedures for characterizing the performance of tissue engineered bone grafts, In: *Methods in Molecular Medicine: Tissue Engineering Methods and Protocols*, Morgan, J.R. and Yarmush, M.L., Eds., The Humana Press, Totowa, NJ, pp. 121 (1999a).

James, K. et al., Small changes in polymer chemistry have a large effect on the bone-implant interface: evaluation of a series of degradable tyrosine-derived polycarbonates in bone defects, *Biomaterials*, **20**, 2203 (1999b).

James, K. and Kohn, J., New biomaterials for tissue engineering, *MRS Bulletin*, **21**, 22 (1996).

James, K. and Kohn, J., Pseudo-poly(amino acid)s: Examples for synthetic materials derived from natural metabolites, In: *Controlled Drug Delivery: Challenges and strategies*, Park, K., Ed., American Chemical Society, Washington, DC, pp. 389 (1997).

Kohn, J., Unpublished results.

Kohn, J., The synthesis and characterization of pseudopoly(amino acids): new polymers for medical applications, *Polym. Prepr.*, **31** (2), 178 (1990).

Kohn, J., Pseudopoly(amino acids), In: *Biodegradable Polymers as Drug Delivery Systems*, Chasin, M. and Langer, R., Eds., Marcel Dekker, New York, pp. 195 (1990).

Kohn, J., Desaminotyrosyl-tyrosine alkyl esters: New diphenolic monomers for the design of tyrosine-derived pseudopoly(amino acids), In: *Polymeric Drugs and Drug Delivery Systems*, Dunn, R.L. and Ottenbrite, R.M., Eds., American Chemical Society, Washington, DC, pp. 155 (1991a).

Kohn, J., Pseudo-poly(amino acids), *Drug News Perspect.*, **4**, 289 (1991b).

Kohn, J., Design, synthesis, and possible applications of pseudo-poly(amino acids), *Trends Polym. Sci.*, **1**, 206 (1993).

Kohn, J., The use of natural metabolites in the design of new materials for tissue engineering, In: *Tissue engineering for therapeutic use*, Ikada, Y. and Yamaoka, Y., Eds., Elsevier Science, New York, pp. 61 (1998).

Kohn, J. and Langer, R., Poly(iminocarbonates) as potential biomaterials, *Biomaterials*, **7**, 176 (1986).

Kohn, J. and Langer, R., Polymerization reactions involving the side chains of α-L-amino acids, *J. Am. Chem. Soc.*, **109**, 817 (1987).

Kohn, J. et al. Bioresorbable and bioerodible materials, In: *Biomaterials Science*, 2nd ed., Ratner, B. et al., Eds., Academic Press, San Diego, CA, pp. 115 (2004).

Lhommeau, C. et al., Preparation of highly interconnected porous, tyrosine-derived polycarbonate scaffolds, *Tissue Eng.*, **4**, 468 (1998).

Mao, H. and Leong, K.W., USA 5912225, 1999, Biodegradable poly(phosphoester-*co*-desaminotyrosyl L-tyrosine ester) compounds, compositions, articles and methods for making and using the same. 04-14-1997.

Pachence, J.M. and Kohn, J., *Biodegradable Polymers*, 2nd ed., Lanza, R.P. et al., Eds., Academic Press, San Diego, CA, pp. 263 (2000).

Pendharkar, S.M. et al. Iodinated derivatives of tyrosine-based polycarbonates: New radio-opaque degradable biomaterials, *Annual Meeting of the Society for Biomaterials*. Society for Biomaterials, San Diego, CA, p. 386 (1998).

Pulapura, S. and Kohn, J., Pseudo-poly(amino acids): An extension of pseudopeptide chemistry to the design of polymeric biomaterials, In: *Peptides-Chemistry and Biology: Proceedings of the 12th american peptide symposium*, Smith, J.A. and Rivier, J.E, Eds., Escom Science Publishers, Leiden, The Netherlands, pp. 539 (1992).

Pulapura, S. and Kohn, J., Tyrosine derived polycarbonates: backbone modified "pseudo"-poly(amino acids) designed for biomedical applications, *Biopolymers*, **32**, 411 (1992).

Schachter, D.M. and Kohn, J., A synthetic polymer matrix for the delayed or pulsatile release of water-soluble peptides, *J. Control. Rel.*, **78**, 143 (2002).

Schachter, D.M. et al. *Controlled Release of an Antithrombic Peptide: The Effect of Peptide–Polymer Miscibility and Phase Separations*, *Advances in Controlled Delivery*, Controlled Release Society, Baltimore, MD, p. 49 (1996).

Sharma, R.I. et al., Poly(ethylene glycol) enhances cell motility on protein based poly(ethylene glycol)-polycarbonate substrates: a mechanism for cell-guided ligand remodeling, *J. Biomed. Mater. Res.*, **69A**, 114–123 (2004).

Sheihet, L. et al., Hydrophobic drug delivery by self-assembling triblock copolymer-derived nanospheres, Submitted for publication.

Sheihet, L. et al., Self-assembled triblock copolymer hollow vesicles for gene and drug delivery, *Mat. Res. Soc. Symp. Proc.*, **EXS-1** (I5), 7 (2003).

Silver, F.H. et al., Tissue compatibility of tyrosine derived polycarbonates and polyiminocarbonates: An initial evaluation, *J. Long-Term Effects Med. Implants*, **1**, 329 (1992).

Tangpasuthadol, V. et al., Hydrolytic degradation of tyrosine-derived polycarbonates, a class of new biomaterials. Part i: Study of model compounds, *Biomaterials*, **21**, 2371 (2000a).

Tangpasuthadol, V. et al., Hydrolytic degradation of tyrosine-derived polycarbonates, a class of new biomaterials. Part ii: 3-yr study of polymeric devices, *Biomaterials*, **21**, 2379 (2000b).

Tschopp, J.F. et al. In vivo resorption profile of matrices from tyrosine-derived polycarbonates with variation in free carboxylate content, *Transactions of the 6th World Biomaterials Congress.* Society for Biomaterials, Kamuela, USA, p. 1334 (2000).

Weber, N. et al., Small changes in the polymer structure influence the adsorption behavior of fibrinogen on polymer surfaces: Validation of a new rapid screening technique, *J. Biomed. Mater. Res.*, **68**, 496 (2004).

Yu, C. and Kohn, J., Tyrosine-peg-derived poly(ether carbonate)s as new biomaterials. Part i: Synthesis and evaluation, *Biomaterials*, **20**, 253 (1999).

Zeltinger, J. et al., Advances in the development of coronary stents, *Biomaterials Forum (Official Newsletter of the Society for Biomaterials)*, **26**, 8 (2004).

# 12

## Poly(Propylene Fumarate)

Xinfeng Shi and Antonios G. Mikos

### CONTENTS

## 12.1 Introduction

Poly(propylene fumarate) (PPF) is a synthetic, unsaturated, linear polyester which can be cross-linked through its fumarate double bonds and degraded by random hydrolytic scission of its ester groups (Figure 12.1) (Temenoff and Mikos, 2000). Its major degradation products, propylene glycol and fumaric acid, are biocompatible and readily removed from the body. When cross-linked, the tight network structure of PPF imparts mechanical strength sufficient for its use in bone replacement scaffolds. Furthermore, porous PPF scaffolds can provide an osteoconductive surface for bone in-growth, making it an attractive biomaterial for orthopaedic and dental applications.

## 12.2 Synthesis

While a variety of schemes have been utilized to synthesize PPF (Sanderson, 1988; Domb, 1989; Gerhart and Hayes, 1989; Kharas et al., 1997; Peter et al., 1999b), a two-step procedure is commonly utilized, involving bis(hydroxypropyl fumarate) as an

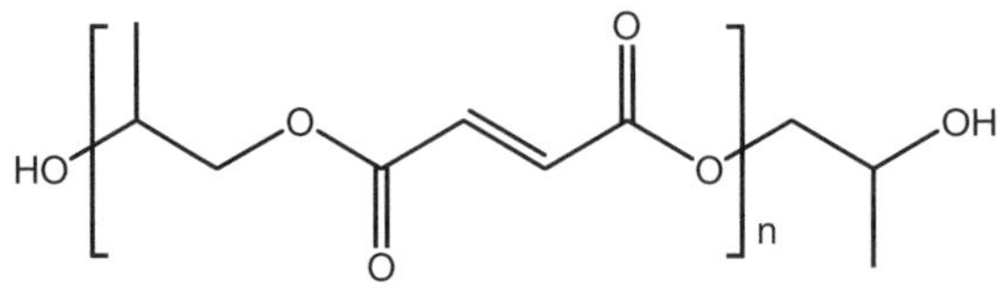

**FIGURE 12.1**
Chemical structure of poly(propylene fumarate) (PPF).

intermediate (Figure 12.2) (Shung et al., 2002). In the first step, diethyl fumarate reacts with excess propylene glycol in a 1:3 molar ratio to produce bis(hydroxypropyl fumarate). Zinc chloride ($ZnCl_2$), an acid catalyst, is added in a 0.01:1 molar ratio with diethyl fumarate. Hydroquinone is also added in a 0.002:1 molar ratio with diethyl fumarate as an inhibitor to restrain undesired thermal cross-linking. This mixture is vigorously mixed by an overhead mechanical stirrer and gradually heated under a

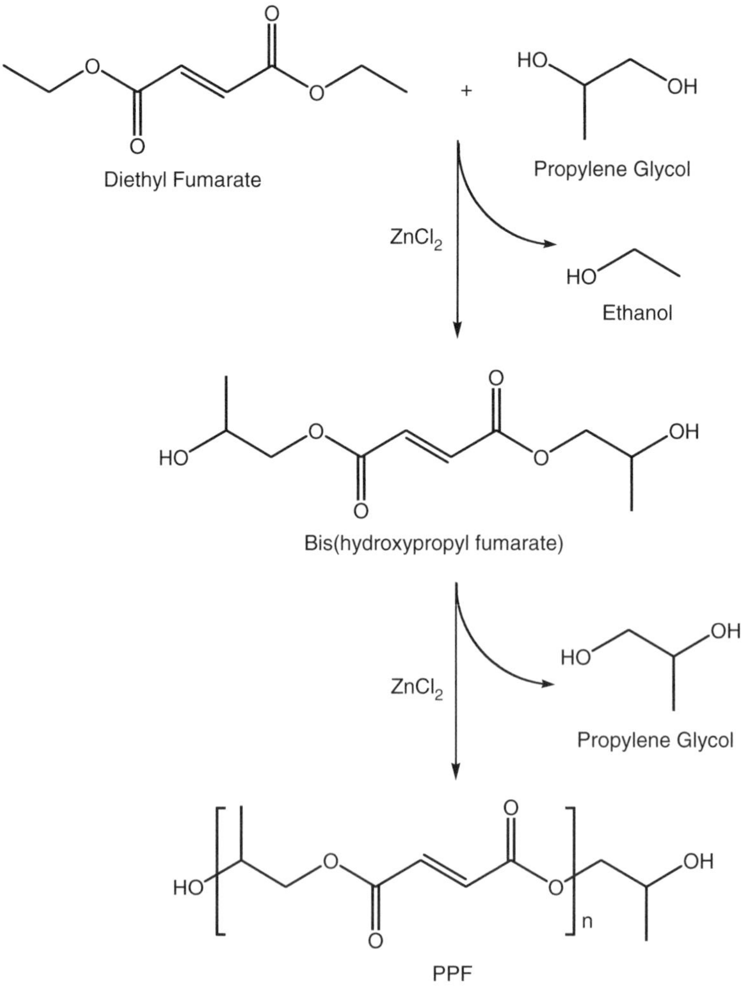

**FIGURE 12.2**
Reaction scheme of the two-step synthesis of PPF from diethyl fumarate and propylene glycol.

nitrogen blanket from 100 to 150°C. The reaction continues until 90% of the theoretical amount of ethanol, a by-product of the reaction, is condensed and collected.

In the second step, the bis(hydroxypropyl fumarate) is transesterified under vacuum (<1 mmHg) while slowly increasing the temperature from 100 to 150°C. PPF is produced in this second step, while propylene glycol is condensed as a by-product. The number average molecular weight, $M_n$, of PPF gradually increases with reaction temperature and time. Therefore, PPF's molecular weight can be monitored by gel permeation chromatography (GPC) as the reaction proceeds.

For purification, the polymer is first dissolved in methylene chloride and then sequentially washed with acid (5 wt% HCl in $H_2O$), water, and brine to remove the $ZnCl_2$ catalyst. After drying with sodium sulfate, methylene chloride is rotary evaporated, and the product is added dropwise to cold ethyl ether to extract the hydroquinone inhibitor. Ethyl ether is then decanted. The remaining product is vacuum dried to remove all organic solvents, leaving a viscous, yellow liquid of purified PPF. Because the only reactant in the second step is the bis(hydroxypropyl fumarate), there is no concern regarding stoichiometric imbalances. Thus, PPF of high purity can be achieved. This synthesis method also ensures that the resulting polymer is hydroxyl-terminated, enabling future peptide functionalization.

## 12.3 Physicochemical Properties

PPF with a few repeat units in length is a viscous yellow liquid at room temperature (Domb, 1989). As the polymer chain length increases, PPF becomes more viscous and eventually exists as a yellow solid plastic. For example, PPF polymer with a $M_n$ of 1460 ± 200 Da and a polydispersity index of 2.6 is a liquid at room temperature and has a glass transition temperature of 11.2°C. Its glass transition has a midpoint of 16.2°C, but there is no melting endotherm due to the amorphous nature of the polymer (Peter et al., 1997b). PPF is soluble in methylene chloride, chloroform, tetrahydrofuran, acetone, ethanol, and ethyl acetate, is partially soluble in toluene, and is not soluble in petroleum ether or water (Domb, 1989).

### 12.3.1 Injectability and Cross-Linking Characteristics

Because PPF is a liquid before cross-linking, it can be easily fabricated into irregularly shaped implants by molding or injection molding. Alternatively, PPF can be injected at a defect site and then cross-linked *in situ*. Injectability makes PPF suitable for bone cements and orthopaedic implants in minimally invasive procedures.

As an unsaturated linear polyester, PPF can be hardened *in situ* via thermal cross-linking or photo cross-linking to form strong polymer networks through its reactive carbon–carbon double bond (Figure 12.3) (Timmer et al., 2003a). This free-radical propagated cross-linking reaction can be achieved without the addition of cross-linking agents. However, cross-linking monomers and macromers, such as methyl methacrylate (MMA), *N*-vinyl pyrrolidone (NVP), diethyl fumarate (DEF), and poly(propylene fumarate)-diacrylate (PPF-DA) are often added to tailor the physical properties of the cross-linked network or to speed the cross-linking reaction (Gerhart and Hayes, 1989; Yaszemski et al., 1995; He et al., 2001; Fisher et al., 2002a).

The choice of cross-linking agent can affect the degradation and mechanical properties of the cross-linked polymer. For instance, NVP can polymerize with itself resulting in nondegradable poly(*N*-vinyl pyrrolidone) (PNVP). However, PNVP is water soluble and

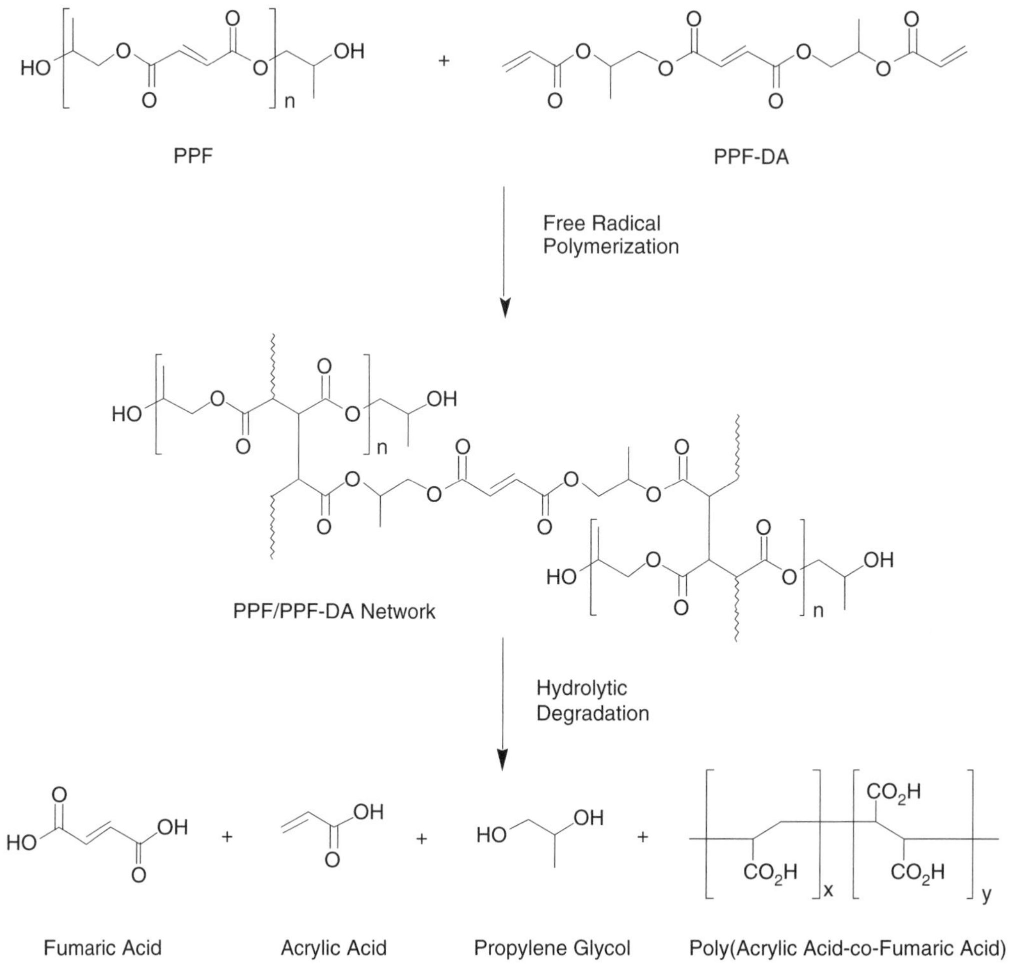

**FIGURE 12.3**
Cross-linking and degradation scheme of PPF/PPF-DA networks. (*Source*: From Timmer, M.D., Shin, H., Horch, R.A., Ambrose, C.G., and Mikos, A.G., *Biomacromolecules*, **4**, 1026 (2003e). With permission.)

may be excreted from the body (Robinson et al., 1990). PPF-DA, a derivative of PPF, contains two acrylate terminal groups, whose double bonds are more reactive than those of the fumarate group. Thus, PPF-DA incorporation may increase the degree of cross-linking of PPF (Timmer et al., 2002). The mechanical properties of highly cross-linked PPF-based networks improve with increasing amounts of PPF-DA, providing a method to tailor the polymer's mechanical properties to correspond to those of the tissue being replaced (He et al., 2001). In addition, the presence of ester groups in PPF-DA and DEF allows for biodegradation of the PPF-based networks into smaller hydrophilic molecules that can be either metabolized or passively excreted by the kidneys (He et al., 2001).

The thermal cross-linking reaction is typically triggered by addition of a suitable free-radical initiator like benzoyl peroxide (BP). The formation of free radicals can be accelerated by mixing with dimethyltoluidene (DMT) at room temperature or by simply increasing the temperature. Photo cross-linking reaction is accomplished by adding a photoinitiator such as bis(2,4,6-trimethylbenzoyl) phenylphosphine oxide (BAPO) followed by irradiation with blue light (14 mW/cm$^2$) or ultraviolet (UV) light (2 mW/cm$^2$) (Fisher et al., 2002a; Timmer et al., 2003c). BAPO absorbs light of wavelengths below 400 nm with a general increase in absorption as the wavelength decreases to 200 nm. Following UV irradiation, BAPO produces a pair of benzoyl and phosphinoyl radicals, which are more efficient in triggering PPF cross-linking and which produce stronger networks than the BP/DMT system (Fisher et al., 2002a). However, the efficiency of photo cross-linking decreases with increasing depth, making photo cross-linking problematic, especially when additives darken PPF's intrinsic yellow color. In these cases, thermal cross-linking or a combination of thermal and photo cross-linking methods can be used.

The cross-linking of PPF is an exothermic reaction, but its curing temperature in both thermal and photo cross-linking never exceeds 48°C. Curing temperatures for a clinically-used poly(methyl methacrylate) (PMMA) bone cement reach as high as 94°C (Peter et al., 1999a; Fisher et al., 2002a). Thus PPF's lower reaction temperature could prevent or reduce the adverse bone tissue responses seen to occur with PMMA at temperatures of 53°C and above (Fisher et al., 2002a).

The curing time of any liquid biomaterials is another critical factor for medical application. The curing period should be long enough to allow surgeons to work with the polymer to mold it or apply it to the appropriate surfaces. Yet, its cure rate should not greatly lengthen the surgery time. The polymerization or solidification period for bone implant fixation typically ranges from 5 to 20 min, with a 10-min curing time being most preferable (Gerhart and Hayes, 1989). Through modulation of various factors, such as type of cross-linker, molecular weight of PPF, and ratio of PPF to cross-linker, initiator, and/or accelerator, the curing time of PPF can be adjusted from less than a minute to over an hour to meet the necessary requirements for most medical applications (Peter et al., 1999a).

## TABLE 12.1

Mechanical Properties of PPF/PPF-DA Networks. The PPF/PPF-DA Double Bond Ratio is Defined as the Mole Fraction of Fumarate Bonds within the PPF Chain to the Acrylate Bonds in PPF-DA. Data Represent Means ± Standard Deviation for $n = 10$.

| Mechanical Property | PPF/PPF-DA Double Bond Ratio | | |
| --- | --- | --- | --- |
| | 0.5 | 1 | 2 |
| Tensile | | | |
| Strength at break (MPa) | 61 ± 4 | 70 ± 6 | 64 ± 4 |
| Yield strength (MPa) | 31 ± 5 | 29 ± 7 | 25 ± 6 |
| Elongation at break (mm/mm) | 0.108 ± 0.014 | 0.113 ± 0.016 | 0.129 ± 0.022 |
| Elongation at yield (mm/mm) | 0.056 ± 0.008 | 0.043 ± 0.009 | 0.043 ± 0.012 |
| Young's modulus (MPa) | 857 ± 57 | 923 ± 43 | 806 ± 84 |
| Compressive | | | |
| Fracture strength (MPa) | 201 ± 51 | 200 ± 39 | 253 ± 81 |
| Yield strength (MPa) | 57 ± 3 | 50 ± 2 | 35 ± 6 |
| Compressive modulus (MPa) | 1854 ± 97 | 1656 ± 215 | 837 ± 109 |
| Flexural | | | |
| Strength at break (MPa) | 100 ± 19 | 103 ± 9 | 92 ± 10 |
| Bending modulus (MPa) | 3124 ± 204 | 2644 ± 236 | 2206 ± 233 |
| Shear | | | |
| Shear strength (MPa) | 43 ± 6 | 40 ± 2 | 37 ± 3 |

*Source*: From Timmer, M.D., Carter, C., Ambrose, C.G., and Mikos, A.G., *Biomaterials*, **24**, 4707 (2003c). With permission.

### 12.3.2  Mechanical Properties

The mechanical properties of cross-linked PPF networks are very promising and vary greatly according to preparation and composition (Table 12.1) (Temenoff and Mikos, 2000; Timmer et al., 2003c). For example, PPF/NVP composite scaffolds with various amounts of beta-tricalcium phosphate (β-TCP) and NaCl porogen exhibited compressive strengths from 6 to 12 MPa and compressive moduli from 76 to 265 MPa (Peter et al., 1999a).

In order to improve these properties for loadbearing applications, such as replacement of cortical bone, PPF may be reinforced with nanomaterials. Nanoscale ceramics and carbon nanotubes are believed to be excellent candidates for reinforcement due to their superb mechanical properties. However, two primary challenges for nanoreinforcement include overcoming dispersion limitations and improving the interface between fillers and the polymer to facilitate load transfer. Surface modification of nanofillers provides an effective method to overcome these challenges. For example, aluminum oxide-based ceramic nanoparticles have been covalently modified with carboxylate groups and acrylate groups to improve both the dispersion of nanoparticles and their cross-linking with PPF/PPF-DA networks (Horch et al., 2004). In particular, a 1 wt% loading of surface-modified nanoparticles improved the flexural modulus of these networks by a factor of 3.5.

---

## 12.4  Biological Properties

### 12.4.1  Biocompatibility

Because PPF is designed as a cross-linkable and degradable biomaterial, all the substances from the implant's lifecycle must be nontoxic. *In vitro* cytotoxicity experiments provide a convenient and reliable method for biocompatibility studies and also serve as an initial screening process for *in vivo* testing (Timmer et al., 2003e). The cytotoxicity of noncross-linked PPF and PPF-DA macromers, cross-linked networks, and degradation products of these networks have been examined using a methyl tetrazolium (MTT) assay (Timmer et al., 2003e). The noncross-linked macromers and the degradation products only displayed a toxic effect to fibroblasts at high concentration (>1000 ppm). However, the cross-linked networks demonstrated high cell viability and attachment. Furthermore, osteoblasts have been shown to attach and proliferate on PPF/NVP/β-TCP composites (Peter et al., 2000).

PPF has also been seen to be biocompatible in several *in vivo* models. In a rat proximal tibia model, osteoblasts, osteoid, and new woven bone were in close apposition to degrading PPF/NVP/β-TCP scaffolds without evidence of an acute or other adverse pathologic inflammatory response (Yaszemski et al., 1995). PPF-based scaffolds implanted subcutaneously in rats elicited a mild initial inflammatory response followed by thin fibrous encapsulation, characteristics of a typical foreign body reaction to biomaterial implantation (Peter et al., 1998). In another experiment, photo cross-linked porous PPF scaffolds were implanted in subcutaneous pockets and cranial defects in a rabbit model to simultaneously examine the soft and hard tissue response to implants (Fisher et al., 2002b). The degradation products from the photo cross-linked networks elicited a mild local tissue response in the soft tissue. However, over time, a progressive reduction in inflammatory cell density and a continued organization of connective tissue within the interstitial space were observed. The hard tissue response was similar to that of the soft tissue, except that bone in-growth was observed, indicating bone biocompatibility. Excellent biocompatibility has also been observed when PPF was implanted into rabbit tooth sockets (Fisher et al., 2004).

## 12.4.2 Biodegradability

Degradation of a polymer is defined as the polymer chain cleavage process that breaks chains down into oligomers and finally into monomers (Gopferich, 1996). The prefix "bio" usually indicates that degradation is mediated by a biological system. PPF is biodegraded through hydrolysis of its ester bonds into its original propylene glycol and fumaric acid subunits (Figure 12.2), both of which are nontoxic and well-tolerated *in vivo*. As a Kreb's cycle intermediate, fumaric acid plays an essential role in the process by which food is converted into energy. Propylene glycol is used throughout the food industry as a food additive and can be metabolized or excreted by the body (Gerhart and Hayes, 1989). During the degradation of networks of PPF and PPF-DA, the hydrophilic degradation product, poly(acrylic acid-*co*-fumaric acid), also occurs. However, its molecular weight is well below the threshold value of 70 kDa, below which hydrophilic polymers can be passively excreted by the kidneys (He et al., 2001).

Cross-linked PPF's degradation rate is dependent on many factors, such as the molecular weight of the PPF macromer, cross-linking agents, cross-linking density of the network, scaffold pore size and pore volume, environmental pH, and the presence of other components in PPF-based composites (Yaszemski et al., 1996; Peter et al., 1997a, 1998; Fisher et al., 2003; Timmer et al., 2003b). For example, the degradation rate of cross-linked networks of PPF and PPF-DA has been shown to increase with decreasing cross-linking densities because fewer chains must be cleaved to disrupt the networks (Timmer et al., 2003b).

For some biodegradable polymers, like poly(lactic-*co*-glycolic acid) (PLGA) copolymers, a phenomenon known as autocatalyzed degradation occurs as their acidic degradation products reduce the local pH and further induce polymer degradation (Suggs and Mikos, 1996). A sudden increased release of acidic degradation products can render the local environment quite acidic, resulting in inflammation or even tissue necrosis. However, autocatalyzed degradation of PPF networks has not been observed. In fact, network cross-linking density was seen to influence PPF's degradation rate to a greater extent than environmental pH (Timmer et al., 2003b). Additional research has demonstrated that β-TCP can be incorporated into PPF to act as a buffering agent, maintaining local pH and preventing accelerated polymer degradation (Peter et al., 1997a, 1998; Timmer et al., 2003b).

According to recent *in vitro* studies, the time needed to degrade 50% of the original weight of the polymer ranged from about 12 weeks for weak thermal cross-linked porous networks of PPF and NVP to more than 52 weeks for strong photo cross-linked solid networks of PPF and PPF-DA (Peter et al., 1997a; Timmer et al., 2003b). Faster PPF degradation has been observed *in vivo* and may result from local cellular activities or enzymatic cleavage of the polymeric networks (Peter et al., 1998; Timmer et al., 2003b). In a rabbit model, histomorphometric analysis indicated a trend of increasing porosity of PPF scaffolds over time due to surface erosion by multinuclear cells (Fisher et al., 2002b). Although PPF undergoes bulk degradation, the PPF/NVP/β-TCP scaffold interior region degraded slower than its surface, allowing the implant interior to maintain its mechanical properties to support the defect for a long period of time (Yaszemski et al., 1995).

Interestingly, all PPF-based scaffolds demonstrate biphasic degradation behavior in both *in vitro* and *in vivo* studies. More specifically, their mechanical properties increase during the first few weeks, and then gradually decrease with degradation time (Yaszemski et al., 1996; Peter et al., 1997a, 1998; Fisher et al., 2003; Timmer et al., 2003b). Although PPF can be hardened within 10 min, its cross-linking reaction continues to proceed at a slow rate during these initial few weeks at physiological conditions (37°C) (Timmer et al., 2003d). Thus, initial mechanical strengthening of PPF networks results as unreacted bonds within these networks continue to undergo cross-linking.

### 12.4.3 Osteoconductivity

PPF has been shown to be osteoconductive, supporting bone cell proliferation and differentiation *in vitro* and bone tissue in-growth *in vivo* (Yaszemski et al., 1995; Peter et al., 2000a,b; Fisher et al., 2002b). Growth factors incorporated into PPF networks have been used to modulate cell functions. In an *in vitro* study, controlled release of transforming growth factor β1 (TGF-β1) resulted in higher cell number, alkaline phosphatase (ALP) activity, and osteocalcin production when marrow stromal cells (MSCs) were cultured on the surface of cross-linked PPF/NVP substrates. These results indicate that cell proliferation and osteoblastic differentiation on PPF networks were enhanced by TGF-β1 release (Peter et al., 2000b). In another study, cross-linked PPF foams with or without preadsorption of TGF-β1 were implanted in rabbit cranial defects. Significantly more bone in-growth was observed on implants coated with TGF-β1 at 8 weeks (Vehof et al., 2002).

Beta-tricalcium phosphate (β-TCP) incorporation into PPF scaffolds has been shown to enhance the mechanical properties and the osteoconductivity of PPF networks. For instance, when porous scaffolds fabricated from PPF alone were implanted *in vivo*, low amounts of bone growth was observed after 8 weeks (Fisher et al., 2002b). However, after only 5 weeks postimplantation, scaffolds fabricated from PPF/β-TCP had promising bone in-growth, beginning at the peripheral surface and progressing towards the center of the defect (Yaszemski et al., 1995). PPF/β-TCP composites also exhibited *in vitro* osteoconductivity similar to or better than that of control tissue culture polystyrene (Peter et al., 2000a). Thus, these results indicate the potential of PPF scaffolds as an osteoconductive carrier of osteoinductive agents to promote bone regeneration.

PPF can also be used to form composite scaffolds incorporating PLGA microspheres for controlled delivery of osteogenic factors to promote bone formation in a rabbit radial defect (Hedberg et al., 2002; Hedberg et al., 2005a–c). Additionally, PPF can be combined with other polymers such as poly(ethylene glycol) (PEG) to construct copolymers, like poly(propylene fumarate-*co*-ethylene glycol) (P(PF-*co*-EG)), which is water soluble (Suggs et al., 1998). Bone cell encapsulation with these PPF-based constructs has been shown to improve the rate and extent of mineralized tissue formation *in vitro* (Payne et al., 1998; Payne et al., 2002a–c). For cell encapsulation within PPF-based networks, microparticles can be utilized as cell carriers. More specifically, marrow stromal cells (MSCs) were encapsulated in gelatin microspheres which were subsequently surface cross-linked to protect cells in the short-term from unfavorable cross-linking conditions, such as the toxic radical species and potential temperature rise (Payne et al., 2002c). These encapsulated MSCs maintained cell viability in cross-linking PPF/NVP (Payne et al., 2002a).

Alternatively, surface modification of PPF-based polymers with biomimetic materials can be used to enhance cellular recognition and to elicit specific cellular responses to aid in tissue growth (Shin et al., 2003). For example, scaffolds covalently attached with a cell attachment ligands such as Arg-Gly-Asp (RGD) peptide increased MSC attachment and migration in a specific and dose-dependent manner (Jo et al., 2000; Behravesh et al., 2003). These attached MSCs retained their ability to differentiate *in vitro* and to produce bone-like, mineralized tissue (Behravesh and Mikos, 2003). Thus, surface modified PPF may be useful for guided tissue regeneration in dental defects where proliferation and migration of specific cell types is desired.

## 12.5 Implant Fabrication

PPF can be easily cast into complex shapes through simple injection into molds with subsequent thermal or photo cross-linking. In a recent study, transparent room temperature vulcanizing (RTV) silicone was used to produce detailed and complex molds that allowed light penetration for rapid photo cross-linking (Timmer et al., 2003c). PPF/PPF-DA polymer was injected into the silicone molds, hardened by photo cross-linking, and then placed at 100°C for 24 h to ensure complete cross-linking. A number of intricate orthopaedic devices, such as an eight-hole adaption plate and a lordotic anterior cervical fusion (ACF) spacer, were successfully fabricated with little shrinkage (Figure 12.4) (Timmer et al., 2003c).

Porous scaffolds are especially important for bone tissue engineering because interconnected pore networks allow vascularization and bone in-growth throughout the scaffolds (Fisher et al., 2002b). They can also serve as carriers for delivery of bioactive factors and/or cells to further promote bone formation (Behravesh et al., 2002; Vehof et al., 2002). PPF-based polymers can be easily fabricated into porous architectures by various methods. One simple method incorporates sodium bicarbonate and acidic agents with P(PF-*co*-EG). When the mixture is dissolved in water, the reaction of sodium bicarbonate

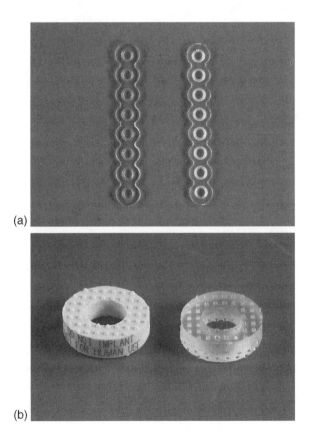

(a)

(b)

**FIGURE 12.4**
(a) 1.5 mm eight-hole adaption plates manufactured with 70:30 Poly(L/DL-lactide) (P(L/DL-LA)) (left) and PPF/PPF-DA (right). (b) Plastic model (left) and PPF/PPF-DA replicate of a 5 mm lordotic ACF spacer. (*Source:* From Timmer, M.D., Carter, C., Ambrose, C.G., and Mikos, A.G., *Biomaterials*, **24**, 4707 (2003c). With permission.)

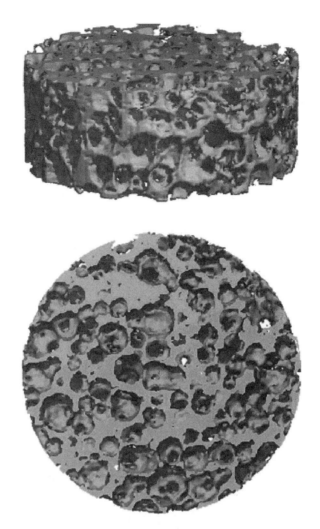

**FIGURE 12.5**
Representative microcomputed tomography ($\mu$CT) scans of P(PF-*co*-EG) macroporous hydrogels (2.5 mm in diameter and 1.5 mm in thickness) with a spatial resolution of 10 $\mu$m. (*Source*: From Behravesh, E., Timmer, M.D., Lemoine, J.J., Liebschner, M.A., and Mikos, A.G., *Biomacromolecules*, **3**, 1263 (2002). With permission.)

and acid produces the porogen, carbon dioxide, making porous hydrogels (Figure 12.5) (Behravesh et al., 2002). Sodium chloride with specific crystal sizes, such as 300–500 $\mu$m, can also be used as a porogen. The salt is mixed with uncross-linked PPF and after cross-linking of the polymer network, sodium chloride is leached out in water, leaving interconnected pores inside PPF (Fisher et al., 2002b). In order to design optimized scaffolds with maximal porosity and suitable mechanical properties, more complex techniques are needed to manufacture three-dimensional architectures. For example, a 3D rapid prototyping system has been used to fabricate wax molds of a topology optimized design in a layer-by-layer printing fashion (Hollister et al., 2002; Taboas et al., 2003). Another 3D printing method is stereolithography that uses an ultraviolet (UV) laser with 325 nm wavelength to photo cross-link PPF/DEF mixtures with a 3D printing resolution of 0.1 mm (Cooke et al., 2003). A 3D solid modeling computer-aided-design (CAD) software package was first used to design a prototype part with features of circular pads, holes, and slots. The resulting geometric data were then used to drive the stereolithographic machine to accurately manufacture the custom-designed PPF/DEF construct with an overall thickness of 4 mm for ultimate use as a biodegradable scaffold to repair a critically-sized human bone defect (Cooke et al., 2003).

## 12.6  Summary

PPF is a synthetic, degradable polymeric biomaterial with suitable physical properties for numerous orthopaedic applications. A liquid polymer at room temperature, PPF can be injected to fill defects or cast into molds of various shapes. Based on its unsaturated carbon–carbon double bonds, PPF can be cross-linked with different cross-linking agents via thermal or photo initiation processes to form strong networks, which can be further reinforced for high loadbearing applications. These PPF-based networks can be degraded by ester hydrolysis into nontoxic small molecules without persistent inflammatory responses. Bone tissue is able to grow into degrading PPF and replace it over time. The properties of PPF can be easily modified with different synthetic and cross-linking conditions, as well as other material additives to satisfy the material property requirements for a specific application. It is the versatility of PPF, stemming from its biocompatibility, *in situ* cross-linking properties, biodegradability, osteoconductivity, and excellent mechanical properties, that makes this polymer a promising candidate for orthopaedic and dental applications.

## Acknowledgments

The work on fumarate-based polymers has been supported by grants from the National Institute of Health (R01-AR48756, R01-DE15164, R01-DE13740).

## References

Behravesh, E. and Mikos, A.G., Three-dimensional culture of differentiating marrow stromal osteoblasts in biomimetic poly(propylene fumarate-*co*-ethylene glycol)-based macroporous hydrogels, *J. Biomed. Mater. Res. A*, **66A**, 698 (2003).

Behravesh, E., Timmer, M.D., Lemoine, J.J., Liebschner, M.A., and Mikos, A.G., Evaluation of the in vitro degradation of macroporous hydrogels using gravimetry, confined compression testing, and microcomputed tomography, *Biomacromolecules*, **3**, 1263 (2002).

Behravesh, E., Zygourakis, K., and Mikos, A.G., Adhesion and migration of marrow-derived osteoblasts on injectable in situ crosslinkable poly(propylene fumarate-*co*-ethylene glycol)-based hydrogels with a covalently linked RGDS peptide, *J. Biomed. Mater. Res. A*, **65A**, 260 (2003).

Cooke, M.N., Fisher, J.P., Dean, D., Rimnac, C., and Mikos, A.G., Use of stereolithography to manufacture critical-sized 3D biodegradable scaffolds for bone ingrowth, *J. Biomed. Mater. Res. B*, **64B**, 65 (2003).

Domb, A.J., Poly(propylene glycol fumarate) compositions for biomedical applications, U.S. Patent 4888413, December 19 (1989).

Fisher, J.P., Dean, D., and Mikos, A.G., Photocrosslinking characteristics and mechanical properties of diethyl fumarate/poly(propylene fumarate) biomaterials, *Biomaterials*, **23**, 4333 (2002a).

Fisher, J.P., Holland, T.A., Dean, D., and Mikos, A.G., Photoinitiated cross-linking of the biodegradable polyester poly(propylene fumarate). Part II. In vitro degradation, *Biomacromolecules*, **4**, 1335 (2003).

Fisher, J.P., Lalani, Z., Bossano, C.M., Brey, E.M., Demian, N., Johnston, C.M., Dean, D., Jansen, J.A., Wong, M.E.K., and Mikos, A.G., Effect of biomaterial properties on bone healing in a rabbit tooth extraction socket model, *J. Biomed. Mater. Res. A*, **68A**, 428 (2004).

Fisher, J.P., Vehof, J.W., Dean, D., van der Waerden, J.P., Holland, T.A., Mikos, A.G., and Jansen, J.A., Soft and hard tissue response to photocrosslinked poly(propylene fumarate) scaffolds in a rabbit model, *J. Biomed. Mater. Res. A*, **59A**, 547 (2002b).

Gerhart, T.N. and Hayes, W.C., Bioerodable implant composition, U.S. Patent 4843112, June 27 (1989).

Gopferich, A., Polymer degradation and erosion: Mechanisms and applications, *Eur. J. Pharm. Biopharm.*, **42**, 1 (1996).

He, S., Timmer, M.D., Yaszemski, M.J., Yasko, A.W., Engel, P.S., and Mikos, A.G., Synthesis of biodegradable poly(propylene fumarate) networks with poly(propylene fumarate)-diacrylate macromers as crosslinking agents and characterization of their degradation products, *Polymer*, **42**, 1251 (2001).

Hedberg, E.L., Kroese-Deutman, H.C., Shih, C.K., Crowther, R.S., Carney, D.H., Mikos, A.G., and Jansen, J.A., Effect of varied release kinetics of the osteogenic thrombin peptide TP508 from biodegradable, polymeric scaffolds on bone formation in vivo, *J. Biomed. Mater. Res. A*, **72A**, 343 (2005a).

Hedberg, E.L., Kroese-Deutman, H.C., Shih, C.K., Crowther, R.S., Carney, D.H., Mikos, A.G., and Jansen, J.A., In vivo degradation of porous poly(propylene fumarate)/poly(DL-lactic-*co*-glycolic acid) composite scaffolds, *Biomaterials*, **26**, 4616 (2005b).

Hedberg, E.L., Shih, C.K., Lemoine, J.J., Timmer, M.D., Liebschner, M.A.K., Jansen, J.A., and Mikos, A.G., In vitro degradation of porous poly(propylene fumarate)/poly(DL-lactic-*co*-glycolic acid) composite scaffolds, *Biomaterials*, **26**, 3215 (2005c).

Hedberg, E.L., Tang, A., Crowther, R.S., Carney, D.H., and Mikos, A.G., Controlled release of an osteogenic peptide from injectable biodegradable polymeric composites, *J. Controlled Release*, **84**, 137 (2002).

Hollister, S.J., Maddox, R.D., and Taboas, J.M., Optimal design and fabrication of scaffolds to mimic tissue properties and satisfy biological constraints, *Biomaterials*, **23**, 4095 (2002).

Horch, R.A., Shahid, N., Mistry, A.S., Timmer, M.D., Mikos, A.G., and Barron, A.R., Nanoreinforcement of poly(propylene fumarate)-based networks with surface modified alumoxane nanoparticles for bone tissue engineering, *Biomacromolecules*, **5**, 1990 (2004).

Jo, S., Engel, P.S., and Mikos, A.G., Synthesis of poly(ethylene glycol)-tethered poly(propylene fumarate) and its modification with GRGD peptide, *Polymer*, **41**, 7595 (2000).

Kharas, G.B., Kamenetsky, M., Simantirakis, J., Beinlich, K.C., Rizzo, A.M.T., Caywood, G.A., and Watson, K., Synthesis and characterization of fumarate-based polyesters for use in bioresorbable bone cement composites, *J. Appl. Polym. Sci.*, **66**, 1123 (1997).

Payne, R.G., McGonigle, J.S., Yaszemski, M.J., Yasko, A.W., and Mikos, A.G., Development of an injectable, in situ crosslinkable, degradable polymeric carrier for osteogenic cell populations. Part 2. Viability of encapsulated marrow stromal osteoblasts cultured on crosslinking poly(propylene fumarate), *Biomaterials*, **23**, 4373 (2002a).

Payne, R.G., McGonigle, J.S., Yaszemski, M.J., Yasko, A.W., and Mikos, A.G., Development of an injectable, in situ crosslinkable, degradable polymeric carrier for osteogenic cell populations. Part 3. Proliferation and differentiation of encapsulated marrow stromal osteoblasts cultured on crosslinking poly(propylene fumarate), *Biomaterials*, **23**, 4381 (2002b).

Payne, R.G., Sivaram, S.A., Babensee, J.E., Yasko, A.W., Yaszemski, M.J., and Mikos, A.G., Temporary encapsulation of rat marrow osteoblasts in gelatin microspheres, *Tissue Eng.*, **4**, 497 (1998).

Payne, R.G., Yaszemski, M.J., Yasko, A.W., and Mikos, A.G., Development of an injectable, in situ crosslinkable, degradable polymeric carrier for osteogenic cell populations. Part 1. Encapsulation of marrow stromal osteoblasts in surface crosslinked gelatin microparticles, *Biomaterials*, **23**, 4359 (2002c).

Peter, S.J., Kim, P., Yasko, A.W., Yaszemski, M.J., and Mikos, A.G., Crosslinking characteristics of an injectable poly(propylene fumarate)/beta-tricalcium phosphate paste and mechanical properties of the crosslinked composite for use as a biodegradable bone cement, *J. Biomed. Mater. Res.*, **44**, 314 (1999a).

Peter, S.J., Lu, L., Kim, D.J., and Mikos, A.G., Marrow stromal osteoblast function on a poly(propylene fumarate)/beta-tricalcium phosphate biodegradable orthopaedic composite, *Biomaterials*, **21**, 1207 (2000a).

Peter, S.J., Lu, L., Kim, D.J., Stamatas, G.N., Miller, M.J., Yaszemski, M.J., and Mikos, A.G., Effects of transforming growth factor β1 released from biodegradable polymer microparticles on marrow stromal osteoblasts cultured on poly(propylene fumarate) substrates, *J. Biomed. Mater. Res.*, **50**, 452 (2000b).

Peter, S.J., Miller, S.T., Zhu, G., Yasko, A.W., and Mikos, A.G., In vivo degradation of a poly(propylene fumarate)/beta-tricalcium phosphate injectable composite scaffold, *J. Biomed. Mater. Res.*, **41**, 1 (1998).

Peter, S.J., Nolley, J.A., Widmer, M.S., Merwin, J.E., Yaszemski, M.J., Yasko, A.W., Engel, P.S., and Mikos, A.G., In vitro degradation of a poly(propylene fumarate)/beta-tricalcium phosphate composite orthopaedic scaffold, *Tissue Eng.*, **3**, 207 (1997a).

Peter, S.J., Suggs, L.J., Yaszemski, M.J., Engel, P.S., and Mikos, A.G., Synthesis of poly(propylene fumarate) by acylation of propylene glycol in the presence of a proton scavenger, *J. Biomater. Sci. Polym. Ed.*, **10**, 363 (1999b).

Peter, S.J., Yaszemski, M.J., Suggs, L.J., Payne, R.G., Langer, R., Hayes, W.C., Unroe, M.R., Alemany, L.B., Engel, P.S., and Mikos, A.G., Characterization of partially saturated poly(propylene fumarate) for orthopaedic application, *J. Biomater. Sci. Polym. Ed.*, **8**, 893 (1997b).

Robinson, B.V., Sullivan, F.M., Borzelleca, J.F., and Schwartz, S.L., *PVP: A Critical Review of the Kinetics and Toxicology of Polyvinylpyrrolidone (povidone)*, Lewis, Chelsea, MI (1990).

Sanderson, J.E., Bone replacement and repair putty material from unsaturated polyester resin and vinyl pyrrolidone, U.S. Patent 4722948, February 2 (1988).

Shin, H., Jo, S., and Mikos, A.G., Biomimetic materials for tissue engineering, *Biomaterials*, **24**, 4353 (2003).

Shung, A.K., Timmer, M.D., Jo, S., Engel, P.S., and Mikos, A.G., Kinetics of poly(propylene fumarate) synthesis by step polymerization of diethyl fumarate and propylene glycol using zinc chloride as a catalyst, *J. Biomater. Sci. Polym. Ed.*, **13**, 95 (2002).

Suggs, L.J., Kao, E.Y., Palombo, L.L., Krishnan, R.S., Widmer, M.S., and Mikos, A.G., Preparation and characterization of poly(propylene fumarate-*co*-ethylene glycol) hydrogels, *J. Biomater. Sci. Polym. Ed.*, **9**, 653 (1998).

Suggs, L.J. and Mikos, A.G., Synthetic biodegradable polymers for medical applications, In: *Physical Properties of Polymers Handbook*, Mark, J.E., Ed., American Institute of Physics, Woodbury, New York, pp. 615 (1996).

Taboas, J.M., Maddox, R.D., Krebsbach, P.H., and Hollister, S.J., Indirect solid free form fabrication of local and global porous, biomimetic and composite 3D polymer-ceramic scaffolds, *Biomaterials*, **24**, 181 (2003).

Temenoff, J.S. and Mikos, A.G., Injectable biodegradable materials for orthopedic tissue engineering, *Biomaterials*, **21**, 2405 (2000).

Timmer, M.D., Ambrose, C.G., and Mikos, A.G., Evaluation of thermal- and photo-crosslinked biodegradable poly(propylene fumarate)-based networks, *J. Biomed. Mater. Res. A*, **66A**, 811 (2003a).

Timmer, M.D., Ambrose, C.G., and Mikos, A.G., In vitro degradation of polymeric networks of poly(propylene fumarate) and the crosslinking macromer poly(propylene fumarate)-diacrylate, *Biomaterials*, **24**, 571 (2003b).

Timmer, M.D., Carter, C., Ambrose, C.G., and Mikos, A.G., Fabrication of poly(propylene fumarate)-based orthopaedic implants by photo-crosslinking through transparent silicone molds, *Biomaterials*, **24**, 4707 (2003c).

Timmer, M.D., Horch, R.A., Ambrose, C.G., and Mikos, A.G., Effect of physiological temperature on the mechanical properties and network structure of biodegradable poly(propylene fumarate)-based networks, *J. Biomater. Sci. Polym. Ed.*, **14**, 369 (2003d).

Timmer, M.D., Jo, S., Wang, C., Ambrose, C.G., and Mikos, A.G., Characterization of the cross-linked structure of fumarate-based degradable polymer networks, *Macromolecules*, **35**, 4373 (2002).

Timmer, M.D., Shin, H., Horch, R.A., Ambrose, C.G., and Mikos, A.G., In vitro cytotoxicity of injectable and biodegradable poly(propylene fumarate)-based networks: unreacted macromers, cross-linked networks, and degradation products, *Biomacromolecules*, **4**, 1026 (2003e).

Vehof, J.W., Fisher, J.P., Dean, D., van der Waerden, J.P., Spauwen, P.H., Mikos, A.G., and Jansen, J.A., Bone formation in transforming growth factor beta-1-coated porous poly(propylene fumarate) scaffolds, *J. Biomed. Mater. Res.*, **60**, 241 (2002).

Yaszemski, M.J., Payne, R.G., Hayes, W.C., Langer, R., Aufdemorte, T.B., and Mikos, A.G., The ingrowth of new bone tissue and initial mechanical properties of a degrading polymeric composite scaffold, *Tissue Eng.*, **1**, 41 (1995).

Yaszemski, M.J., Payne, R.G., Hayes, W.C., Langer, R., and Mikos, A.G., In vitro degradation of a poly(propylene fumarate)-based composite material, *Biomaterials*, **17**, 2127 (1996).

# 13

## Hyaluronan as a Biomaterial

John H. Brekke and Kipling Thacker

## CONTENTS

## 13.1   Introduction

Recent developments in production of recombinant, human morphogens, as well as in tissue specific differentiation of adult and fetal stem cells, have unlocked therapeutic potentials that not long ago would have been consigned to tales of science fiction. Nevertheless, the very real healing benefits of these advances will not become clinical realities until tissue engineers develop the means for presenting exogenous biologic agents and pluripotent cells to damaged tissues in a manner consistent with innate wound healing and embryonic tissue development and cognizant of existing surgical, medical, and regulatory parameters. Central to this endeavor is the ancient, and much misunderstood, compound known by two monikers: hyaluronan (HY), its modern term, and hyaluronic acid, its archaic name (Balazas et al., 1986).

In its native tissue form, the compound is a salt, and as such cannot be specified; it is given the name hyaluronan. When Karl Meyer discovered hyaluronan in 1934, he coined the term hyaluronic acid from hyaloid (vitreous) + uronic acid, one of its constituents (Meyer and Palmer, 1934). Hyaluronan is a linear polysaccharide, composed of alternating units of N-acetyl-D-glucosamine and a salt of glucuronic acid (Figure 13.1), and found in

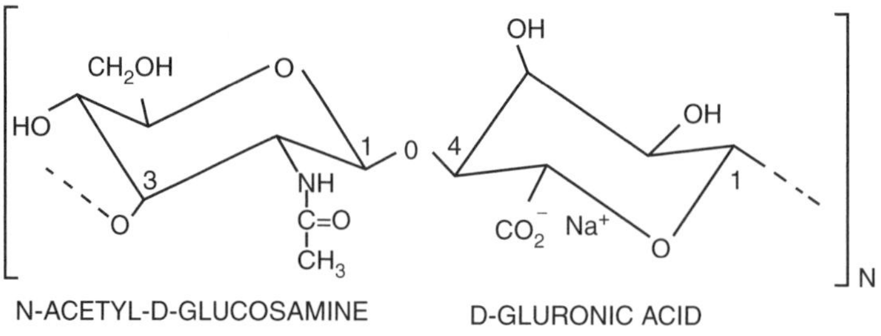

**FIGURE 13.1**
Hyaluronan. Molecular schematic of hyaluronan.

tissues of all chordates and in certain bacterial species. Darke et al. (1975) in studies of sodium haluronate solutions by proton nuclear magnetic resonance (NMR), confirmed the accepted covalent structure of the molecule which was worked out by Rapport et al. (1951). In mammals, hyaluronan is found at high concentration in synovial fluid, vitreous humor, skin, and *in utero* in the umbilical cord. It plays significant structural roles in the extracellular matrix (ECM) of adult tissues as diverse as articular cartilage, the cervix, and the glycocalyx of endothelial cells. The fact that hyaluronan is synthesized in large but carefully titrated quantities by epidermal keratinocytes, peritoneal mesothelial cells, fibroblasts, and other cells of the early wound healing milieu is of particular interest to tissue engineers (Weigel et al., 1986; Oksala et al., 1995; Bowen et al., 2004; Pasonen-Seppänen et al., 2004).

By definition and NMR studies, the chemical identity of hyaluronan is the same across all species (Welti et al., 1979; Bociek et al., 1980; Rosner et al., 1992; Lifecore, personal communication). Consequently, appropriately purified hyaluronan from one species does not stimulate an immunologic response in tissues of another. Hyaluronan is the simplest of ECM glycosaminoglycans and is the only member of this group that is not sulfonated. Commercially, it is most commonly available as the sodium salt, Na-hyaluronate, in molecular weight ranges between 5000 Da and greater than 6 million Da. Oligosacharides from the disaccharide to 25 disaccharide units (molecular weight $(M_w) = <10$ kDa), are less readily available. Pharmaceutical grade sodium hyaluronate is presently produced as an extract from cock's combs, and by bacterial fermentation processes. With several manufacturers producing hyaluronan for ophthalmic and orthopedic injectable applications, the tissue engineer should consider sourcing experimental hyaluronan directly from producers who thoroughly characterize their product rather than from chemical supply houses. A recently published ASTM standard can serve as a starting point for characterization and testing of hyaluronan used in tissue engineering applications.

This deceptively simple compound is possessed of multiple, diverse biochemical and physical properties fundamental to new tissue development in the embryo, as well as to tissue regeneration and repair in adult organisms (Chen et al., 1999; Toole, 2004). Physical characteristics of HY impacting tissue regeneration are focused on its capacity to govern physical location and concentration of growth factors and morphogens as well as its ability to expand the volume of intercellular spaces by acquiring and sequestering large volumes of water (Papini et al., 1993; Takigami and Takifami, 1993; Sasaki and Watanabe, 1995; Masuda et al., 2001). Its biochemical properties function through chemotaxis for cell migration, cell differentiation, signals stimulating angiogenesis and direct signaling to the genome by interaction with cell surface receptors and via HY oligosaccharides generated within the cytosol (West et al., 1985; Samuel et al., 1993; Rooney et al., 1995; Rao et al., 1997; Oliferenko et al., 2000; Savani et al., 2001; Nicoll et al., 2002; Turley et al., 2002;

Yasuda et al., 2002; Aziz, 2003; Heldin, 2003). Consequently, HY is emerging as an important tissue engineering material.

## 13.2   Chemical and Physical Properties

The physical properties of hyaluronan are, as with all polymers, determined by the chemistry of the basic building block, a disaccharide (β1-3 linked cation glucuronic acid and *N*-acetyl-*d*-glucosamine) in the present case, and the $M_w$ of the molecule.

Hyaluronan solutions are rheologically pseudoplastic viscoelastics with both viscous and elastic components that can be measured with a dynamic rheometer, a basic description of which can be found in Wik (1991). Viscosity is the internal resistance to flow by a fluid and is often measured with a "cone on plate" or rotational viscometer. For hyaluronan solutions a number of factors must be specified and reported in order to make interlaboratory comparisons meaningful; concentration and $M_w$ are the most obvious and critical, pH, ionic strength, temperature, and shear rate (shear — the ratio of stress applied laterally and strain resulting from that force) are also important. Elasticity is the ability of a material to recover its original shape after a deforming force has been removed. Hyaluronan in solution exhibits the property of elasticity that is measured by applying low frequency oscillating forces to the solution in the rheometer and is $M_w$ dependent. At a frequency of 1.0 Hz, the predominant behavior is viscous for hyaluronan molecules under 1 million Da. Above 1 million the elastic component progressively dominates (Wik, 1991).

Hyaluronan's viscoelastic behavior is not in dispute, however, there is an active discussion of the underlying mechanism responsible for this behavior. Gribbon et al. (2000) have argued that there is no evidence for HY chain association. "The results suggest that the effects of electrolytes and solvent are determined primarily by their effect on HY chain flexibility, with no evidence for association between chain segments contributing significantly to the major properties." Scott (1989) has suggested that hydrophobic regions of the molecule contribute to its viscoelastic behavior. In studies of the hyaluronan and phospholipid interactions designed to learn more about the lubricating property of synovial fluid, Pasquali-Ronchetti showed a high degree of interaction adding support to the concept of hydrophobic interactions (Pasquali-Ronchetti et al., 1997).

Most hyaluronan solutions are pseudoplastic (shear thinning — apparent viscosity drops with increased shear force) allowing them to be injected through narrow gauge needles. "High intrinsic viscosity values for high $M_w$ hyaluronan implies large hydrodynamic volume with considerable water included with the molecular domain" (Cowman and Matsouka, 2002). At sufficient concentration, hyaluronan molecules are crowded enough to entangle, creating increasingly viscous solutions. However, pure native hyaluronan never forms a true gel. In concert with link proteins and other components of the ECM, deformable gel structures are generated. The reader with more interest in the rheological properties of NaHy is directed to the dissertation of Wik (1991).

Molecular weight determination of hyaluronan larger than oligosaccharides is commonly performed by measuring intrinsic viscosity (using either an Ubbelohde capillary viscometer or a Viscotek differential pressure viscometer) and converting the values to $M_w$ using the Mark–Houwink equation (Laurent et al., 1960; Wik, 1991). Alternatively, many labs are now measuring $M_w$ directly from size exclusion chromatography (SEC) column(s) with a multiangle laser light scattering (MALLS) detector (Soltes et al., 2002; Hokputsa et al., 2003). SEC-MALLS has the added advantage of being able to determine the molecular weight number average ($M_n$) as well as molecular weight average ($M_w$) from which one can calculate the polydispersity index; $I = M_n/M_w$, quantifying the heterogeneity of the preparation. There is no formal definition for oligosaccharides with respect to number of basic units and $M_w$ for hyaluronan. For practical purposes of large scale preparation by chromatographic means, $\sim$26 disaccharides ($\sim$10 kDa) is the upper limit (Tawada et al., 2002). The classical techniques of chromatography and mass spectrometry are used for measuring molecular weight of oligosaccharides.

Cowman and Matsouka (2002) describe an inflection point in the relationship between intrinsic viscosity and $M_w$ at 37.5 kDa (Wik (1991) describes another inflection point at a $M_w$ of about 1 million Da). They also showed that at approximately 37,500 Da, or 93 disaccharide units, hyaluronan can act as a free-draining chain (in which solvent flows undisturbed through the coil) rather than a nonfree-draining ball-like coil. They also describe this as the shortest HY molecule that can make a complete circle. Mammalian hyaluronidase-2 (Hyal-2) cleaves hyaluronan to a molecule of approximately 20 kDa ($\sim$50 disaccharide units) suggesting this length is physiologically important (Lepperdinger et al., 1998).

When handling HY, or any biological material destined for incorporation into a tissue engineering matrix, consideration must be given to depolymerization, which is loss of $M_w$, and decomposition or degradation, which is a change in the chemical structure of the molecule. Significant depolymerization of hyaluronan solutions occurs at all temperatures above 80°C (Lowry and Beavers, 1994). The molecular weight values were not reported, but a decrease of viscosity by 50% was noted at 15 h. At 90°C those same changes occurred in $\sim$45 min.

At autoclave temperatures of 128°C for times beyond standard times of 15 to 30 min for sterilization, decomposition, in addition to deplymerization, become obvious as the solution yellowed (Lifecore, personal communication, Wik, 1991). Wik (1991) starting with HY of $M_w = 4.3 \times 10^6$ Da at 128°C, showed $M_w$ decreases of 42% after 5 min, 56% after 10 min and 75% after 30 min. As a dry powder, some depolymerization takes place over several days at room temperature accelerating to a rapid rate above 90°C. At 100°C, an $\sim$25% loss of $M_w$ occurred in 2 h with some decomposition over an extended period of time.

Because of hyaluronan's heat sensitivity, chemical reactivity, and sensitivity to radiation, classical means of sterilization for medical devices have to be approached with appropriate caution. Post-sterilization validation by the tissue engineer is essential.

Most sterile pharmaceutical preparations of HY solutions are prepared in one of the three ways:

(i) Filter sterilization of relatively dilute solutions (up to 1%) or low viscosity (5 to 10 kcps) solutions. (A subset of this is a proprietary filtration technique for solutions up to 100 kcps.)

(ii) Preparations from sterile powder that have been prepared aseptically from filtered dilute solutions.

(iii) Heat (autoclave) sterilization with resultant loss of $M_w$. The product designers start with solutions of higher $M_w$ than the final product requires, thus compensating for subsequent depolymerization.

Under some circumstances, plasma gas or ethylene oxide gas (ETO) are used to sterilize medical devices containing hyaluronan. Unfortunately, these processes expose HY to oxides or atomic oxygen, both of which are powerful agents of depolymerization and decomposition (Al-Assaf et al., 2003). Because HY is so vulnerable to depolymerization it should be stored at temperatures of $-20°C$ or less.

Hadler et al. looked at the effect of a hyaluronan matrix on the permeability or diffusion of small molecules, modulating it with different concentrations of calcium or contaminating protein (Napier and Hadler, 1978; Carr and Hadler, 1980; Hadler, 1980). Glucose and sucrose (glucose–fructose disaccharide) are small molecules in the Mw range of 200 Da. They diffuse through agarose at equivalent rates, but in a 2.5% sodium hyaluronate matrix, the rate of diffusion of glucose was twice that of sucrose. Hadler concluded that hyaluronan solutions can alter diffusion rates of small molecules, acting as a selectively permeable membrane. These results suggest that one of the roles of the hyaluronan-containing ECM is to regulate the transport and flow of molecules to and from the cell surface. It is possible that this structure is regulated by such things as calcium ions, pH and concentration, and $M_w$ of the hyaluronan. Since tissue engineering constructs are often designed as vehicles for delivery of biologically active proteins (i.e., compounds of 30 to 60 kDa), composition of the substance that is serving the role of an artificial ECM must take these interactions into account.

Laurent demonstrated that large molecules, such as myoglobin, albumin, and gamma globulin, were largely excluded from hyaluronan gels and solutions (Laurent, 1964, 1977). By extension, one can envision entrapment of biologically active proteins such as bone morphogenetic protein (BMP), basic fibroblast growth factor (bFGF), insulin-like growth factor (IGF) etc., by viscoelastic gels of HY.

## 13.3  Biologic Properties of Hyaluronan

### 13.3.1  The Cytoskeleton and Cellular Tensegrity

Tissue engineering devices may be viewed as three-dimensional cell culture systems whether used *in vivo* as tissue implants or *in vitro* as cell culture matrices. If these constructs are to succeed in fostering undifferentiated stem cells to pursue a specific phenotypic pathway, those who fabricate them must understand that the cells populating these materials are subject to a kaleidoscope of messages originating independently from a variety of sources. While soluble signaling proteins (i.e., morphogens, growth factors, and hormones) exert powerful phenotypic influences upon pluripotent cells, the tissue engineering devices delivering these proteins are, themselves, generators of information influencing cell differentiation by mechanical mechanisms independent from those employed by soluble signaling factors (Brekke and Toth, 1998). The means by which cells perceive mechanical forces within their microenvironments and translate this information into biochemical signals capable of influencing gene expression is known as mechanochemical signal transduction and is studied under the rubric of cellular tensegrity (Ingber, 1997; Chen et al., 2004).

Tensegrity is an engineering term referring to an organization of structural elements capable of mechanically stabilizing itself by continually balancing and redistributing compressive and tensional forces throughout the entire construct. Tensegrity structures can be found in the geodesic domes of Buckminster Fuller, the sculptures of Kenneth Snelson, and in all eucaryotic cells. Tensegrity structures of the latter two examples are prestressed such that all members of the unit are under tension or compression before any external forces might be applied (Ingber, 1998). Dynamic balancing and redistribution of mechanical forces within cells of living tissues are accomplished by elements of the cyotskeleton. The resulting changes in cell shape can have profound effects on its behaviors. While a detailed discussion of the cytoskeleton is beyond the scope of this chapter, a conversational knowledge of its most important components is necessary to understand cellular tensegrity, mechanochemical signal transduction and the biologic properties of hyaluronan.

Three cytoskeletal elements, critical for maintaining the cell's tensegrity structure are depicted in Figure 13.2:

   (i) Microtubules, composed of the protein tubulin, are the intracellular elements capable of withstanding compressive forces. They are, in fact, polymers of tubulin that can polymerize and depolymerize quickly.

  (ii) Intermediate filaments connect microtubules and actin filaments to each other, to the plasma and nuclear membranes as well as to subcellular organelles.

 (iii) Actin filaments (also known as microfilaments) are contractile proteins that generate tensile forces resisted by microtubules. Though microfilaments are found throughout the cytosol, they are concentrated in the cell cortex, just beneath the plasma membrane (Wang et al., 2001; Alberts et al., 2002).

Integrins are transmembrane glycoprotein heterodimers, composed of 24 types of α-subunits and 9 types of β-subunits (Figure 13.3). Their extracellular domains engage ECM proteins while the intracellular tail of the β subunit binds microfilaments (α-actin) of the cytoskeleton. Because their affinity for ECM proteins (e.g., fibronectin, laminin, collagen IV) is relatively weak, multiple integrins cluster together as focal adhesion complexes (FAC) in order to successfully engage the ECM. Binding of β-subunits to microfilaments is mediated by anchorproteins (talin, α-actinin, and filamin) which also attract tyrosine-phosphorylated proteins such as the focal adhesion kinase (FAK) to the

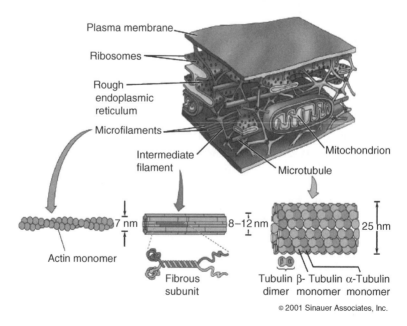

© 2001 Sinauer Associates, Inc.

**FIGURE 13.2**
Representation of major cytoskeletal elements. Found via Dogpile/cytoskeleton/images/Figure 13.16.

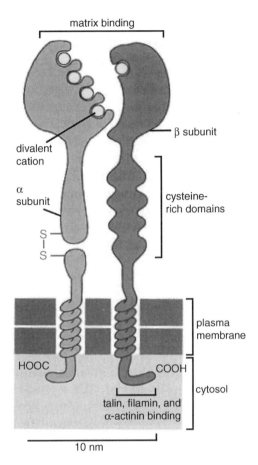

**FIGURE 13.3**

Integrin. (Taken from Alberts, B., Johnson, A., Lewis, J., Raff, M., Roberts, K., and Walter, P., *The Molecular Biology of the Cell*, 4th ed., Garland Science, Taylor & Francis Group, New York. With permission.)

β-subunit. Another anchor protein, paxillin, binds FAK to the α-subunit (Ingber, 1999; Wang et al., 2001; Goessler et al., 2004).

This network of structural proteins transmits mechanical forces generated within a cell's microenvironment throughout the cyctoskeleton to affect changes in cell shape and initiate cascades of intracellular signaling kinases. Cell shape is a critical determinant of cell behavior. Among adherent cells, those that are fully rounded (unattached) undergo apoptosis. Those that are retracted, but not fully rounded, undergo differentiation to a specific phenotype. Those that are attached to a rigid substratum and spread (flattened) proliferate. Phosphorylated intracellular kinases ultimately activate transcription factors that influence expression of the genome and selection of a specific phenotypic pathway (Clark and Brugge, 1995; Ingber, 2003; Millward-Sadler and Salter, 2004). The effect of cell shape on phenotype selection has been shown by Cancedda et al. who studied the influence of cell morphology on phenotype selection of chick hypertrophic chondrocytes and mature human articular chondrocytes. They demonstrated pluripotent mesenchymal cells must be cultured within a malleable three-dimensional substratum that permits them to remain rounded and nonadherent if they are to develop along the chondrocyte pathway. If these cells are cultured on an anchorage dependent substratum, they transdifferentiate to the osteoblast phenotype (Tacchetti et al., 1987; Cancedda et al., 1992; Gentili et al., 1993; Malpeli et al., 2004).

### 13.3.2 HY–CD44 Interactions and Consequences

While insoluble glycoproteins of the ECM engage integrins, hyaluronan polysaccharide binds to several plasma membrane receptors, known as hyaladherins, including the receptor for hyaluronic acid mediated motility (RHAMM), liver endothelial cell (LEC) receptor, intercellular adhesion molecule-1 (ICAM-1), lymph vessel endothelial hyaluronan receptor-1 (LYVE-1), hyaluronan receptor for endocytosis (HARE) and the CD44 glycoprotein (Knudson and Knudson, 1993; McCourt et al., 1994; Banerji et al., 1999; Zhou et al., 2000; Knudson, 2003; Nedvetzki et al., 2004).

Because CD44 is the primary receptor interacting with HY, and the principal instrument by which hyaluronan's many and varied biologic effects are produced, it is important to understand how CD44 binds HY and the intracellular consequences of this union (Aruffo et al., 1990; Day and Prestwich, 2002; Thorne et al., 2004). Though differences exist at the molecular level, all HY receptors engage the HY ligand via a common binding motif consisting of two basic amino acids (arginine and lysine) separated by seven nonacidic amino acids (Yang et al., 1994; Wang et al., 1996). The CD44 receptor has two such amino acid groupings, known as the $B(X_7)B$ motif. Both are located in its distal extracellular domain; one in the region that is homologous with the link protein that binds aggrecan, a proteoglycan, to hyaluronan in articular cartilage ECM (Figure 13.4). The other is positioned more proximal to the plasma membrane (Peach et al., 1993; Knudson and Knudson, 1999). CD44 engages its HY ligand by forming polyelectrolytic complexes (PEC) between the negatively-charged carboxylic acid group of HY's glucuronic acid moiety (the anion) and positively charged amino acids of its $B(X_7)B$ motif (the cation) (Kahmann et al., 2000). Binding of HY to an individual CD44 receptor is weak, in spite of the fact that a single CD44 receptor can bind a single HY molecule at two different locations. In a manner similar to integrins, multiple CD44 receptors cluster together so that many receptors can

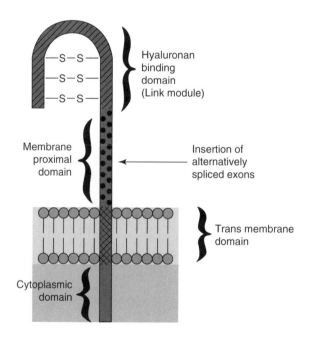

**FIGURE 13.4**
Major components of CD44. (*Source*: Toole B., Hyaluronan in morphogenesis and tissue remodeling, *Glycoforum* #8, (December 15, 1998). With permission.)

interact with a single HY chain producing a union of high binding affinity (Knudson and Knudson, 1999).

Ten isoforms of CD44 have been identified since the standard form (CD44s) was first isolated from hematopoetic cells (and termed CD44H). These variations on the standard CD44 theme are located in the receptor's membrane-proximal domain and are produced by various messenger ribonucleic acids (mRNA) generated by alternative splicing of exons 6 through 15 of the CD44 gene (Figure 13.4 and Figure 13.5) (Knudson and Knudson, 1999). Each variant is responsible for different biochemical properties and has different affinities for binding HY (Toole, 1998). For example, CD44v3 binds heparin sulfate, a sulfonated glycosaminoglycan, producing a proteoglycan complex capable of binding basic growth factors and presenting them to appropriate receptors (Knudson and Knudson, 2005). The membrane-proximal domain of CD44v3 and other isoforms also functions as an attachment site for matrix metalloproteinases (MMP), enzymes responsible for catabolism of ECM proteins (Bourguignon et al., 1998; Knudson and Knudson, 2005).

The 70 amino acid cytoplasmic domain is highly conserved among CD44 variants. In contrast to the integrins, the CD44 "tail" has no kinase or phosphatase activity. The extracellular clustering of CD44 is the inductive signaling event, mediated by components which are predominantly in lipid rafts (Knudson and Knudson, 2005). Its attachment to actin filaments of the cytoskeleton is mediated by anchor proteins of the ankyrin and ERM (ezrin, radixin, moesin, and merlin) families binding to a 20 to 30 amino acid sequence of CD44's cytoplasmic tail adjacent to the plasma membrane (Figure 13.5) (Tsukita et al., 1994; Bourguignon et al., 1998; Yonemura et al., 1998; Brown et al., 2005).

This brief review of the cytoskeleton and its associated integrins and receptors provides a foundation for understanding those biologic properties of hyaluronan of greatest importance to the tissue engineer. These include hyaluronan's role in cell migration,

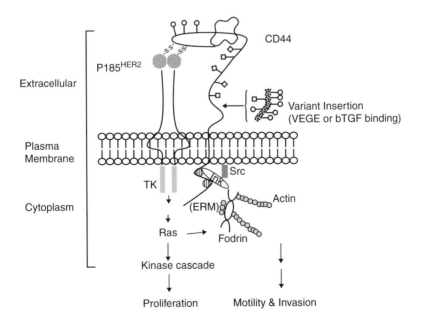

**FIGURE 13.5**
Functioning of the CD44 receptor. (*Source*: Bourguignon, L.Y.W., Zhu D., and Zhu H., CD44 isoform–cytosceleton interaction in oncogenic signaling and tumor progression, *Front. Biosci.*, 3 (July 1, d637–d649, (1998), www. bioscience.org. With permission.)

angiogenesis, signaling to the genome, modulation of signals produced by growth factors/morphogens, cell differentiation and its mechanisms of synthesis and metabolism. We begin with hyaluronan's role in cell migration.

### 13.3.3 Chemotaxis and Cell Migration

Success of tissue engineering devices depends upon their ability to attract undifferentiated host cells into the space of tissue regeneration and into intimate contact with the device itself. Hyaluronan facilitates migration of undifferentiated cells of the embryo as well as migration of pluripotent host cells into adult tissue defects. HY's ability to mediate three-dimensional cell migration is a function of both its physical and biochemical properties (Nehls and Hayen, 2000).

As noted above, hyaluronan is capable of maintaining a large hydrated volume. In developing tissues, the large spaces created by HY's hydrated volume provide a low resistance environment favorable for cell migration (Nathanson, 1990). Molecular weight of HY also plays a role in its ability to support cell migrations. Ito et al. (2004) found HY specimens of $2.0 \times 10^6$ Da weight-average molecular weight were more effective in promoting cell migrations than were HY examples of $5.4 \times 10^4$ Da.

Hyaluronan's performance as a chemotactic ground substance is enhanced by its association with compounds already recognized for their chemotactic properties, such as collagen IV, plasma fibronectin, laminin, and fibrin (Kielty et al., 1992; Nakamura et al., 1994; Hayen et al., 1999).

Cell motility, using HY as a chemotactic ground substance, is accomplished through the interaction of CD44 and RHAMM cytoplasmic domains with ankyrin, ezrin, radixin, moesin, merlin, and other anchorage proteins related to actin and myosin, contractile filaments of the cytoskeleton found in the cell cortex (Liu et al., 1996; Peck and Isacke, 1996; Legg et al., 2002). This fundamental mechanism for cell migration is employed by primary cells of the embryo, adult pluripotent stromal and mesenchymal stem cells (MSC), macrophages and fibroblasts of wound healing tissues, and by metastatic cells of malignant tumors (Toole et al., 1989; Underhill, 1993; Deplech et al., 1997; Knudson, 1998; Toole, 2001; Brown, 2004).

HY activated CD44 receptors produce two additional biochemical consequences important for cell migrations. In the first instance, clusters of HY activated CD44 receptors are able to colocalize with enzymes, known as matrix metalloproteases (MMP), responsible for degradation of ECM components (Bourguignon et al., 1998; Knudson and Knudson, 2005). Specifically, clusters of HY-activated CD44 receptors increase the concentration of MMP-2 and MMP-9 at particular locations on the plasma membrane, thus providing the means for creating a migratory pathway through the ECM (Murphy and Gavrilovic, 1999; Isacke and Yarwood, 2002). In the second instance, HY binding to CD44v3 promotes an intracellular signaling cascade resulting in tumor cell migration (Bourguignon et al., 2000).

Hyaluronan has many attributes of a material the tissue engineer needs to incorporate into an artificial matrix for the role of enhancing migration of undifferentiated cells from the surrounding host tissue and/or from the circulation.

### 13.3.4 Angiogenesis Induced by Hyaluronan Oligosaccharides

In 1985, West et al. demonstrated that oligosaccharides of hyaluronan (o-HY) in the length range of 4 to 25 disaccharides (1500 to 10,000 Da) induce an angiogenic response in the chick chorioallantoic membrane and native (high molecular weight) HY inhibited the angiogenic response (West et al., 1985). Since then, it has been learned that 6 to 10 disaccharides (2400 to 4000 Da) is the minimum chain length of HY required for binding to a single CD44 receptor and activation of CD44 receptors by HY oligosaccharides in endothelial cells (EC) initiates expression of immediate early response genes (ERG), resulting in EC proliferation and migration (Knudson, 1993; Rooney et al., 1995; Lesley et al., 2000; Asari, 2005).

Proliferation of ECs in response to CD44 activation by o-HY results from activation of a number of kinases (an intracellular phosphorylation cascade) culminating in activation of the mitogen-activated protein kinase (MAP-kinase) which translocates into the nucleus and turns on the ERG complex (Deed et al., 1997; Slevin et al., 1998). Migration of endothelial cells is as important to the process of angiogenesis as is their proliferation. EC migration through an ECM is facilitated by HY's hygroscopic property to enlarge acellular space and is accomplished by interaction of its transmembrane RHAMM receptors with high molecular weight HY of the ECM (Savani et al., 2001).

The biochemical role of o-HY in angiogenesis is not limited to EC proliferation and migration. Oligosaccharides of HY operate synergistically with vascular endothelial growth factor (VEGF) to amplify the angiogenic response beyond that attainable with either substance individually. The exact mechanism of action for this phenomenon is not yet understood, but may involve mutual activation of intracellular signaling pathways employed by both compounds (Montesano et al., 1996; Peattie et al., 2004). Another interesting possibility centers on a CD44 variant (CD44v3,8–10) that preferentially binds VEGF at its heparin binding site (in the membrane proximal domain of the extracellular region). Bourguignon et al. (1998) speculate that CD44v3,8–10 serves as modified receptor for VEGF capable of communicating with a transmembrane tyrosine kinase linked to it by disulfide bonds. Such an arrangement could activate two different angiogenic signaling pathways simultaneously, thus amplifying the end result.

The reader is directed to an excellent review of angiogenesis by Liekens et al. (2001) for a detailed description of this complicated process that must be directed and controlled by the components of any engineered matrix.

### 13.3.5 Hyaluronan as an Agent for Signaling to the Genome and as a Modulator of Soluble Signaling Factors

The complex intracellular signaling cascades initiated by HY binding to CD44, its variants, and to RHAMM will not be discussed here, but may be studied in excellent reviews by Kundson, Bourguignon, Turley, and others (Bourguignon et al., 1998; Knudson and Knudson, 1999; Turley and Harrison, 1999; Bourguignon et al., 2000; Lynn et al., 2001; Thorne et al., 2004; Knudson and Knudson, 2005). Some examples are offered to illustrate the role of HY oligosaccharides and macromolecular hyaluronan in initiating and modulating intracellular signaling to the genome.

Stimulation of angiogenesis by o-HY is an excellent example of "outside-in" signaling achieved by hyaluronan acting as a signaling agent to the genome through the CD44 receptor. Activation of CD44 by o-HY leads to other gene signals governing diseases such as cancer, osteoarthritis, and rheumatoid arthritis, as well as apoptosis (Bourguignon et al., 1998; Ishiwatari-Haysaka et al., 1999; Lee and Spicer, 2000; Yasuda et al., 2002; Knudson and Knudson, 2005). Common to these apparently diverse signaling activities is a release of CD44 binding to macromolecular HY, consequent disassociation of CD44 clusters in the plasma membrane and subsequent binding of individual CD44 receptors with HY oligosaccharides (Bourguignon et al., 1998).

In 1998, Reddi anticipated signal transduction interactions between those signals initiated by soluble morphogens/growth factors (i.e., BMPs) and signals received by the cell from its ECM (Reddi, 1998). This concept has now been verified by Peterson et al. (2004), who demonstrated that binding of CD44s to macomolecular hyaluronan of the chondrocyte pericellular matrix is required for translocation of BMP-7 signal transduction proteins SMAD-1 and SMAD-4 to the nucleus. With the observation by Evanko and Wight (1999) that hyaluronan is in the nucleus of smooth muscle cells and fibroblasts, internalization of endogenous HY may be an additional and direct route of signal transduction by HY effecting nucleolar function, chromosomal rearrangement, or other events in proliferating cells.

### 13.3.6 Bioynthesis and Metabolism of Hyaluronan

Tissues of a 70 kg person contain about 15 g of hyaluronan, 5 g of which are turned over every 24 h. Half of the body's total HY is found in the skin and in this location has a half-life of 24 h. In articular cartilage the half-life of HY is 1 to 3 weeks, while in the bloodstream its half-life is only 2 to 5 min (Stern and Csóka, 2000). Clearly, synthesis and degradation of HY are finely balanced and tightly controlled.

Hyaluronan is synthesized on the cytosol surface of the plasma membrane, unlike other glycosaminoglycans that are produce in roughened endoplasmic reticulum and expressed via the golgi apparatus. The latter are synthesized covalently bound to protein and are sulfonated, whereas HY is not (Lebel, 1991; Laurent and Fraser, 1992; Lee and Spicer, 2000). Synthesis of HY is under the direction of three glycosyl-transferases: hyaluronan synthase-1 (Has1), Has2 and Has3. These enzymes reside within the lipid layer of the plasma membrane with their uridine diphospho-$N$-acetylglucosamine (UDP-GlcNAc) and uridine diphospho-glucuronic acid (UDP-GlcA) transferase domains penetrating into the cytosol (Spicer and McDonald, 1998; Weigel, 1998). While it is clear that Has2 is the principal enzyme responsible for HY synthesis during embryogenesis, specific roles played by Has1 and Has3 are as yet unclear (Camenisch et al., 2000; Tammi et al., 2002).

The growing number of hyaluronan synthases has recently been categorized into two classes. Class I enzymes splice the alternating $N$-acetyl-D-glucosamine and glucuronic acid components to the reducing end of the growing HY chain as it is being extruded through the plasma membrane to the extracellular space (Figure 13.6). The single member of Class II splices the monomers at the nonreducing end of the chain (Weigel, 2004).

Catabolic processes by which macromolecular hyaluronan is digested are not completely understood. Yet enough is known to construct a general scheme for HY's clearance from tissue and ultimate catabolism to ammonia, acetate, lactate, and $CO_2$ (McCourt, 1999).

In mammals, enzymatic degradation of high molecular weight hyaluronan begins in somatic tissues, continues in regional lymph nodes, and is completed in the liver and to lesser extents in the kidney and spleen (Jackson, 2004). Six genes, located on two chromosomes, have been identified that code for mammalian-type hyaluronidases. Genes for hyaluronidase-1 (*HYAL-1*), *HYAL-2* and *HYAL-3* are clustered together on one chromosome while the gene for *HYAL-4*, a pseudogene for an inactive version of *HYAL-1* (*PHYAL-1*) and the gene for sperm adhesion molecule-1 (SPAM1 — aka PH-20) are clustered together on the other chromosome (Stern and Csóka, 2000). The role played by *HYAL-3* has not been identified. *HYAL-4* is thought to be a specific chondroitinase. *PHYAL-1* is not translated into an active enzyme in humans. PH-20 facilitates penetration of sperm through the HY cumulus of the ovum (Stern, 2003). Therefore, our attention will be directed toward the functions of *HYAL*-1 and *HYAL*-2.

*HYAL*-2 is anchored to the plasma membrane and, in cooperation with CD44, binds HY to the cell surface (Stern, 2003). It has been known for some time that endocytosis of CD44,

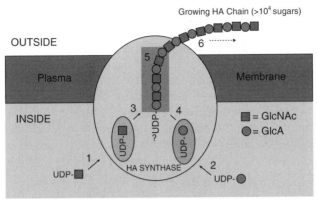

Growing HA Chain (>$10^4$ sugars)

OUTSIDE

6 ........→
5

Plasma | Membrane

INSIDE

3    4

■ = GlcNAc
● = GlcA

1

UDP-■

HA SYNTHASE

2

UDP-●

Multiple Functions of Hyaluronan Synthases

1) UDP-GlcNAc Binding Site     4) beta (1,3) GlcA Transferase
2) UDP-GlcA Binding Site        5) HA (acceptor) Binding Site
3) beta (1,4) GlcNAc Transferase   6) HA Transfer (translocation)

**FIGURE 13.6**

Hyaluronan synthase. (*Source*: Weigel, P.H., Bacterial hyaluronan synthases, *Glycoforum*, #6(August 15), (1998). With permission.)

together with any HY ligand that may be bound to it, is the first step of HY catabolism (Aguiar et al., 1999; Knudson et al., 2002). More details of this process have recently been reported. Invagination of HY-CD44 also involves *HYAL-2* and its bound HY. This complex represents a specialized microdomain within the plasma membrane known as a lipid raft and, under the influence of a sodium–hydrogen exchanger (NHE1), becomes an acidic enclave favorable for *HYAL-2* cleavage of HY to its limit of 20-kDa fragments (Ishiwatari-Haysaka et al., 1999; Yasuda et al., 2002; Bourguignon et al., 2004). Once fully incorporated into the cytosol, these endocytic vesicles fuse to lysosomes for further digestion of HY to mono- and disaccharides by *HYAL-1*. These small HY fragments leave the lysosome to be completely digested through the Krebs cycle to $CO_2$, $H_2O$, and $NH_3$ or to participate in intracellular signaling mechanisms (Knudson et al., 2002).

Stern has proposed a new miniorganelle specialized for simultaneous synthesis and catabolism of HY termed the "hyaluronasome." If such a structure is proved, it would explain the cell's ability to rapidly and precisely control molecular size and quantity of hyaluronan in response to changing conditions both extra- and intracellularly (Stern, 2004).

Degradation of macromolecular hyaluronan begins within its tissue of origin through attack by free radicals such as nitric oxide (NO) and MMP (Murphy and Gavrilovic, 1999; Isacke and Yarwood, 2002; Al-Assaf et al., 2003). However, only a small quantity is digested by cells within its tissue of origin. Once freed from its ECM attachments, high molecular weight HY (i.e., up to 1000 kDA) is conducted to regional lymph nodes where about 85% of the 5 g daily catabolic load is removed by endothelial cells of lymph sinusoids. About 15% of the daily catabolic load, now in the form of lower molecular weight HY fragments, enters the general circulation for removal by LECs and to a lesser extent by endothelial cells of the spleen and kidney (Jackson, 2004). Endocytosis of hyaluronan by these organs is facilitated by two recently identified endocytic receptors: LYVE-1 and HARE (Zhou et al., 2003; Jackson, 2004). LYVE-1 appears to be specific for hyaluronan while HARE can bind HY as well as chondroitin sulfate. Once incorporated within the cytosol, both the receptor and its attached HY molecule are degraded by lysosomal enzymes and metabolized through the Krebs cycle (Harris et al., 2004).

### 13.3.7  HY Role in Cell Differentiation

Providing clinicians with materials and devices capable of regenerating damaged or missing tissues is the goal of tissue engineers. A defect undergoing regeneration recapitulates many of the morphogenetic events observed in embryonic tissue development (Caplan, 2003). Since hyaluronan is the embryo's first ECM material, it is only reasonable that tissue engineers would look to HY to facilitate migration and targeted differentiation of pluripotent cells within their constructs (Nader et al., 1996).

Hyaluronan influences proliferation and differentiation of a wide variety of cells in diverse tissues. These include lymphocytes and dendritic cells of the immune system, hematopoietic progenitor cells of bone marrow, keratinocytes of the epidermis as well as induction of connective tissue MSC to osteoblasts and chondrocytes (Kujawa et al., 1986; Sasaki and Watanabe, 1995; Rafi et al., 1997; Termeer et al., 2002; Yang et al., 2002; Nilsson et al., 2003; Bourguignon et al., 2004). The latter two cell types are particularly important to tissue engineers, and will be the focus of our attention.

Pilloni and Bernard (1998) studied the effect of hyaluronan at various molecular weights and concentrations on the differentiation of fetal mouse calvarial mesenchymal cells *in vitro* (on two-dimensional, rigid substrata). They found that HY of 30 to 40 kDa (at 1.0 and 2.0 mg/ml) dramatically increased the number of bone forming colonies vs. untreated controls, but high molecular weight HY (e.g., >550 kDa) had no such effect. In a similar *in vitro* study, Huang et al. (2003) investigated the effect of low and high molecular weight HY, at 0.5, 1.0, and 2.0 mg/ml concentrations, on differentiation of cells derived from neonatal rat calvarium. They found that 60 kDa HY, at all concentrations studied, stimulated cell growth and production of mRNA for osteocalcin, an ECM marker of the osteoblast phenotype. However, synthesis of alkaline phosphatase and subsequent calcification within bone forming colonies were not affected by presence of 60 kDa in the media. By contrast, HY at 900 kDa and 2300 kDa up-regulated all responses studied, especially at the 2.0 mg/ml dose concentration.

An explanation for these seemingly contradictory results may be found by comparing (i) molecular weights of HY employed, (ii) culture media used in each study, (iii) reported cell population densities, and (iv) the protocol used for cell exposure to HY. Both studies employed fetal bovine serum (FBS) in the media, but Pillioni used heat inactivated FBS at 10% while Huang used active FBS, initially at 20 and 10% after cells reached confluence. It is impossible to compare cell population densities since Pillioni reports his cell concentration in terms of volume at $1 \times 10^4$ cells/ml, and Huang reports his cell population in terms of area at $1 \times 10^4$ cells/cm$^2$. In Pillioni's study, HY was added only once to the media during the first plating. Huang, on the other hand, exposed his cells to HY intermittently; initially, during the first plating, followed in 48 h by a change to HY-free media. Between 10 and 14 days prior to each experimental observation, the cells were once again exposed to various molecular weights and concentrations of HY.

bFGF (also known as FGF-2) is a powerful mitogen, found in FBS, that plays an important role in connective tissue repair. High molecular weight hyaluronan has no such effect (Radomsky et al., 1997). Radomsky et al. have demonstrated that bFGF delivered to osteotomy wounds in rabbit and baboon fibulas dramatically accelerates callous development and bone-wound healing (Radomsky et al., 1998, 1999). It is likely, therefore, that osteoblast differentiation and bone colony formation observed by Huang et al. were the result of HY's interaction with bFGF and other agents of FBS used to supplement the nutrient media. This theory is supported by Sasaki and Watanabe (1995) who found that a viscoelastic gel of HY at 1900 kDa accelerated osteogenesis in rat femoral defects. They speculate that the HY gel sequestered endogenous osteoinductive morphogens and maintained them within the wound environment at elevated concentrations.

From these studies it is clear that the effect hyaluronan has on differentiation of the osteoblast phenotype is dependent on its molecular weight and the timing of its exposure to developing cells, and is strongly influenced by growth factors and morphogens it might be carrying. However, interpretation of these findings must be considered in light of the fact that all these *in vitro* studies were conducted using two dimensional, rigid substrata; i.e., cell culture plates. We will now examine the effect of hyaluronan on pluripotent connective tissue cells grown on malleable, three-dimensional substrata containing hyaluronan.

The viscoelastic gel created by hyaluronan is a richly hydrated, malleable, three-dimensional environment conducive to maintaining the chondrocyte's rounded morphology. As we have already seen, cell shape is intimately involved with the cell's phenotype expression and biosynthetic activities (Tacchetti et al., 1987; Cancedda et al., 1992; Gentili et al., 1993; Malpeli et al., 2004). Additionally, HY's interactions with CD44 and RHAMM cell surface receptors impact activation of intracellular signaling molecules that are believed to govern phenotype expression and biosynthetic activities as well as modifying transduction of signals initiated by morphogens and growth factors (Knudson, 1998; Peterson et al., 2004). These physicochemical and biochemical properties of hyaluronan are particularly important to development and expression of the chondrocyte phenotype.

Miralles et al. (2000) observed that three-dimensional, malleable sponges of alginate support the chondrocyte phenotype and reasoned that this is due to preservation of the rounded morphology favored by chondrocytes. This conclusion is supported by the work of Kawasaki et al. (1999) and Knudson (2003).

Several recent *in vitro* studies provide evidence that HY in the microenvironment of cells expressing the chondrocyte phenotype stimulates synthesis of chondroitin-6-SO$_4$, collagen type II and aggrecan; all markers of chondrocyte biosynthesis (Kawasaki et al., 1999; Ehlers et al., 2000; Allemann et al., 2001; Miralles et al., 2001). These studies have several critical elements in common. (i) They all employed already differentiated chondrocytes from diverse species (rat, rabbit, bovine, and human sources). (ii) Where reported, HY weight-average molecular weights used were $4.8 \times 10^5$, $8.0 \times 10^5$ and (estimated) $1.5 \times 10^6$; all considered "high" molecular weight. (iii) All used a malleable, three-dimensional substratum (composed of collagen type I, alginate, a composite of collagens I and III, or a colyophilized composite of collagen I and HY). (iv) All studies used culture media supplemented with active fetal bovine (calf) serum at concentrations of 10 to 12%.

None of the four studies observed evidence of the osteoblast phenotype, even though they all employed hyaluronan and FBS in the culture system. Comparison of the Pillioni and Huang studies with the four described here leads one to conclude that physical properties of the substratum strongly influence selection of phenotype. Plasticity of expression between the osteoblast and chondrocyte phenotypes is a recognized phenomenon shown by Cancedda et al. to depend on the mechanical properties of culture substratum (Cancedda et al., 1992; Gentili et al., 1993; Caplan, 2003; Malpeli et al., 2004). The investigations described above comport well with those reported by Cancedda.

Though none of these four studies comment specifically on the effect of HY molecular weight, three (Kawasaki et al., Ehlers et al., and Allemann et al.) agree that lower concentrations of HY in the system are more effective than higher concentrations for stimulating chondrocyte differentiation and expression of phenotype specific ECM markers. Kawasaki and Ehlers arrived at the same optimum hyaluronan concentration of 100 μg/100 ml. Clearly HY has a dose response effect independent of whatever contributions might be added by its association with bFGF and other biologically active agents resident in FBS.

It has recently been shown that SMAD-1, a signal transduction protein for the BMP family (specifically BMP-7), interacts with the cytoplasmic tail of CD44. Furthermore, binding of CD44 to high molecular weight HY increases cell responses to BMP-7 (rhOP-1) such as SMAD-1 phosphorylation and nuclear translocation (Peterson et al., 2004). Furthermore, BMP-7 has been has been shown to amplify synthesis of collagen type II and aggrecan by mature chondrocytes and expression of HAS-2 and CD44 mRNA (Flechtenmacher et al., 1996; Nishida et al., 2000a, 2000b). Thus, there exists a mutually synergistic relationship between a soluble signaling factor, BMP-7, and HY of the cell's microenvironment. One might speculate that similar mechanisms exist between exogenous HY added to a culture media and soluble signaling factors present with FBS (e.g., bFGF). Furthermore, the ability of a single molecule of high molecular weight HY to bind more than one CD44 receptor results in clustering of CD44 receptors within the plasma membrane, thus promoting a geometric ordering of functional receptors, increase of intracellular communication and amplification of signals initiated by soluble factors (Knudson and Knudson, 2001; Knudson, 2003; Goodstone et al., 2004).

## 13.4  Hyaluronan Applications in Tissue Engineering

Hyaluronan's physical and biochemical properties are beginning to be recognized as attributes valuable to tissue engineers and drug delivery specialists. A manufactured substitute for bone grafts was fabricated by incorporating sodium hyaluronan within a three-dimensional, open-cell structural polymer (D,D-L,L-polylactic acid; OPLA) as a dry filamentous velour (Figure 13.7 and Figure 13.8) (Brekke, 1996). When hydrated with a solution of BMP it embodies all the critical elements of bone graft: (i) structural/ architectural competence of specific geometry to maintain space for denovo bone, (ii) a viscoelastic gel capable of retaining BMP within the boundaries of the device at its effective dose concentration, (iii) chemotactic substance facilitating invasion of the device by MSC and vascular pericytes, (iv) angiogenic stimulus produced by HY oligosaccharides released into the wound milieu, and (v) osteoinductive potential provided by BMP.

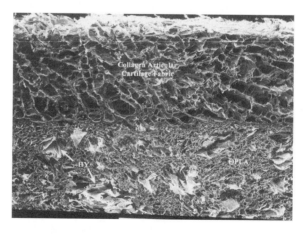

**FIGURE 13.7**
Scanning electron micrograph of OPLA structural polymer, cancellous bone architecture, Na−HY invested as a dry velour. Original magnification = 20 × .

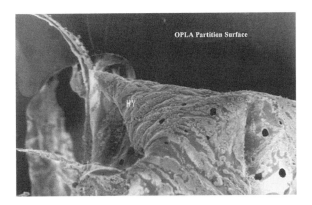

**FIGURE 13.8**
SEM image of a single pour in OPLA invested with a leaflet of Na–HY. Original magnification $= 1.03k \times$.

This device proved an effective bone graft substitute in the dog intertransverse process, spinal fusion model, as a matrix for ectopic prefabrication of viable bone, as a bone graft substitute in the rat femur and as the subchondral bone component of an articular cartilage regeneration device (Figure 13.7) (Brekke and Toth, 1998; Vögelin et al., 2000, 2002, 2005; Frenkel et al., 2005).

More recently, sodium hyaluronan has been joined to chitosan (CT) as a polyelectrolytic complex (HY–CT–PEC) to form a dry, porous, insoluble fabric that can be joined to the OPLA/HY subchondral bone construct, forming a biphasic device for regeneration of articular cartilage (Figure 13.9) (Brekke et al., 2005). In this formulation, HY, the anion, interacts with CT, the cation, to form an insoluble coacervate that can be processed into a dry fabric (Denuziere et al., 1996, 1998, 2000). Each region of this device can be independently hydrated with solutions of growth factors or morphogens at concentrations appropriate for inducing the target tissue. Upon hydration, the HY–CT–PEC articular cartilage fabric assumes some qualities of a hydrogel (i.e., swelling) even though it is composed exclusively of insoluble HY–CT–PEC coacervate. We speculate that high

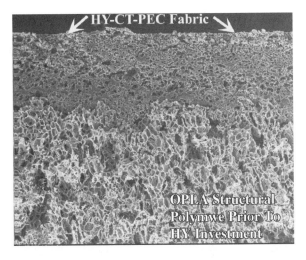

**FIGURE 13.9**
HY–CT–PEC articular cartilage regeneration fabric, joined to OPLA structural polymer prior to investment of HY microstructure. Original magnification $= 50 \times$.

molecular weight HY interacts with the chitosan cation at intervals dictated by steric hindrance. If this is correct, a random loop morphology for unreacted regions of both macromolecules could interact with water of hydration as viscoelastic gel or hydrogel.

A malleable, three-dimensional hydrogel composed of unreacted HY, unreacted CT, and a network of self-assembled HY–CT–PEC microfibers has been employed recently for culture multipotent, adult progenitor cells (MAPC) (Jiang et al., 2002; Brekke et al., 2005). Hydrated by a cell seeding fluid, a "cocoon" forms, composed of HY viscoelastic gel, CT hydrogel, and a network of HY–CT–PEC microfibers penetrating both the HY viscoelastic gel and the CT hydrogel (Figure 13.10 and Figure 13.11). The microfibers provide structural support for the construct as a whole as well as a fabric for cell attachment. Figure 13.12 depicts cells originating as porcine MAPCs after being cultured for 25 days in an HCP-h "cocoon" and engaged with HY–CT–PEC microfibers.

### 13.4.1 Derivatives of Hyaluronan Used as Tissue Engineering Materials

In an effort to create tissue engineering devices of hyaluronan, two interesting formulations have been developed involving esterification of HY's carboxylic acid group located on the glucuronic acid moiety (Fidia Biopolymers, Padova, Italy). One formulation produces an auto-cross-linked polysaccharide (ACP) in which the carboxylic acid groups of glucuronic acid are esterified with hydroxyl groups on the same or neighboring molecules. The other formulation esterifies the carboxylic acid groups of glucuronic acid with an alcohol, preferably benzyl alcohol (Campoccia et al., 1998). All esterification formulations of HY reduce its negative charge (e.g., hydrophilic properties) and increase its hydrophobicity, thus rendering the compound insoluble in aqueous media and imparting novel mechanical properties. The best characterized material emanating from these formulations is a benzyl alcohol esterification of HY in which 100% of its glucuronic acid carboxylic acid groups are joined to a molecule of benzyl alcohol (HYAFF® 11; Fidia Biopolymers, Padova, Italy) (Milella et al., 2002). Soluble growth factors and morphogens have been successfully delivered to bone defects by HYAFF® 11 sponges. In one study, HYAFF® 11 was the vehicle used to deliver bone marrow stromal cells (BMSC) and basic fibroblast growth factor to segmental defects in the rat radius (Lisignoli et al., 2002). In another study, HYAFF® 11 was compared with the absorbable collagen sponge (ACS) typically used to deliver an osteoinductive protein, recombinant human, bone morphogenetic protein-2 (rhBMP-2), at a dose concentration of 200 μg/100 μl (Hunt et al., 2001). These investigators report that defects treated with HYAFF® 11/rhBMP-2 sponges grow significantly greater quantities of de novo bone than did those treated with the ACS/rhBMP-2 formulations. They attribute this superior performance of HYAFF® 11 sponges to

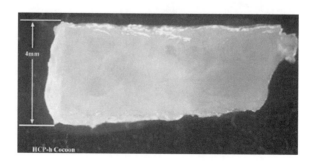

**FIGURE 13.10**
HCP-h "cocoon."

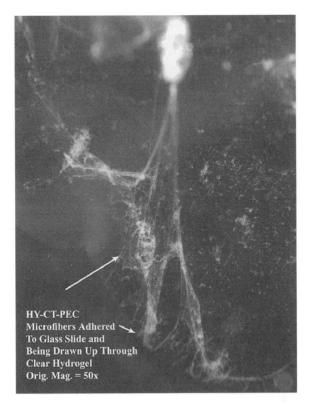

**FIGURE 13.11**
HT–CT–PEC microfibers being drawn up though HCP-h hydrogel. Steresocope, original magnification = 50 ×.

its ability to maintain space for new bone development. HYAFF® 11, of varying gross configurations, has proved to be useful for both *in vitro* and *in vivo* culturing of MSC, chondrocytes and endothelial cells (Grigolo et al., 2002; Girotto et al., 2003; Turner et al., 2004; Cristino et al., 2005).

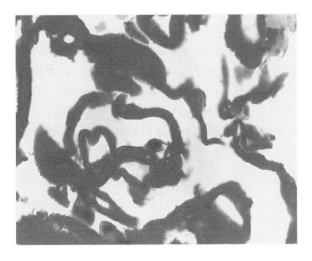

**FIGURE 13.12**
Cells originating as porcine MAPCs attached to HY–CT–PEC microfibers at culture day 25. H&E stain. Original magnification = 1000 ×.

In spite of the impressive results reported for HYAFF® 11, the fact that 100% of HY's carboxylic acid groups are occupied by benzyl alcohol ester is troubling for the present authors, since it is the $-COO^-$ group of HY's glucuronic acid moiety that engages the hyaluronan binding domains of its primary receptors, CD44 and RHAMM. Milella et al. (2002) report evidence for hydrolysis of the ester bond when HYAFF® 11 is incubated at 37°C in Dulbecco Modified Eagle's Medium (DMEM) beginning on the first day of incubation. However, only approximately 23% of the total benzyl alcohol in the HYAFF® 11 sample is recovered in media by day 11. Since most of the important wound-healing events that would benefit from biologically active hyaluronan take place within the first 7 days, it is difficult to imagine how HYAFF® 11, or any of the other HY derivatives employing the carboxylic acid group of the glucuronic acid moiety can contribute to cell motility, cell differentiation, or angiogenesis. Though materials of the HYAFF® group are clearly excellent biocompatible cell substrata, they may not possess many of the biological properties described earlier in this chapter.

Allogeneic, freeze-dried, demineralized bone (FDDB) has been used for decades in treatment of bone defects, either alone or in conjunction with autologous bone. In order to improve handling characteristics, FDDB particles have recently been blended with sodium hyaluronan (Gertzman and Sunwoo, 2001). Since HY in these preparations is not reacted with any other compound, its positive biology properties (e.g., angiogenesis and chemotaxis) are thought to contribute to the osteoinductive effect of FDDB particles (Yee et al., 2003).

---

## Ten Questions and Answers

1. **Question:**  When employing hyaluronan as a tissue engineering material, what precautions are required to ensure its usefulness in the final construct?
   **Answer:**
   (a) HY must be sourced from a manufacturer who thoroughly characterizes the material according to ASTM standards.
   (b) HY should be filter sterilized and aseptically packaged.
   (c) HY should be stored at temperatures of $-20$°C or less.
   (d) HY chemical properties must be validated following device fabrication and sterilization.

2. **Question:**  Identify two qualities of HY that distinguish it from all the other glycosaminoglycans (GAG).
   **Answer:**
   (i) HY is the only GAG that is not sulfonated.
   (ii) HY is synthesized within the plasma membrane and directly extruded into the ECM. All the other GAGs are synthesized on the rough endoplasmic reticulum and secreted into the ECM via the golgi apparatus.

3. **Question:**  Why is HY's capacity to exclude large molecules from its hydrated domain important for tissue engineers?

**Answer:**
Theoretically, this exclusionary property of high molecular weight HY can be used to temporarily retain soluble growth factors and morphogens within the boundaries of a tissue-engineering construct if the dry device is hydrated with a solution of the biologically active compounds.

4. **Question:** Identify the primary cell surface receptors for hyaluronan (HY) and describe the molecular mechanism by which they engage the HY ligand.
   **Answer:**
   The primary receptors for hyaluronan are CD44 and RHAMM. They engage the HY ligand by forming a polyelectrolytic complex between their $B(X_7)B$ motifs and the carboxylic acid group of HY's glucuronic acid component.

5. **Question:** What are the physical and biologic consequences of reacting HY's $-COO^-$ group (glucuronic acid component) with alcohols, or esterifying it with other pendants on the HY molecule?
   **Answer:**
   Hydration of HY-esters is inversely proportional to the degree of esterification. At 100% esterification, the HY-ester is insoluble and its rate of biodegradation is prolonged. By masking HY's carboxylic acid group with alcohols, one is removing its primary mechanism for engaging its cell surface receptors.

6. **Question:** At the molecular level, how do cells use HY as a chemotactic ground substance?
   **Answer:**
   CD44 and RHAMM receptors engage HY of the ECM via their $B(X_7)B$ motifs. These activated receptors are bound to then contractile elements (actin and myosin) of the cytoskeleton by anchorage proteins. Once a sufficient number of these receptors are clustered in one region of the plasma membrane, the cell can pull itself through the ECM.
   Clustering of HY activated CD44 receptors also concentrates certain MMP (e.g., MMP-2 and MMP-9) which enzymatically digest ECM components, creating a pathway for cell movement.

7. **Question:** Outline how HY operates as an angiogenic stimulus.
   **Answer:**
   Oligosaccharides of HY activate CD44 receptors resulting in expression of immediate early response genes (ERG) and endothelial cell proliferation. Also, oligosaccharides of HY operate synergistically with vascular endothelial growth factor (VEGF) using mechanisms that are not yet completely understood.

8. **Question:** Give at least one example of high molecular weight HY impacting signal transduction of a soluble signaling protein.
   **Answer:**
   In the chondrocyte, binding of CD44s to macromolecular HY is required for translocation of SMAD-1 and SMAD-4 to the nucleus.

9. **Question:** By what mechanism is HY synthesized?
   **Answer:**
   A glycosyltransferase, Has2, is the principle enzyme responsible for HY synthesis. It is located in the lipid portion of the plasma membrane. This enzyme adds glucuronic acid alternately to N-acetyl-D-glucosamine at the reducing end of the growing HY polymer; this taking place within the cytosol just beneath the plasma membrane. As each component is added to the HY

chain, the complete molecule is extruded through the plasma membrane into the ECM.

10. **Question:** What are the mechanisms by which hyaluronan is degraded and metabolized?

   **Answer:**

   (i) Within its tissue of origin, HY is degraded by free radicals and MMPs found in the ECM and endocytosed via the CD44 receptor or reduced to fragments of approximately 20 kDa by Hyal-2, a hyaluronidase anchored to the plasma membrane. Once fully incorporated into the cytosol, the HY-CD44 complex and the Hyal-2-HY complex fuse to lysosomes which further digest the HY to mono- and disaccharides suitable for complete degradation to ammonia, carbon dioxide and water via the Krebs cycle.

   (ii) The majority of partially digested HY leaves its tissue of origin and is sequestered in regional lymph nodes where it is completely metabolized by endothelial cells of the lymph sinusoids by mechanisms outlined in (i). The only difference is that lymph endothelial cells utilize LYVE-1 and HARE receptors rather than CD44 to HY endocytosis.

   (iii) Small quantities of HY escape to the general circulation from which they are dispatched by endothelial cells of the liver, spleen, and kidney.

# References

Aguiar, D., Knudson, W., and Knudson, C., Internalization of the hyaluronan receptor CD44 by chondrocytes, *Exp. Cell Res.*, **252**, 292–302 (1999).

Al-Assaf, S.,. Navaratnam, S., Parsons, B.J., and Phillips, G.O., The chain scission of hyaluronan by peroxynitrite, *Arch. Biochem. Biophys.*, **411** (1), 73–82 (2003).

Alberts, B., Johnson, A., Lewis, J., Raff, M., Roberts, K., and Walter, P., Molecular biology of the cell, 4th ed., *The Cytoskeleton*. Garland Science — Taylor & Francis Group, New York (2002), pp. 907–982.

Allemann, F., Mizuno, S., Eid, K., Yates, K.E., Zaleske, D., and Glowacki, J., Effects of hyaluronan on engineered articular cartilage extracellular matrix gene expression in 3-dimensional collagen scaffolds, *J. Biomed. Mater. Res.*, **55**, 13–19 (2001).

Aruffo, A., Stamenkovic, I., Meinick, M., Underhill, C.B., and Seed, B., CD44 is the principal cell surface receptor for hyaluronate, *Cell*, **61**, 1303–1313 (1990).

Asari, A., Novel functions of hyaluronan oligosaccharides, *Glycoscience, Science of Hyaluronan*, **29** (February 24) (2005).

ASTM. Standard guide for characterization and testing of hyaluronan as starting materials intended for use in biomedical and tissue engineered medical product applications, ASTM 2347-03.

Aziz, K.A., CD44 mediates polymorphonuclear leukocyte motility on hyaluronan, *Saudi Med. J.*, **24** (8), 827–831 (2003).

Balazas, E.A., Laurent, T.C., and Jeanloz, R.W., Nomenclature of hyaluronic acid, *Biochem. J. Lett.*, **235**, 903 (1986).

Banerji, S., Ni, J., Clasper, S., Su, J., Tammi, R., Jones, M., and Jackson, D.G., LYVE-1, a new homologue of the CD44 glycoprotein, is a lymph-specific receptor for hyaluronan, *J. Cell Biol.*, **144** (4), 789–801 (1999).

Bociek, M., Darke, A.H., Welti, D., and Rees, D.A., The 13C-NMR spectra of hyaluronate and chondroitin sulphates, *Eur. J. Biochem.*, **109**, 447–456 (1980).

Bourguignon, L.Y.W., Singleton, P.A., and Diedrich, F., Hyaluronan-CD44 interaction with RAC1-dependent protein kinase N-γ promotes phospholipase Cγ1 activation, $Ca^{2+}$ signaling, and cortactin-cytoskeleton function leading to keratinocyte adhesion and differentiation, *J. Biol. Chem.*, **279** (28), 29654–29669 (2004).

Bourguignon, L.Y., Singleton, P.A., Diedrich, F., Stern, R., and Gilad, E., CD44 interaction with Na$^+$ and H$^+$ exchanger (NHE1) creates acidic microenvironments leading to hyaluronidase-2 and cathepsin B activation and breast tumor cell invasion, *J. Biol. Chem.*, **279** (26), 26991–27007 (2004).

Bourguignon, L.Y.W., Zhu, H., Shao, L., and Chen, Y.W., CD44 interaction with TIAM-1 promotes rac1 signaling and hyaluronic acid-mediated breast tumor cell migration, *J. Biol. Chem.*, **275** (3), 1829–1838 (2000).

Bourguignon, L.Y.W., Zhu, D., and Zhu, H., CD44 isoform-cytoskeleton interaction in oncogenic signaling and tumor progression, *Front. Biosci.*, **3**, d637–d649 (1998).

Bowen, T., Davies, M., and Williams, J.D., Variations of hyaluronan synthesis and migration of human peritoneal mesothelial cells following mechanical wounding and cytokine stimulation. In: *Hyaluronan: Structure, Metabolism, Biological Activities, Therapeutic Applications* (Balazs, E.A. and Hascall, V.C., Eds). Winmar Enterprises, Edgewater, NJ (in press).

Brekke, J.H., A rationale for delivery of osteoinductive proteins, *Tissue Eng.*, **2** (2), 97–114 (1996).

Brekke, J.H., Bradica, G., Goldman, S.M., Kroengold, R., Coutts, R.D., and Frenkel, S.R., *Biphasic polyelectrolytic device to regenerate articular cartilage, Poster 426, Society for Biomaterials Annual Meeting, Memphis, TN*, (2005).

Brekke, J.H., Perkins, E., Holy, J., Sandquist, L.J., Rahmann, E.P., and O'Brien, T.D., *A biomimetic, three-dimensional cell culture matrix, 5th Regenerate Conference & Exposition, Atlanta, GA*, (2005).

Brekke, J.H. and Toth, J.M., Principles of tissue engineering applied to programmable osteogenesis, *J. Biomed. Mater. Res (Appl. Biomater.)*, **43**, 380–398 (1998).

Brown, J.A., The role of hyaluronic acid in wound healing's proliferative phase, *J. Wound Care*, **13** (2), 48–51 (2004).

Brown, K.L., Birkenhead, D., Lai, J.C.Y., Li, L., Li, R., and Johnson, P., Regulation of hyaluronan binding by F-actin and colocalization of CD44 and phosphorylated ezrin/radixin/moesin (ERM) proteins in myueloid cells, *Exp. Cell Res.*, **303**, 400–414 (2005).

Camenisch, T.D., Spicer, A.P., Brehm-Gibson, T., Biesterfeldt, J., Augustine, M.L., Calabro, J.r.A., Kubslsk, S., Klewwer, S.E., and McDonald, J.A., Disruption of hyaluronan synthase-2 abrogates normal cardiac morphogenesis and hyaluronan-mediated transformation of epithelium to mesenchyme, *J. Clin Inves*, **106** (3), 349–360 (2000).

Campoccia, D., Doherty, P., Radice, M., Brun, P., Abatangelo, G., and Williams, D., Semisynthetic resorbable materials from hyaluronan esterification, *Biomaterials*, **19**, 2101–2127 (1998).

Cancedda, F.D., Gentili, C., Manduca, P., and Cancedda, R., Hypertryphic chondrocytes undergo further differentiation in culture, *J. Cell Biol.*, **117** (2), 427–435 (1992).

Caplan, A., Embryonic development and the principles of tissue engineering, In: *Tissue Engineering of Cartilage and Bone, Novartis Foundation Symposium, 249*, Bock, G. and Goode, J., Eds., pp. 17–33 (2003).

Carr, M.E. and Hadler, N.M., Permeability of hyaluronic acid solutions. The effects of matrix concentration, calcium and pH, *Arthritis Rheum.*, **23**, 1371–1375 (1980), Abstract.

Chen, J., Abatangelo, W.Y., and Abatangelo, G., Functions of hyaluronan in wound repair, *Wound Repair Regen.*, **7**, 79–89 (1999).

Chen, C.S., Tan, J., and Tien, J., Mechanotransduction at cell–matrix and cell–cell contacts, *Annu. Rev. Biomed. Eng.*, **6**, 275–302 (2004).

Clark, E.A. and Brugge, J.S., Integrins and signal transduction pathways: the road taken, *Science*, **268**, 233–239 (1995).

Cowman, M.K. and Matsouka, S., *The Intrinsic Viscosity of Hyaluronan, Hyaluronan: Volume 1 — Chemical, Biochemical and Biological Aspects*, Woodhead Publishing Ltd, Cambridge, pp. 75–78 (2002).

Cristino, S., Grassi, F., Toneguzzi, S., Piacentini, A., Grigolo, B. et al., Analysis of mesenchymal stem cells grown on a three-dimensional HYAFF® 11-based ligament scaffold, *J. Biomed. Mater. Res.*, **73A**, 275–283 (2005).

Dark, A., Finer, E.G., Moorhouse, R., and Rees, D.A., Studies of hyaluronate solutions by nuclear magnetic relaxation measurements. Detection of covalently-defined, stiff segments within the flexible chains, *J. Mol. Biol.*, **99**, 477–486 (1975).

Day, J.A. and Prestwich, G.D., Hyaluronan-binding proteins: tying up the giant, *J. Biol. Chem.*, **277** (7), 4585–4588 (2002).

Deed, R., Rooney, P., Kumar, P., Norton, J.D., Smith, J., Freemont, A.J., and Kumar, S., Early-response gene signaling is induced by angiogenic oligosaccharides of hyaluronan in endothelial cells. Inhibition by non-angiogenic, high-molecular-weight hyaluronan, *Int. J. Cancer*, **71**, 251–256 (1997).

Denuziere, A., Ferrier, D., Damour, O., and Domard, A., Chitosan-chondroitin sulfate and chitosan-hyaluronate polyelectrolytic complexes: biological properties, *Biomaterials*, **19** (14), 1275–1285 (1998).

Denuziere, A., Ferrier, D., and Domard, A., Chitosan-chondroitin sulfate and chitosan-hyaluronate polyelectrolyte complexes. Physio-chemical aspects, *Carbohydr. Polym.*, **29** (4), 317–323 (1996).

Denuziere, A., Ferrier, D., and Domard, A., Interactions between chitosan and glycosaminoglycans (chondroitin sulfate and hyaluronic acid): physicochemical and biological studies, *Ann. Pharm. Fr.*, **58** (1), 47–53 (2000).

Deplech, B., Girard, N., Bertrand, P., Courel, M.-N., Chauzy, C., and Delpech, A., Hyaluronan: fundamental principles and applications in cancer, *J. Int. Med.*, **242**, 41–48 (1997).

Ehlers, E.-M., Behrens, P., Wünsch, L., Kühnel, W., and Russlies, M., Effects of hyaluronic acid on the morphology and proliferation of human chondrocytes in primary cell culture, *Ann. Anat.*, **183**, 13–17 (2000).

Evanko, S.P. and Wight, T.N., Intracellular localization of hyaluronan in proliferating cells, *J. Histochem. Cytochem.*, **47**, 1331–1342 (1999).

Flechtenmacher, J., Huch, K., Thonar, E.J.M.A., Mollenhauer, J., Davis, S.R. et al., Recombinant human osteogenic protein 1 is a potent stimulator of the synthesis of cartilage proteoglycans and collagens by human articular chondrocytes, *Arthritis Rheum.*, **39**, 478–488 (1996).

Frenkel, S.R., Bradica, G., Brekke, J.H., Goldman, S.M., Ieska, K., Issack, P., Bong, M.R., Tian, H., Gokhale, J., Coutts, R.D., and Kronengold, R.T., Regeneration of articular cartilage — evaluation of osteochondral defect repair in the rabbit using multiphasic implants, *Osteoarthritis and Cartilage*, 13 (9), 798–807 (2005).

Gentili, C., Bianco, P., Neri, M., Malpeli, M., Campanile, G., Castagnola, P., Cancedda, R., and Cancedda, F.D., Cell proliferation, extracellular matrix mineralization, and ovotransferrin transient expression during in vitro differentiation of chick hypertrophic chondrocytes into osteoblast-like cells, *J. Cell Biol.*, **122** (3), 703–712 (1993).

Gertzman, A.A. and Sunwoo, M.H., A pilot study evaluating sodium hyaluronate as a carrier for freeze-dried demineralized bone powder, *Cell Tissue Bank.*, **2**, 87–94 (2001).

Girotto, D., Urbani, S., Brun, P., Renier, D., Barbucci, R., and Abatangelo, G., Tissue-specific gene expression in chondrocytes grown on three-dimensional hyaluronic acid scaffolds, *Biomaterials*, **24**, 3265–3275 (2003).

Goessler, U.R., Hörmann, K., and Riedel, F., Tissue engineering with chondrocytes and function of the extracellular matrix (Review), *Int. J. Mol. Med.*, **13**, 505–513 (2004).

Goodstone, N.J., Cartwright, A., and Ashton, B., Effects of high molecular weight hyaluronan on chondrocytes cultured within a resorbable gelatin sponge, *Tissue Eng.*, **10** (3/4), 621–631 (2004).

Gribbon, P., Heng, B.C., and Hardingham, T.E., The analysis of intermolecular interactions in concentrated hyaluronan solutions suggest no evidence for chain-chain association, *Biochem. J-London*, **350**, 329–335 (2000).

Grigolo, B., Lisignoli, G., Piacentini, A., Fiorini, M., Gobbi, P. et al., Evidence for redifferentiation of human chondrocytes grown on a hyaluronan-based biomaterial (HYAFF® 11): molecular, immunohistochemical and ultrastructural analysis, *Biomaterials*, **23**, 1187–1195 (2002).

Hadler, N.M., Enhanced diffusivity of glucose in a matrix of hyaluronic acid, *J. Biol. Chem.*, **255**, 3532–3535 (1980).

Harris, E.N., Weigel, J.A., and Weigel, P.H., Endocytic function, glycosaminoglycan specificity, and antibody sensitivity of the recombinant human 190-kDa hyaluronan receptor for endocytosis (HARE), *J. Biol. Chem.*, **279** (35), 36201–36209 (2004).

Hayen, W., Goebeler, M., Kumar, S., Rleßen, R., and Nehls, V., Hyaluronan stimulates tumor cell migration by modulating the fibrin fiber architecture, *J. Cell. Sci.*, **112**, 2241–2251 (1999).

Heldin, P., Importance of hyaluronan biosynthesis and degradation in cell differentiation and tumor formation, *Braz. J. Med. Biol. Res.*, **36** (8), 967–973 (2003).

Hokputsa, S., Jumel, K., Alexander, C., and Harding, S.E., A comparison of molecular mass determination of hyaluronic acid using SEC/MALLS and sedimentation equilibrium, *Eur. Biophys. J.*, **32**, 450–456 (2003).

Huang, L., Cheng, Y.Y., Koo, P.L., Lee, K.M., Qin, L., Cheng, J.C.Y., and Kumta, S.M., The effect of hyaluronan on ostoblast proliferation and differentiation in rat calvarial-derived cell cultures, *J. Biomed. Mater. Res.*, **66A**, 880–884 (2003).

Hunt, D.R., Jovanovic, S.A., Wikesjö, U.M.E., Wozney, J.M., and Bernard, G.W., Hyaluronan supports recombinant human bone morphogenetic protein-2 induced bone reconstruction of advanced alveolar ridge defects in dogs. A pilot study, *J. Periontol.*, **72** (5), 651–657 (2001).

Ingber, D.E., Tensegrity: The architectural basis of cellular mechanotransduction, *Annu. Rev. Physiol.*, **59**, 575–599 (1997).

Ingber, D.E., The architecture of life, *Sci. Am.*, **January**, 48–57 (1998).

Ingber, D., How cells (might) sense microgravity, *FASEB J.*, **13**, S3–S15 (1999).

Ingber, D., Tensegrity II. How structural networks influence cellular information processing networks, *J. Cell Sci.*, **116** (8), 1397–1408 (2003).

Isacke, C.M. and Yarwood, H., The hyaluronan receptor, CD44, *Int. J Biochem. Cell Biol.*, **34**, 718–721 (2002).

Ishiwatari-Haysaka, H., Fujimoto, T., Osawa, T., Hirama, T., Toyama-Sorimachi, N., and Miyasaka, M., Requirements for signal delivery through CD44: analysis using CD44-Fas chimeric proteins, *J. Immunol.*, **163**, 1258–1264 (1999).

Ito, T., Williams, J.D., Al-Assaf, S., Phillips, G.O., and Phillips, A.O., Hyaluronan and proximal tubular cell migration, *Kidney Int.*, **65**, 823–833 (2004).

Jackson, D.G., The lymphatic endothelial hyaluronan receptor LYVE-1, *Glycoforum, Glycoscience, Science of Hyaluronan*, **#28** (April 22) (2004).

Jiang, Y., Jahagirdar, B.N., Reinhardt, R.L., Schwartz, R.E., Keene, C.D. et al., Pluripotency of mesenchymal stem cells derived from adult marrow, *Nature*, **418**, 41–49 (2002).

Kahmann, J.D., O'Brien, R., Werner, J.M., Heinegård, D., Ladbury, J.E., Cambell, I.K., and Day, A.J., Localization and characterization of the hyaluronan-binding site on the link module from human TSG-6, *Structure*, **8** (7), 763–774 (2000).

Kawasaki, K., Ochi, M., Uchio, Y., Adachi, N., and Matsusaki, M., Hyaluronic acid enhances proliferation and chondroitin sulfate synthesis in cultured chondrocytes embedded in collagen gels, *J. Cell. Physiol.*, **179**, 142–248 (1999).

Kielty, C.M., Whittaker, S.P., Grant, M.E., and Shuttleworth, C.A., Type IV collagen microfibrils: evidence for a structural association with hyaluronan, *J. Cell Biol.*, **118** (4), 979–990 (1992).

Knudson, C.B., Hyaluronan receptor-directed assembly of chondrocyte pericellular matrix, *J. Cell Biol.*, **120** (3), 825–834 (1993).

Knudson, W., The role of CD44 as a cell surface hyaluronan receptor during tumor invasion of connective tissue, *Front. Biosci.*, **3**, d604–d615 (1998).

Knudson, C.B., Hyaluronan-cell interactions during chondrogenesis and matrix assembly, *Cell. Mater.*, **8**, 33–56 (1998).

Knudson, C.B., Hyaluronan and CD44: strategic players for cell–matrix interactions during chondrogenesis and matrix assembly, *Birth Defects Res (Part C)*, **69**, 174–196 (2003).

Knudson, C.B. and Knudson, W., Hyaluronan-binding proteins in development, tissue homeostasis and disease, *FASEB J.*, **7**, 1233–1241 (1993).

Knudson, W., and Knudson, C.B., The hyaluronan receptor, CD44, *Glycoforum, Glycoscience, Science of Hyaluronan*, **10**, 15 (1999).

Knudson, C.B. and Knudson, W., Cartilage proteoglycans, *Cell. Dev. Biol.*, **12**, 69–78 (2001).

Knudson, W. and Knudson, C.B., The hyaluronan receptor, CD44 — an update, *Glycoforum, Glycoscience, Science of Hyaluronan*, **#10a** (January 13) (2005).

Knudson, W., Chow, G., and Knudson, C., CD44-mediated uptake and degradation of hyaluronan, *Matrix Biol.*, **21**, 15–23 (2002).

Kujawa, M.J., Carrino, D.A., and Caplan, A.I., Substrate-bonded hyaluronic acid exhibits a size-dependent stimulation of chondrogenic differentiation of stage 24 limb mesenchymal cells in culture, *Dev. Biol.*, **114**, 519–528 (1986).

Laurent, T.C., The interaction between polysaccharides and other macromolecules, *Biochem. J.*, **93**, 106–112 (1964).

Laurent, T.C., Interaction between proteins and glycosaminoglycans, *Fed. Proc.*, **36**, 24–27 (1977).

Laurent, T.C. and Fraser, R.E., Hyaluronan, *FASEB J.*, **6**, 2397–3404 (1992).

Laurent, T.C., Ryan, M., and Pietruszkiewicz, A., Fractionation of hyaluronic acid: the polydispersity of hyaluronic acid from the bovine vitreous body, *Biochim. Biophys. Acta*, **42**, 476–485 (1960).

Lebel, L., Clearance of hyaluronan from the circulation, *Adv. Drug Delivery Rev.*, **7**, 221–235 (1991).

Lee, J.Y. and Spicer, A.P., Hyaluronan: a multifunctional, megaDalton, stealth molecule, *Curr. Opin. Cell Biol.*, **12**, 581–586 (2000).

Legg, J.W., Lewis, C.A., Parsons, M., Ng, T., and Isacki, C.M., A novel PKC-regulated mechanism controls CD44-ezrin association and directional cell motility, *Nat. Cell Biol.*, **4**, 399–407 (2002).

Lepperdinger, G.B., Strobl, B., and Kreil, G., HYAL2, a human gene expressed in many cells, encodes a lysosomal hyaluronidase with a novel type of specificity, *J. Biol. Chem.*, **273**, 22466–22470 (1998), (Abstract).

Lesley, J., Hasxall, V.C., Tammi, M., and Hyman, T., Hyaluronan binding by cell surface CD44, *J. Biol. Chem.*, **275** (35), 26967–26975 (2000).

Liekens, S., De Clercq, E., and Neyts, J., Angiogenesis: regulators and clinical applications, *Biochem. Pharm.*, **61**, 253–270 (2001).

Lisignoli, G., Fini, M., Giavaresi, G., Aldini, N.N., Toneguzzi, S., and Facchini, A., Osteogenesis of large segmental radius defects enhanced by basic fibroblast growth factor activated bone marrow stromal cells grown on non-woven hyaluronic acid-based polymer scaffold, *Biomaterials*, **23**, 1043–1051 (2002).

Liu, D., Zhang, D., Mori, H., and Sy, M.-S., Binding of CD44 to hyaluronic acid can be induced by multiple signals and requires the CD44 cytoplasmic domain, *Cell. Immunol.*, **174**, 73–83 (1996).

Lowry, K.M. and Beavers, E.M., Thermal stability of sodium hyaluronate in aqueous solution, *J. Biomed. Mat. Res.*, **28**, 1239–1244 (1994).

Lynn, B.D., Li, X., Cattini, P.A., Turley, E.A., and Nagy, J.I., Identification of sequence, protein isoforms, and distribution of the hyaluronan-binding protein RHAMM in adult and developing brain, *J. Comp. Neurol.*, **439**, 315–330 (2001).

Malpeli, M., Randazzo, N., Cancedda, R., and Dozin, B., Serum-free growth medium sustains commitment of human articular chondrocyte through maintenance of sox-9 expression, *Tissue Eng.*, **10** (1/2), 145–155 (2004).

Masuda, A., Ushida, K., Koshino, H., Yamashita, K., and Kluge, A., Novel distance dependence of diffusion constants in hyaluronan aqueous solution resulting from its characteristic nano-microstructure, *J. Am. Chem. Soc.*, **123**, 11468–11471 (2001).

McCourt, P.A.G., How does the hyaluronan scrap-yard operate?, *Matrix Biol.*, **18**, 427–432 (1999).

McCourt, P.A.G., Eks, B., Forsberg, N., and Gustafson, S., Intercellular adhesion molecule-1 is a cell surface receptor for hyaluronan, *J. Biol. Chem.*, **269** (48), 30081–30084 (1994).

Meyer, K. and Palmer, J.W., The polysaccharide of vitreous humor, *J. Biol. Chem.*, **107**, 629–634 (1934).

Milella, E., Brescia, E., Massaro, C., Ramires, P.A., Miglietta, M.R., Fiori, V., and Aversa, P., Physico-chemical properties and degradability of non-oven hyaluronan benzylic esters as tissue engineering scaffolds, *Biomaterials*, **23**, 1053–1063 (2002).

Millward-Sadler, S.J. and Salter, D.M., Integrin-dependent signal cascades in chondrocyte mechanotransduction, *Ann. Biomed. Eng.*, **32** (3), 435–446 (2004).

Miralles, G., Baudoin, R., Dumas, D., Baptiste, D., Hubert, P. et al., Sodium alginate sponges with or without sodium hyaluronate: in vitro engineering of cartilage, *J. Biomed. Mater. Res.*, **57**, 268–278 (2001).

Montesano, R., Kumar, S., Orci, L., and Pepper, M.S., Synergistic effect of hyaluronan oligosaccharides and vascular endothelial growth factor on angiogenesis in vitro, *Lab. Invest.*, **75** (2), 249–262 (1996).

Murphy, G. and Gavrilovic, J., Proteolysis and cell migration: creating a path?, *Curr. Opin. Cell Biol.*, **11**, 614–621 (1999).

Nader, H.B., Oliveira, F.W., Jerônimo, S.M.B., Chavante, S.F., Sampaio, L.O., and Dietrich, C.P., Synchronized order of appearance of hyaluronic acid (or acidic galactan) → chondroitin C-6 sulfate → chondroitin C-4/C-6 sulfate, heparan sulfate, dermatan sulfate → heparin during morphogenesis, differentiation and development, *Braz. J. Med. Biol. Res.*, **29**, 1221–1226 (1996).

Nakamura, M., Mishima, H., Nishida, T., and Otori, T., Binding of hyaluronan to plasma fibronectin increases the attachment of corneal epithelial cells to a fibronectin matrix, *J. Cell. Physiol.*, **159**, 415–422 (1994).

Napier, M.A. and Hadler, N.M., Effect of calcium on structure and function of a hyaluronic acid matrix: carbon-13 nuclear magnetic resonance analysis and the diffusional behavior of small solutes, *Proc. Natl Acad. Sci.*, **75**, 2261–2265 (1978).

Nathanson, M.A., Hyaluronates in developing skeletal tissues, *Clin. Orthop. Rel. Res.*, **251**, 275–289 (1990).

Nedvetzki, S., Gonen, E., Assayag, N., Reich, R., Williams, R.O. et al., RHAMM, a receptor for hyaluronan-mediated motility, compensates for CD44 in inflamed CD44-knockout mice: a different interpretation of reduncancy, *PNAS*, **101** (52), 18081–18086 (2004).

Nehls, V. and Hayen, W., Are hyaluronan receptors involved in three-dimensional cell migration, *Histol. Histopathol.*, **15**, 629–636 (2000).

Nicoll, S.B., Barak, O., Csoka, A.B., Bhatnagar, R.S., and Stern, R., Hyaluronidases and CD44 undergo differential modulation during chondrogenesis, *Biochem. Biophys. Res. Commun.*, **292** (4), 819–825 (2002).

Nilsson, S.K., Haylock, D.N., Johnston, H.M., Occhiodoro, T., Brown, T.J., and Simmons, P.J., Hyaluronan is synthesized by primitive hemopoietic cells, participates in their lodgment at the endosteum following transplantation, and is involved in the regulation of their proliferation and differentiation in vitro, *Blood*, **101** (3), 856–862 (2003).

Nishida, Y., Knudson, C.B., Eger, W., Kuettner, K.E., and Knudson, W., Oseogenic protein-1 stimulates cell-associated matrix assembly by normal human articular chondrocytes, *Arthritis Rheum.*, **43**, 206–214 (2000).

Nishida, Y., Knudson, C.S., Kuettner, K.E., and Knudson, W., Oseogenic protein-1 promotes the synthesis and retention of extracellular matrix within bovine articular cartilage and chondrocyte cultures, *Osteoarthr. Cartilage*, **8**, 127–136 (2000).

Oksala, O., Salo, T., Tammi, R., Häkkinen, H., Jalkanen, M., Inki, P., and Larjava, H., Expression of proteoglycans and hyaluronan during wound healing, *J Histochem Cytochem*, **43**, 125–135 (1995).

Oliferenko, S., Kaverina, I., Small, J.V., and Huber, L.A., Hyaluronic acid (HA) binding to CD44 activates Rac1 and induces lamellipodia outgrowth, *J. Cell Biol.*, **148** (6), 1159–1164 (2000).

Papini, D., Stella, V.J., and Topp, E.M., Diffusion of macromolecules in membranes of hyaluronic esters, *J. Controlled Release*, **27**, 47–57 (1993).

Pasonen-Seppänen, S., Hyttinen, J., Kolehmaninen, E., Tammi, M., and Tammi, R., Wounding-induced upregulation of Has-2/Has-3 expression and hyaluronan synthesis in adult mouse epidermis correlates with keratinocytes migration and proliferation. In: *Hyaluronan: Structure, Metabolism, Biological Activities, Therapeutic Applications* (Balazs, E.A. and Hascall, V.C., Eds). Winmar Enterprises, Edgewater, NJ (in press).

Pasquali-Ronchetti, I., Quaglino, D., Mori, G., Bacchelli, B., and Ghosh, P., Hyaluronan–phospholipid interactions, *J. Struct. Biol.*, **120**, 1–10 (1997), (Abstract).

Peach, R.J., Hollenbaugh, D., Stamenkovic, I., and Aruffo, A., Identification of hyaluronic acid binding sites in the extracellular domain of CD44, *J. Cell Biol.*, **122** (1), 257–264 (1993).

Peattie, R.A., Nayate, A.P., Firpo, M.A., Shelby, J., Fisher, R.J., and Prestwich, G.D., Stimulation of in vivo angiogenesis by cytokine-loaded hyaluronic acid hydrogel implants, *Biomaterials*, **25**, 2789–2798 (2004).

Peck, D. and Isacke, C.M., CD44 phosphorylation regulates melanoma cell and fibroblast migration on, but not attachment to, a hyaluronan substratum, *Curr. Biol.*, 6(7), 884–890 (1996).

Personal communication, Lifecore Biomedical.

Peterson, R.S., Andhare, R.A., Rousche, K.T., Kundson, W., Wang, W., Grossfield, J.B., Thomas, R.O., Hollingsworth, R.E., and Knudson, C.B., CD44 modulates Smad 1 activation in the BMP-7 signaling pathway, *J. Cell Biol.*, **116** (7), 1081–1091 (2004).

Pilloni, A. and Bernard, G.W., The effect of hyaluronan on mouse intramembranous osteogenesis in vitro, *Cell Tissue Res.*, **294**, 323–333 (1998).

Radomsky, M.L., Aufdemorte, T.B., Swain, L.D., Fox, W.C., Spiro, R.C., and Poser, J.W., Novel formulation of fibroblast growth factor-2 in a hyaluronan gel accelerates fracture healing in nonhuman primates, *J. Orthop. Res.*, **17**, 607–614 (1999).

Radomsky, M., Merck, A., Gonsalves, M., Anudokem, G., and Poser, J., *Basic Fibroblast Growth Factor in a Hyaluronic Acid Gel Stimulates Intramembranous Bone Formation*, Orthopaedic Research Society 43rd Annual Meeting, San Fransisco, (1997).

Radomsky, M.L., Thompson, A.Y., Spiro, R.C., and Poser, J.W., Potential role of fibroblast growth factor in enhancement of fracture healing, *Clin. Orthop. Rel. Res.*, 355S, S283–S293 (1998).

Rafi, A., Nagarkatti, M., and Nagarkatti, P.S., Hyaluronate-CD44 interactions can induce murine B-cell activation, *Blood*, **89** (8), 2901–2908 (1997).

Rao, C.M., Deb, T.B., Gupta, S., and Datta, K., Regulation of cellular phosphorylation of hyaluronan binding protein and its role in the formation of second messenger, *Biochem. Biophys. Acta*, **1336**, 387–393 (1997).

Rapport, M.M., Weissmann, B., Linker, A., and Meyer, K., Isolation of a crystalline disaccharide, hyalobiuronic acid, from hyaluronic acid, *Nature*, **168**, 996–997 (1951).

Reddi, A.H., Role of morphogenetic proteins in skeletal tissue engineering and regeneration, *Nat. Biotechnol.*, **16**, 247–252 (1998).

Rooney, P., Kumar, S., Ponting, J., and Wanf, M., The role of hyaluronan in tumour neovascularization (review), *Int. J. Cancer*, **60**, 632–636 (1995).

Rosner, H., Grimmecke, H.D., Knirel, Y.A., and Shashkov, A.S., Hyaluronic acid and a $(1 \rightarrow 4)$-beta-D-xylan, extracellular polysaccharides of pasteurella-multocida (Carter type-A) strain-880, *Carbohydr. Res.*, **223**, 329–333 (1992).

Samuel, S.K., Hurta, R.A.R., Spearman, M.A., Wright, J.A., Turley, E.A., and Greenberg, A.H., TGF-$\beta_1$ stimulation of cell locomotion utilizes the hyaluronan receptor RHAMM and hualuronan, *J. Cell Biol.*, **123** (3), 749–758 (1993).

Sasaki, T. and Watanabe, C., Stimulation of osteoinduction in bone wound healing by high-molecular hyaluronic acid, *Bone*, **16** (1), 9–15 (1995).

Savani, R.C., Cao, G., Pooler, P.M., Zaman, A., Zhou, Z., and DeLisser, H.M., Differential involvement of the hyaluronan (HA) receptors CD44 and receptor for HA-mediated motility in endothelial cell function and angiogeneis, *J. Biol. Chem.*, **276** (39), 36770–36778 (2001).

Scott, J.E., Secondary structures in hyaluronan: chemical and biological implications, *The Biology of Hyaluronan*, Ciba Foundation Symposium No. 143, pp. 6–20 (1989).

Slevin, M., Krupinski, J., Kumsar, S., and Gaffney, J., Angiogenic oligosaccharides of hyaluronan induce protein tyrosine kinase activity in endothelial cells and activate a cytoplasmic signal transduction pathway resulting in proliferation, *Lab. Invest.*, **78** (8), 987–1003 (1998).

Soltes, L., Mendichi, R., Lath, D., Mach, M., and Bakos, D., Molecular characteristics of some commercial high-molecular-weight hyaluronans, *Biomed. Chromatogr.*, **16**, 459–462 (2002), (Abstract).

Spicer, A.P. and McDonald, J.A., Eukaryotic hyaluronan synthases, *Glycoforum, Glycoscience, Science of Hyaluronan*, #7 (September 15) (1998).

Stern, R. and Csóka, A.B., Mammalian hyaluronidases, *Glycoforum, Glycoscience, Science of Hyaluronan*, 15 (June 23) (2000).

Stern, R., Devising a pathway for hyaluronan catabolism: are we there yet?, *Glycobiology*, **13** (12), 105R–115R (2003).

Stern, R., Hyaluronan catabolism: a new metabolic pathway, *Eur. J. Cell Biol.*, **83**, 317–325 (2004).

Tacchetti, C., Quarto, R., Nitsch, L., Hartmann, D.J., and Canceeda, R., In vitro morphogenesis of chick embryo hypertrophic cartilage, *J. Cell Biol.*, **105**, 999–1006 (1987).

Takigami, S. and Takifami, M., Hydration characteristics of the cross-linked hyaluronan derivative hylan, *Carbohydrate Polymers*, **22**, 153–160 (1993).

Tammi, M.I., Day, A.J., and Turley, E.A., Hyaluronan and hemostasis: a balancing act, *J. Biol. Chem.*, **277** (7), 4581–4584 (2002).

Tawada, A.T., Masa, T., Oonuki, Y., Watanabe, A., Matsuzaki, Y., and Asari, A., Large-scale preparation, purification, and characterization of hyaluronan oligosaccharides from 4-mers to 52-mers, *Glycobiology — Oxford*, **12**, 421–426 (2002).

Termeer, C., Nenedix, F., Sleeman, J., Fieber, C., Voith, U. et al., Oligosaccharides of hyaluronan activate dentritic cells via toll-like receptor 4, *J. Exp. Med.*, **195** (1), 99–111 (2002).

Thorne, R.F., Legg, J.W., and Isacke, C.M., The role of CD44 transmembrane and cytoplasmic domains in co-ordinating adhesive and signaling events, *J. Cell Sci.*, **117**, 373–380 (2004).

Toole, B., Hyaluronan in morphogenesis and tissue remodeling, *Glycoforum, Glycoscience, Science of Hyaluronan*, **#9** (December 15) (1998).

Toole, B.P., Hyaluronan in morphogenesis, *Cell Dev. Biol.*, **12**, 79–87 (2001).

Toole, B.P., Hyaluronan: from extracellular glue to pericellular cue, *Nature*, **4**, 528–539 (2004).

Toole, B.P., Munaim, S.I., Welles, S., and Knudson, C.B., Hyaluronate–cell interactions and growth factor regulation of hyaluronate synthesis during limb development, *The Biology of Hyaluronan*. Wiley, Chichester, Ciba Foundation Symposium 143, pp. 138–149 (1989).

Tsukita, S., Oishi, K., Sato, N., Sagara, J., Kawai, A. et al., ERM family members as molecular linkers between the cell surface glycoprotein CD44 and actin-based cytoskeletons, *J. Cell Biol.*, **126**, 391–401 (1994).

Turley, E. and Harrison, R., RHAMM, a member of the hyaladherins, *Glycoforum, Glycoscience, Science of Hyaluronan*, **#11** (July 25) (1999).

Turley, E.A., Noble, P.W., and Bourguignon, T.W., Signaling properties of hyaluronan receptors, *J. Biol. Chem.*, **277** (7), 4589–4592 (2002).

Turner, N.J., Kielty, C.M., Walker, M.G., and Canfield, A.E., A novel hyaluronan-based biomaterial (HYAFF® 11) as a scaffold for endothelial cells in tissue engineered vascular grafts, *Biomaterials*, **25**, 5955–5964 (2004).

Underhill, C.B., Hyaluronan is inversely correlated with the expression of CD44 in the dermal condensation of the embryonic hair follicle, *J. Invest. Dermatol.*, **101**, 820–826 (1993).

Vögelin, E., Jones, N.F., Huang, J.I., Brekke, J.H., and Lieberman, J., Healing of a critical-sized defect in the rat femur with use of a vascularized periosteal flap, a biodegradable matrix, and bone morphogenetic protein, *J. Bone Joint Surg. Am.*, **87-A** (6), 1323–1331 (2005).

Vögelin, E., Jones, N.F., Huang, J.I., Brekke, J.H., and Toth, J.M., Practical illustrations in tissue engineering: surgical considerations relevant to the implantation of osteoinductive devices, *Tissue Eng.*, **6** (4), 449–460 (2000).

Vögelin, E., Jones, N.F., Lieberman, J., Baker, J.M., Tsingotjidou, A.S., and Brekke, J.H., Prefabrication of bone by use of a vascularized periosteal flap and bone morphogenetic protein, *Plast. Reconstr. Surg.*, **109**, 190–198 (2002).

Wang, C., Entwistle, J., Hou, G., Li, Q., and Turley, E.A., The characterization of a human RHAMM cDNA: conservation of the hyaluronan-binding domains, *Gene*, **174**, 299–306 (1996).

Wang, N., Naruse, K., Stamenovic, D., Fredberg, J.J., Mijailovice, S.M. et al., Mechanical behavior in living cells consistent with the tensegrity model, *PNAS*, **98** (14), 7765–7770 (2001).

Weigel, P.H., Bacterial hyaluronan synthases, *Glycoforum, Glycoscience, Science of Hyaluronan*, **#6** (August 15) (1998).

Weigel, P.H., Bacterial hyaluronan syntheses — an update, *Glycoforum, Glycoscience, Science of Hyaluronan*, **#6a** (April 15) (2004).

Weigel, P.H., Fuller, G.M., and LeBoeuf, R.D., A model for the role of hyaluronic acid and fibrin in the early events during the inflammatory response and wound healing, *J. Theor. Biol.*, **119**, 219–234 (1986).

Welti, D., Rees, D.A., and Welsh, E.J., Solution conformation of glycosaminoglycans: Assignment of the 300-MHz 1H-magnetic resonance spectra of chondroitin 4-sulphate, chondroitin 6-sulphate and hyaluronate, and investigation of an alkali-induced conformation change, *Eur. J. Biochem.*, **94**, 505–514 (1979).

West, D.C., Hampson, I.N., Arnold, F., and Kumar, S., Angiogenesis induced by degradation products of hyaluronic acid, *Science*, **228**, 1324–1326 (1985).

Wik, H.B., Rheological studies of sodium hyaluronate in pharmaceutical preparations, *Acta Universitatis Upsaliensis*, **3** (4), 256 (1991).

Yang, R., Yan, Z., Chen, F., Hansson, G.K., and Kiessling, R., Hyaluronic acid and chondroitin sulphate: a rapidly promote differentiation of immature DC with upregulation of costimulatory and antigen-presenting molecules, and enhancement of NF-κB and protein kinase activity, *Scand. J. Immunol.*, **55**, 2–13 (2002).

Yang, B., Yang, L.Y., Savani, R.C., and Turley, E.A., Identification of a common hyaluronan binding motif in the hyaluronan binding proteins RHAMM, CD44 and link protein, *EMBO J.*, **13** (2), 286–296 (1994).

Yasuda, M., Nakano, K., Yasumoto, K., and Tanaka, Y., CD44: functional relevance to inflammation and malignancy, *Histol. Histopathol.*, **17** (3), 945–950 (2002).

Yee, A.J.M., Bae, H.W., Friess, D., Robbin, M., Johnstone, B., and Yoo, J.U., Augmentation of rabbit posterolateral spondylodesis using a novel demineralized bone matrix-hyaluronan putty, *Spine*, **29** (21), 2435–2440 (2003).

Yonemura, S., Hirao, M., Doi, Y., Takahashi, N., Kondo, T., Tsukita, S., and Tsukita, S., Ezrin/radixin/moesin (ERM) proteins bind to a positively charged amino acid cluster in the juxta-membrane cytoplasmic domain of CD44, CD43 and ICAM-2, *J. Cell Biol.*, **140** (4), 885–895 (1998).

Zhou, B., McGary, C.T., Weigel, J.A., Saxena, A., and Weigel, P.H., Purification and molecular identification of the human hyaluronan receptor for endocytosis, *Glycobiology*, **13** (5), 339–349 (2003).

Zhou, B., Weigel, J.A., Fauss, L., and Weigel, P., Identification of the hyaluronan receptor for endocytosis (HARE), *J. Biol. Chem.*, **275** (48), 37733–37741 (2000).

# 14

## *Chitosan*

Frank Rauh and Michael Dornish

## 14.1  Introduction

The history of the development of chitosan is a story 200 years in the making. The first isolation of chitin was performed by Braconnot (1811). Chitin is a structural polymer found in the shells of crabs and shrimp (lobster, squid, some yeast and mold). A chemical description of chitosan was given by Rouget (1859). Chitosan is a high molecular weight, cationic polysaccharide derived from crustacean shells by deacetylation of naturally occurring chitin. Chitosan is a linear polysaccharide that is composed of randomly distributed D-glucosamine (D-units) and N-acetyl glucosamine (**A**-units) linked in a $\beta(1 \rightarrow 4)$ manner (Figure 14.1). The ratio between glucosamine and N-acetyl glucosamine is referred to as the degree of deacetylation. The deacetylated monomers (glucosamine) are randomly distributed along the polymer chain. The amino groups of chitosan can act as a polyelectrolyte and can carry a positive charge ($-NH_3^+$), thereby becoming a cationic biopolymer. Thus, in aqueous media at acidic pH, the chitosan molecule will be highly positively charged. The dissociation constant of this conjugate acid ($pK_a$) will depend on the charge density of the polymer and therefore also depend on the extent of neutralization of the charged groups (Roberts, 1992). A detailed study has been carried out by Domard (1987) using potentiometric and CD measurements. He reported that the

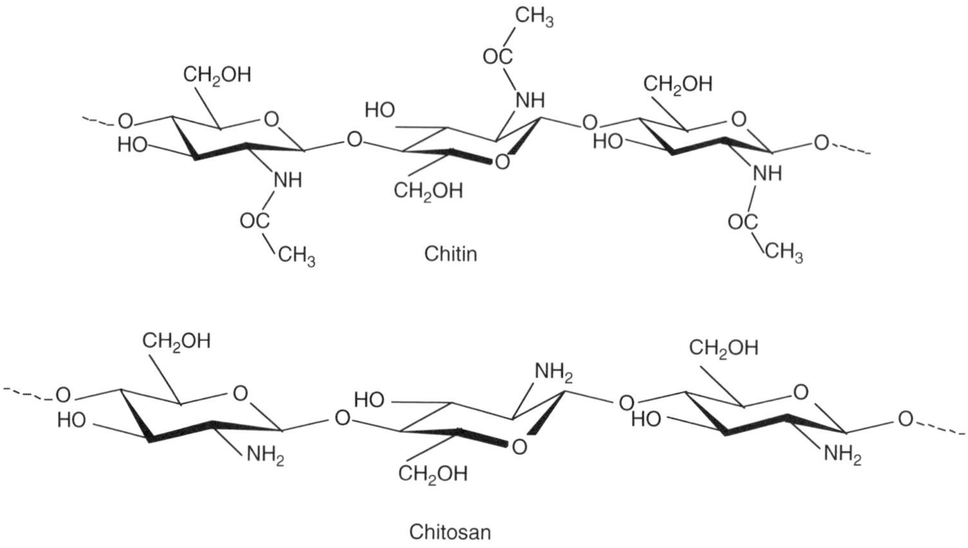

**FIGURE 14.1**
Chemical structure of chitin and chitosan.

amino group in chitosan has an apparent $pK_a$-value of about 6.5. The $pK_a$ of the amino group of chitosan has been reported by others to be 6.2 to 7 (Muzzarelli et al., 1980; Rinaudo and Domard, 1989; Vårum et al., 1994), depending on chain length and composition (FA). In solutions where pH < $pK_a$, chitosan is a polycation and has a more expanded structure because of electrostatic repulsion between the charged D-units, which gives most chitosans a rather high intrinsic viscosity.

Chitosan is soluble in aqueous media at acidic pH, where the polysaccharide will become positively charged. High molecular weight chitosans with a degree of deacetylation (DA) of between 40 and 60% have been shown to be fully soluble at neutral pH because of the irregular sequence of the monomers. Chitosans have shown increasing solubility at higher pH values with decreasing DA (Vårum et al., 1994). Also, by depolymerizing chitosans with DA above 60%, their water solubilities at neutral pH values can be increased. The functional properties of chitosan are primarily decided by the degree of deacetylation and molecular weight.

Chitosan is a linear biodegradable polysaccharide comprised of randomly distributed β-(1 → 4) bound N-acetylglucosamine (A-units) and D-glucosamine (D-units), and is considered to be nontoxic after oral administration to humans (Arai et al., 1968). It has been approved as a food additive and has been incorporated into wound-healing products (Illum, 1998). Chitosan with a degree of acetylation less than 35% (Köping-Höggård et al., 2001) and as low molecular weight as 4,700 Da (Köping-Höggård et al., 2003) was recently optimized to form stable complexes with plasmid DNA (pDNA) that mediates gene expression both *in vitro* and *in vivo*.

## 14.2   Characterization

There are several physicochemical factors that affect the functionality of chitosan. These are: viscosity (or molecular weight), ionic strength, degree of deacetylation, chitosan concentration (in solution), and finally stability. So it is important to work with well-characterized chitosan products.

- Viscosity/molecular weight
- Ionic strength
- Degree of deacetylation
- Chitosan concentration (for solutions)
- Stability
- Purity

### 14.2.1 Composition and Sequential Structure

The composition of chitosan can be determined by high resolution $^1$H- and $^{13}$C-nuclear magnetic resonance spectroscopy (NMR). For chitosan, the degree of deacetylation can be detected by $^1$H- and $^{13}$C-NMR (Vårum et al., 1991). Quantitative $^1$H NMR spectroscopy reports directly on the relative concentration of chemically distinct protons in the sample, consequently only the determination of relative signal intensity ratios is necessary. The degree of deacetylation can directly be determined from the intensity ratios between the relevant protons from the acetylated (**A**) and deacetylated (**D**) units.

### 14.2.2 Molecular Weight

Chitosan is polydisperse with chains of different lengths. The molecular weight represents an average value, generally expressed as a number average ($M_n$) or a weight average ($M_w$). The ratio $M_w/M_n$ is referred to as the polydispersity index. The molecular weight ($M_w$) is determined by size exclusion chromatography with multiple-angle laser light scattering and refractive index detection.

### 14.2.3 Solubility

The solubility of chitosan depends, to a certain extent, on the molecular weight and degree of deacetylation. Dissolution of the chitosan base requires an acidic environment. Chitosan base is soluble at concentrations of 1% in many acids. Most often chitosan is dissolved in 0.15% HCl or in 1% acetic acid. Chitosan base is marginally soluble in $H_3PO_4$ and is insoluble in $H_2SO_4$. There are water-soluble chitosan salts commercially available. In aqueous media at acidic pH, the chitosan molecule will be highly positively charged.

In Figure 14.2, chitosans having various degrees of deacetylation were first made up as aqueous acidic solutions. The pH was then adjusted towards neutrality and the amount of insoluble chitosan determined. As can be seen, a 40% deacetylated chitosan was more soluble at pH 7 than chitosan having a degree of deactylation of 63 or 83%.

### 14.2.4 Viscosity

Viscosity is a function of the molecular weight of the biopolymer and its conformation in solution. Under different conditions the flow characteristic (rheology) of the chitosan solution will vary as, for example, on varying the ionic strength of the polymer solution (Figure 14.3). The viscosity of a chitosan solution is dependent upon the ionic strength. There is, however, a plateau in ionic strength equivalent to between about 0.15 and 0.3 $M$ NaCl wherein the viscosity of a chitosan solution changes little. Therefore, it is important

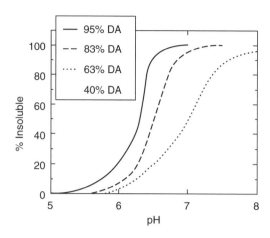

**FIGURE 14.2**
Solubility of chitosans with varying degrees of deacetylation.

in the formulation of chitosan solutions that one should consider the ionic strength and preferably have a formulation with an ionic strength within the plateau area. At very high ionic strengths chitosan precipitates due to a salting out effect.

The viscosity of a chitosan solution is dependent upon several factors in addition to the ionic strength: the concentration of the chitosan in the solution and the molecular weight of the chitosan. Figure 14.4 illustrates the dependency of viscosity following increases in concentration for two chitosan salts. Protasan "113" (trademark FMC BioPolymer AS, Norway) is a lower molecular weight (shorter polymer molecule) than the "213." One can say, in general, that doubling the chitosan concentration results in a tenfold increase in solution viscosity. Increases in viscosity can have profound effects on, for example, spraying patterns from an atomizer used for nasal administration.

### 14.2.5  Polyelectrolytic Properties of Chitosan

The apparent $pK_a$-value of the amino group of the glucosamine moiety is 6.5. In aqueous media at acidic pH, the chitosan molecule will be highly positively charged. The repelling effect of each positively-charged deacetylated unit on neighboring glucosamine units will result in an extended conformation of the polymer in solution. The addition of salt will reduce this effect, resulting in a more random coil conformation of the molecule. At higher ionic strength a salting-out effect will occur, precipitating the chitosan from the solution. This is shown as a reduction in solution viscosity in Figure 14.3.

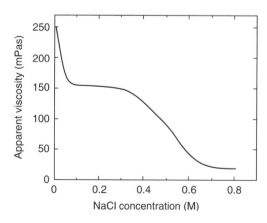

**FIGURE 14.3**
The effect of ionic strength on the viscosity of chitosan solutions.

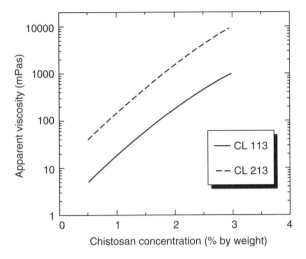

**FIGURE 14.4**
The dependency of viscosity on the concentration of two chitosan salts.

## 14.2.6  Stability

Stability issues are also important to consider. As for all biopolymers, chitosan is subjected to depolymerization (degradation) over time. The glycosidic bonds are subjected to free radical attack. Bond breakage leads to shortening of the chitosan polymer chain which results in a reduction in viscosity measured over a period of time for chitosan (both as solid powder and as a solution). Normally chitosan in the powder form is stable for several years if stored at 25°C or below. Solutions of chitosan, however, may need to be stored at 5°C in order to avoid a reduction in viscosity (or molecular weight).

## 14.2.7  Impurity

The term impurity relates to the presence of extraneous substances and materials in the biopolymer sample. Most chitosan is produced from crustacean shells recovered as a by-product of food production. These shells generally have a high bioburden including protein and bacterial contamination. Processing the chitin into chitosan can remove many of these contaminants, however chitosans cationic nature makes purification to high purity grades suitable for biomedical use difficult. Most chitosan produced is used in industrial and food applications where high purity is not particularly critical. It is therefore important to use high purity, well-characterized chitosan for biomedical applications (see Regulatory section, below). Some of the critical purity factors are:

1. *Endotoxin content*: The endotoxin level in chitosan will ultimately be critical to its use in biomedical applications where there are regulatory limits to the amount of endotoxin that can be implanted into humans. For example, for implantable devices the endotoxin level must be below 5 EU/kg of body weight.

2. *Protein content*: Residual protein in chitosan could cause allergic reactions such as hypersensitivity. The biopolymer supplier should demonstrate protein removal and protein quantitative methods of satisfactory sensitivity.

3. *Heavy metals*: The marine source of chitosan indicates that possible heavy metal contaminates such as lead and mercury should be analyzed.

4. *Microbiological burden*: The presence of bacteria, yeast, and mould are also impurities that can arise in processed material. The presence of bacteria may also contribute to the presence of endotoxins.

## 14.3   Uses of Chitosan

Despite the fact that chitin and chitosan have been known for at least 100 years, and that there are hundreds of patents filed over the last 10 to 15 years, commercial use still resides in technical applications such as water treatment, treatment of agricultural products, paper manufacture, and small niches of the food and healthcare markets. Over the past few years there has been a boom in chitosan use as a weight-reducing aid. The use of chitin and chitosan in applications such as drug-delivery and tissue-engineering matrices is still awaiting commercialization. Chitosan is used in several commercial bandage formulations where its bioadhesive and hemostatic properties are used to advantage (Table 14.1).

### 14.3.1   Tissue Engineering

Chitosan has shown an interesting potential for use as scaffolds in tissue engineered medical products (Madihally and Matthew, 1999; Seong et al., 2000), as a component of a drug delivery system (Genta et al., 1997; Illum, 1998; Paul and Sharma, 2000; Sabnis and Block, 2000), and as an encapsulating matrix for the immobilization of living cells (Kim and Rha, 1989; Zielinski and Aebischer, 1994). Reactivity with negatively charged surfaces is a direct function of the positive charge density of chitosan. The cationic nature of chitosan gives this polymer good bioadhesive and hemostatic properties which find use in drug-delivery, bandage and wound-healing products (Allan, 1984; Li et al., 1992; Skaugrud, 1995).

**TABLE 14.1**

Commercial Uses of Chitosan

| *Water Treatment* | *Food* | *Cosmetic and Toiletry* |
|---|---|---|
| Flocculant | Preservative | Hair care |
| Filtration | Color stabilization | Face, hand and body creams |
| Removal of metal ions | Animal feed additive | Moisturizer |
| | | Nail polish |
| | | Toothpaste |
| *Pulp and Paper* | *Agriculture* | *Pharmaceutical and Medical* |
| Surface treatment | Seed coating | Drug delivery |
| Photographic paper | Agrochemical release | Wound treatment |
| Carbonless copying paper | Fertilizer | Cholesterol reduction |
| *Membranes* | *Biotechnology* | Artificial skin |
| Reverse osmosis | Enzyme immobilization | Contact lens |
| Permeability control | Protein separation | Bandages and sponges |
| Solvent separation | Cell recovery | Dental plaque inhibitor |
| | Cell immobilization | Tumor inhibitor |
| | | Bone matrix |

### 14.3.2 Gene Delivery with Chitosan

Gene therapy is the treatment and prevention of disease by gene transfer. Generally, there are three main types of gene delivery vectors: viral, physical and nonviral. The first group includes all use of viruses for accomplishing the gene transfer, where retrovirus, adenovirus and adeno-associated virus are some of the more advanced. Physical methods involve needle-free injectors and electroporation. Nonviral gene delivery systems involve the use of naked DNA, DNA complexed with cationic lipids, and particles comprising DNA condensed with cationic polymers. To date, gene delivery systems using viruses have been the most successful in obtaining gene expression, however there are several disadvantages and risks involved with the use of viral gene transfer, thereby making the development of efficient nonviral systems interesting. There are several advantages with nonviral therapies including their apparent safety and cost of manufacture.

The ability of chitosan to condense DNA to form complexes is the basis for its use in nonviral gene delivery. Polycations can make complexes (polyplexes) with DNA, and in such a way protect it from degradation by nucleases and in some cases work as a vehicle for gene delivery. Chitosan, as a polycation, can bind DNA to form polyplexes. These polyplexes can be about 50 nm in size. These DNA/chitosan polyplexes will actually be taken up into cells, and genetic material expressed. Several researchers have shown that chitosan/DNA polyplexes lead to increased gene expression in cultured cells and *in vivo* in rats (Erbacher et al., 1998; Richardson et al., 1999; Köping-Höggård et al., 2001; Mao et al., 2001).

### 14.3.3 Biological Effects

One example of chitosan's biological activity is its effect on tight junctions. CaCo-2, and other cells, can form tight junctions between cells when grown on membranes. Tight junctions are contact areas between cells that effectively form ion- and drug-impermeable barriers. For the CaCo-2 cell line, culturing over a period of time causes cells to polarize and form tight junctions, usually after about 2 to 3 weeks following seeding on to membranes.

Figure 14.5 shows results from an experiment showing the effect of chitosan on tight junction integrity as measured by changes in transepithelial electrical resistance (TEER). One of the mechanisms of action of chitosan is the opening of tight junctions between cells in an epithelial cell layer. In this experiment the electrical resistance was measured over a multicellular membrane. The higher the TEER value, the tighter the cell junctions are. Control cells have established tight junctions and therefore a high TEER value (measured in resistance units of Ohms). However, when the cell layer is exposed to chitosan on one side (usually the upper or apical side), the TEER decreases almost immediately and remains low during the duration of the treatment period. Lower TEER means that there is a greater ion flux across the cell layer, thus indicating that junctions are open (Smith et al., 2004). This experiment was performed using radiolabelled chitosan ($^3$H-labelled). This was done to determine if chitosan could pass through the open junction. From our studies chitosan remains outside the cells, i.e., on the apical side and is not transported or diffuse between cells to the basolaterial side.

The formation of tight junctions reduces ion flux and increases electrical resistance over a cell monolayer. On the addition of chitosan, the tight junctions are opened and ions can flow, thereby reducing resistance and decreasing TEER. This is also the basis for the drug enhancing effect induced by chitosan, the drug can pass through the open tight junctions. Figure 14.6 shows the results from an experiment where chitosan chloride having various degrees of deacetylation was tested using the Caco-2 cell line. Caco-2 cells were allowed to form a confluent and polarized cell layer. All chitosans

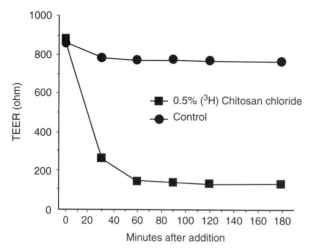

**FIGURE 14.5**
The effect of chitosan on tight junction integrity as measured by transepithelial electrical resistance (TEER).

induced an initial decrease in TEER, i.e., they opened tight junctions between cells. On removal of the chitosan solution, tight junctions were reestablished and electrical resistance increased (TEER increased), the reversibility being somewhat dependent upon the degree of deacetylation of the chitosan. The reversibility of chitosan is important and separates this biopolymer from other enhancing agents such as bile salts and detergents (Holme et al., 2000). It appears that chitosan may affect the translocation of protein kinase C (Smith et al., 2004).

## 14.4 Regulatory Standards

Weiner (Weiner, 1992) has previously published an overview of the regulatory status of chitosan (In the 10 + years since this publication, there have been some important developments in the regulatory approach and status of these biopolymers. Chitosan can still be found on the list of inert ingredients for pesticides (U.S. Environmental Protection Agency Fact Sheet 128930; U.S. Environmental Protection Agency Fact Sheet 128991) as

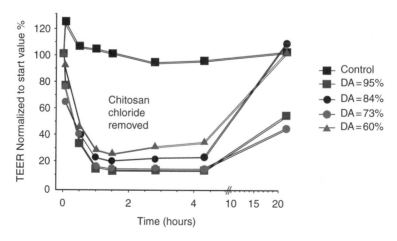

**FIGURE 14.6**
The effect of chitosans with varying degrees of deacetylation on TEER of CaCo-2 cells.

well as exemptions from the requirement of a tolerance of residues when used as a seed treatment as referenced in the Code of Federal Regulations (CFR).

Chitosan has been included in the Codex Alimentarius Inventory of Processing Aids (Codex, 1990). This listing indicates that chitosan may be used as flocculating agents, clarifying agents, or filtration aids in processing foods. However, this listing does not indicate approval for the use of chitosan in pharmaceutical and/or biomedical applications.

Within the pharmaceutical area, a monograph for chitosan hydrochloride does appear in the European Pharmacopoeia (2002: 1774). This monograph, however, does not distinguish purity or special grades for biomedical applications. The monograph does give tests for heavy metals as a contaminant, but issues of microbial contamination (bioburden), sterility and bacterial endotoxins are not addressed.

In 2001 the guide entitled "Standard Guide for Characterization and Testing of Chitosan Salts as Starting Materials Intended for Use in Biomedical and Tissue-Engineered Medical Products Application" was published in the ASTM Book of Standards under the designation F 2103 (Anonymous, 2004). The aim of the guide is to identify key parameters relevant for the functionality and characterization of chitosan salts for the development of new commercial applications of chitosan-containing tissue-engineered medical products for the biomedical and pharmaceutical industries. The American Society for Testing and Materials (ASTM) is making a concerted effort to establish standards and guidelines for TEMPs. Safety, consistency, and functionality of chitosan used in TEMPs are a concern. Critical parameters such as degree of deacetylation, molecular weight and viscosity as well as dry matter, heavy metal, bioburden, and endotoxin content are described in the ASTM document. The protein content, and hence, potential for allergic reactions and hypersensitivity, will be an issue in chitosan preparations for TEMPs (Dornish et al., 2001).

Further information regarding chitosan's regulatory status can be found in (Dornish and Kaplan, 2004).

---

## Study Questions

1. What two properties determine the functional behaviour of chitosan?
   Molecular weight and degree of deacetylation.

2. Describe briefly the relationship between chitosan concentration and viscosity
   Doubling the concentration of chitosan will cause a tenfold increase in solution viscosity

3. Why is chitosan bioadhesive?
   Chitosan's cationic charge is responsible for its bioadhesive properties

4. Describe how chitosan functions in gene delivery.
   The ability of chitosan to condense DNA to form complexes is the basis for its use in nonviral gene delivery. These polyplexes have been shown to be taken up by cells and lead to gene expression.

5. Why is chitosan potentially a better permeation enhancer than bile slats or detergents?
   Chitosan will open tight junctions reversibly.

6. What analytical method is used for determining chitosan's degree of deacetylation?
   High resolution NMR

7. Which acids are commonly used to dissolve chitosan base?

Dilute HCl or acetic acid. Chitosan base is marginally soluble in phosphoric and sulphuric acids.

8. Why would chitosan salts be advantageous over base in formulation of nasal drug delivery systems?

The salts are soluble at physiological pH. Many drugs will be degraded by the acidic pH required to dissolve the chitosan base.

9. What are the four key purity considerations for biomedical grade chitosan?

Endotoxins, protein, heavy metals, and bioburden.

10. What differences in purity would you expect between chitosan salts and chitosan base?

Production of chitosan salts generally requires putting the starting chitosan base in solution. This solution can be easily filtered to remove insolubles and other impurities. Chitosan base production does not generally include this dissolution step.

---

## References

Allan, G.G. et al., Biomedical applications of chitin and chitosan, In: *Chitin, Chitosan and Related Enzymes*, Zikakis, J.P., Ed., Academic Press, New York, pp. 119 (1984).

Anonymous, F2103 Standard guide for characterization and testing of chitosan salts as starting materials intended for use in biomedical and tissue-engineered medical product applications, *Annual Book of ASTM Standards*, Vol. 13. ASTM International, West Conshohocken (2004), p. 1191.

Arai et al., Toxicity of Chitosan, *Bull. Tokai Reg. Fish. Lab.*, 43, 89–94 (1968).

Braconnot, H., Sue la natrue ces champignons, *Ann. Chim. Phys.*, **79**, 265 (1811).

CFR Part 180.1072.

Codex Alimentarius Inventory of Processing Aids Document CAC/MISC 3 ALINORM 91/12, §104; 22nd Session of the Codex Committee on Food Additives and Contaminants, Hague, 20 March 1990, available at www.codexalimentarius.net.

Domard, A., pH and c.d. measurements on a fully deacetylated chitosan: application to $Cu^{II}$-polymer interactions, *Int. J. Biol. Macromol.*, **9**, 98 (1987).

Dornish, M. and Kaplan, D., Regulatory aspects and standardization of chitin and chitosan, *Adv. Chitin Sci.*, **7**, 152–156 (2004).

Dornish, M., Kaplan, D., and Skaugrud, Ø., Standards and guidelines for biopolymers in tissue engineered medical products — ASTM alginate and chitosan standard guides, *Ann. N.Y. Acad. Sci.*, **944**, 388 (2001).

Erbacher, P., Zou, S., Bettinger, T., Steffan, A.-M., and Remy, J.-S., Chitosan-based vector/DNA complexes for gene delivery: biophysical characteristics and transfection ability, *Pharm. Res.*, **15**, 1332–1339 (1998).

Genta, I. et al., Preparation methods for chitosan microparticulate drug delivery systems, In: *Chitin Handbook*, Muzzarelli, R.A.A. and Peter, M.G., Eds., Atec Edizioni, Grottammare, pp. 391 (1997).

Holme, H.K., Hagen, A., and Dornish, M., Influence of chitosans on permeability of human intestinal epithelial (Caco-2) cells: the effect of molecular weight, degree of deacetylation and exposure time, *Adv. Chitin Sci.*, **4**, 256 (2000).

Illum, L., Chitosan and its use as a pharmaceutical excipient, *Pharm. Res.*, **15**, 1326 (1998).

Kim, S-K. and Rha, C., Chitosan for the encapsulation of mammalian cell culture, In: *Chitin and Chitosan: Sources, Biochemistry, Physical Properties and Applications*, Skjåk-Bræk, G., Anthonsen, T., and Sandford, P., Eds., Elsevier Science Publishers, Barking, pp. 17 (1989).

Köping-Höggård, M. et al., Chitosan as a non-viral gene delivery system. Structure property relationships and characteristics compared with polyethylenimine *in vitro* and after lung administration *in vivo*, *Gene Ther.*, **8**, 1108 (2001).

Köping-Höggård, M. et al., Relationship between the physical shape and the efficiency of oligomeric chitosan as a gene delivery system *in vitro* and *in vivo*, *J. Gene Med.*, **5** (2), 130–141 (2003).

Li, Q. et al., Applications and properties of chitosan, *J. Bioact. Compat. Polym.*, **7**, 370 (1992).

Madihally, S.V. and Matthew, H.W., Porous chitosan scaffolds for tissue engineering, *Biomaterials*, **20**, 1133 (1999).

Mao, H.-Q. et al., Chitosan-DNA nanoparticles as gene carriers: synthesis, characterization and transfection efficiency, *J. Controlled Release*, **70**, 399 (2001).

Muzzarelli, R.A.A. et al., The chelation of cupric ions by chitosan membranes, *J. Appl. Biochem.*, **2**, 380 (1980).

Paul, W. and Sharma, C.P., Chitosan, a drug carrier for the 21st century: a review, *S.T.P. Pharma Sci.*, **10**, 5 (2000).

Richardson, S.C.W., Kolbe, H.V.J., and Duncan, R., Potential of low molecular mass chitosan as a DNA delivery system: biocompatibility, body distribution and ability to complex and protect DNA, *Int. J. Pharm.*, **178**, 231 (1999).

Rinaudo, M. and Domard, A., Solution properties of chitosans, In: *Chitin and Chitosan*, Skjåk-Bræk, G., Anthonsen, T., and Sandford, P.A., Eds., Elsevier Applied Science, London, pp. 71 (1989).

Roberts, G.A.F., *Chitin Chemistry*, The Macmillan Press, Basingstoke, UK, p. 203 (1992).

Rouget, C., Des substances amylacees dans le tissue des animux, specialement les Articules (Chitine), *Compt. Rend.*, **48**, 792 (1859).

Sabnis, S. and Block, L.H., Chitosan as an enabling excipient for drug delivery systems, *Int. J. Biol. Macromol.*, **27**, 181 (2000).

Seong, H. et al., Chitosan macroporous scaffolds for cell culture, *Polym. Prepr.*, **41**, 1687 (2000).

Skaugrud, Ø., Drug delivery sytems with alginate and chitosan, In: *Excipients and Delivery Systems for Pharmaceutical Formulations* (Spec. Publ. Royal Soc. Chem. No 161), Karsa, D.R. and Stephenson, R.A., Eds., Royal Society of Chemistry, Cambridge, pp. 96 (1995).

Smith, J.M., Dornish, M., and Wood, E.J., Involvement of protein kinase C in chitosan glutamate-medicated tight junction disruption, *Biomaterials*, **26**, 3269 (2004).

Smith, J., Wood, E. and Dornish, M., Effect of chitosan on epithelial cell tight junctions, *Pharm. Res.*, **21**, 43 (2004).

U.S. Environmental Protection Agency Fact Sheet 128930, Chitosan; Poly-D-glucosamine issued 3/01 (http://www.epa.gov).

U.S. Environmental Protection Agency Fact Sheet 128991, Chitin; Poly-N-acetyl-D-glucosamine issued 3/01 (http://www.epa.gov).

Vårum, K.M., Ottøy, M.H., and Smidsrød, O., Water-solubility of partially N-acetylated chitosans as a function of pH: effect of chemical composition and depolymerisation, *Carbohydr. Polym.*, **25**, 65 (1994).

Vårum, K.M. et al., Determination of the degree of N-acetylation and the distribution of N-acetyl groups in partially N-deacetylated chitins (chitosans) by high-field n.m.r. spectroscopy, *Carbohydr. Res.*, **211**, 17–19 (1991).

Weiner, M.L., An overview of the regulatory status and of the safety of chitin and chitosan as food and pharmaceutical ingredients, In: *Advances in Chitin and Chitosan*, Brine, C.J., Sandford, P.A., and Zikakis, J.P., Eds., Elsevier Applied Science, London, pp. 663 (1992).

Zielinski, B.A. and Aebischer, P., Chitosan as a matrix for mammalian cell encapsulation, *Biomaterials*, **15**, 1049 (1994).

# 15

## Alginate

Michael Dornish and Frank Rauh

**CONTENTS**

## 15.1 Introduction

Alginate, first described by the British chemist Stanford in 1881 (Stanford, 1883), exists in brown algae as the most abundant polysaccharide. Alginate occurs in the cell walls and intercellular spaces of brown algae (seaweed and kelp). Its main function is to give flexibility and strength to the plants, necessary properties adapted to the growth conditions in a marine environment. The alginate in brown algae can be compared to cellulose found in trees and plants. Although some soil bacteria (*Azotobacter* and *Pseudomonas* species) produce alginate as an exocellular polymeric material, most commercial alginates are extracted from algal sources.

Alginate has numerous functional properties that can be utilized in a large number of applications (Table 15.1). You have no doubt already been "exposed" to alginate used as a thickener in salad dressings and as a component in ice cream where it reduces ice crystal formation. Other restructured food products, as well as pet food, utilize alginate and alginate gels. Alginate fibers have been used for many years in various wound-dressing products to absorb wound fluid while protecting the injury sites with an oxygen-permeable gel layer. Finally, alginate is used as a disintegrant in some tablet formulations and as a coating material. The biomedical and pharmaceutical industries are continually searching for functional materials in their development

**TABLE 15.1**

Characteristics and Functionality of Alginate and Potential Applications

| Characteristics | Functionality | Benefits | Applications |
|---|---|---|---|
| Molecular weight | Viscosity | Thickening, film-forming | Suspensions, coatings |
| Composition and sequence | Cross-linking | Gelling | Immobilization, encapsulation |
| Dissociation, $pK_a$ | Soluble at pH, precipitate at pH, swelling capability | Solutions, fibers, films, absorption | Solutions/pastes, scaffolds, dressings, membranes, tablet disintegration |
| Polyanion | Cation affinity | Chelation | Gelation, drug/metal binding |

of improved devices and drug delivery systems. Alginate (and chitosan, see separate chapter) have shown potential for use as scaffolds in tissue engineered medical products (TEMPs) (Rowley et al., 1999a; Kim et al., 2000), as drug-containing materials for depot delivery (Ramdas et al., 1999; Miyazaki et al., 2000) and as an encapsulating matrix for immobilization of living cells (Uludag et al., 2000). However, the ability of alginate to form gels at physiological conditions and without the use of heat has created a unique possibility for immobilizing cells for both *in vitro* and *in vivo* applications.

### 15.1.1   What Is Alginate?

Alginates are a family of nonbranched binary copolymers of $(1 \rightarrow 4)$ glycosidically linked β-D-mannuronic acid (M) and α-L-guluronic acid (G) monomers (Figure 15.1). The relative amount of the two uronic acid monomers and their sequential arrangement along the polymer chain vary widely, depending on the origin of the alginate (see Table 15.2). The uronic acid residues are distributed along the polymer chain in a pattern of blocks, where homopolymeric blocks of G residues (G-blocks), homopolymeric blocks of M residues (M-blocks) and blocks with alternating sequence of M and G units (MG-blocks) coexist. Thus, the alginate molecule cannot be described by the monomer composition alone.

Alginate can be produced from several types of algae (Table 15.2). Algae is harvested, milled, washed, extracted with base, precipitated with calcium chloride and reacted with acid to produce alginic acid. The desired salt (alginate) is produced by neutralization by the appropriate cation. In spite of this multi-step process, endotoxins, polyphenols and other impurities are carried along with the alginate and contaminate the final product. This has significant implications for the use of alginate in tissue engineering and other biomedical applications, discussed below.

M-blocks will be flexible while G-blocks represent the calcium binding sites in alginate. Chelating calcium, for example, in the G-blocks leads to gelling. Binding of calcium to alginate is cooperative, i.e., the longer the G-blocks, the tighter the successive binding of calcium — and the stronger the gel becomes. The functional properties of alginate are primarily influenced by the G content, the average number G's in a G-block length and the molecular weight.

The length of the polymer chain is rather long in native form, but will decrease during the process of manufacture. Depolymerization is a natural process for biopolymers, but the rate at which it will happen depends on the mechanisms involved, which again is influenced by the environmental conditions. The molecular weight of commercial alginates will seldom be higher that 500,000 g/mol, similar to a degree of polymerization (DP) of approximately 2500.

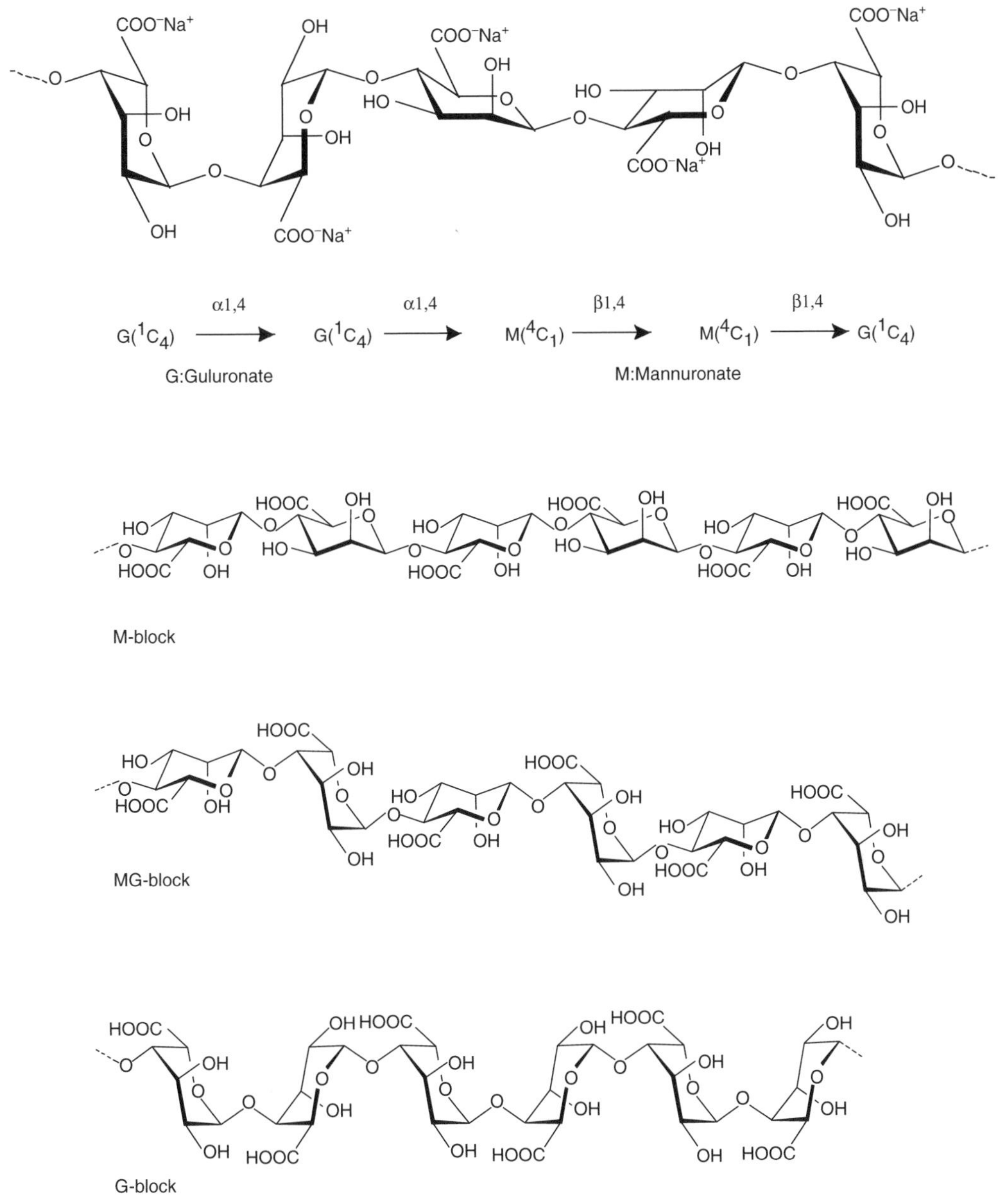

**FIGURE 15.1**
Chemical structures of sodium alginate.

## 15.2 Innate Characteristics of Alginate

### 15.2.1 Composition and Sequential Structure

Composition and sequential structure together with molecular weight and molecular conformation are the key characteristics of alginate in determining its properties and functionality (Smidsrød and Draget, 1996). The composition and sequential structure

**TABLE 15.2**

Typical M/G Composition and Structural Sequences of Alginate from Various Species of Brown Algae

| Alginate Source | M/G | %M | %G | %MM | %GG | %GGG | %MGM | $N_{G>1}$ |
|---|---|---|---|---|---|---|---|---|
| *Laminaria hyperborea* (stem) | 0.45 | 30 | 70 | 18 | 52 | 48 | 7 | 15 |
| *L. hyperborea* (leaf) | 1.22 | 55 | 45 | 36 | 31 | 25 | 13 | 8 |
| *Laminaria digitata* | 1.22 | 55 | 45 | 39 | 25 | 20 | 11 | 6 |
| *Macrocystis pyrifera* | 1.50 | 60 | 40 | 40 | 20 | 16 | 17 | 6 |
| *Lessonia nigrescens* | 1.50 | 60 | 40 | 43 | 22 | 17 | 14 | 6 |
| *Ascophyllum nodosum* | 1.86 | 65 | 35 | 56 | 23 | 17 | 9 | 5 |
| *Durvillea antarctica* | 2.45 | 71 | 29 | 58 | 16 | 11 | 12 | 4 |

of M and G residues in the alginate chain can be determined by high-resolution [1]H- and [13]C-nuclear magnetic resonance spectroscopy (NMR). Techniques have been developed to determine the monad frequencies as well as diads and triads. Based upon such measurements, parameters like $M/G$ ratio, G-content with consecutive $G > 1$ blocks, M-content with consecutive $M > 1$ blocks, and average length of blocks of G and M, respectively, can be calculated and are useful parameters in the characterization of the polymer. It has also been shown by NMR spectroscopy that alginate has no regular repeating unit (Grasdalen et al., 1979; Grasdalen, 1983). Figure 15.2 shows the difference in NMR spectrum of a G-rich ($G > 65\%$) sodium alginate denoted Pronova™ LVG and an M-rich ($M > 50\%$) sodium alginate denoted Pronova™ LVM (FMC BioPolymer AS/NovaMatrix, Oslo, Norway). The term "LV" indicates "low viscosity" and represents the manufacturer's specification of a product having a viscosity of between 20 and 200 mPa.

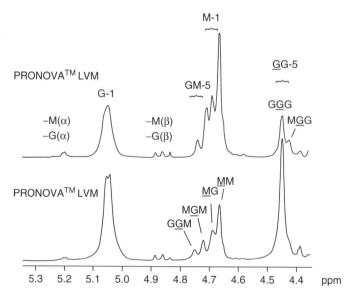

**FIGURE 15.2**
[1]H-NMR spectra of two sodium alginate samples. Pronova™ LVG (low viscosity G-rich) and Pronova™ LVM (low viscosity M-rich) alginate were analyzed by NMR at a field strength of 400 MHz.

## 15.2.2 Molecular Weight

Commercial alginates, like polysaccharides in general, are polydisperse with respect to molecular weight ($M_w$). Therefore, the given $M_w$ of an alginate always represent an average of all of the molecules in the population. The most common ways to express the $M_w$ are as the number average ($\overline{M}_n$) and the weight average ($\overline{M}_w$). The two averages are defined by the following equations

$$\overline{M}_n = \frac{\sum_i N_i M_i}{\sum_i N_i}$$

and

$$\overline{M}_w = \frac{\sum_i w_i M_i}{\sum_i w_i} = \frac{\sum_i N_i M_i^2}{\sum_i N_i M_i}$$

where $N_i$ = number of molecules having a specific molecular weight $M_i$, and $w_i$ = weight of molecules having a specific molecular weight $M_i$.

In a polydisperse molecular population the relation $\overline{M}_w > \overline{M}_n$ is always valid. The coefficient $\overline{M}_w/\overline{M}_n$ is referred to as the polydispersity index, and will typically be in the range 1.5 to 3.0 for commercial alginates.

Molecular weight can be determined by more than one method. The most common methods in general use are calculations based upon intrinsic viscosity (Mark–Houwink–Sakurada equation), and size-exclusion chromatography with light-scattering measurement. A size-exclusion chromatogram showing the refractive index and multiple angle laser light scatter profile of alginate is shown in Figure 15.3. It should be noted that the calculation based on intrinsic viscosity only gives an estimate of the molecular weight. This is important, as most producers blend alginates to target a given viscosity-specification product with the same intrinsic viscosity which may (probably will) have different molecular weight populations. This is important in biomedical applications as "equivalent products" may have differing cellular interactions. In addition to average molecular weight, expressed as number average and weight average, the ratio between

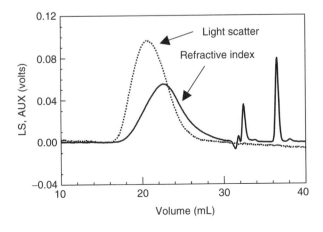

**FIGURE 15.3**
Chromatogram of alginate analyzed by size-exclusion chromatography with refractive index and multiple-angle laser light scatter detection.

the two, referred to as the polydispersity index, is often used to describe the molecular weight distribution within a population.

## 15.3 Biomedical and Pharmaceutical Applications of Alginate

Commodity alginates are well-known to the biomedical and pharmaceutical industry for their traditional uses in the treatment of topical wounds (Thomas, 2000a–c), as an antireflux remedy (Hagstam, 1986; Mandel et al., 2000), and as a tablet excipient (Onsøyen, 1995). The purity level and the current method of manufacture make it unlikely, however, that commodity alginates will find a use in implantable devices and drug formulations for parenteral administration.

Major differences between commodity and ultrapure alginate are: reduction in the level of endotoxin contamination, reduced protein and polyphenol content, reduced ash content and often reduced heavy metal content. Commodity alginates will often have an excess of salt or free alginic acid as a consequence of dry blending. Ultrapure alginates made in accordance with GMP/ISO 9000 guidelines and with a high level of purity, have been successfully utilized for applications inside the human body, and several products containing ultrapure alginate are in the process of being clinically evaluated. Ultrapure alginate should have a stoichiometric amount of counter ion integrated into the product (i.e., no free acid). Normally ultrapure alginates will also be analyzed with respect to composition, sequence and molecular weight. Table 15.3 lists some potential applications where ultrapure alginate could play a role as a biostructure.

## 15.4 Functional Properties and Applications of Alginate

The functional properties of alginate mostly utilized are: viscoelasticity, as a gelling agent through cross-linking with calcium, and as a thickener (viscosifiers) in aqueous solutions. Solubility, "swellability," and film-forming properties are other capabilities utilized in biomedical and pharmaceutical applications.

**TABLE 15.3**

Biomedical and Pharmaceutical Applications of Ultrapure Alginate

| Matrices and Scaffolds | Directed Drug Delivery | Artificial Organs |
|---|---|---|
| Bone regeneration (Kenley et al., 1994; Maruyama et al., 1995) | Covalent attachment (Morgan et al., 1995) | Artificial pancreas (Sun et al., 1984) |
| Nerve regeneration (Suzuki et al., 1999; Kataoka et al., 2000) | Endostatin producing cells (Joki et al., 2001; Read et al., 2001) | Artificial liver (Wong and Chang, 1986; Sun et al., 1987) |
| Bulking agent (Atala et al., 1994; Diamond and Caldamone, 1999; Gentile, 1999) | Hormones and growth (Chang et al., 1994; Peirone et al., 1998; Stockley et al., 2000) | Artificial kidney (Chang and Malave, 2000) |
| Anti-reflux (Hagstam, 1986; Mandel et al., 2000) | Parkinson's disease (Emerich et al., 1992) | |
| Soft tissue implant (Brunstedt et al., 1996) | CNS (Chen and Mohr, 1996; Visted et al., 2001) | |

### 15.4.1 Solutions

The rheological properties of a pure alginate solution are strongly dependent on the molecular weight of the alginate, while the structural composition may play only a minor role, such as with viscosity. By adding other components to the solution, it is well known that various physicochemical interactions will occur, of which some could make a dramatic change to the final properties of the solution. Changes in the molecular conformation as a result of increased ionic strength, and building of an artificial viscosity due to interactions with cations are probably the most common effects of adding other components. In the case of chemical interaction with cations, the structural composition will play an important role.

*Solubility* of alginate is related to the rate of dissociation of the alginate molecule. At pH < 3, both M-structures and G-structures will precipitate as alginic acid, while alternating structures will still remain in solution even though fully protonized. In pharmaceutical applications, the change from a soluble alginate to an insoluble alginic acid at low pH is actually the property behind the volume-wise largest product, namely an antireflux remedy which, when swallowed, forms an alginic acid raft on the top of the stomach contents.

*Thickening properties* of alginate are a function of the molecular weight and the conformation of the alginate molecule in solution. Interaction with other molecules in the solution as well as competition for water at high concentrations will also have an impact on the flow properties. If calcium or other cross-linking materials are present in small quantities, an artificial viscosity higher than the real one will be the result. Such solutions will have thixotropic flow properties. To separate artificial viscosity from real viscosity, a sequestrant can be added to bind the cross-linking agent.

*Swellability* of alginate is related to the rate of hydration, and will strongly depend on the form in which alginate will be presented to water. Cross-linked alginates will, for instance, swell slower than a pure sodium alginate. Swellability of alginate is utilized in sustained release tablets, while swellability of partly neutralized alginic acid has a long tradition as a tablet disintegrant.

*Film-forming properties* of alginate can be considered as entanglement of the alginate molecules during drying of a solution, or simply just removal of water from a cross-linked gel. The molecular weight needs to be above a certain lower limit in order to achieve film formation and avoid brittleness. Films can easily be formed *in situ* by spraying an alginate solution on to a binding surface.

### 15.4.2 Cross-Linked Gels

*Gelling properties* of alginate are a function of the M/G composition and the sequential structure of M and G along the alginate chain. Alginate forms gels with most di- and multivalent cations, although calcium is most widely used (Smidsrød and Skjåk-Bræk, 1990). Consecutive guluronic residues forming a G-block structure have the ability to cross-link with multivalent cations, with the exception of magnesium (Figure 15.4). In general terms, an increase in G-content (measured as $G_{N>1}$) as well as in molecular weight will give a stronger gel (Smidsrød and Skjåk-Bræk, 1990). The process of making a gel, however, will also be of importance. In practice, the gelling can take place through diffusing of the cross-linking agent from the outside (external gelling), or the cross-linking agent can be released homogenously from the inside of the gelling solution (internal gelling). Several methods exist to measure gel strength, where an important issue is to distinguish between the elastic modulus and the viscous one, where the later often is misinterpreted as gel strength, for high viscosity solutions in particular.

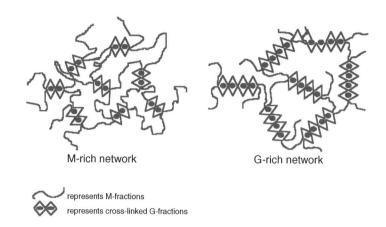

M-rich network                                    G-rich network

represents M-fractions
represents cross-linked G-fractions

**FIGURE 15.4**
Schematic representation of cross-linking of alginate with calcium.

Skjåk-Bræk et al. (1989) have shown how the presence of nongelling ions such as NaCl will influence the homogeneity of the final gel at external gelling. With no NaCl present the concentration of alginate at the outer part of the gel, closest to the interface with the gelling bath, will be higher than in the center due to alginate diffusion from the center to the gelling zone. By adding NaCl in the process, a relatively homogenous gel can be achieved. Figure 15.5 illustrates the differences in alginate concentrations that can be obtained inside a cylindrical gel when $Ca^{2+}$ diffuses, with and without NaCl present.

For internal gelling, the ratio between the alginate and the cross-linking agent has been shown to be of importance. Internal gelling can be induced by first preparing a solution of $CaCl_2$ in EDTA where the pH is adjusted to 7 to 7.5. $Ca^{2+}$ ions are effectively chelated and not available for cross-linking with alginate. Sodium alginate is added to the $CaCl_2$–EDTA solution in varying amounts as indicated in Figure 15.6. Gluconic acid δ-lactone (GDL) is then added. GDL will, over time, induce a reduction in pH that leads to release of $Ca^{2+}$ from the chelated complex. Calcium ions are now available for cross-linking with alginate and internal gelling occurs over a period of several hours. Gel strength is determined, in this case, by measuring the force (in grams) needed to rotate a metal plate immersed into the gel by 30°. For high-G alginates ($G > 60\%$) cross-linked with $Ca^{2+}$, the strongest gels, i.e., maximum gel strength, are achieved when the amount of calcium stoichiometrically matches the amount of calcium-binding guluronic acid blocks ($G_{N>1}$).

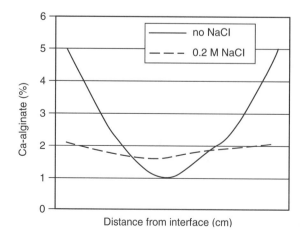

**FIGURE 15.5**
The effect of external gelling with and without NaCl present on alginate concentration in a gel cylinder.

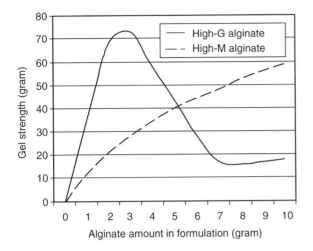

**FIGURE 15.6**
The effect of alginate concentration on gel strength for internal gelling of high-G and high-M alginate at constant calcium concentration.

When a surplus of alginate is present in the gelling formulation, $Ca^{2+}$ will not bind to the available G-sites in an optimal manner and the gel formed, therefore, will have a lower gel strength. For high-M alginates a continuous increase in gel strength is observed. This is due to the fact that M-rich alginates have fewer, and shorter, guluronic acid blocks. Increasing the alginate concentration presents additional calcium ion binding sites to the mixture resulting in increased gel strength. Figure 15.6 shows a comparison in gel strength for a high-G and a high-M alginate as a function of the alginate amount in a gelling formulation. Alginates can also be cross-linked covalently by a number of strategies. A good overview is contained in *The Biomedical Engineering Handbook* (Park, 1999).

## 15.5 Cell Immobilization with Alginate

The technique to immobilize cells, particularly pancreatic islet cells, in calcium alginate matrices was developed by Lim at the end of the 1970s (Lim and Sun, 1980). By coating the alginate gel bead with polycations like poly-L-lysine, poly-L-ornithine, or chitosan, the strength of the surface coating as well as the capsule porosity can be controlled (Figure 15.7) (Skjåk-Bræk and Espevik, 1996).

One important characteristic of alginates is their very limited inherent cell adhesion and cellular interaction. This is an advantage for cell encapsulation applications, but can be a disadvantage for tissue engineering applications. However, alginate can be modified by the addition of cell attachment peptides or other biologically active molecules (Rowley et al., 1999b).

## 15.6 Pharmacokinetics

Pharmacokinetic studies of alginate have been carried out following administration of a [14C] radiolabeled alginate purified from *Pseudomonas aeruginosa* (Hagen et al., 1996; Skaugrud et al., 1999). The pharmacokinetics in mice following an intravenous (IV) bolus injection of 100 $\mu$g [14C] alginate indicates a two-compartment model. The data show an initial rapid elimination of alginate from the blood (0 to 5 h) followed by a slower elimination (5 to 48 h). The initial half-life ($t_{1/2}\alpha$) is approximately 4 h, while the secondary half-life ($t_{1/2}\beta$) appears to be about 22 h (Figure 15.8, left panel).

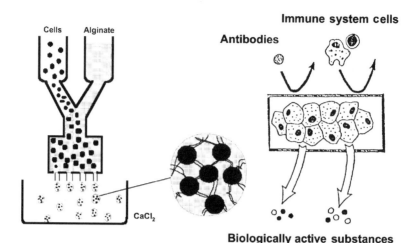

**FIGURE 15.7**
Schematic representation of encapsulation of cells within alginate gel beads.

The pharmacokinetics in mice following an intraperitoneal (IP) bolus injection of 100 $\mu$g [$^{14}$C] alginate shows that absorption reaches a maximum after 5 to 6 h (Figure 15.8, right panel). Thereafter, the serum concentration declines with an apparent half-life of about 12.5 h. The elimination following IP administration may also occur in a biphasic fashion, similar to IV administration. Alginate was not absorbed into the blood following oral administration. Studies using a radioiodinated tyrosinamide-derivatized alginate support the pharmacokinetic data produced with the bacterial alginate (Al-Shamkhani and Duncan, 1995).

## 15.7 Regulatory Standards

Sodium alginate is listed on the list of materials affirmed Generally Recognized as Safe (GRAS) by the US Food and Drug Administration (FDA) (21CFR184.1724). This permits sodium alginate (but not other salts such as magnesium) to be used in foods as a thickener or gelling agent. That sodium alginate is listed on the GRAS list does not indicate approval

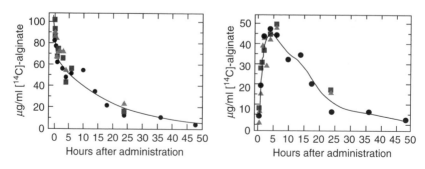

**FIGURE 15.8**
Pharmacokinetics of sodium alginate. Mice were administered either intravenous (left panel) or intraperitoneal (right panel) bolus injections of [$^{14}$C] alginate. Each data point represents the amount of alginate in blood serum (calculated from radioactivity) from one individual animal.

for the use of alginate in pharmaceutical and/or biomedical applications. Each application or product must go through its own regulatory approval process. Alginate is also referenced in the United States Pharmacopoeia as well as the European Pharmacopoeia. In order to assist in the development of alginate-containing applications, a guide for the characterization and testing of alginates as starting materials intended for use in biomedical and TEMP applications has been approved by the American Society for Testing and Materials (ASTM) under designation F2064 (Anonymous, 2004). This guide is meant to provide information concerning what parameters (both analytical and regulatory) need to be addressed either by the alginate supplier or the developer when using alginate in pharmaceutical and biomedical applications, such as TEMPs.

# References

Al-Shamkhani, A. and Duncan, R., Radioiodination of alginate via covalently-bound tyrosinamide allows monitoring of it fate *in vivo*, *J. Bioact. Compat. Polym.*, **10**, 4 (1995).

Anonymous, *F 2064 Standard guide for characterization and testing of alginates as starting materials intended for use in biomedical and tissue-engineered medical products application*, Annual Book of ASTM Standards, Vol. 13. ASTM International, West Conshohocken (2004), 1126.

Atala, A. et al., Endoscopic treatment of vesicoureteral reflux with a chondrocyte-alginate suspension, *J. Urol.*, **152**, 641 (1994).

Brunstedt, M. et al., Filling material for soft tissue implant prostheses and implants made therewith, EP 0 727 232 A2 (1996).

Chang, T.M. and Malave, N., The development and first clinical use of semipermeable microcapsules (artificial cells) as a compact artificial kidney. 1970 [classical article], *Ther. Apher.*, **4**, 108 (2000).

Chang, P.L. et al., Growth of recombinant fibroblasts in alginate microcapsules, *Biotechnol. Bioeng.*, **43**, 925 (1994).

Chen, Z.P. and Mohr, G., Microencapsulation for cell implants into the central nervous system: the importance of alginate viscosity and related factors, *Stereot. Funct. Neuros.*, **66**, 141 (1996).

Diamond, D.A. and Caldamone, A.A., Endoscopic correction of vesicoureteral reflux in children using autologous chondrocytes: preliminary results, *J. Urol.*, **162**, 1185 (1999).

Emerich, D.F. et al., A novel approach to neural transplantation in Parkinson's disease: use of polymer-encapsulated cell therapy, *Neurosci. Biobehav. Rev.*, **16**, 437 (1992).

Gentile, F.T., Vesicourethral reflux, *Sci. Med.*, **Nov./Dec.**, 6 (1999).

Grasdalen, H., $^1$H-N.M.R. spectroscopy of alginate: sequential structure and linkage conformations, *Carbohydr. Res.*, **118**, 255 (1983).

Grasdalen, H., Larsen, B., and Smidsrød, O., An N.M.R. study of the composition and sequence of uronate residues in alginates, *Carbohydr. Res.*, **68**, 23 (1979).

Hagen, A., Skjåk-Bræk, G., and Dornish, M., Pharmacokinetics of sodium alginate in mice, *Eur. J. Pharm. Sci.*, **4**, S100 (1996).

Hagstam, H., Alginates and heartburn — evaluation of a medicine with a mechanical mode of action, In: *Gums and Stabilizers in the Food Industry*, Phillips, G.O., Ed., Elsevier, Amsterdam, pp. 363 (1986).

Joki, T. et al., Continuous release of endostatin from microencapsulated engineered cells for tumor therapy, *Nat. Biotechnol.*, **19**, 35 (2001).

Kataoka, K. et al., Alginate, a bioresorbable material derived from brown seaweed, enhances elongation of amputated axons of spinal cord in infant rats, *J. Biomed. Mater. Res.*, **54**, 373 (2000).

Kenley, R. et al., Osseous regeneration in the rat calvarium using novel delivery systems for recombinant human bone morphogenetic protein-2 (rhBMP-2), *J. Biomed. Mater. Res.*, **28**, 1139 (1994).

Kim, B.S., Bacz, C.E., and Atala, A., Biomaterials for tissue engineering, *World J. Urol.*, **18**, 2 (2000).

Lim, F. and Sun, A.M., Microencapsulated islets as bioartificial endocrine pancreas, *Science*, **210**, 908 (1980).

Mandel, K.G. et al., Review article: alginate-raft formulations in the treatment of heartburn and acid reflux, *Aliment. Pharm. Therap.*, **14**, 669 (2000).

Maruyama, M. et al., Hydroxyapatite clay for gap filling and adequate bone ingrowth, *J. Biomed. Mater. Res.*, **29**, 329 (1995).

Miyazaki, S., Kubo, W., and Attwood, D., Oral sustained delivery of theophylline using in-situ gelation of sodium alginate, *J. Controlled Release*, **67**, 275 (2000).

Morgan, S.M. et al., Alginates as drug carriers: covalent attachment of alginates to therapeutic agents containing primary amino groups, *Int. J. Pharm.*, **122**, 121 (1995).

Onsøyen, E., Hydration induced swelling of alginate based matrix tablets at GI-tract pH conditions, In: *Excipients and Delivery Systems for Pharmaceutical Formulations*, Karse, D.R. and Stephenson, R.A., Eds., The Royal Society of Chemistry, Cambridge, pp. 108 (1995).

Park, J.B., Biomaterials, In: *The Biomedical Engineering Handbook*, Vol. 1, Bronzino, J.D., Ed., CRC Press, Boca Raton (1999).

Peirone, M.A. et al., Delivery of recombinant gene product to canines with nonautologous microencapsulated cells, *Hum. Gene Ther.*, **9**, 195 (1998).

Ramdas, M. et al., Alginate encapsulated bioadhesive chitosan microspheres for intestinal drug delivery, *J. Biomater. Appl.*, **13**, 290 (1999).

Read, T.-A. et al., Local endostatin treatment of gliomas administered by microencapsulated producer cells, *Nat. Biotechnol.*, **19**, 29 (2001).

Rowley, J.A., Madlambayan, G., and Mooney, D.J., Alginate hydrogels as synthetic extracellular matrix materials, *Biomaterials*, **20**, 45 (1999a).

Rowley, J.A., Madlambayan, G., and Mooney, D.J., Alginate hydrogels as synthetic extracellular matrix materials, *Biomaterials*, **20**, 45 (1999b).

Skaugrud, Ø. et al., Biomedical and pharmaceutical applications of alginate and chitosan, *Biotechnol. Genet. Eng. Rev.*, **16**, 23 (1999).

Skjåk-Bræk, G. and Espevik, T., Application of alginate gels in biotechnology and biomedicine, *Carbohydr. Eur.*, **14**, 19 (1996).

Skjåk-Bræk, G., Grasdalen, H., and Smidsrød, O., Inhomogeneous polysaccharide ionic gels, *Carbohydr. Res.*, **10**, 31 (1989).

Smidsrød, O. and Draget, K., Chemistry and physical properties of alginates, *Carbohydr. Eur.*, **14**, 6 (1996).

Smidsrød, O. and Skjåk-Bræk, G., Alginate as immobilization matrix for cells, *TIBTECH*, **8**, 71 (1990).

Stanford, E.E.C., On algin: a new substance obtained from some of the commoner species of marine algae, *Chem. News*, 254 (1883).

Stockley, T.L. et al., Delivery of recombinant product from subcutaneous implants of encapsulated recombinant cells in canines, *J. Lab. Clin. Med.*, **135**, 484 (2000).

Sun, A.M., O'shea, G.M., and Goosen, M.F., Injectable microencapsulated islet cells as a bioartificial pancreas, *Appl. Biochem. Biotechnol.*, **10**, 87 (1984).

Sun, A.M. et al., Microencapsulated hepatocytes: an in vitro and in vivo study, *Biomater. Artif. Cells Artif. Organs*, **15**, 483 (1987).

Suzuki, K. et al., Regeneration of transected spinal cord in young adult rats using freeze-dried alginate gel, *Neuroreport*, **10**, 2891 (1999).

Thomas, S., Alginate dressings in surgery and wound management — part 1, *J. Wound Care*, **9**, 56 (2000a).

Thomas, S., Alginate dressings in surgery and wound management: part 2, *J. Wound Care*, **9**, 115 (2000b).

Thomas, S., Alginate dressings in surgery and wound management: part 3, *J. Wound Care*, **9**, 163 (2000c).

Uludag, H., DeVos, P., and Tresco, P.A., Technology of mammalian cell encapsulation, *Adv. Drug Deliv. Rev.*, **42**, 29 (2000).

Visted, T., Bjerkvig, R., and Enger, P.Ø., Cell encapsulation as a therapeutic strategy for CNS malignancies, *Neuro-Oncology*, **July**, 201 (2001).

Wong, H. and Chang, T.M., Bioartificial liver: implanted artificial cells microencapsulated living hepatocytes increases survival of liver failure rats, *Int. J. Artif. Organs*, **9**, 335 (1986).

# 16

## *Polyphosphazenes*

**Lakshmi S. Nair, Yusuf M. Khan, and Cato T. Laurencin**

## CONTENTS

## 16.1   Inorganic Polymers

The rapid technological development in the latter half of the twentieth century demanded the development of a wide range of specialty polymers for various applications. Even though a large number of organic polymers have been developed to meet these demands by synthesizing a wide range of monomeric molecules and varying the polymerization techniques, it has been found that organic polymers alone cannot provide the property profiles required for all these applications. This has led to the development of a wide range of inorganic and organometallic polymers with versatile properties.

Inorganic polymers can be broadly defined as polymers having inorganic repeating units in the backbone (Archer, 2001). This clearly distinguishes them from organic polymers where the polymer backbones are mainly composed of carbon atoms along with oxygen or nitrogen. Inorganic polymers form a unique class of materials with unusual physical, chemical and biological properties. This can be attributed to their distinctive structure which combines the macromolecular architecture with the unusual properties of inorganic elements. The macromolecular structure imparts inorganic polymers with properties such as chain entanglement and increased intermolecular interactions which significantly increase the strength, toughness and processibility of these materials. Incorporation of inorganic elements into the macromolecular structure imparts unique

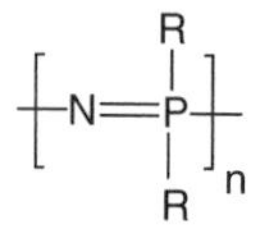

$$\left[ -N = \underset{\underset{R}{|}}{\overset{\overset{R}{|}}{P}} - \right]_n \qquad \text{R = Organic groups, Organometallic groups}$$

**SCHEME 16.1**
Structure of polyphosphazene.

thermal, electrical and optical properties, electrolytic conductivity, electroactivity, high oxidative stability and biocompatibility to these materials.

The first commercially developed inorganic polymers were polysiloxanes; a class of polymers having versatile chemical physical and electrical properties, low temperature flexibility, thermal stability and excellent biocompatibility (Jones et al., 2000). Due to these excellent properties, polysiloxanes rapidly found a wide range of commercial applications as elastomers, coatings, wire insulation and biomaterials. They demonstrated, for the first time, the unique advantages of inorganic polymers. The development of polysiloxanes was followed by the development of several other inorganic polymers such as polysilazanes, polycarboranes, polysilanes and polyphosphazenes, with polysilanes and polyphosphazenes being the most two rapidly developing classes of inorganic polymers. Polysilanes are linear polymers having a backbone of silicon atoms with two organic groups attached to each silicon atom. These polymers are known to exhibit unusual properties such as thermochrism, photoreactivity, liquid crystal properties, nonlinear optical properties and semiconductive properties, making them interesting candidates for developing novel electronic and optical devices (Jones et al., 2000).

Polyphosphazenes, on the other hand, can be considered the most chemically versatile and diverse class of inorganic polymers. Polyphosphazenes, previously referred to as polyphosphonitriles, are polymers having a phosphorus nitrogen backbone with each phosphorous–nitrogen atom attached to two organic or organometallic groups (Allcock, 2003) (Scheme 16.1).

In addition to a phosphoros–nitrogen backbone, very few polyphosphazenes having a phosphoros–nitrogen–sulfur or a phosphoros–nitrogen–carbon backbone have also been synthesized (Allcock, 2003). However, polymers having alternate phosphorus and nitrogen atoms form the largest member of the polyphosphazene family. In fact, almost 750 different types of polyphosphazenes with the $-P=N-$ backbone possessing a wide spectrum of properties have been developed simply by varying the type of the side groups (R) linked to the phosphoros atom.

## 16.2  Polyphosphazene Synthesis

Two different polymerization routes have been developed to synthesize polyphosphazenes in which the side groups are attached to the phosphoros atoms by P–N, P–O or P–C bonds. They are the ring opening polymerization of unsubstituted or substituted cyclic trimers and the condensation polymerization of N-silylphosphor-animines.

### 16.2.1  Ring Opening Polymerization

The first and most extensively investigated route for polyphosphazene synthesis is the two-step thermal ring-opening polymerization followed by nucleophilic substitution of

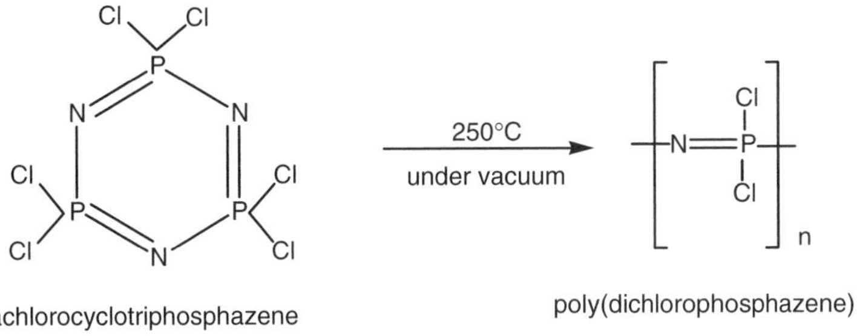

**SCHEME 16.2**
Ring opening polymerization of hexachlorocyclotriphosphazene.

the macromolecular intermediate developed by Allcock and coworkers during the later half of 1960s (Allcock and Kugel, 1965; Allcock, 2003). The first step involves the thermal ring-opening polymerization of hexachlorocyclotriphosphazene at 250°C for approximately 8 h under vacuum to form a highly reactive macromolecular intermediate, poly(dichlorophosphazene) (PDCP) at approximately 70% yield (Scheme 16.2).

The PDCP is a highly unstable polymer due to the high reactivity of P–Cl bonds, and rapidly hydrolyzes upon exposure to atmospheric moisture breaking down into phosphate, ammonia and hydrochloric acid. Allcock and coworkers used the high reactivity of P–Cl bonds in PDCP to develop hydrolytically stable, soluble, high molecular weight polyphosphazenes by replacing chlorine atoms of PDCP with organic or organometallic groups (Scheme 16.3).

The availability of a wide range of nucleophiles, coupled with the flexibility of the substitution reaction, which allows the incorporation of more than one type of substituent along the PDCP chain by simultaneous or sequential substitution reactions, enabled the synthesis of hundreds of polyphosphazenes from the same macromolecular precursor (Allcock, 2003). Due to the high reactivity of P–Cl bonds and high stability of the –P=N– backbone, completely-substituted polyphosphazenes could be developed using a wide range of alkoxides, aryloxides and amines (Allcock et al., 1966). The only exception to this is the reaction of PDCP with organometallic reagents to form poly[(alkyl/aryl)phosphazenes] where the reaction is sometimes hindered by the coordination of the metal to the backbone nitrogen atoms (Allcock and Chu, 1979).

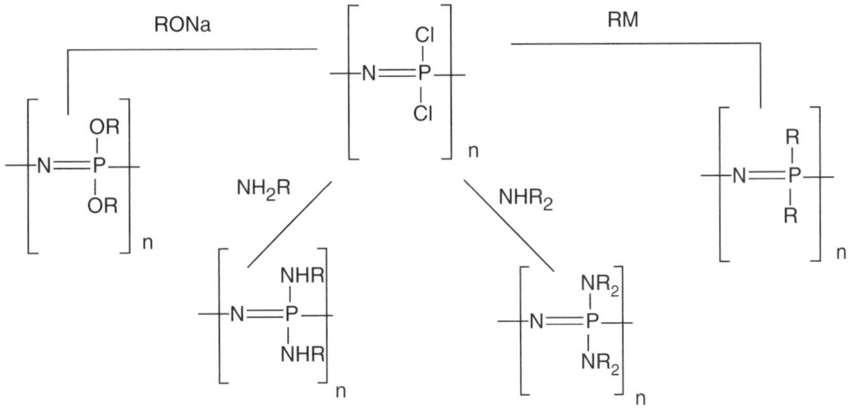

**SCHEME 16.3**
Macromolecular substitution route to form polyphosphazenes.

The mechanism of ring-opening polymerization of the cyclic trimer has been extensively investigated (Allcock and Best, 1964; Allcock, 1980; Hagnauer, 1981). The generally accepted mechanism of the ring-opening polymerization reaction involves the ionization of a P–Cl bond of the trimer to yield a cationic species called phosphazenium cation. This cation then attacks and cleaves another phosphazene ring resulting in the transfer of the cationic charge to the terminal phosphorous atom. The chain propagation then continues from that site to form a linear PDCP.

The synthetic procedure outlined above for polyphosphazenes is thus quite different from the synthesis of organic macromolecules, which mainly depends on the development of specific monomers that could undergo polymerization at a feasible rate. The unusual synthetic versatility of the macromolecular substitution route for polyphosphazenes has led to the development of an unprecedented array of novel inorganic macromolecules with a wide spectrum of properties. In addition to the macromolecular substitution route a cyclic trimer substitution/polymerization route was also attempted as an alternative approach to develop polyphosphazenes (Scheme 16.4). However, it has been found that except for few cases, the complete substitution of the halogen atoms of the cyclic trimer by organic units fully inhibited ring-opening polymerization (Allcock and Patterson, 1977). This has been attributed to the lack of a halogen atom to initiate the polymerization as well as to the steric interferences in the case of bulky R groups. It has been found that the ring opening polymerization of substituted cyclic trimers takes place when only one or two of the chlorine atoms were replaced by these groups and the tendency to polymerize decreases with an increase in the number of organic groups present. However, the presence of strain-inducing transannular metallocene bridging groups, such as ferrocinyl groups, along with other R groups has been reported to undergo polymerization even when completely substituted (Allcock et al., 1985).

Even though the ring-opening polymerization route led to the development of polyphosphazenes as a class of novel inorganic polymers, the synthetic route suffers from various disadvantages particularly as a commercially feasible polymerization route, such as the long polymerization time, high polymerization temperature, poor control over the molecular weight and polydispersity of the polymers, and the difficulty in preparing fully alkylated or arylated polyphosphazenes.

Therefore, several catalytic systems have been developed to accelerate the rate of ring opening polymerization as well as to reduce the temperature of polymerization with some success. These include Lewis acid catalysts such as $BCl_3$, $PCl_3$ and $Cl_3B \cdot OP(OPh)_3$, traces of water, various sulfur acids and organic acids (Allcock, 2003).

### 16.2.2 Condensation Polymerization

The condensation polymerization route has recently attracted great interest as a unique method to both overcome many of the disadvantages of ring opening polymerization

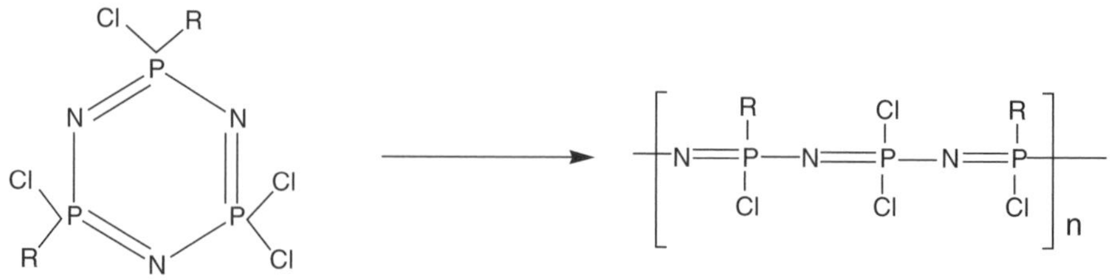

**SCHEME 16.4**
Ring opening polymerization of substituted cyclic trimers.

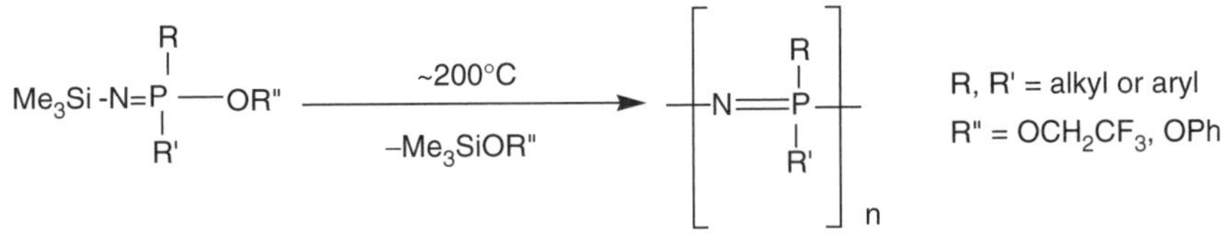

**SCHEME 16.5**
Condensation polymerization of *N*-silyl phosphoranimines.

as well as to develop polyphosphazenes with novel architectures. The first condensation process reported involved the condensation of phosphorous pentachloride with ammonium chloride in a chlorinated organic solvent to generate linear oligomers (Allen et al., 1970). The oligomers were then heated to high temperature in the presence of excess ammonium chloride to form PDCP. However, this process resulted in the formation of low to moderate molecular weight polymers with broad polydispersities.

Research in the late 1970s showed the possibility of developing cyclic phosphazenes and polyphosphazenes from *N*-silylphosphoranimines. Neilson and Wisian-Neilson (1988) and Wisian-Neilson and Neilson (1989) performed an extensive investigation to develop poly[(alkyl/aryl)phosphazene]s by this route since it is difficult to synthesize fully substituted alkyl/aryl polyphosphazenes by the ring-opening polymerization route (Scheme 16.5). The possibility of forming copolymers by the co-thermolysis of two or more different phosphoranimines was also demonstrated by the same group. This thermal uncatalyzed condensation polymerization route led to the development of a series of alkyl or aryl polyphosphazenes with high yields of 90 to 100%. Polymers with molecular weight in the range of 25,000 to 200,000 were obtained by this process.

A living cationic condensation polymerization route was developed by Allcock and coworkers in 1995 as a novel route to develop poly(dichlorophosphazene) and poly(organophosphazene)s at ambient temperature (Scheme 16.6) (Manners et al., 1989; Allcock et al., 1991; Honeyman et al., 1995).

The living cationic polymerization route presents several advantages compared to other polymerization routes developed so far for polyphosphazenes. Here the polymerization takes place at room temperature compared to the high temperature requirement for the ring opening polymerization. The process also allowed the possibility of precisely controlling the molecular weight of the polymer by changing the ratio of $PCl_5$ to monomer. Moreover the polydispersity of the polymers formed by the living polymerization route was found to be very low. Furthermore, since the condensation reaction takes place by a living polymerization process, this route introduced the possibility of developing novel polyphosphazenes with unique structures such as block copolymers, star polymers, telechelic polymers and comb polymers (Scheme 16.7). Thus, the living cationic polymerization route led to the development of wide range of novel polyphosphazenes having well defined and well controlled architectures.

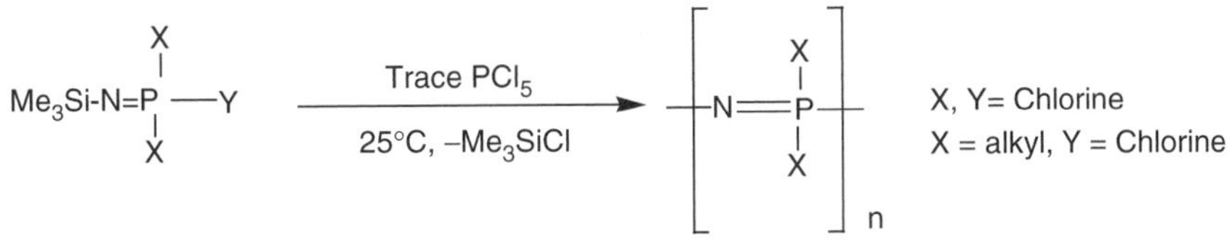

**SCHEME 16.6**
Living cationic polymerization of phosphoranimines.

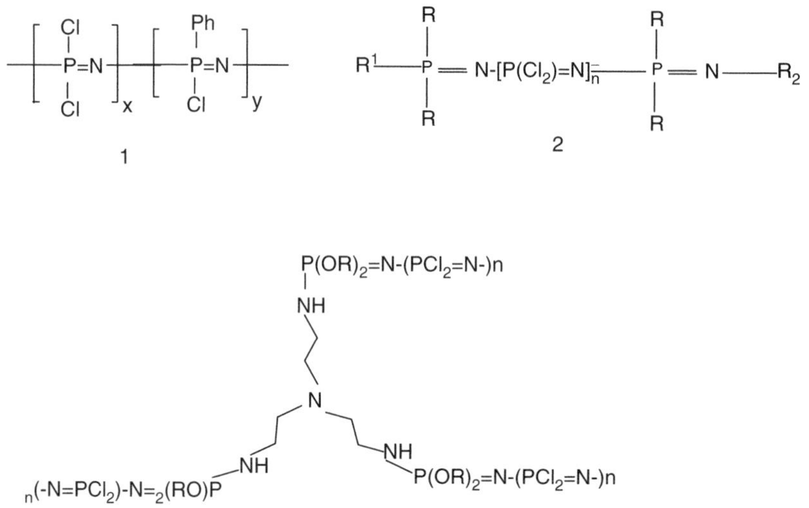

**SCHEME 16.7**
Polyphosphazenes having different architectures by living cationic polymerization. 1. Block copolymer, 2. Ditelechelic polymer, 3. Star polymer.

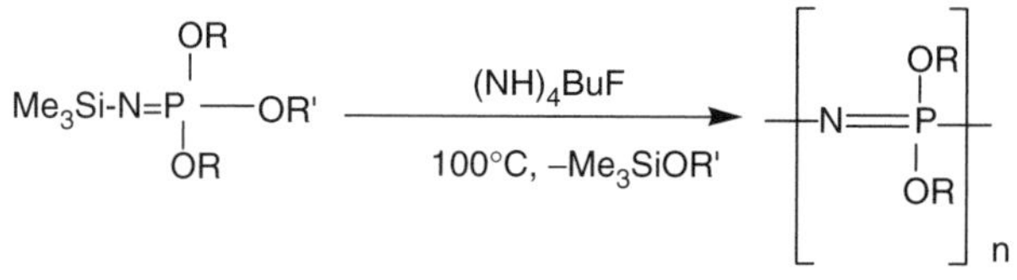

**SCHEME 16.8**
Living anionic polymerization of phosphoranimines.

In addition to the living cationic polymerization route, an anionic living polymerization route was developed as a means of synthesizing alkoxy polyphosphazenes as well as random and block copolymers from two different phosphoranimine monomers by Montague and Matyjaszewski (1990) (Scheme 16.8). These block copolymers showed mono model molecular weight distributions and had physical and thermal properties which were dependent on the repeating unit ratios. The properties of these block copolymers were found to be quite different from the corresponding random copolymers.

Matyjaszewski et al. (1992) also refined a phosphorous azide based method as an alternative route to synthesize poly(aryl/alkyl)polyphosphazene.

## 16.3   Different Classes of Polyphosphazene

The various synthetic routes developed so far thus led to the synthesis of almost 750 different types of polyphosphazenes having different types and different combinations of side groups and thereby different property profiles. Based on the side groups, polyphosphazenes can be broadly classified into alkoxy/aryloxy polyphosphazenes, aminated polyphosphazenes and alkyl/arylpolyphosphazenes.

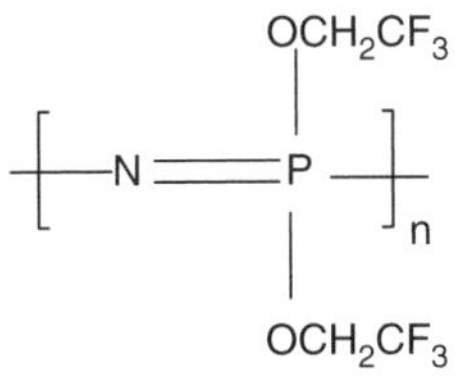

$$\left[ N = P \right]_n$$
OCH$_2$CF$_3$ (top)
OCH$_2$CF$_3$ (bottom)

**1**

**SCHEME 16.9**

### 16.3.1 Alkoxy/Aryloxy Polyphosphazenes

The largest class of polyphosphazenes that are synthesized and commercially developed are the alkoxy/aryloxy polyphosphazenes. The mostly commonly used route to develop poly[(alkoxy/aryloxy)phosphazenes] is the ring-opening polymerization route followed by macromolecular substitution of the chlorine atoms of PDCP by alkoxy or aryloxy groups. The wide range of alkoxy or aryloxy groups available led to the development of a large number of alkoxy/aryloxy polyphosphazenes. Recently the condensation polymerization route has been explored to develop various alkoxy/aryloxy polyphosphazenes.

The first stable polyphosphazene synthesized was a fluorinated alkoxy polymer poly[bis(trifluoro ethoxy)phosphazene] (PTFEP) (Scheme 16.9) and therefore it has been extensively investigated. PTFEP is a microcrystalline, thermoplastic, hydrophobic (contact angle 109°) polymer with a glass transition temperature of $-66°C$. This polymer is currently used for various applications which make use of its excellent water-repellency, fire-resistance and fiber-forming properties. Various mixed substituent fluoroalkoxy polyphosphazenes were also developed with unique elastomeric properties. The presence of two different fluoroalkoxy groups markedly reduced the microcrystallinity of homopolymers while the mixed substituent polymers have become known for their high performance elastomeric properties (Scheme 16.10). They form one of the most commercially exploited classes of polyphosphazenes due to their low temperature (as low as $-55°C$) elastomeric properties, high temperature and radiation stability and solvent resistance (Allcock, 2003).

In addition to fluorinated alkoxy polyphosphazenes, a wide range of nonfluorinated alkoxy polyphosphazenes were also developed mainly by Allcock and coworkers. Most of these polymers form amorphous elastomers with very low glass-transition temperature ($T_g$) (as low as $-104°C$) (Scheme 16.11). However, compared to fluorinated alkoxy polyphosphazenes, these polymers show lower temperature and radiation stability. A series of hydrolytically sensitive alkoxy polyphosphazenes was developed by Allcock and coworkers as candidates for various biomedical applications. These include polyphosphazenes having glycolic acid and lactic acid ester side groups (Scheme 16.12), glyceryl substituted polyphosphazenes (Scheme 16.13) and glucosyl substituted

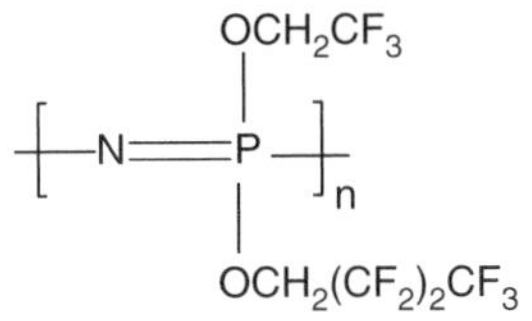

$$\left[ N = P \right]_n$$
OCH$_2$CF$_3$ (top)
OCH$_2$(CF$_2$)$_2$CF$_3$ (bottom)

**2**

**SCHEME 16.10**

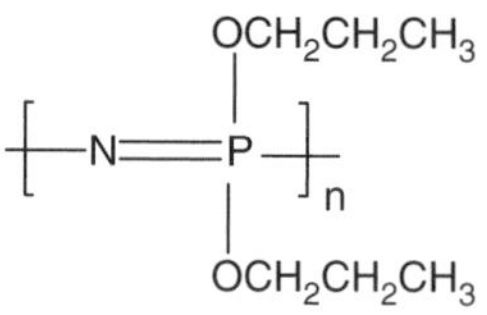

OCH$_2$CH$_2$CH$_3$

−N═P−

OCH$_2$CH$_2$CH$_3$

**3**

**SCHEME 16.11**

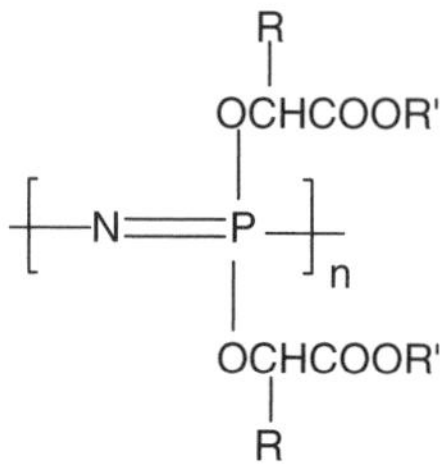

R

OCHCOOR'

−N═P−

OCHCOOR'

R

R = H/Me , R' = Et/Bz

**4**

**SCHEME 16.12**

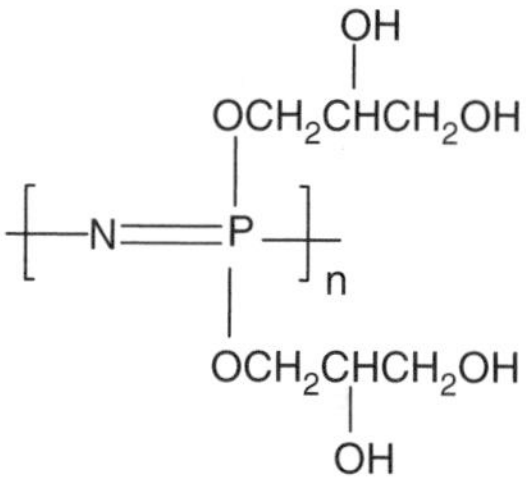

OH

OCH$_2$CHCH$_2$OH

−N═P−

OCH$_2$CHCH$_2$OH

OH

**5**

**SCHEME 16.13**

polyphosphazenes (Scheme 16.14) (Allcock and Kwon, 1988; Allcock and Pucher, 1991; Allcock et al., 1994b). These polymers undergo hydrolytic degradation to form corresponding side groups, phosphates, and ammonia and the degradation rate of the polymers was found to vary with the type of side groups present.

Nonfluorinated alkoxy polymers having ethyleneoxy side groups (Scheme 16.15) form another extensively investigated group of polyphosphazenes due to their versatile properties. These polymers have low $T_g$s and those with short chains (less than four repeating units) and branched side groups are amorphous. However, these polymers exhibit crystallinity as the side groups become larger. Ethyleneoxy polyphosphazenes are attractive candidates for biomedical applications mainly due to their water solubility, ability to be cross-linked by chemical and radiation processes, and the ability of some of them to undergo thermosensitive transitions. The lower critical solution temperatures (LCST) of these polymers are found to depend on the length of the ethyleneoxy side chain length and the presence of branching. Some of these polymers show transitions near physiological temperature which makes them a potential candidate for injectable delivery systems.

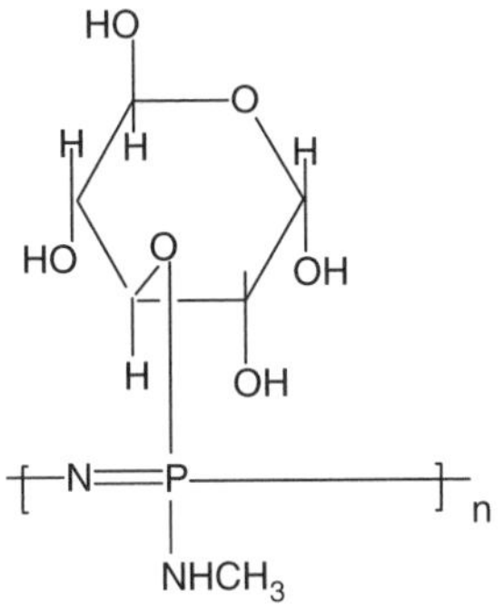

**6**

**SCHEME 16.14**

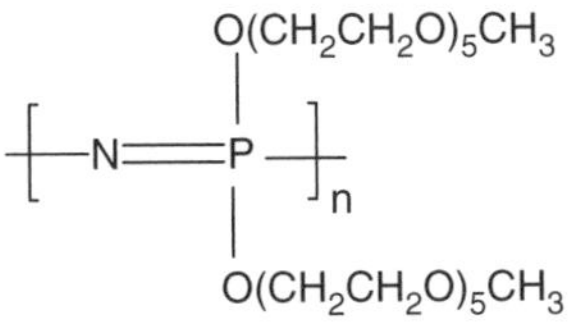

**7**

**SCHEME 16.15**

A wide range of aryloxy polyphosphazenes have been developed and they form the most versatile class of specialty polymers due to their unusual properties. This class of polyphosphazenes comprises a range of high refractive index polymers, liquid crystalline polymers, ferroelectric polymers, polymers with nonlinear optical properties and photochromic properties. Most of these polymers have $T_g$s at or above 0°C. The first synthesized poly[(aryloxy)phosphazene] is poly(diphenxoy phosphazene) (PDPP) (Scheme 16.16) which is a microcrystalline polymer having a $T_g$ near 0°C and is the most extensively investigated aryloxy polyphosphazene.

A wide range of halogen, alkyl, aryl or other functional group-substituted PDPPs have been developed for various applications. The incorporation of bulky groups on the aryl groups imposes steric restrictions which significantly affect the physical properties of the resulting polymers, depending on the size of the groups and position of substitution. Thus, incorporation of a phenyl group in the *para* position, as in the case of poly[bis(4-phenyl phenoxy)phosphazene] (Scheme 16.17), increases the $T_g$ of PDPP by approximately 90°C. The functionalization of the aromatic rings can lead to the development of interesting polymers as in the case of poly[bis (carboxy phenoxy)

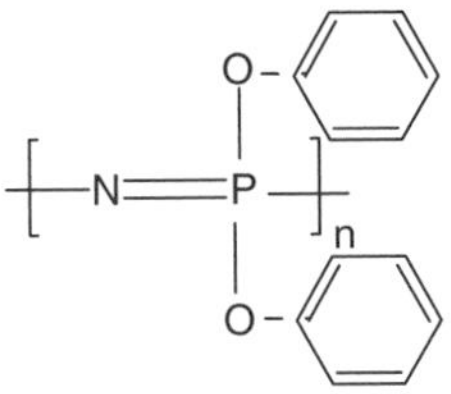

**8**

**SCHEME 16.16**

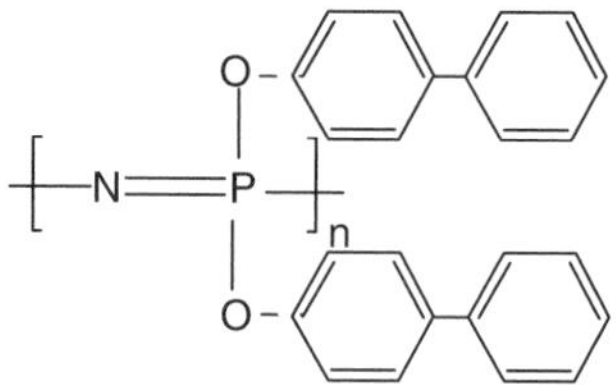

**9**

**SCHEME 16.17**

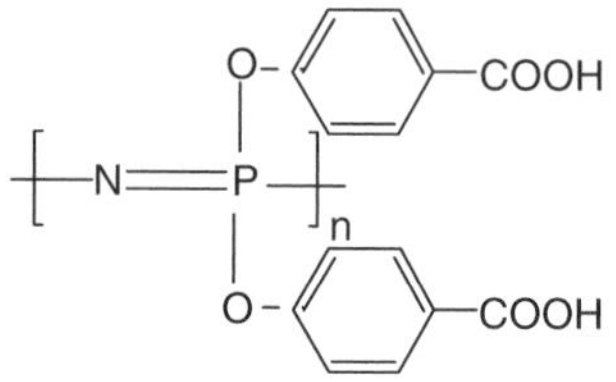

**10**

**SCHEME 16.18**

phosphazene], which is a pH sensitive polymer and is found to form cross-links in the presence of di- or trivalent cations. This polymer has been extensively investigated for various biomedical applications such as drug delivery devices and as adjuvants for vaccine delivery (Scheme 16.18).

Even though the homosubstituent aryloxypolyphosphazenes are microcrystalline, incorporation of two different aryloxy groups randomly along the main chain by a simultaneous or sequential macromolecular substitution reaction results in amorphous elastomers that have been extensively investigated (Scheme 16.19). In a similar way to mixed substituent fluoroalkoxy polymers, these polymers form another of the most commercially exploited classes of polyphosphazenes due to their comparatively low cost, fire-resistance and insulating properties.

In addition to aryloxy polyphosphazenes a wide range of arylalkoxy polyphosphazenes were also developed where the aryl groups are connected to the phosphoros atoms via alkoxy or ethoxy groups. The incorporation of alkyl groups in arylalkoxy polyphosphazenes significantly increases the flexibility of the polymers as evidenced by the decrease in $T_g$ and the absence of crystallinity in these polymers (Scheme 16.20).

Another versatile method to modulate the properties of alkoxy/aryloxy polyphosphazenes is to develop mixed substituent polyphosphazenes having aryloxy and alkoxy (fluorinated and nonfluorinated) side groups. These polymers are

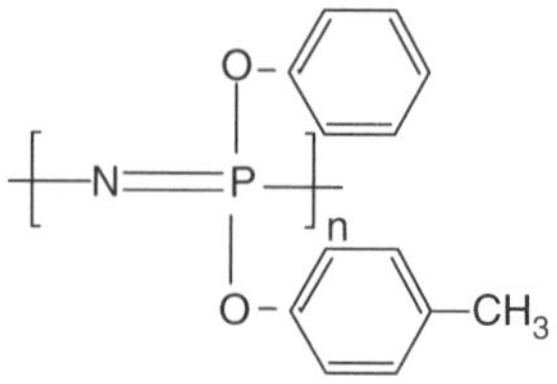

**11**

**SCHEME 16.19**

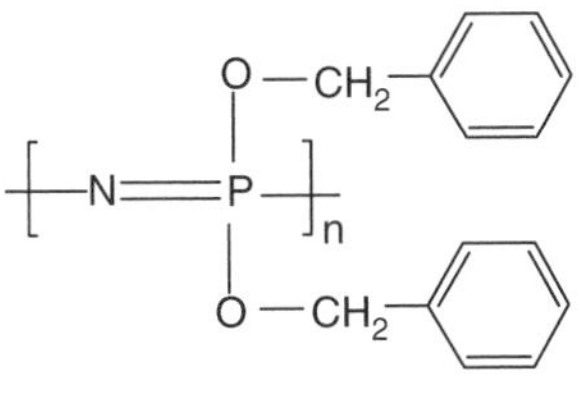

**12**

**SCHEME 16.20**

mainly developed by the sequential or simultaneous macromolecular substitution reaction. Here, the properties of the resulting polymers vary depending on the ratio of the two side groups along the polymer chain.

### 16.3.2 Aminated Polyphosphazenes

The high nucleophilicity of aminated compounds makes them effective substituent groups for developing novel polyphosphazenes. Therefore, various amines (alkyl and aryl amines) have been investigated as side groups for polyphosphazene synthesis. The synthesis of aminated polyphosphazenes was first reported by Allcock and coworkers. They were developed from PDCP by sequential or simultaneous substitution of chlorine atoms using various amines or substituted amines (Allcock et al., 1977). The aminated polyphosphazenes showed higher $T_g$s compared to their alkoxy or aryloxy derivatives as the thermal transitions of these polymers depends on the size of the side groups as well as the hydrogen bonding ability of the groups. Thus the alkoxy analog poly[(bis methoxy) phosphazene] is an amorphous, hydrophobic polymer having a $T_g$ of $-74°C$ whereas the corresponding aminated polymer poly[bis(methyl amino)phosphazene] is a crystalline polymers with a $T_g$ of $+14°C$ (Scheme 16.21). Unlike alkyl/aryl polyphosphazenes, aminated polyphosphazenes are a class of polyphosphazenes extensively investigated for biomedical applications, mainly as hydrolytically degradable materials. Among these, the amino acid ester polyphosphazenes form the most extensively investigated polymers for biomedical applications (Scheme 16.22). The $T_g$ of these polymers has been found to depend on the size of the groups (R) attached to the α-carbon atom as well as the ester group (R'). All these polymers are hydrolytically sensitive and degrade to form the corresponding amino acid, alcohol, phosphate and ammonia, thereby resulting in neutral and nontoxic degradation products (Welle et al., 1998). The degradation rate of these polymers also depends on the nature of the R and R' (Scheme 16.22); the larger the alkyl group, the lower the degradation rate. It has been found that the degradation rates of these polymers can be effectively modulated by developing mixed substituent amino acid ester polyphosphazenes or more effectively by developing mixed substituent amino acid ester and aryl/alkoxy polyphosphazenes (Scheme 16.23).

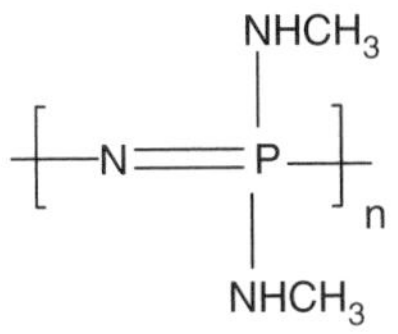

**13**

**SCHEME 16.21**

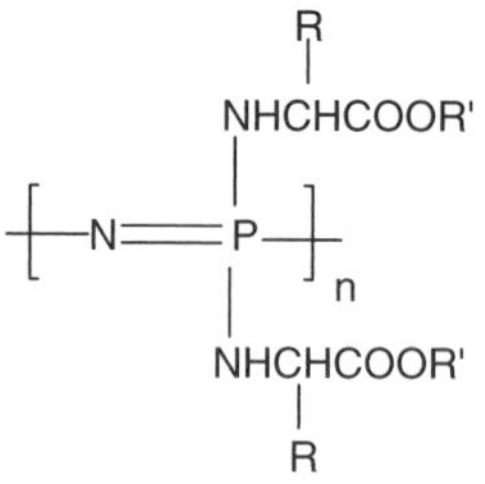

$$\begin{array}{c} R \\ | \\ NHCHCOOR' \\ | \\ \left[ -N\!\!=\!\!P- \right]_n \\ | \\ NHCHCOOR' \\ | \\ R \end{array}$$

R = H, CH$_3$, CH$_2$ CH(CH$_3$)$_2$ or
CH$_2$C$_6$H$_5$ and R' = CH$_2$CH$_3$

**14**

**SCHEME 16.22**

In addition to alkyl amino polyphosphazenes, a wide range of arylamino polyphosphazenes have been developed. These form brittle, glassy polymers with $T_g$s in the range of 50 to 100°C.

### 16.3.3  Alkyl/Aryl Phosphazenes

The alkyl/aryl polyphosphazenes are interesting polymers with a structure similar to polysilanes. Extensive research has been done to synthesize these polymers. Although Allcock and coworkers demonstrated as early as the 1970s the feasibility of developing aryl and alkyl polyphosphazenes by the reaction of PDCP with organometallic reagents, most of these polymers came from the condensation polymerization routes developed by Weison and Nelson's group and living cationic polymerization by Allcock's group. The most extensively investigated poly(alkylphosphazene) is poly[(bis methyl) phosphazene] (Scheme 16.24) which has been found to be a microcrystalline polymer with very low $T_g$.

Thus, the range of physical and chemical properties that can be obtained from polyphosphazenes is enormous. Thus, the class of polyphosphazenes encompasses very low $T_g$, amorphous elastomers ($-90$°C) to highly crystalline glasses, water soluble and organic soluble polymers, hydrophilic (0° contact angle) and hydrophobic (110° contact angle) polymers, hydrolytically stable and unstable polymers.

The versatility of polyphosphazenes comes from the combined effect of the unique backbone structure and the wide range of side groups that are attached to alternate atoms along the polymer backbone. The polyphosphazene backbone presents a structure with considerable torsional and angular freedom (Allcock, 2003). Several models have been postulated to describe the free rotation of the –P=N– backbone in polyphosphazenes.

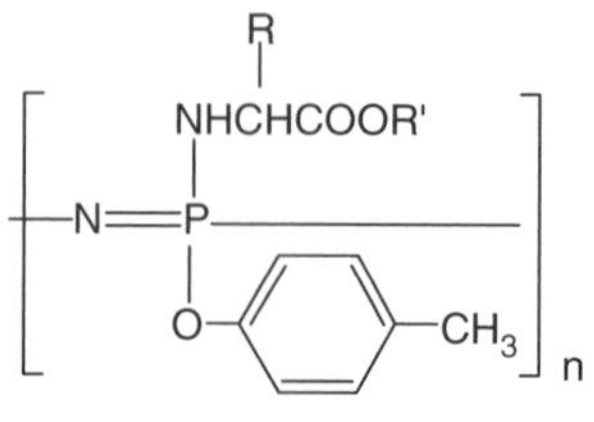

$$\begin{array}{c} R \\ | \\ NHCHCOOR' \\ | \\ \left[ -N\!\!=\!\!P- \right. \\ | \\ \left. O\!-\!\!\langle C_6H_4 \rangle\!-\!CH_3 \right]_n \end{array}$$

**15**

**SCHEME 16.23**

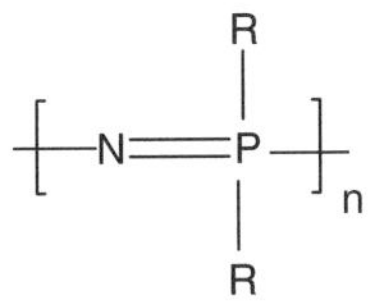

R
|
$\left[ -N{=\!=}P \right]_n$
|
R

R = CH$_3$

R = alkyl or aryl groups

**16**

**SCHEME 16.24**

After the sigma-bond formation, each −P=N− repeating unit will be left with four electrons; two of them will form a lone-pair orbital of nitrogen, which is responsible for the basicity and coordinating ability of the polyphosphazene backbone. The remaining 2p electron of nitrogen pairs with an electron in the 3D orbital of the phosphoros atom to form a 3d$\pi$−2p$\pi$ bond. However unlike organic d$\pi$−p$\pi$ bonds, here any one of the five 3D orbitals at each phosphoros atom can $\pi$ bond to the nitrogen 2p orbital thereby providing an unrestricted rotation about the −P=N− bond.

In addition to the inherent chain flexibility, the side groups in polyphosphazenes play an important role in determining the properties of the corresponding polymers. The inherent flexibility of the chain will be manifested only in the presence of small/flexible side groups resulting in elastomeric properties. Large/stiff side groups or polar or hydrogen bonding units can significantly affect the torsional freedom of the polymers, resulting in the formation of crystalline polymers.

This clearly shows the broad opportunities available with polyphosphazenes as a polymer system where the synthetic flexibility enables the design and synthesis of polymers with well controlled architecture and properties for specific applications.

## 16.4 Biomedical Applications of Polyphosphazenes

The ability to control the chemistry and thereby the properties of polyphosphazenes by simple macromolecular substitution makes them attractive candidates for various applications including biomedical applications. The inorganic nature of these polymers has also raised their interest, since the previously developed inorganic polymers such as "polysiloxanes" were found to be highly biocompatible and are currently used for various biomedical applications.

### 16.4.1 Hydrolytically Stable Polyphosphazenes

The first polyphosphazenes to be developed, fluoroalkoxy polymers and aryloxy polymers were the first polyphosphazenes investigated as biomaterials. These polymers, being elastomeric, were evaluated as potential candidates for cardiovascular applications. Well et al. demonstrated by *ex vivo* experiments that fluoroalkoxy polymers promote the adhesion of albumin once it comes into contact with blood and showed very low platelet adhesion, identifying them as compatible polymers for blood-contacting applications (Welle et al., 1998). The *in vivo* biocompatibility of various fluoroalkoxy and aryloxy polyphosphazenes was demonstrated by intramuscular implantation in a rat model showing minimal tissue response (Wade et al., 1978).

The ability to surface modify materials with bioactive molecules is highly favorable for biomedical applications since surfaces control most of the initial biological response to an implant. Polyphosphazenes are ideal candidates in this respect due to their high reactivity, chemical and radiation stability, and the ease with which polymers with suitable functional groups to tether biologically active molecules can be developed. Most of the initial studies in this direction were aimed at improving the blood compatibility of polyphosphazenes. These include ionic immobilization of biologically active heparin on the surface of quaternized aryloxy polyphosphazenes (Neenan and Allcock, 1982), as well as radiation grafting of hydrophilic polymers on the surface followed by heparin immobilization (Lora et al., 1991). Both the modification processes were found to significantly reduce blood-clotting time on polyphosphazene films. Chemical modification of aryloxy polyphosphazenes such as incorporation of sulfonyl groups were also made to improve the blood compatibility and cytocompatibility of polyphosphazenes. Further, these polymers were found to exhibit antibacterial activity towards *Salmonella typhimirium* (Allcock and Fitzpatrick, 1991).

Various aminated and hydrophilic alkoxy polyphosphazenes have been investigated for ophthalmologic applications due to their good high oxygen permeability, refractive index and low protein adsorption (Allcock, 2003). Similarly fluoroalkoxy polyphosphazenes have been investigated for developing maxillofacial reconstruction prostheses as well as elastomeric denture liners due to their excellent tear-resistance, elasticity, impact-dampening and enhanced resistance to bacterial colonization (Allcock, 2003).

The ease of functionalization makes polyphosphazenes suitable candidates for developing substrates for the immobilization of bioactive molecules. Thus, immobilization of proteins, such as glucose 6-phosphate dehydrogenase and trypsin, were performed on surface-modified poly(diphenoxy phosphazene). The immobilized enzymes were found to have high storage stability and retained their activity through numerous reaction cycles (Allcock and Kwon, 1986). Similarly a protein A immobilized substrate was developed from poly[bis(methyl phenoxy)phosphazene]. The immobilized protein A was found to bind specifically to immunoglobulins (IgG) and has been investigated to develop blood dialysis systems that selectively remove IgG from the blood (Allcock et al., 1994a).

Prototypical polymer-bound chemotherapeutic or herbicidal systems have been synthesized in which bioactive molecules were linked to polyphosphazenes via hydrolytically sensitive bonds as depots for drug delivery. Thus Allcock and coworkers immobilized several bioactive molecules, such as 2,4-dinitrophenylhydrazine, sulfadiazine, 3-hydroxytyramine, 2-amino-4-picoline and citral via Schiff base linkages (Allcock, 2003; Lakshmi et al., 2003). Polyphosphazenes with pendent primary amino groups used to immobilize acetic, propionic, benzoic, acrylic and nicotinic acids, N-acetylglycine, N-acetyl-DL-penicillamine, *p*-(dipropylsulfamoyl)benzoic acid, and 2,4-dichlorophenoxyacetic acid were coupled using dicyclohexylcarbodiimide (DCC) (Allcock, 2003; Lakshmi et al., 2003). Similarly, steroidal residues, such as dexoestrone, estrone, 17β-estradiol, 17α-ethynylestradiol, estradiol 3-methyl ether, and 1,4-dihydro estradiol 3-methyl ether were attached to the polyphosphazene backbone via the sodium salt of steroidal hydroxy function vial alkoxy group to develop a system that slowly releases the steroid by the cleavage of P–O bonds (Allcock, 2003; Lakshmi et al., 2003). Attempts were made to improve the biological activity of local anesthetics such as procaine, benzocaine, chloroprocaine, butyl *p*-aminobenzoate and 2-amino-4-picoline by attaching them to a polyphosphazene backbone by direct aminolysis (Allcock, 2003; Lakshmi et al., 2003).

Polyphosphazenes have also been investigated as a matrix for developing anticancer drug conjugates by the reaction of aminated polyphosphazenes with $K_2PtCl_4$ (Sohn et al., 1997).

### 16.4.2 Hydrolytically Sensitive Polymers

The ability to develop polyphosphazenes that can undergo hydrolytic degradation significantly increased the potential of polyphosphazenes as a biomaterial for transient medical applications. Several studies are currently underway using hydrolytically sensitive polyphosphazenes to develop devices for the controlled delivery of pharmaceutical agents and to develop scaffolds for tissue engineering applications.

The most extensively investigated hydrolytically sensitive polyphosphazenes for biomedical applications are aminated polyphosphazenes. The initial studies were performed by Allcock using a series of aminated polyphosphazenes and demonstrated that rate of degradation of these polymers depend on the nature of the amino groups present. In these compounds hydrolysis is presumed to be triggered either by protonation of the nitrogen atoms in the polymer skeleton or the nitrogen atoms of the side groups (Allcock et al., 1982). Imidazole substituted polyphosphazenes were found to be the most hydrolytically sensitive aminated polyphosphazenes (Scheme 16.25). The study also demonstrated the ability to control the degradation rate of imidazole substituted polymer by cosubstituting them with less hydrolytically sensitive methyl amino groups or methyl phenoxy groups.

Among the aminated polyphosphazenes, the amino acid ester polyphosphazenes are the most preferred candidates for biomedical applications. Allcock and coworkers performed a detailed study on the effects that different amino acid ester side groups have on the rate of degradation of polyphosphazenes (Scheme 16.22) (Allcock et al., 1994c). The ability to form mixed substituent polymers demonstrated the feasibility of controlling the rate of degradation of polymers for specific applications as demonstrated by Laurencin and coworkers using ethylglycinato cosubstituted polyphosphazenes (Figure 16.1) (Laurencin et al., 1993).

Initial studies of amino acid ester polyphosphazenes as biomaterials were carried out to develop controlled drug delivery devices due to the ability to fine control the rate of degradation of the polymers, their excellent biocompatibility and ease of processibility. Thus Grolleman and coworkers developed a system consisting of 65 to 90% of glycine ethyl ester with 10 to 35% of an antiinflammatory agent, naproxen, attached to the polymer backbone via a spacer group such as L-lysine ethyl ester (Allcock, 2003; Lakshmi et al., 2003). Laurencin and coworkers explored the feasibility of imidazole cosubstituted polyphosphazenes (poly[(imidazolyl)(p-methyl phenoxy)phosphazene] as a monolithic controlled drug delivery system (Allcock, 2003; Lakshmi et al., 2003). The *in vitro* studies showed a diffusion-controlled release profile, independent of the initial loading of

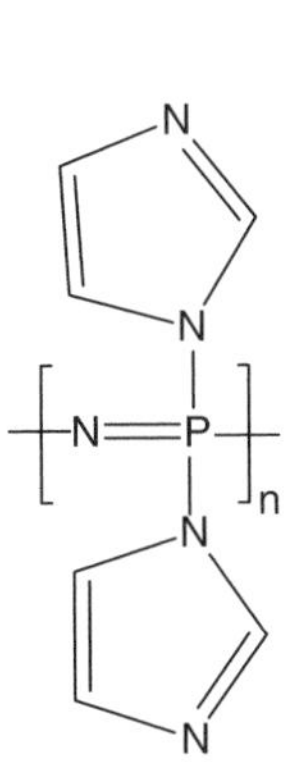

17

**SCHEME 16.25**

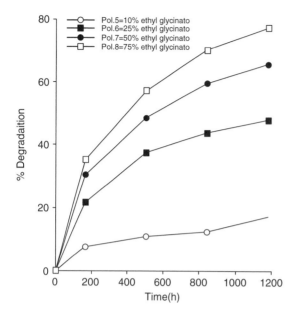

**FIGURE 16.1**
Variation in degradation rates of poly[(ethyl glycinato)(methyl phenoxy)phosphazene] with different ratios of the side groups.

the drug. Caliceti and coworkers used copolymers of amino acid ester with imidazoly to develop matrices for the controlled release of drugs (Allcock, 2003; Lakshmi et al., 2003). The study showed that the release of model drugs such as naproxen, nariclasine and acetyl tryptophanamide depends on polymer composition as well as the rate of polymer degradation. The pharmacological efficacy of the system was demonstrated *in vivo* in acute inflammation and chronic arthritis models in rats. In addition to polymer films, microspheres of these polymers were also formed to encapsulate the drug to develop novel delivery devices ( Allcock, 2003; Lakshmi et al., 2003). The release of insulin from these microsphere matrices showed a bimodal behavior with a burst release followed by a slow release in the range of 2 to 70 h and subcutaneous administration of microspheres to diabetic mice resulted in rapid reduction of glucose levels. The study shows the potential of polyphosphazene matrices for the development of one-shot vaccines.

In addition to aminated polyphosphazenes, several alkoxy-, ethoxy- or aryloxy-substituted polyphosphazenes were investigated as drug delivery devices due to the ability of these polymers to form hydrogels via chemical or radiation cross-linking. The most extensively studied polymer in this class is poly[bis(carboxylato phenoxy)phosphazene] (PCPP) (Scheme 16.18). The polymer becomes water soluble when ionized in neutral or basic solution due to the presence of two carboxyl groups per repeating unit. The ability of PCPP to form hydrogels in the presence of divalent ions such as calcium ions under mild physiological conditions makes it an attractive candidate for microencapsulation technology (Allcock, 2003). Also it has been found that PCPP in its soluble state is a powerful immunostimulant and could form a potential candidate for vaccine delivery (Payne et al., 1998).

The amino acid ester polyphosphazenes were also investigated extensively as candidates for tissue engineering applications due to their biocompatibility and their ability to be processed into two- and three-dimensional matrices (Figure 16.2). Laurencin and coworkers investigated glycine- and alanine-substituted polyphosphazenes as matrices for regenerating musculoskeletal tissues. Thus the glycine cosubstituted polyphosphazenes showed very high adhesion and proliferation of osteoblasts (bone cells) compared to poly(lactide-*co*-glycolide) the most extensively-used hydrolytically sensitive organic polymer (Laurencin et al., 1993). Porous matrices of polyphosphazenes

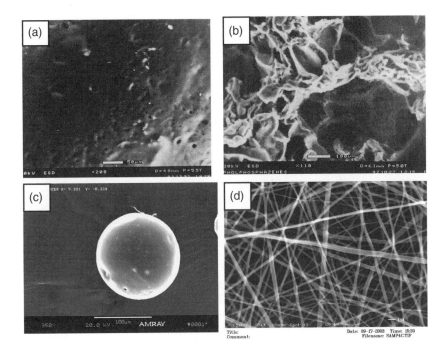

**FIGURE 16.2**
Different structures developed from hydrolytically sensitive polyphosphazenes for biomedical applications.
(a) Thin films, (b) porous sponges, (c) microsphere, (d) nanofibers.

support the proliferation of osteoblast cells demonstrating the ability of these matrices to form tissue constructs (Laurencin et al., 1996). The excellent osteocompatibility of these polymers was also demonstrated by implanting these polymers to augment *in vivo* bone repair in New Zealand White rabbits (Laurenicin et al., 1998).

The amino acid ester-substituted polyphosphazenes were investigated as conduits for peripheral nerve repair due to their flexibility, suturability, translucence and degradation into nontoxic byproducts (Allcock, 2003). Amino acid ester polyphosphazenes were also investigated for guided-tissue regeneration of deep periodontal tissues by Veronese et al. (1999).

All these studies reveal the excellent biocompatibility of polyphosphazenes which make them preferred candidates for a variety of biomedical applications.

## References

Allcock, H.R., *Polymer*, **21**, 673 (1980).
Allcock, H.R., *Chemistry and Applications of Polyphosphazenes*, Wiley, Hoboken, NJ (2003).
Allcock, H.R. and Best, R.J., Phophonitrile compounds I, *Can. J. Chem.*, **42**, 447 (1964).
Allcock, H.R. and Chu, C.T.W., *Macromolecues*, **12**, 551 (1979).
Allcock, H.R., Dodge, J.A., Manners, I., and Riding, G.H., *J. Am. Chem. Soc.*, **113**, 9596–9603 (1991).
Allcock, H.R. and Fitzpatrick, R.J., *Chem. Mater.*, **3**, 1120 (1991).
Allcock, H.R., Fuller, T.J., Mack, D.P., Matsumura, K., and Smeltz, K.M., *Macromolecules*, **10**, 824–830 (1977).
Allcock, H.R., Fuller, T.J., and Matsumura, K., *Inorg. Chem.*, **21**, 515 (1982).

Allcock, H.R. and Kugel, R.L., *J. Am. Chem. Soc.*, **87**, 4216 (1965).

Allcock, H.R., Kugel, R.L., and Valan, K.J., *Inorg. Chem.*, **5**, 1709 (1966).

Allcock, H.R. and Kwon, S., *Macromolecules*, **19**, 1502–1508 (1986).

Allcock, H.R. and Kwon, S., *Macromolecules*, **21**, 1980 (1988).

Allcock, H.R., Lavin, K.D., and Riding, G.H., *Macromolecules*, **18**, 1340 (1985).

Allcock, H.R., Nelson, C.J., and Coggio, W.D., *Chem. Mater.*, **6**, 516–524 (1994a).

Allcock, H.R. and Patterson, D.B., *Inorg. Chem.*, **16**, 197 (1977).

Allcock, H.R. and Pucher, S.R., *Macromolecules*, **24**, 23 (1991).

Allcock, H.R., Pucher, S.R., and Scopelianos, A.G., *Macromolecules*, **27**, 1 (1994b).

Allcock, H.R., Pucher, S.R., and Scopelianos, A.G., *Macromolecules*, **27**, 1071–1075 (1994c).

Allen, G., Lewis, C.J., and Todd, S.M., *Polymer*, **11**, 31 (1970).

Archer, R.D., *Inorganic and Organometallic Polymers*, Wiley, New York (2001).

Hagnauer, G.L., *J. Macromol. Sci. Chem.*, **A16**, 385 (1981).

Honeyman, C.H., Manners, I., Morrissey, C.T., and Allcock, H.R., *J. Am. Chem. Soc.*, **117**, 7035 (1995).

Jones, R.G., Ando, W., and Chojnowski, J., Eds., *Silicon-Containing Polymers: The Science and Technology of their Synthesis and Applications*, Kluwer, Boston, MA (2000).

Lakshmi, S., Katti, D.S., and Laurencin, C.T., *Adv. Drug Deliv. Rev.*, **55**, 467–482 (2003).

Laurenicin, C.T., Ambrosio, A.M.A., Bauer, T.W., Allcock, H.R., Attawia, M.A., Borden, M.D., Gorum, W.J., and Frank, D. *Proceedings of the Society for Biomaterials 24th Annual Meeting in Conjunction with the 30th International Symposium*, San Diego, CA (1998).

Laurencin, C.T., El-Amin, S.F., Ibim, S.E., Willoughby, D.A., Attawia, M., Allcock, H.R., and Ambrosio, A.A., *J. Biomed. Mater. Res.*, **30**, 1338 (1996).

Laurencin, C.T., Norman, M.E., Elgendy, H.M., El-Amin, S.F., Allcock, H.R., Pucher, S.R., and Ambrosio, A.A., *J. Biomed. Mater. Res.*, **27**, 963–973 (1993).

Lora, S., Carenza, M., Plama, G., Pezzin, G., Calceti, P., Battaglia, P., and Lora, A., *Biomaterials*, **12**, 275 (1991).

Manners, I., Riding, G.H., Dodge, J.A., and Allcock, H.R., *J. Am. Chem. Soc.*, **111**, 3067 (1989).

Matyjaszewski, K., Montague, R., Dauth, J., and Nuyken, O., *J. Polym. Sci.*, **30**, 813 (1992).

Montague, R.A. and Matyjaszewski, K., *J. Am. Chem. Soc.*, **112**, 6721 (1990).

Neenan, T.X. and Allcock, H.R., *Biomaterials*, **3**, 78 (1982).

Neilson, R.H. and Wisian-Neilson, P., *Chem. Rev.*, **88**, 541 (1988).

Payne, L.G., Jenkins, S.A., Woods, A.L., Grund, E.M., Geribo, W.E., Loebelenz, J.R., Andrianov, A.K., and Robers, B.E., *Vaccine*, **16**, 92 (1998).

Sohn, Y.S., Baek, H.G., Cho, Y.H., Lee, Y.A., Jung, O.S., Lee, C.O., and Kim, Y.S., *Int. J. Pharm.*, **153**, 79 (1997).

Veronese, F.M., Marsilio, F., Lora, S., Caliceti, P., Passi, P., and Orsolini, P., *Biomaterials*, **20**, 91 (1999).

Wade, C.W.R., Gourlay, S., Rice, R., Hegyeli, A., Singler, R., and White, J., *Organometallic Polymers*, Carraher, C.E., Sheats, J.E., and Pittman, C.U., Eds., Academic Press, New York, pp. 283 (1978).

Welle, A., Grunze, M., and Tur, D., *J. Colloid Interface Sci.*, **197**, 263 (1998).

Wisian-Neilson, P. and Neilson, R.H., *Inorg. Synth.*, **25**, 69 (1989).

# 17

## Metallic Biomaterials

Henry R. Piehler

## CONTENTS

## 17.1   Introduction

Metals and alloys have been and continue to be very widely used in implantable medical devices. The following data, extracted from Table 2 of Ratner et al. (2004), serve to illustrate this point:

| Device | Annual Number of Devices (U.S.) |
|---|---|
| Intraocular lenses (2003) | 2,500,000 |
| Vascular grafts | 300,000 |
| **Heart valves | 100,000 (some) |
| **Pacemakers | 400,000 |
| Breast prostheses | 250,000 |
| *Coronary stents | 1,500,000 |
| *Hip prostheses (2002) | 250,000 |
| *Knee prostheses (2002) | 250,000 |
| *Dental implants (2000) | 910,000 |

* indicates all or predominantly metal; ** indicates metal containing.

These data indicate that metals and alloys are widely used, not only in more traditional devices such as hip and knee prostheses, but also in newer devices such as cardiovascular stents, which are widely recognized as the most important cardiovascular device introduced in the last decade.

The history and use of much of the current use of metallic materials in implantable medical devices has been extensively described previously (Bechtol et al., 1959; Park, 1984; Helsen and Breme, 1998; Brunette et al., 2001; Grimm, 2002; Shrivastava, 2003; Ratner et al., 2004). Following a brief review of the standards for traditional metallic biomaterials, the focus of this review is on:

- Microstructural influences on metallic implant performance, including failure
- Recent innovations in microstructure and configuration of metallic biomaterials
- New or revisited uses of metallic biomaterials in implantable medical devices
- Modeling of metallic implant performance
- Future developments for enhancing metallic or hybrid implant performance

The range of devices considered will be limited to orthopedic and cardiovascular implants.

Metallic biomaterials for implantable medical devices, as other biomaterials for the same applications, have fundamental mechanical integrity and biocompatibility requirements. The mechanical integrity requirements include resistance to permanent deformation under monotonic loading, resistance to crack initiation and propagation, and resistance to wear. The biocompatibility requirements include those that focus on the effects of the physiological environment on the *in vivo* performance of the implant itself as well as the effects of the implant on local and systemic tissue. Examples of the former include the influences of the physiological environment on mechanical integrity and surface degradation by processes such as corrosion; examples of the latter include allergic response to metallic ions liberated from the metallic implants and local and/or systemic responses to wear debris, either from the implant itself or from the material on which the metallic implant articulates, which could be a polymer.

## 17.2   Standards for Metallic Biomaterials

Metallic biomaterials can be conveniently grouped in the following categories (Lemons and Freese, 2002):

1. Specialty steels
2. Cobalt base alloys
3. Titanium alloys
4. Specialty metallic alloys

Standards for these metallic biomaterials (with ASTM, ISO, and UNS designations) are referenced in Table 17.1 (Lemons and Freese, 2002) below.

Several metallic biomaterials included in Table 17.1 will be examined subsequently in more detail.

Several points need to be emphasized regarding the standards included in Table 17.1. The first is that these standards focus on properties (or performance in laboratory test)

**TABLE 17.1**

Metallic Biomaterials for Medical and Surgical Implants

| Material Designation | Common Name or Trade Name | UNS Designation | ASTM Standard | ISO Standard |
|---|---|---|---|---|
| *Speciality Steel Biomaterials* | | | | |
| Fe–18Cr–14Ni–2.5Mo | 316 L Stainless Steel | S31673 | ASTM F 138 | ISO 5832-1 |
| Fe–18Cr–12.5Ni–2.5Mo, Cast | 316 L Stainless Steel | Unassigned | ASTM F 745 | — |
| Fe–21Cr–10Ni–3.5Mn–2.5Mo | "REX 734" | S31675 | ASTM F 1586 | ISO 5832-9 |
| Fe–22Cr–12.5Ni–5Mn–2.5Mo | "XM-19" | S20910 | ASTM F 1314 | — |
| Fe–23Mn–21Cr–1Mo–1N | "108" | Unassigned | F-04.12.35 | — |
| *Cobalt Base Biomaterials* | | | | |
| Co–28Cr–6Mo Casting Alloy | Cast CoCrMo | R30075 | ASTM F 75 | ISO 5832-4 |
| Co–28Cr–6Mo Wrought Alloy #1 | Wrought CoCrMo, Alloy 1 | R31537 | ASTM F 1537 | ISO 5832-12 |
| Co–28Cr–6Mo Wrought Alloy #2 | Wrought CoCrMo, Alloy 2 | R31538 | ASTM F 1537 | ISO 5832-12 |
| Co–28Cr–6Mo Wrought Alloy #3 | Wrought CoCrMo, "GADS" | R31539 | ASTM F 1537 | — |
| Co–20Cr–15W–10Ni–1.5Mn | "L-605" | R30605 | ASTM F 90 | ISO 5832-5 |
| Co–20Ni–20Cr–5Fe–3.5Mo–3.5W–2Ti | "Syncoben" | R30563 | ASTM F 563 | ISO 5832-8 |
| Co–19Cr–7Ni–14Fe–7Mo–1.5Mn | Grade 2 "Phynox" | R30008 | ASTM F 1058 | ISO 5832-7 |
| Co–20Cr–15Ni–15Fe–7Mo–2Mn | Grade 1 "Elgiloy" | R30003 | ASTM F 1058 | ISO 5832-7 |
| Co–35Ni–20Cr–10Mo | "35N" | R30035 | ASTM F 562 | ISO 5832-6 |
| *Titanium Base Biomaterials* | | | | |
| Ti CP-1 | CP-1 (Alpha) | R50250 | ASTM F 67 | ISO 5832-2 |
| Ti CP-2 | CP-2 (Alpha) | R50400 | ASTM F 67 | ISO 5832-2 |
| Ti CP-3 | CP-3 (Alpha) | R50550 | ASTM F 67 | ISO 5832-2 |

*(continued)*

**TABLE 17.1**  (Continued)

| Material Designation | Common Name (Alloy Classification) | UNS Designation | ASTM Standard | ISO Standard |
|---|---|---|---|---|
| Ti CP-4 | CP-4 (Alpha) | R50700 | ASTM F 67 | ISO 5832-2 |
| Ti–3Al–2.5V | Ti–3Al–2.5W (Alpha/Beta) | R56320 | ASTM F 2146 | — |
| Ti–5Al–2.5Fe | Tikrutan (Alpha/Beta) | Unassigned | — | ISO 5832-10 |
| Ti–6Al–4V | Ti–6Al–4V (Alpha/Beta) | R56400 | ASTM F 1472 | ISO 5832-3 |
| Ti–6Al–4V, Cast | Ti–6Al–4V (Alpha/Beta) | R56406 | ASTM F 1108 | — |
| Ti–6Al–4V ELI | Ti–6Al–4V ELI (Alpha/Beta) | R56401 | ASTM F 136 | ISO 5832-3 |
| Ti–6Al–7Nb | Ti–6Al–7Nb (Alpha/Beta) | R56700 | ASTM F 1295 | ISO 5832-11 |
| Ti–15Mo | Ti–15Mo (Metastable Beta) | R58150 | ASTM F 2066 | — |
| Ti–12Mo–6Zr–2Fe* | "TMZF" (Metastable Beta) | R58120 | ASTM F 1813 | — |
| Ti–11.5Mo–6Zr–4.5Sn | "Beta 3" (Metastable Beta) | R58030 | AMS-T-9046 | — |
| Ti–13Nb–13Zr* | Ti–13Nb–13Zr (Metastable Beta) | R58130 | ASTM F 1713 | — |
| Ti–45Nb | Ti–45Nb (Metastable Beta) | R58450 | F-04.12.44 | — |
| Ti–35Nb–7Zr–5Ta* | "TiOsteum" (Metastable Beta) | R58350 | F-04.12.23 | — |
| *Specialty Metallic Biomaterials* | | | | |
| Ta, Unalloyed, Cast | Unalloyed Tantalum (Alpha) | R05200 | ASTM F 560 | — |
| Zr–2.5Nb | "Zircadyne" 705 | R60705 | F-04.12.45 | — |
| Ni–45Ti | "Nitinol" (Intermetallic) | N01555 | ASTM F 2063 | — |

*Notes and references:* Material designations with asterisks are patented. Common names in quotation marks may be proprietary or registered trademarks. Information in italics refers to ASTM task groups (standards "in progress") or other standards organizations such as SAE. *Annual Book of ASTM Standards* (2001). Vol. 13.01, ASTM, West Conshohocken, PA, www.astm.org. *Metals and Alloys in the Unified Numbering System* (2001). 9th ed., ASTM, West Conshohocken, PA, www.astm.org. *Stelachaussel* (Key to Steels). Verlag Stelachaussel Wegst GmbH, Marbach, Germany.

rather than for performance in actual clinical use. Hence conformance to these property standards does not guarantee an acceptable level of clinical performance for a given implant. The second is that there is no such thing as an FDA-approved biomaterial. The FDA focuses exclusively on devices, not materials. The prior successful use of a material in a similar device will aid in the acceptance of a new device; the prior use of a material in a different device application will have virtually no influence on the approval of the fundamentally different new device. Teflon provides an excellent example of this drastically different performance in different applications. Teflon is a widely and successfully used as an implantable fabric; its use in mandibular implants has been a total disaster (ironically, as was its prior use in acetabular cups). There is also often a considerable variability in clinical performance obtainable for materials that all fall within a standard's compositional limits for both essential and tramp elements. Device manufacturers often specify materials at the boundaries of these compositional limits to enhance fabricability and/or clinical performance. Finally, the laboratory and clinical performance of a metallic biomaterial that conforms to specific compositional requirements can be altered by changing its microstructure through changes in its processing history.

## 17.3  Microstructural Influences on Metallic Implant Performance

The ASTM standards in Table 17.1 were promulgated by ASTM Committee F04 on Medical and Surgical Materials and Devices, subcommittee F04.12 on Metallurgical Materials. This committee was established in 1962; its activities are available on the web (www.astm.org). In the early 1970s there was considerable debate concerning how to proceed with fatigue performance testing of orthopedic implants. Fracture mechanics at that time was dominated by the aircraft industry, where fatigue-crack propagation rather than fatigue-crack initiation was of primary concern. It was not entirely clear that this should be true for the fatigue of orthopedic implants. Another issue was the role, if any, of the physiological environment on fatigue performance. Laboratory performance testing and microstructural characterization were extremely helpful in addressing both these issues.

Sloter (1979) and Sloter and Piehler (1979) performed fatigue and corrosion-fatigue performance tests on several orthopedic hip nails configured to simulate a nonunion, the common precursor to implant fatigue failure. His load vs. number of cycles to failure data showed that the presence of the simulated physiological environment (Ringers solution) reduced the number of cycles to failure at a given load. This clearly indicated the need to perform fatigue testing in a physiological environment. Microstructural and fractographic characterization using optical and scanning electron microscopy confirmed this need for environmental testing and answered the fatigue-crack initiation/propagation question as well. Since the laboratory fatigue crack was not damaged, the origin of the crack could be determined optically. A scanning electron micrograph of the area at and near the fracture origin is shown in Figure 17.1. Both the fracture surface (top) and the surface of the implant itself (bottom) are shown; the crack origin is in the center of the micrograph at the intersection of these two surfaces. The parallel lines on the implant surface are intrusions and extrusions formed during fatigue loading. Their role in initiating the fatigue crack is apparent. Noteworthy also is the staining from corrosion in the area where intrusions and extrusions have formed, indicating an association between corrosion and fatigue-crack initiation. Hence this figure shows both that the fatigue crack is initiated as a result of fatigue loading (rather than being present initially) and that corrosion is associated with the deformation-induced fatigue-crack initiation. Whether corrosion preceded, followed, or occurred contemporaneously with intrusion/extrusion formation cannot be determined

20 μm

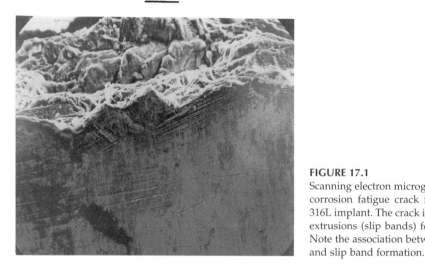

**FIGURE 17.1**
Scanning electron micrograph at the origin of a corrosion fatigue crack in a laboratory-tested 316L implant. The crack initiated at intrusions/extrusions (slip bands) formed during testing. Note the association between surface corrosion and slip band formation.

from this micrograph alone. However, the reduction in fatigue life of the implants tested in Ringers solution compared to that of the devices tested in air indicates that corrosion occurred prior to or contemporaneously with intrusion/extrusion formation.

Gilbert (1982), Gilbert and Piehler (1989) studied the corrosion-fatigue behavior of Ti–6Al–4V hip prostheses that were fabricated by machining, conventional forging, and flashless forging. Optical micrographs of the flashlessly forged material in three orientations were used to create the three-dimensional representation of the microstructure shown in Figure 17.2. The microstructure consists of lamellar colonies of the α- and β-phases in a matrix of α. (It should be noted that there are current efforts to use sectioning and computerized tomographic techniques to display actual three-dimensional microstructures (Lanzagazorta et al., 1998)). Such efforts have provided new insights into the relationships among processing, structure, and performance in test and/or service. To the best of my knowledge, no such three-dimensional microstructural representation has been created for an implant material. Gilbert identified the onset

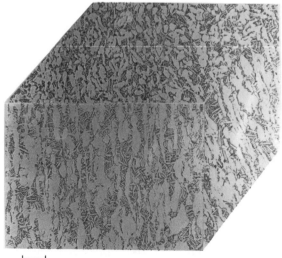

20 μm

**FIGURE 17.2**
Three-dimensional representation of the microstructure of a flashlessly-forged Ti–6Al–4V hip prosthesis.

of fatigue-crack initiation by monitoring the corrosion potential of the implant during corrosion-fatigue testing. The initiation of a fatigue crack broke down the passive layer on the implant surface, resulting in a marked increase in corrosion potential which was used to shut down the test. Scanning electron micrographs of the likely crack-initiation site are shown in Figure 17.3(a) and (b) (the fatigue crack is vertical). Several important observations can be made from these figures:

1. Crack initiation did not occur at any of the surface imperfections evident in Figure 17.3(a).
2. The crack initiation site is similar in topography to the microstructure shown in Figure 17.1.
3. Early shutdown of the test preserved the crystallographic nature of the crack-initiation site; continued exposure to the corrosive environment would have turned this initiation site into a "corrosion pit", thus obscuring its microstructural origin.

Hence reducing the surface roughness of the implant compared to that shown in Figure 17.3 will have no noticeable effect on delaying fatigue-crack initiation; any attempt to delay fatigue-crack initiation must focus on the microstructural origin of the crack-initiation process.

The use of welds in metallic implantable devices has had a long and varied history. Perhaps the most glaring example is the fatigue failure of the Björk-Shiley 60° convexo-concave tilting disc heart valve (U.S. Congress, 1990). This heart valve had an outlet strut that was welded to the annulus, both of which were of the cobalt base alloy Haynes 25 or L-605. This valve was implanted in 86,000 people worldwide; there were approximately 1500 failures and 1000 deaths. All investigators agree that the failure involved an inherent design flaw which caused an abnormal loading on the tip of the outlet strut. The role of the single-pass tungsten inert gas autogenous unannealed weld is widely debated. There have been numerous metallurgical analyses which point to weld flaws as a conjoint cause of outlet-strut fracture, a view bolstered by the statistical conclusion that weld date and welder identity are two of the four criteria used when considering valve explantation. Some of these metallurgical analyses appeared in medical journals, which lack the expertise to conduct an adequate peer review. An example of the consequences of this inadequate review is the misinterpretation of Figure 4(a) of Böcklein et al. (1989), where

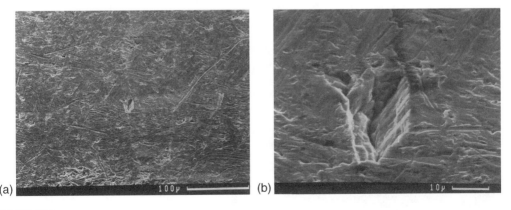

**FIGURE 17.3**
(a) Scanning electron micrograph of the surface of a flashlessly-forged Ti–6Al–4V hip prosthesis showing the initiation of a laboratory-produced fatigue crack (vertical). The crack-initiation site is at the center. Note that the crack did not appear to initiate at surface scratches. (b) Higher magnification micrograph of area shown in (a).

abrasion is incorrectly identified as cleavage This incorrect observation would lead to inappropriate microstructural amelioration efforts.

Not all welds in fatigue-critical areas are necessarily inadequate, however. Some cardiovascular stents are successfully fabricated using inert gas shielded multiple-pass autogenous laser welding. Final annealing results in an equiaxed microstructure where the weld is indistinguishable from the parent metal (personal communication).

## 17.4   Recent Innovations in Microstructure and Configuration of Metallic Biomaterials

*Trabecular Metal (Porous Tantalum):*   Trabecular metal is a porous tantalum biomaterial with an interconnected porosity of approximately 75% and a mean tetrakaidodecahedral pore size of approximately 430 $\mu$m, A scanning electron micrograph of Trabecular metal is shown in Figure 17.4. It is similar in appearance and stiffness to dense cancellous bone. The surface also has a pronounced microtexture on the individual struts which results from the crystallographic nature of the deposition process. This Ta strut surface promotes rapid tissue in-growth and strong fixation. Trabecular metal can be used as an implant itself or as an in-growth material on a substrate such as in hip and knee prostheses.

The fabrication process involves the pyrolysis of a thermosetting polymer foam precursor to form a skeletal structure on to which tantalum is deposited by chemical vapor deposition/infiltration. A typical Ta coating thickness is 40 to 60 $\mu$m. This porous structure has a compressive elastic modulus of 2.5 to 3.9 GPa, an ultimate compressive strength of 50 to 70 MPa, and a 10-million cycle endurance limit in four-point bending of 18 to 20 MPa (Bobyn et al., 1999b).

Animal studies revealed that trabecular metal facilitated rapid bone (Bobyn et al., 1999a) and vascularized soft tissue (Hacking et al., 2000) in-growth. The soft tissue attachment strength to porous tantalum was three to sixfold greater than that measured previously for porous samples created using sintered Co–Cr beads (Bobyn et al., 1982).

A porous tantalum acetabular cup with a direct compression molded polyethylene insert, in use since 1997, is shown in Figure 17.5. This creates an integral polyethylene/porous tantalum interface and a low stiffness component. This device is designed to

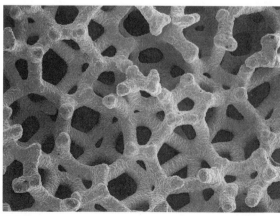

200 µm

**FIGURE 17.4**
Scanning electron micrograph of porous tantalum (Trabecular metal).

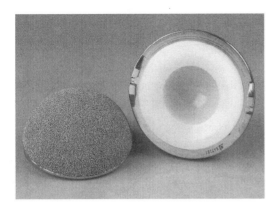

**FIGURE 17.5**

Acetabular cup with porous tantalum backing inter-locked into compression molded polyethylene.

reduce the articular stress and wear and eliminate backside wear entirely. A multicenter clinical study with a follow-up of 2 to 5 years (Gruen et al., 2005) revealed that 412 of 414 cups were osseointegrated; there was no lysis in any of the 414 cases.

*β-Titanium Alloys*:  The interest in β-titanium alloys for biomedical applications is driven by their lower modulus compared to alpha-beta alloys, the most common of which is Ti–6Al–4V, the workhorse of the aerospace industry. Various β-alloys, such as Ti–15Mo, have been around for decades, but their difficulty in manufacture and lack of biocompatibility information limited their introduction to the marketplace. Hence device manufacturers had to choose between biocompatibility testing of existing alloys or developing entirely new alloys and then testing for their biocompatibility. ASTM standards were published for the Ti–15Mo in 2000(F 2066) and for two new alloys in 1997 (F 1713 and F 1813). Data for all these alloys along with Ti–6Al–4V are shown in Table 17.2 below.

Hence there is the opportunity to reduce the modulus by about one third compared to that of Ti–6Al–4V. Yield strengths are comparable or substantially below that of Ti–6Al–4V.

Additional new β-alloys, such as Ti–35Nb–7Zr–5Ta (Gruen et al., 2005), are currently being evaluated for use as biomaterials. This same alloy demonstrated superior bone filling characteristics than CP Ti, Ti–6Al–4V, and Ti–15Mo–2.8Nb–Si-3O (Hawkins et al., 2000). The adhesive strengths of this alloy were also markedly superior to those of the other alloys.

*Nickel Free Stainless Steel*:  Nickel serves to stabilize the (nonmagnetic) austenitic phase in stainless steels used as biomaterials (316L contains >11.5% Ni). Although metal sensitivity is a problem in only 5% of the patient population, nickel accounts for about 90% of these adverse reactions (Hierholzer and Hierholzer, 1992). One approach to Ni removal in implant-quality stainless steels has been to add substantial amounts of manganese and nitrogen to stabilize the austenitic phase. A nickel-free 108 alloy containing 21.59 Cr,

**TABLE 17.2**

Selected Mechanical Properties for Selected ASTM Material Specifications (annealed condition)

| Alloy Designation | Elastic Modulus (GPa) | ASTM Standard | Yield Strength (MPa) |
| --- | --- | --- | --- |
| Ti–15Mo | 77.7 | F 2066 | 483 |
| Ti–13Nb–13 Zr | 64–77 | F 1713 | 345 |
| Ti–12Mo–6Zr–2Fe | 74–85 | F 1813 | 897 |
| (Ti–6Al–4V | 110 | F 1472 | 860 |

0.74 Mo, 23.91 Mn, 0.97 N, and 0.02 Ni was evaluated for its corrosion resistance and compared to that of CP Ti and 316L stainless steel (Desigi et al., 2000). The results indicated that the corrosion resistance of this nickel-free alloy was superior to that of 316L stainless steel but inferior to that of CP titanium. Results for the physical, mechanical, and metallurgical properties of the nickel-free alloy 108 indicated that these properties were generally comparable to those of the nickel containing alloys 316L and an alloy conforming to ASTM 1314 (Roach et al., 2001).

*Microclean Co–Ni–Cr–Mo Alloy*:  Metal cleanliness improves both fabricability and service performance. This is especially true for wires, which undergo substantial deformation during thermomechanical processing. Nonmetallic inclusions typically form in the melt and may or may not be broken up during processing. Those which do not break up become increasingly dangerous as deformation proceeds, since they occupy an increasingly larger fraction of the cross-sectional area, either on the surface or in the interior of the wire. Recent advances in second-phase particle control have led to substantial improvements in fabricability, wear resistance, and fatigue lifetime compared to a less clean alloy that still conforms to the specifications for ASTM F 562. This improved alloy has been designated 35N LT and is described in several patents to Fehring et al. (2001, 2003, 2004). The optimization of the melt chemistry and properties of 35N LT has been reported by Bradley et al. (2004), and is summarized below.

The principal changes in chemistry have been directed at removing carbide, nitride, and sigma second phase particles. This was accomplished by:

1. Reducing the tramp elements P and S virtually to 0
2. Reducing the Fe content by a factor of 10
3. Reducing the elements C, Si,, Mn, B, and Ti essentially to 0

Surface visualization analysis revealed that the surface performance of 35N LT was increased anywhere from 46 to 65% over that of the ASTM F 562 alloy.

The tensile yield stress, ultimate tensile stress, and percentage elongation of 35N LT were nearly identical to those for the ASTM F 562 alloy. The fatigue behavior of 35N LT, on the other hand, is substantially improved over that of the ASTM F 562 alloy, as is shown in Table 17.3 below.

These results indicate that the endurance limit of 35N LT is at least 10,000 psi larger that that of the ASTM F 562 alloy, which adds a healthy increment that will be appreciated by designers.

*Equal Channel Angular Extrusion*:   Equal channel angular extrusion (ECAE) is a forming process that was developed in Russia by Segal (1995) among others. It is a pure-shear

**TABLE 17.3**

Average Number of Cycles to Failure

| Stress (ksi) | ASTM F 562 Alloy | 35N LT |
| --- | --- | --- |
| 250 | 11,130 | 9,550 |
| 200 | 27,070 | 33,780 |
| 150 | 86,530 | 144,900 |
| 125 | 218,700 | 9,835,000 |
| 110 | 1,154,000 | 33,470,000 |
| 100 | 6,774,000 | 54,000,000 |
| 90 | 17,610,000 | (not tested) |

process that is capable of imposing enormous strains during processing, especially if multiple passes are used. Among the microstructural benefits obtainable by ECAE is a substantial degree of grain refinement compared to that obtainable by conventional thermomechanical processing. This grain refinement has been useful to enhance subsequent superplastic deformation and has also been shown to improve high-cycle fatigue resistance (Chung et al., 2002).

This severe plastic deformation (SPD) technique has been used by Valiev et al. (2004) to improve the properties of CP Ti for use in medical applications. This process, especially when coupled with subsequent thermomechanical processing, can produce mechanical properties which are comparable to those of annealed Ti–6Al–4V. For example, various SPD and subsequent thermomechanical processing routes for CP Ti can lead to yield stresses ranging from 625 to 915 MPa, compared to 380 for coarse-grained CP Ti. For comparison, the yield stress of Ti–6Al–4V is 875 MPa. The fatigue limit for SPD CP Ti was found to be 403 to 500 MPa. Again, the comparable fatigue-limit values for coarse-grained CP Ti and Ti–6Al–4V are 238 and 515 MPa, respectively. Hence SPD CP Ti is a viable candidate to replace Ti–6Al–4V in implantable medical devices, thus avoiding any potential biocompatibility problems associated with V and/or Al.

## 17.5 New or Revisited Uses of Metallic Biomaterials in Implantable Medical Devices

*Metal-on-Metal Articulation of Hip Prostheses*: Metal-on-metal articulation of hip prostheses was commonplace until the mid-1970s. The change to metal-on-polyethylene was prompted largely by the occurrence of early cup loosening in metal-on-metal prostheses, which was probably influenced by both the metal-on-metal wear process and the fundamental implant design configuration. In the late 1980s Sulzer Orthopedics in Switzerland introduced its metal-on-metal articulating Metasul prosthesis design that provided increased space between the femoral head and the acetabular component to encourage both fluid film lubrication and wear debris clearance. Recent interest in a return to metal-on-metal articulation of hip prostheses has been rekindled largely as a result of the occurrence of bone lysis associated with polyethylene wear debris (Schmalzried et al., 1992). Linear wear rates of more than 0.2 mm/year were observed in cemented prostheses and linked to bone changes and loosening (Willert et al., 1990); in addition, similar observations that osteolysis and loosening occurred at a greater rate when linear wear rates exceeded 0.2 mm/year were made for uncemented prostheses (Wan and Dorr, 1996). Further impetus for the return to metal-on-metal articulation was provided by Jantsch et al. (1991), who reported an average wear rate on three retrieved metal-on-metal articulating prostheses of only 0.001 mm/year over an average of 14 years.

Dorr et al. (2000) have presented 4- to 7-year clinical results with the Metasul metal-on-metal (Co–Cr) articulating hip prostheses. Seventy patients had a total hip replacement with a Metasul prosthesis and a cemented Weber cup from 1991 to 1994. The study group was 56 of these 70 patients for which complete clinical and radiographic data for periods of 4 to 6.8 years were available. Of these 56 patients, three required revision surgery: one for a loose cup and two because of dislocation. The average Harris total hip score for the 53 remaining patients was 89.6. No patient had a loose or revised femoral component. Based on the results of this study Dorr et al. concluded that the clinical results using metal-on-metal articulation are similar to those using metal-on-polyethylene articulation over a similar 4- to 7-year time frame.

A number of metal-on-metal wear studies have been performed to assess the extent of wear particle and ion generation and its clinical consequences. These include laboratory *in vitro* wear tests (Bader et al., 2005; Bowsher et al., 2005a, 2005b; Williams et al., 2005) and numerical modeling (Jin and Fisher, 2005) as well as clinical studies (Heisel et al., 2005; Skipor et al., 2005) of metal ion concentrations under a variety of conditions. The results of these studies are often contradictory. Laboratory simulations of wear (Bowsher et al., 2005a) indicate that "severe" patient activity substantially increases wear particle surface. Clinical results from patients with metal-on-metal bearing hip prostheses (Heisel et al., 2005) revealed no correlation between Co and Cr ion concentration and patient activity. Results from patients with metal-on-metal bilateral surface or total hip arthroplasty (Skipor et al., 2005) showed a general increase in metal ion concentration over the unilateral levels following the second surface or total hip arthroplasty. However, some patients had second prosthesis-related increases that were significantly more than twice the unilateral levels. These authors pointed out that the clinical significance of their ion concentration measurements remains unknown, since there are no reliable threshold values for the toxicity of degradation products of metal orthopedic implants. Theoretical and experimental studies of the effects of different lubrication regimes and lubricants on the friction of metal-on-metal and ceramic-on-ceramic bearings (Williams et al., 2005) indicated that increases in concentration of the bovine serum used in wear testing decreased the coefficient of friction of metal-on-metal bearings but increased it in ceramic-on-ceramic bearings. Another laboratory simulation of vibrational effects in metal-on-polyethylene, metal-on-metal, and ceramic-on-ceramic implants (Bader et al., 2005) indicated that the amplitude and range of vibration increased dramatically when the femoral head was separated from the acetabular cup during impact conditions. The hard metal-on-metal and ceramic-on-ceramic conditions also resulted in the largest magnitude of the dominant frequency and led to larger impulse signals generated on impact, which could damage the implants or bones in clinical use. Another laboratory simulation (Bowsher et al., 2005b) found that larger prosthesis head diameters have the potential to reduce ion release from metal-on-metal wear. The result of all these tests and simulations is that the mechanical performance and local biocompatability response of metal-on-metal prostheses appears promising; the long-term systemic effects remain unanswered and must await the results of implant retrieval analyses.

Several metal-on-metal articulating prostheses are currently in use in the United States. These include the Metasul and the Ultamet prostheses. The Ultamet cobalt–chromium metal-on-metal articulating prosthesis is shown in Figure 17.6. This prosthesis has a metal acetabular liner that articulates on the metal femoral head.

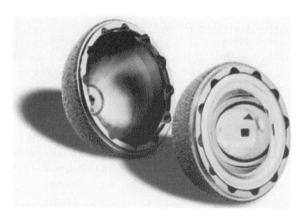

**FIGURE 17.6**
Ultamet metal-on-metal articulating prosthesis.

*Hybrid Metallic Implants:*   While the ultimate clinical goal is clearly to move from tissue replacement to tissue regeneration and total resorption of scaffolds, there are existing and potential hybrid applications involving metallic materials that make sense to pursue until this ultimate goal is achieved. A hybrid metallic device will be taken here to contain a mechanically functioning metallic component in addition to a biologic or pharmacologic component. These latter components must actively promote tissue development not only at the metallic interface but in areas removed from the metallic interface as well. This definition excludes coatings such as HA, which behave more like a surface catalyst rather than a bulk reactant. Two examples of such hybrid devices are bone morphogenetic protein containing spinal cages and drug eluting cardiovascular stents.

The Infuse spinal cage is the first hybrid device approved by the FDA that contains recombinant bone morphogenetic protein (rhBMP-2) in a threaded Ti spinal cage (metallic plus biologic component). This FDA approval, along with the approval for reimbursement by the Center for Medicare and Medicaid Services, was based on the results of a multicenter, prospective, randomized, nonblinded, 2-year study which involved 279 patients with degenerative lumbar disc disease (Burkus et al., 2002). In addition to a tapered-thread Ti spinal fusion cage, the investigational group of 143 patients were given rhBMP-2 in an absorbable sponge of collagen. The control group of 136 patients were given an autogenous iliac bone graft instead. Fusion was evaluated at 6, 12, and 24 months after surgery. Mean operative times for the investigative and control groups were 1.6 and 2.0 h, respectively; the corresponding blood losses were 109.8 and 153.1 ml. After 24 months the fusion rate of the investigational was 94.5% compared to 88.7% for the control group. Various pain measures and neurologic status improved in both groups with similar outcomes. Eight adverse events occurred in the control group related to the iliac crest harvest (5.9%). At 24 months 32% of the control patients reported bone graft site discomfort and 16% were bothered by its appearance. Clearly this hybrid device using rhBMP-2 and a tapered Ti fusion cage can result in a solid union while at the same time obviating the need for harvesting the iliac crest bone graft.

*Drug Eluting Cardiovascular Stents:*   Drug eluting cardiovascular stents are the latest hybrid device (metallic plus pharmacologic components) used to treat stenosed blood vessels percutaneously rather than by open heart bypass surgery. The first percutaneous transluminal angioplasty was balloon angioplasty, which typically resulted in a restenosis rate at the same site of the order of 50% over 5 years. The restenosis rate with balloon angioplasty was approximately halved with the introduction of cardiovascular stents, which served as permanent scaffolds to assist in maintaining vessel patency. These metallic scaffolds are crimped on to an angioplasty balloon that is then delivered transluminally to the lesion site and expanded. The balloon is then deflated and removed, leaving the stent permanently embedded in the vessel wall. The stent is intended to be endotheliolized, thus removing it from direct contact with the bloodstream. Most cardiovascular stents are fabricated from 316L stainless steel which is softened by annealing to facilitate deployment. 316L is an attractive choice for a stent material because it can be softened to be expandable under moderate balloon pressures while at the same time work hardening substantially to resist the subsequent pulsatile stresses imposed by the vessel.

The restenosis rate after stenting was approximately halved again by the use of drug eluting stents. There are currently three drug eluting stents on the market. These are Cordis' Cypher stent, which elutes the drug sirolimus from polymer coating, Boston Scientific's Taxus stent, which elutes the drug paclitaxel, and Medtronic's Endeavor stent, which elutes the drug ABT-578. The Cypher and Taxus stents themselves are fabricated from 316L, the Endeavor stent is fabricated from a cobalt chromium alloy. The long term effectiveness of the drug eluting stents is still being evaluated.

## 17.6  Modeling of Metallic Implant Performance

The enormous improvement in computing capabilities has made it possible to model implant performance to a level which was previously unimaginable. What has not occurred is a concomitant improvement in the material models such as those needed for input into finite element programs.

One of the first serious attempts to model medical device fatigue performance is that of Ritchie and Lubock, (1986). They evaluated fatigue using both stress/life and damage-tolerant analyses. The stress/life approach relates the total fatigue life (crack initiation plus propagation) to the applied stress and seeks to achieve local stresses which are below the fatigue limit below which fracture should never occur. The damage-tolerant approach, on the other hand, focuses exclusively on crack propagation to failure from the largest undetected crack, predicting either the number of cycles or time-to-failure. The fundamental material data for the stress/life approach comes from traditional $S/N$ curve; the damage-tolerant approach requires data relating the crack advance per cycle ($da/dN$) to the cyclic variation in the stress intensity factor ($\Delta K$), which combines the influence of both the current crack size and the cyclic stress amplitude. $da/dN$ is then integrated to predict the critical crack size for fracture, from which the number of cycles to failure can then be predicted. Experimentally it is often found that there is a threshold value of $\Delta K$ for which no crack propagation occurs.

It is often difficult, if not impossible, to measure the local stresses which are needed as input to both these fatigue-life estimation procedures, especially if the maximum stress is located at a notch. This difficulty has been dealt with historically by making use of data for stress concentration factors associated with various notch conditions. Nowadays numerical procedures such as finite element analysis can be used to calculate local stresses at complex geometries knowing the global loads and local geometry. Ritchie and Lubock used this approach to calculate stresses in the Björk-Shiley monostrut heart valve. They predicted that the peak physiological stress was 0 to 76 MPa in the inlet strut and 0 to 34 MPa in the outlet strut. Since the fatigue limit obtained experimentally for the Haynes 25 material tested in air and saline solution was estimated to be 366 MPa, the design is extremely conservative from a stress/life approach. Calculations for $\Delta K$ using the same maximum stresses and a crack size of up to 50% of the cross-sectional area indicated that the resulting $\Delta K$s were below the measured threshold. This means that cracks of up to 50% of the cross sectional area will never grow, again indicating a conservative design.

## 17.7  Future Developments for Enhancing Metallic or Hybrid Implant Performance

1. New and existing fabrication processes will be used to optimize the performance of traditional and specialty metallic biomaterials such as nitinol. New processing techniques designed to engineer the orientations of grains as well as grain boundaries appear particularly attractive.

2. Hybrid metallic medical devices will continue to expand into new clinical applications.

3. Emphasis will shift from focusing primarily on bulk to surface and interfacial properties.

4. Analytical techniques such as finite element analysis will find expanded use in controlling both the processing and performance of metallic biomaterials

5. New characterization techniques such as confocal and environmental scanning electron microscopy will facilitate our deeper understanding of biomaterial/cellular interactions.

6. Cellular/metallic biomaterial interactions will be understood and controlled on a more fundamental scientific basis.

7. Implant retrieval and analysis, bolstered by new observational and computational techniques, will continue to be an essential tool in validating as well as improving the performance of metallic and hybrid biomaterials.

## Acknowledgments

Many people provided information for this chapter. I would especially like to thank Matthew Birdsall of Medtronic Vascular, Howard L. Freese of ATI Allvac, and Robert A. Pogie of Zimmer Trabecular Metal.

## HRP Questions

1. The presence of a metallic orthopedic implant results in stress shielding, which is generally thought to be deleterious. The level of compressive stress in an implant containing bone, $\sigma_b$ is affected by the bone cross-sectional area fraction, $a_b$, and the stiffnesses of the bone and implant, $E_b$ and $E_i$. Assuming that the bone and implant are loaded in uniaxial compression and that the compressive normal strain is the same in both the bone and implant, show that

$$\sigma_b = \frac{\overline{\sigma}}{a_b + \frac{E_i}{E_b}a_i} \qquad \text{where } a_i + a_b = 1$$

where $\overline{\sigma}$ is the compressive stress averaged over the area of both the bone and implant.

2. If the stiffness of the metallic implant is orders of magnitude larger than the stiffness of the bone and the area fractions of the bone and implant are approximately equal, show that the result in problem 1 reduces to

$$\sigma_b = \frac{\overline{\sigma}}{a_i \frac{E_i}{E_b}}$$

How do changes in $a_i$ and $E_i/E_b$ affect the compressive stress applied to the bone?

3. The assumption that the normal strains in the bone and implant are equal (isostrain) results in an upper bound to the stresses in the bone and implant. A lower bound to these stresses is found if one assumes that the stresses in the

bone and implant are equal (isostress). This results in a strain ($\varepsilon$) mismatch at the bone/implant interface. Show that this mismatch ratio is

$$\frac{\varepsilon_b}{\varepsilon_i} = \frac{E_i}{E_b}$$

which of these assumptions, isostress or isostrain, appears to be more realistic?

4. Calculate that heart valves and stents experience roughly $10^8$ cycles of stress every 3 years. How does this compare to the number of cycles commonly used to determine the endurance limit of metallic biomaterials?

5. It is commonly accepted that the fatigue behavior of metallic biomaterials must be tested in a physiologically appropriate environment. Many corrosion-fatigue experiments are conducted at 30 cycles/second and higher. Do corrosion-fatigue data obtained under these conditions overestimate or underestimate *in vivo* corrosion-fatigue behavior?

6. Show that the stress/life analysis performed by Ritchie and Lubock (Burkus et al., 2002) for the monostrut heart valve resulted in a safety factor of 4.8 for the inlet strut and 10.8 for the outlet strut.

7. Use the data for PTFE rod given in ASTM 1710-02 and Ti–6Al–4V given in ASTM F 136-02 to show that the ultimate tensile stress of metallic biomaterials is typically more than 50 times greater than that of polymeric biomaterials.

8. Compare the potential for stiffness reduction in metallic biomaterials by changes in chemistry and processing (see Table 17.2) and the use of porosity such as in Trabecular metal.

9. Many metal-on-metal articulating orthopedic prostheses contain a polymer layer as part of the backing to the metal articulating surface. What benefits are there to using such a polymeric component layer?

10. What is the microstructural mechanism by which the endurance limit of 35N LT is at least 10,000 psi higher than a typical ASTM F 562 material?

**HRP Answers**

1. The load

$$P_{total} = P_{bone} + P_{implant} = \sigma_b + A_b + \sigma_i A_i$$

$$\frac{P_{total}}{A_b + A_i} = \overline{\sigma} = \sigma_b a_b + \sigma_i A_i \qquad \text{where } a_b + a_i = 1$$

$$\varepsilon_b = \varepsilon_i = \frac{\sigma_b}{E_b} = \frac{\sigma_i}{E_i} .$$

or

$$\sigma_i = \sigma_b \frac{E_i}{E_b}$$

$$\overline{\sigma} = \sigma_b a_b + \sigma_b \frac{E_i}{E_b} a_i$$

$$\sigma_b = \frac{\overline{\sigma}}{a_b + \dfrac{E_i}{E_b}a_i}$$

2.

$$\sigma_b = \frac{\overline{\sigma}}{1 - a_i + \dfrac{E_i}{E_b}a_i} = \frac{\overline{\sigma}}{1 + a_i\left(\dfrac{E_i}{E_b} - 1\right)}$$

For

$$\frac{E_i}{E_b} \gg 1 \quad \text{and} \quad a_i \approx a_b$$

$$\sigma_b = \frac{\overline{\sigma}}{a_i \dfrac{E_i}{E_b}}$$

The stress in the bone $\sigma_b$ by decreasing $a_i$ and decreasing $E_i/E_b$ (increasing $E_b/E_i$)

3. Isotress Care

$$\sigma_b = \sigma_i = \overline{\sigma}$$

$$E_b \varepsilon_b = E_i \varepsilon_i$$

Since $E_i/E_b \gg 1$ there is a huge normal strain mismatch. $\therefore$ Isostrain seems more realistic.

4. Assuming 70 heartbeats/minute

$$\frac{70 \text{ beats}}{\text{min}} \times \frac{10 \text{ min}}{\text{h}} \times \frac{24 \text{ h}}{\text{day}} \times \frac{365 \text{ days}}{\text{year}} = 36.8 \times 10^6 \frac{\text{beat}}{\text{year}}$$

$\sim 10^8$ beats/3 years
Most fatigue experiments are terminated after $10^7$ cycles.

5. Physiological processes typically occur at 1 cycle/second or lower. Since this is substantially below 30 cycles/second, there is more time for corrosion *in vivo* than *in vitro*. Hence the laboratory tests tend to overestimate fatigue lifetimes.

6. The fatigue limit for Haynes 25 is given as 366 MPa. The maximum stress is 76 MPa at the inlet strut and 34 MPa at the outlet strut. This gives safety factors of 4.8 and 10.8, respectively.

7. ASTM 1710-02 specifies a minimum ultimate tensile stress of 15.2 MPa for extruded PTFE rod. ASTM F 136-02 specifies a minimum ultimate tensile stress of 825 MPa for wrought Ti–6Al–4V. This gives a ratio of 54.2.

8. Table 17.2 shows a maximum reduction in stiffness of 110 to 64 GPa. The modulus of fully dense tantalum is 185 GPa; that of trabecular bone, 2.5–3.9 GPa. Increasing porosity is clearly more effective in reducing stiffness than alloying or thermomechanical processing.

9. The presence of a polymeric liner in a metal-on-metal system serves to dampen impact loading. It might also enhance alignment by differentially creeping under load.

10. The principal microstructural changes in 35N LT have been directed atremoving carbide, nitride, and sigma second-phase particles. This was accomplished by

   - reducing the tramp elements P and S virtually to 0
   - reducing the Fe content by a factor of ten
   - reducing the elements C, Si, Mn, B, and Ti essentially to 0.

## References

Bader, J.S., Komistek, R.D., Wasserman, J.F., and Haas, B.D., *Clinical Significance of Hip Separation in Metal on Polyethylene, Metal on Metal, and Ceramic on Ceramic THA due to Resonant and Energy Dispersion Effects*, Poster No: 1606, 51st Annual Meeting of the Orthopaedic Research Society (2005).

Bechtol, C.O., Ferguson, Jr. A.S., and Laing, P.G., *Metals and Engineering in Bone and Joint Surgery*, Williams & Wilkins, Baltimore, MD (1959).

Bobyn, J.D., Hacking, S.A., Chan, S.P., Tanzer, M., and Krygier, J.J., Tissue response to porous coated acetabular cups: a canine model, *J. Arthroplast.*, **14**, 347–354 (1999a).

Bobyn, J.D., Hacking, S.A., Chan, S.P., Toh, K.-K., Krygier, J.J., and Tanzer, M., Characterization of a new porous biomaterial for reconstructive orthopaedics, *Trans. American Academy of Orthopaedic Surgeons 66th Annual Meeting*, AAOS, Anaheim, CA (1999b).

Bobyn, J.D., Wilson, G.J., MacGregor, D.C., Pilliar, R.M., and Weatherly, G.C., Effect of pore size on the peel strength of attachment of fibrous tissue to porous-surfaced implants, *J. Biomed. Mater. Res.*, **16**, 571–584 (1982).

Böcklein, G., Breme, J., and von der Emde, J., Lethal blockage of a Björk-Shiley artificial heart valve caused by strut fracture — the metallurgical aspect, *Thorac. Cardiovasc. Surg.*, **37**, 47–51 (1989).

Bradley, D., Kay, L., Lippard, H., and Stephenson, T., *Optimization of Melt Chemistry and Properties of 35Cobalt–35Nickel–20Chromium–10Molybdenum Medical Grade Wire*, Proceedings from the Materials and Processes for Medical Devices Conference, ASM International, The Netherlands pp. 301–307 (2004).

Brunette, D.M., Tengvall, P., Textor, M., and Thomsen, P., *Titanium in Medicine*, Springer, Berlin (2001).

Bowsher, J.G., Hussain, A., Nevclos, J., Williams, P.A., and Shelton, J.C., I 'severe' patient activity substantially increased wear particle surface area in metal-on-metal hip simulation, Paper No: 1626, *51st Annual Meeting of the Orthopaedic Research Society* (2005a).

Bowsher, J.G., Hussain, A., Nevclos, J., Williams, P.A., and Shelton, J.C., *Large Head Diameters Have the Potential to Reduce Ion Release in Metal-on-Metal Hip Wear Simulation*, Poster No: 1626, 51st Annual Meeting of the Orthopaedic Research Society (2005b).

Burkus, J.K., Gornet, M.F., Dickman, C.A., and Zdeblick, T.A., Anterior lumbar interbody fusion using rhBMP-2 with tapered interbody cages, *J. Spinal Disord. Tech.*, **15** (5), 337–349 (2002).

Chung, C.S., Kim, J.K., Kim, H.K., and Kim, W.J., Improvement of high-cycle fatigue life in a 6061 Al alloy produced by equal channel angular pressing, *Mater. Sci. Eng. A*, **337** (1 & 2), 39–44 (2002).

Desigi, J.A., Zardiackas, L.D., and Mitchell, D.W., *Anodic Polarization of Nickel-Free Implant Quality Stainless Steel*, Sixth World Biomaterials Congress Transactions, Society for Biomaterials, p. 816 (2000).

Dorr, L.D., Wan, Z., Longjohrn, D.B., DuBois, B., and Murken, R., Total hip arthroplasty with use of the metasul metal-on-metal articulation, *J. Bone Joint Surg.*, **82-A** (6), 789–798 (2000).

Fehring, T.K., Chaffin III, H., and Kennedy, R.L., Enhanced Biocompatible Implants and Alloys, U.S. Patents 6,187,045 B1 (2001), 6,539,607 B1 (2003), and 6,773,520 (2004).

Gilbert, J.L., The corrosion-fatigue behavior of Ti–6Al–4V hip prostheses: fabrication effects and *in-vitro* performance, Ph.D. Thesis, Carnegie Mellon University (1982).

Gilbert, J.L. and Piehler, H.R., Grain egression: a new mechanism of fatigue-crack initiation in Ti–6Al–4V, *Metall. Trans. A*, **20A**, 1715–1725 (1989).

Grimm, M.J., Selection of materials for biomedical applications, In *Handbook of Materials Selection*, Kutz, M., Ed., John Wiley & Sons, New York, pp. 1165–1194 (2002).

Gruen, T., Christie, M., Eilers, V., Hanssen, A., Lewallen, D., Lewis, R., Keefe, T.O., Stulberg, S.D., Sutherland, C., Unger, A., and Poggie, R.A., Radiographic evaluation of a monoblock acetabular component-a multi-center study with 2 to 5 year results, *J. Arthroplast.*, **20** (3), 369–378 (2005).

Hacking, S.A., Bobyn, J.D., Koh, K.-K., Tanzer, M., and Krygier, J.J., Fibrous tissue ingrowth and attachment to porous tantalum, *J. Biomed. Mater. Res.*, **52**, 631–638 (2000).

Hawkins, M.J., Ricci, J.L., Kaufman, J., and Jaffee, W., *Osseointegration of a New Beta Titanium Alloy as Compared to Standard Orthopaedic Implant Materials*, Sixth World Biomaterials Congress Transactions, Society for Biomaterials, p. 1083 (2000).

Heisel, C., Skipor, A.K., Jacobs, J.J., and Schmalzreis, T.P., *The Relationship between Activity and Ions in Patients with Metal–Metal Bearing Hip Implants*, 51st Annual Meeting of the Orthopaedic Research Society, (2005).

Helsen, J.A. and Breme, H.J., *Metals as Biomaterials*, Wiley, New York (1998).

Hierholzer, S. and Hierholzer, G., *Internal Fixation and Metal Allergie*, Thieme Medical Publishers, New York (1992).

Jantsch, S., Schwagerl, W., Lenz, P., Semlitsch, M., and Fertschak, W., Long-term results after implantation of McKee-Ferrar total hip prostheses, *Arch. Orthop. Trauma Surg.*, **110**, 230–237 (1991).

Jin, Z.M. and Fisher, J., *Effect of Running in on Contact Mechanics and Lubrication in Metal-on-Metal Hip Implants*, Paper No: 0895, 51st Annual Meeting of the Orthopaedic Research Society (2005).

Lanzagazorta, M., Kral, M.V., Swan, J.E. II, Spanos, G., Rosenberg, R., and Kuo, E., Three-dimensional visualization of microstructures, *IEEE Vis.*, 487–490 (1998).

Lemons, J. and Freese, H., Metallic biomaterials for surgical implant devices, *BONE Zone, Fall*, pp. 5, 7, 9 (2002).

Park, J.B., *Biomaterials Science and Engineering*, Plenum Press, New York (1984).

Personal communication, Matt Birdsall, Medtronic Vascular.

Ratner, B.D., Hoffman, A.S., Schoen, F.J., and Lemons, J.E., *Biomaterials Science: An Introduction to Materials in Medicine*, 2nd ed., Elsevier Academic Press, San Diego, CA (2004).

Ritchie, R.O. and Lubock, P., Fatigue life estimation procedures for the endurance of a cardiac valve prosthesis: stress/life and damage-tolerant analyses, *J. Biomed. Eng.*, **108**, 153–160 (1986).

Roach, M.D., Zardiackas, L.D., Brown, R.S., and Gebeau, R.C., *Physical, Metallurgical, and Mechanical Comparison of a Low-Alloy Stainless Steel*, Transactions of the 27th Annual Meeting of the Society for Biomaterials, p. 343 (2001).

Schmalzried, T.P., Jasty, M., and Harris, W.H., Periprosthetic bone loss in total hip arthroplasty, *J. Bone Joint Surg.*, **74A**, 849–863 (1992).

Segal, V.M., Materials processing by simple shear, *Mater. Sci. Eng. A*, **A197** (2), 157–164 (1995).

Shrivastava, S., Ed., *Medical Device Materials, Proceedings of the Materials and Processes for Medical Devices Conference*, ASM International, The Netherlands (2003).

Skipor, A.K., Campbell, P.A., Gitelis, S., Berger, R.A., Schmalzreid, T.P., Amstutz, H.C., and Jacobs, J.J., *Metal Ion Levels in Patients with Metal Bilateral Surface and Total Hip Arthroplasty*, Poster No: 0834, 51st Annual Meeting of the Orthopaedic Research Society (2005).

Sloter, L.E., *The Performance of Surgical Implants: An Engineering and Policy Analysis*, Ph.D. thesis, Carnegie Mellon University (1979).

Sloter, L.E. and Piehler, H.R., Corrosion-fatigue performance of hip Nails–Jewett type, In *Corrosion and Degradation of Implant Materials*, ASTM STP684, pp. 173–195 (1979).

U.S. Congress, The Björk-Shiley Heart Valve: "Earn While You Learn", Committee Print 101-R, Subcommittee on Oversight and Investigation, Committee on Energy and Commerce, U.S. House of Representatives (1990) February.

Valiev, R.Z., Stolyarov, V.V., Rack, H.J., and Lowe, T.C., *SPD Processed Ultra-Fine Grained Materials for Medical Application, Proceedings from the Materials and Processes for Medical Devices Conference*, ASM International, The Netherlands, pp. 362–367 (2004).

Wan, Z. and Dorr, L.D., Natural history of femoral osteolysis with proximal ingrowth smooth stem implant, *J. Arthroplast.*, **11**, 718–725 (1996).

Willert, H.-G., Bertram, H., and Buchhorn, G.H., Osteolysis in alloarthroplasty of the hip. The role of ultra-high molecular weight polyethylene particles, *Clin. Orthop.*, **282**, 95–107 (1990).

Williams, S., Jin, Z.M., Stone, M.H., Ingham, E., and Fisher, J., *The Effect of Different Lubricant Regimes and Lubrication on the Friction Hard-on-Hard Bearings*, Poster No: 0894, 51st Annual Meeting of the Orthopaedic Research Society (2005).

# 18

## Ceramic Biomaterials

**Prashant N. Kumta**

## CONTENTS

*Brief History*: As recently as 30 years ago, the notion of ceramics as biomaterials was not common. For a long time, ceramic materials have been studied for applications in the electronic, optical, magnetics, steel, and glass industries. The field has witnessed an evolution from ceramics being regarded solely as objects of art, pottery, and ornaments in the early 1900s to a resurgence of interest with the onset of new processing techniques such as the sol–gel approach in the mid-1900s. This has resulted in research in ceramics applications never seen before, in the areas of nonlinear optics, infrared windows, ferroelectrics, dielectrics, capacitors, superconductors, and magnetics.

The high-temperature capabilities of ceramics, known from their use as refractory linings in furnaces, resulted in their implementation as heat sinks and tiles in spacecrafts and shuttles by NASA. With the ever-increasing popularity of ceramics brought about by new synthetic methods and characterization technologies in the optical and electronic fields, subsequent interest in their application for biological uses also grew.

Interest in bioceramics has increased dramatically over the past two decades and the intense activity has led to a widespread belief that they could be one of the materials of choice for many orthopedic, otologic, maxillofacial, and dental applications. A number of ceramics have been researched over the past three decades as viable materials for a number of implants and in the newly evolving field of tissue engineering. Alumina, the most traditional of ceramics apart from silica, has been extensively studied for use as articulating components in total joint prostheses, and dental and maxillofacial applications (Ravaglioli, 1992). Other materials and systems have also evolved over the years.

The use of extraneous materials as implants has been known since the pre-Christian era where paper was used for replacing extensively damaged bony parts in the body. By the mid-19th century, science had made progress in exploring the use of metals and in the latter half of the century, ceramics systems were also intensely explored. The identification of ceramics as potential biocompatible and bioresorbable materials makes them a good candidate for chemically bonding with tissue, unlike metals, making them strong candidates for long-term implantation inside a living organism. In 1963, Smith used ceramics for bone substitution for the first time. Many subsequent studies have highlighted the use of these materials for clinical applications (Hulbert and Young, 1969). The wide chemical and functional characteristics of ceramics enabling them to be bioinert, biocompatible and even bioactive have widened their use considerably in recent years. The major limitations of ceramics are their brittle nature and the difficulty in processing these materials into the desired shape and form under physiological conditions. Subsequent microstructural changes make them susceptible to displaying varying mechanical and biological properties. Both positive and negative attributes can, therefore, be assigned to this fascinating class of materials. The negative properties limit their use, while the positive attributes undoubtedly offer a plethora of biofunctional applications ranging from implants to scaffolds and, more recently, drug, protein and gene delivery.

## 18.1   Definition of Ceramics

Ceramics, in general, can be defined as the art and science of making and using solid articles composed of inorganic and nonmetallic materials for functional applications. Typically, ceramics are fabricated by synthesizing powders, followed by shaping and consolidation processes which enable the fabrication of objects of different shapes and sizes. Ceramics are refractory, inorganic compounds made of metals and nonmetals such as O, N, C, S. Exceptions to this general category include diamond, graphite, carbon nanotubes, and pyrolized carbons (Kingery et al., 1976).

In recent years, we have realized that ceramics and composites can also be used to augment or replace various parts of the body, particularly bone. Ceramics used for the body are called bioceramics. Their relative inertness to body fluids, high compressive strength, and pleasing esthetic appearance has led to the use of ceramics in dentistry as dental crowns. Some carbons have been used as implants for blood interfacing applications such as heart valves. Due to their high specific strength as fibers and to their biocompatibility, ceramics are also used as reinforcing components of composite implant materials and for tensile loading applications such as tendons and ligaments.

Unlike metals and polymers, ceramics do not shear plastically due to the ionic nature of the bonding and a minimum number of slip systems. Thus ceramics are nonductile and are responsible for almost zero creep at room temperature. Ceramics are susceptible to notches or cracks (microcracks) since they do not undergo plastic deformation; they fracture elastically on initiation of cracks. At the crack tip, stress could be many times higher than the stress in the material away from the tip, leading to stress concentration weakening the material (Billotte, 2000).

Ceramics, in general, are hard; diamond is the hardest, with a hardness index of 10 on the Moh's scale; followed by alumina (hardness 9); quartz ($SiO_2$) (hardness 8); and apatite ($Ca_5P_3O_{12}F$; hardness 5). Other characteristics are: (1) high melting temperatures and (2) low conductivity of electricity and heat.

The desired properties of bioceramics are

1. Nontoxic
2. Noncarcinogenic
3. Nonallergic
4. Noninflammatory
5. Biocompatible
6. Biofunctional for its lifetime in the host

Ceramics used in fabricating implants can be classified as nonresorbable (relatively inert), bioactive or surface reactive (semi-inert) and biodegradable or resorbable (noninert). $Al_2O_3$, $ZrO_2$, $Si_3N_4$, and carbons are inert bioceramics. Certain glass-ceramics and dense hydroxyapatite (HA) are semi-inert (bioreactive) and calcium phosphates are resorbable ceramics. Some Ca-phosphates also contain alumina (ALCAP) which can be bioresorbable.

## 18.2 Nonabsorbable or Relatively Bioinert Bioceramics

These ceramics maintain their physical and mechanical properties while in the host. They resist corrosion and wear and have all the attributes necessary. Typical examples of bioinert ceramics include: pyrolitic carbon-coated devices, dense and nonporous $Al_2O_3$, porous $Al_2O_3$, $ZrO_2$-related ceramics, dense hydroxyapatite, and calcium aluminates. Relatively bioinert ceramics are typically used as structural-support implants, for example, bone plates, bone screws, and femoral heads. Nonstructural supports are ventilation tubes, sterilization devices, and drug delivery devices. A more detailed list of the various applications is as follows: reconstruction of acetabular cavities, bone plates and screws, ceramic–ceramic composites, ceramic–polymer composites, drug delivery devices, femoral heads, middle ear ossicles, reconstruction of orbital rims, components of total and partial hips, sterilization and ventilation tubes, and repair of cardiovascular area.

### 18.2.1 Alumina ($Al_2O_3$)

The main sources of high purity alumina are bauxite and native corundum. The most ubiquitous form of alumina is the alpha form, $\alpha$-$Al_2O_3$ which can be obtained by calcining the hydroxide, $Al(OH)_3$. The typical chemical composition of $Al_2O_3$ is given in Table 18.1.

**TABLE 18.1**

Chemical Composition of Calcined Alumina Powder
(Billotte, 2000)

| Ingredients | Chemical Composition (wt%) |
|---|---|
| $Al_2O_3$ | 99.6 |
| $SiO_2$ | 0.12 |
| $Fe_2O_3$ | 0.03 |
| $Na_2O$ | 0.04 |

$\alpha$-$Al_2O_3$ has a rhombohedral structure ($a = 4.758$ Å, $c = 12.991$ Å). Natural alumina is also known as sapphire or ruby depending on the impurity, particularly $Cr_2O_3$ which gives the ruby red color. Alumina can be made in single crystal form or polycrystalline form. Single crystals are made by pulling molten $Al_2O_3$ over a seed crystal using an electric arc or an oxy-hydrogen flame as the fused powder builds up. Single crystals have been used successfully to form implants (Park, 1991). The strength of polycrystalline alumina depends on its grain size and porosity. Generally, the smaller the grain size, the lower the porosity and the higher the strength of the ceramic. ASTM standards require a flexural strength $>400$ MPa and elastic modulus 380 GPa (see Table 18.2).

Alumina has been used in orthopedics for more than 25 years. Single crystal $Al_2O_3$ has been used in orthopedics and dental surgery for almost 20 years. Alumina is usually quite a hard material, its hardness varying from 20 to 30 Gpa; its high hardness allows it to be used as an abrasive. Its high hardness is accompanied by low friction and wear and inertness to the *in vivo* environment. These properties make $Al_2O_3$ an ideal material for use in joint replacements. Aluminum oxide implants in bones of rhesus monkeys have shown no signs of rejection or toxicity for 350 days. One of the popular uses of polycrystalline $Al_2O_3$ is in total hip prostheses. $Al_2O_3$ hip prostheses with an ultrahigh molecular weight (UHMW) polyethylene (PE) socket have been claimed to be a better device than a metal prosthesis with an UHMWPE socket (Hench, 1991).

### 18.2.2   Zirconia ($ZrO_2$)

Pure $ZrO_2$ can be obtained from chemical conversion of zircon ($ZrSiO_4$), which is an abundant mineral deposit. $ZrO_2$ has a $T_m = 2953$K and chemical stability with $a = 5.145$ Å, $b = 0.521$ Å, $c = 5.311$ Å, and $\beta = 99°14'$. A major problem is its huge volume change during phase changes at high temperature in pure form, i.e., the monoclinic to tetragonal phase transformation. A dopant such as $Y_2O_3$ is, therefore, used to stabilize the cubic form at high temperature. $Y_2O_3$ (6 mol%) is used as a dopant to fabricate zirconia for implantation in bone known as *partially stabilized zirconia* (Drennen and Steele, 1991). The physical properties are, however, slightly inferior compared to $Al_2O_3$ as can be seen in Table 18.2 above.

**TABLE 18.2**

Physical Property Needs of Alumina and Partially Stabilized Zirconia (Billotte, 2000)

| Properties | Alumina (3 mol%-$Y_2O_3$) | Zirconia (3 mol%-$Y_2O_3$) |
|---|---|---|
| Elastic modulus (GPa) | 380 | 190 |
| Flexural strength (GPa) | $>0.4$ | 1.0 |
| Hardness (Mohs) | 9 | 6.5 |
| Density (g/cm$^3$) | 3.8–3.9 | 5.95 |
| Grain size ($\mu$m) | 4.0 | 0.6 |

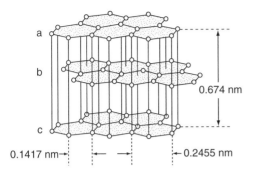

**FIGURE 18.1**
Hexagonal layered structure of graphite showing the basal and c-direction arrangement of the carbon–carbon bonds.

High density $ZrO_2$ has also shown excellent compatibility with autogenous rhesus monkey bone and was found to be completely nonreactive to the body environment for a period of 350 days. It has shown excellent biocompatibility and good wear and friction when combined with UHMWPE.

### 18.2.3 Carbons

Carbons can be made in many allotropic forms namely, graphite, crystalline diamond, nanocrystalline glassy carbon, and quasicrystalline pyrolitic carbon. Recently, there are also the new variations of nanotubes and bucky-balls of carbon. However, the one most commonly used for implants is pyrolitic carbon. It is normally used as a surface coating. Surface coatings of diamond, though possible, have not been commercially produced yet.

The crystalline structure of carbon used in implants is similar to graphite (Figure 18.1). The planar hexagonal arrays comprises covalently bonded C–C bonds while between the layers the bonding is mainly nondirectional and of van der Waals type. This leads to the anisotropic electrical conductivity known to graphite, although good lubricating properties are displayed by the system.

The poorly crystalline carbons are thought to contain unassociated or nonoriented carbon atoms resulting in slightly disordered arrays of randomly oriented crystallites (Figure 18.2). These randomly dispersed aggregates, however, become isotropic. The mechanical properties of carbon, particularly pyrolitic carbon, are largely dependent on its density (Figure 18.3 and Figure 18.4; Kaae, 1971). Higher density translates to better

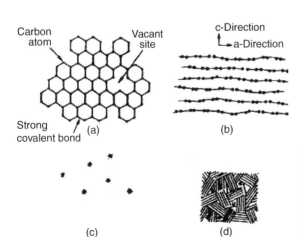

**FIGURE 18.2**
Schematic representation of various forms of poorly crystalline carbons. (a) Single layer plane of defective carbon; (b) parallel layers of carbon in a crystallite; (c) unassociated carbon; (d) aggregates of crystallites, single layers and unassociated carbons.

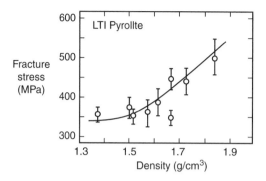

**FIGURE 18.3**
Fracture stress plotted against density for unalloyed low temperature isotropic pyrolitic carbons. (*Source*: Kaae, J.L., *J. Nucl. Mater.*, **38**, 42–50 (1971). With permission.)

mechanical properties, thus implying the influence of the aggregate structure and the random dispersion of the crystallites (Park, 1992).

Graphite and glassy carbon have a much lower mechanical strength than pyrolitic carbon (Table 18.3). The average modulus of elasticity appears to be the same for all carbons. The strength of pyrolitic carbon is high compared to graphite and glassy carbon. The main reason is the low number of flaws and unassociated carbons in the aggregate. Composites of carbon reinforced with carbon fiber have been considered as a potential implant. However, the carbon–carbon composite is highly anisotropic, and its density is in the range of 1.4–1.45 g/cm$^3$ with a porosity of 35–38% (see Table 18.4) (Adams and Williams, 1978).

Carbons exhibit good compatibility with body tissue. Hence these materials have been used extensively for repairing diseased heart valves and blood vessels. Pyrolitic carbon can be deposited onto finished implants from hydrocarbon gas in a fluidized bed at controlled temperature and pressure. The microstructure and crystallinity of carbon can be controlled by adjusting the process parameters. It is also possible to introduce dopants such as Si into the reactor to the extent of 10–20 wt% to increase hardness for applications requiring abrasion resistance in heart-valve discs.

Recently, it has been possible to fabricate ultra low temperature isotropic carbon by deposition onto surfaces of blood vessel implants made of polymers. These materials are

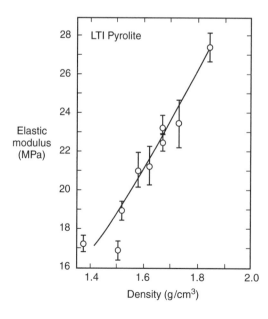

**FIGURE 18.4**
Plot of elastic modulus and density for unalloyed LTI pyrolitic carbons. (*Source*: Kaae, J.L., *J. Nucl. Mater.*, **38**, 42–50 (1971). With permission.)

**TABLE 18.3**

Physical and Mechanical Properties of Various Types of Carbons for Biofunctional Applications

| | Various Types of Carbon | | |
|---|---|---|---|
| Properties | Graphite | Glassy | Pyrolytic[a] |
| Density (g/cm$^3$) | 1.5–1.9 | 1.5 | 1.5–2.0 |
| Elastic modulus (GPa) | 24 | 24 | 28 |
| Compressive strength (MPa) | 138 | 172 | 517(575[a]) |
| Toughness (mN/cm$^3$)[b] | 6.3 | 0.6 | 4.8 |

*Source*: Park, J.B. and Lakes, R.S. Ceramic implant materials, *Biomaterials: An Introduction*, 2nd ed., p. 133, Plenum Press, New York (1992).

[a]   1.0 w/o Si-alloyed pyrolytic carbon, Pyrolite™ (Carbomedics, Austin, TX).

[b]   1 mN/cm$^3$ = $1.45 \times 10^{-3}$ in.-lb/in.$^3$.

better than low temperature isotropic (LTI) carbons and are known to exhibit excellent compatibility with blood. They are also thin enough not to interfere with the flexibility of the grafts (Sharma, 1984; Billotte, 2000).

Vitreous or glassy carbons are made by controlled pyrolysis of polymers such as phenolformaldehyde, Rayon and polyacrylonitrile (PAN) at high temperature in a controlled environment. This approach is used to make carbon fibers and textiles.

## 18.3   Biodegradable or Resorbable Ceramics

The concept of resorbable ceramics as bone substitutes was introduced in 1969 by Hentrich. However, long before this *Plaster of Paris* was already being used (since 1892) as a bone substitute. *Resorbable ceramics*, as the name implies, degrade upon implantation in the host. The resorbed material is replaced by endogenous tissues. The rate of degradation does, however, vary from material to material. Most bioresorbable ceramics except Biocoral and Plaster of Paris (calcium sulfate dihydrate) are essentially variations of calcium phosphate. Examples of biodegradable bioceramics include: aluminum–calcium–phosphorus oxides (ALCAP) (Mattie and Bajpai, 1988), glass fibers and their composites (Alexander et al., 1987), corals (Guillemin et al., 1989; Khavari and Bajpai,

**TABLE 18.4**

Mechanical Properties of Carbon Fiber-Reinforced Carbon

| | Fiber Lay-Up | |
|---|---|---|
| Property | Unidirectional | 0–90° Crossply |
| Flexural modulus (GPa) | | |
| Longitudinal | 140 | 60 |
| Transverse | 7 | 60 |
| Flexural strength (MPa) | | |
| Longitudinal | 1200 | 500 |
| Transverse | 15 | 500 |
| Interlaminar shear strength (MPa) | 18 | 18 |

*Source*: Adams, D. and Williams, D.F., Carbon fiber-reinforced carbon as a potential implant materials. *J. Biomed. Mater. Res.*, **12**, 35–42 (1978). With permission.

1993), calcium sulfates, including plaster of Paris (Peltier, 1961), ferric calcium phosphorus oxides (Stricker et al., 1992; Larrabee et al., 1993), hydroxyapatites (HAs) (Ravaglioli, 1992), tricalcium phosphate (TCP) (LeGeros, 1991), zinc–calcium–phosphorus oxides (Arrar and Bajpai, 1992), and zinc-sulfate–calcium–phosphorus oxides (Scheidler and Bajpai, 1992). Typical uses of biodegradable ceramics are as drug delivery devices (Abrams and Bajpai, 1994), for repair of damaged bone due to disease or trauma (Scheidler and Bajpai, 1992; Khavari and Bajpai, 1993), for repair and fusion of spinal and lumbo-sacral vertebrae, for repair of herniated discs, and maxillofacial and dental defects, and hydroxyapatite ocular implants (Billotte, 2000).

### 18.3.1 Calcium Phosphates

There are several forms of calcium phosphate. They typically form a family of compounds called "apatites." This term describes a family of compounds having similar structure (hexagonal system, space group, $P6_3/m$) in spite of a wide range of composition. The similarity of the x-ray diffraction maps of enamel, dentin, and bone to those of mineral apatites (HA, fluorapatite, FA) along with the chemical analyses showing calcium and phosphate as principal constituents led to the belief that the inorganic components of bone and teeth are essentially calcium hydroxyapatite (HA) represented by the chemical formula $Ca_{10}(PO_4)_6(OH)_2$. However, the exact structure of biological apatites is not clear. This is because of the myriad forms of their morphology and variations in nonstoichiometry (LeGeros, 1991).

Apatite was first named as a mineral by Werner in 1786. The name was derived from "apataw," the Greek word to deceive, since it was confused with several other similar looking minerals until chemical analysis conducted in 1788 proved that it is a calcium phosphate similar to bone (Kumta, 2004).

Apatite mineral is essentially fluorapatite, the highest symmetry possessing mineral. Its composition is given as $Ca_5(PO_4)_3F$. Apatite minerals are all based on the fluorapatite structure which gives the structural formula $X_3Y_2(TO_4)Z$.

The structure allows for easy substitution in natural apatites where

X and Y = Ca, Sr, Ba, Re, Pb, U, Mn and, rarely, Na, K, Y and Cu;

T = P, As, V, Si, S, and C (as $CO_3$);

Z = F, Cl, OH, and O.

As a biomaterial, the apatites of interest are those where X = Y = Ca, T = P and Z = F, OH. When Z = F, i.e., $Ca_5(PO_4)_3F$, the apatites are called fluorapatite (FAp); when Z = Cl, the apatites are likewise called chloroapatite (ClAp); while apatites wherein T = P and Z = OH are called hydroxyapatite (Hap or HA), i.e., $Ca_5(PO_4)_3OH$.

#### 18.3.1.1 Substituted Apatites

##### 18.3.1.1.1 Carbonate Apatites

Synthetic $CO_3$ apatites have been classified as type A or type B depending on the mode of $CO_3$ substitution:

$CO_3$-for-OH (type A), or $CO_3$-for-$PO_4$ (type B).

Type A carbonate apatites are prepared by passing dry $CO_2$ gas over HA at temperatures of 1000°C.

Type B carbonate apatites are prepared in aqueous conditions by reacting $CaHPO_4$ with $NaHCO_3$.

There are several types of calcium phosphates as indicated below:
Main calcium phosphate compounds having biological use (Elliott, 1994) are:

1. Monocalcium phosphate monohydrate (MCPM)

*Chemical formula*: $Ca(H_2PO_4)_2 \cdot H_2O$

*Atomic ratio*: $Ca/P = 0.5$

*Structure*: Triclinic; unit cell, $a = 5.62615$ Å, $b = 11.8892$ Å, $c = 6.47318$ Å, $\alpha = 98.6336°$, $\beta = 118.2626°$ and $\gamma = 83.3446°$.

*Preparation*: Can be grown as well-formed crystals by lowering the temperature of an acidic solution with appropriate composition.

*Stability*: stable in air but loses water above 108°C to form the anhydrous form or the pyrophosphate $Ca_2P_2O_7$.

2. Monocalcium phosphate anhydrous (MCPA)

*Chemical formula*: $Ca(H_2PO_4)_2$

*Atomic ratio*: $Ca/P = 0.5$

*Structure*: Also triclinic; unit cell, $a = 7.55775$ Å, $b = 8.25316$ Å, $c = 5.55043$ Å, $\alpha = 109.871°$, $\beta = 93.681$ Å, $\gamma = 109.51°$.

*Preparation*: Can be grown under conditions from solution similar to the monohydrate form. The anhydrous form can be crystallized over a four day period from a solution of $Ca(OH)_2$ or CaO and $H_3PO_4$ at 130°C.

*Stability*: MCPA transforms to $CaH_2P_2O_7$ and calcium polyphosphates above 186°C.

3. Dicalcium phosphate dihydrate (DCPD)

*Chemical formula*: $CaHPO_4 \cdot 2H_2O$

*Mineral name*: Brushite

*Atomic ratio*: $Ca/P$ ratio $= 1.0$

*Structure*: Monoclinic, space group $Ia$; $a = 5.8122$ Å, $b = 15.1803$ Å, $c = 6.2392$ Å, and $\beta = 116°25'$

*Preparation*: Direct precipitation by the simultaneous addition during stirring of a solution containing $Na_2HPO_4 \cdot 2H_2O$ and $KH_2PO_4$ and $CaCl_2 \cdot 6H_2O$ to a solution of $KH_2PO_4$ at pH $= 4$–5.

*Stability*: Brushite decomposes upon heating to 900°C to form $Ca_2P_2O_7$. The sequence of the decomposition reaction can be indicated as follows

$$DCPD \rightarrow DCPA \text{ at } 180°C \rightarrow \gamma\text{-}Ca_2P_2O_7 \text{ at } 320\text{–}340°C \rightarrow \beta\text{-}Ca_2P_2O_7 \text{ at } 700°C$$

$$\rightarrow \alpha\text{-}Ca_2P_2O_7 \text{ at } 1200°C$$

4. Dicalcium phosphate anhydrous (DCPA)

*Chemical formula*: $CaHPO_4$

*Mineral name*: Monetite

*Atomic ratio*: $Ca/P = 1.0$

*Structure*: Triclinic, space group $P\bar{1}$; $a = 6.9101$ Å, $b = 6.6272$ Å, $c = 6.9982$ Å; $\alpha = 96.342°$, $\beta = 103.822°$, and $\gamma = 88.332°$.

*Preparation*: The preparation protocol is similar to the preparation of DCPD by the addition of phosphate and calcium solutions to $KH_2PO_4$ solution but at 100°C.

*Stability*: The stability of monetite is very similar to that described for brushite as described above in DCPD.

## 5. Octacalcium phosphate (OCP)

*Chemical formula*: $Ca_8(HPO_4)_2(PO_4)_4 \cdot 5H_2O$

*Other names*: Octacalcium bis(hydrogenphosphate)tetrakis(phosphate)pentahydrate, tetracalcium hydrogen triphosphate trihydrate

*Atomic ratio*: $Ca/P = 1.33$

*Structure*: Triclinic, space group $P\bar{1}$; $a = 19.6924$ Å, $b = 9.5232$ Å, $c = 6.8352$ Å; $\alpha = 90.152°$, $\beta = 92.542°$, and $\gamma = 108.651°$.

*Preparation*: OCP is known to be obtained by the slow hydrolysis of $CaHPO_4 \cdot 2H_2O$ in $CH_3COONa$ renewed when the pH falls to 6.1. It can also be prepared by the hydrolysis of DCPD at 80–85°C in dilute $HNO_3$ at pH 5 for 30 min.

*Stability*: The decomposition of the OCP follows a complex path with partial loss of water of hydration and formation of collapsed OCP, DCPA, HAp, $\beta$-$Ca_2P_2O_7$ and tripolyphosphate with increase in temperature. Initial loss of water occurs at 180°C followed by the formation of DCPA and HAp at 220°C. Between 325 and 600°C, the major products are HAp and $\beta$-$Ca_2P_2O_7$. Between 650 and 900°C, the products were $\beta$-$Ca_3(PO_4)_2$ and $\beta$-$Ca_2P_2O_7$ (Elliott, 1994).

## 6. Tricalcium phosphate (TCP)

*Chemical formula*: $Ca_3(PO_4)_2$ ($\alpha$ and $\beta$ phases)

*Other names*: Tricalcium diorthophosphates and TCP

*Mineral name*: Whitlockite

*Atomic ratio*: $Ca/P = 1.5$

*Structure*: $\alpha$-TCP crystallizes in the monoclinic space group, $P2_1/a$ with lattice parameters: $a = 12.8872$ Å, $b = 27.2804$ Å, $c = 15.2192$ Å and $\beta = 126.201°$. $\beta$-TCP crystallizes in the rhombohedral space group $R3c$ with unit cell $a = 10.4391$ Å, $c = 37.3756$ Å.

*Preparation*: $\beta$-TCP is the low-temperature phase in the $CaO$–$P_2O_5$ phase diagram. $\beta$-TCP transforms to $\alpha$-TCP at 1125°C. $\beta$-TCP is prepared by heating an intimate mixture of stoichiometric amounts of DCPA and $CaCO_3$. $\beta$-TCP does not form in aqueous systems under normal laboratory conditions except with the introduction of small amounts of $Mg^{2+}$ ions.

*Stability*: $\beta$-TCP is stable up to 1125°C and above this, up to 1430°C, $\alpha$-TCP is the stable phase. Beyond 1430°C, the super-$\alpha$-TCP form becomes stable until the melting point of 1756°C.

## 7. Tetracalcium phosphate monoxide (TCPM)

*Chemical formula*: $Ca_4(PO_4)_2O$

*Mineral name*: Hilgenstockite

*Other names*: TetCP, tetracalcium diphosphate monoxide

*Atomic ratio*: Ca/P = 2.0

*Structure*: Monoclinic with space group $P2_1$ with unit cell parameters,
$a = 7.0231$ Å, $b = 11.9864$ Å, $c = 9.4732$ Å, $\beta = 90.901°$.

*Preparation*: Solid-state reactions at high temperatures, usually between DCPA and $CaCO_3$ carried out in a dry atmosphere or vacuum with rapid cooling to prevent formation of HAp.

*Stability*: TetCP is stable in dry air but rapidly converts to HA in the presence of water according to the following reaction

$$Ca_4(PO_4)_2O + H_2O \rightarrow Ca_{10}(PO_4)_6(OH)_2 + 2CaO \tag{18.1}$$

## 8. Hydroxyapatite (HA or HAp or OHAp)

*Chemical formula*: $Ca_{10}(PO_4)_6(OH)_2$

*Atomic ratio*: Ca/P = 1.67

*Structure*: Stoichiometric HA is monoclinic with space group $P2_1/b$, with lattice parameters, $a = 9.42148$ Å, $b = 2a$, $c = 6.88147$ Å, $\gamma = 120°$. Earlier studies showed that it could exhibit the hexagonal structure with space group $P6_3/m$.

*Preparation*: Pure and stoichiometric HA similar to TCP cannot be synthesized under aqueous conditions. HA is obtained by solid-state reactions or under hydrothermal (high pressure–high temperature) conditions at 375°C or at temperatures above 900°C. In aqueous solution environments, HA can be obtained by precipitation under very basic conditions (pH > 11). This is done by reacting $Ca(OH)_2$ with $H_3PO_4$ at pH 12. Another reaction often followed is the reaction of $Ca(NO_3)_2 \cdot 4H_2O$ with $(NH_4)_2HPO_4$ in an aqueous solution at pH > 7. At pH less than 8, other phases are stabilized and at pH < 12, the Ca/P ratio is altered giving Ca-deficient HA. The pH of the solution is extremely important for the stability and formation of stoichiometric HA. At pH < 5, DCPA and DCPD are the stable phases, while HA begins to be stable only above pH 6 (see Figure 18.5).

*Stability*: The decomposition temperatures and stability correspondingly depend on the ratio of Ca/P. Typically, the lattice hydroxide if present is lost at 400°C along with loss of acid phosphate $(HPO_4)^{2-}$ by the formation of the pyrophosphate in the temperature range of 400–700°C. Above 700°C, the pyrophosphate reacts with HA to give β-TCP. The formation of β-TCP at 900°C is an indicator of the Ca/P ratio and the formation of a composition with a Ca/P ratio less than stoichiometry. Above 1000°C and higher, HA decomposes to α-TCP and TetCP as is known from the $CaO$–$P_2O_5$ phase diagram (Elliott, 1994).

## 9. Amorphous calcium phosphates (ACP)

*Chemical formula*: $Ca_x(PO_4)_y$, where $x$ and $y$ depend on the reaction conditions and stoichiometry of the reacting reagents.

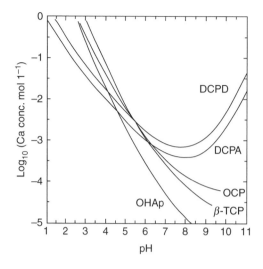

**FIGURE 18.5**
Solubility isotherms of CaP phases in the Ca(OH)$_2$–H$_3$PO$_4$–H$_2$O system shown at 37°C. The solubility curves are calculated using known software. (*Source:* Elliott, J.C., *Structure and Chemistry of the Apatites and other Calcium Orthophosphates*, Elsevier, Amsterdam (1994). With permission.)

*Preparation*: Prepared at room temperature by the rapid addition of Ca(NO$_3$)$_2$·4 H$_2$O to a solution of (NH$_4$)$_2$HPO$_4$ to give a final Ca/P ratio of 1.71. Other reactions conducted by varying the concentrations, stoichiometry and pH can yield ACP with Ca/P ratios of ≈1.5.

*Stability*: The Ca/P ratio remains unchanged under dry conditions while in aqueous conditions there could be rapid transformation and crystallization to Ca-deficient forms of apatite.

   When heated to ≈530°C, volatiles escape, the material remains amorphous, but further heating above 650°C produces crystalline α-TCP and/or β-TCP. Thus α-TCP can be produced at temperatures lower than its equilibrium transformation temperatures.

HA and TCP are the two forms of apatites that are very tissue compatible and are used as bone substitutes in a granular form or a solid block. The apatite form of calcium phosphate is considered to be closely related to the mineral phase of bone and teeth. Polycrystalline HA has a high elastic modulus (40–117 GPa; see Table 18.5). Hard tissue such as bone, dentin, and dental enamel are natural composites which contain HA as well as protein, other organic materials and water. Enamel is the stiffest hard tissue with an elastic modulus of 74 GPa, and contains the most mineral. Dentin ($E = 21$ GPa) and

**TABLE 18.5**

Physical Properties of Calcium Phosphate

| Properties | Values |
|---|---|
| Elastic modulus (GPa) | 4.0–117 |
| Compressive strength (MPa) | 294 |
| Bending strength (MPa) | 147 |
| Hardness (Vickers, GPa) | 3.43 |
| Poisson's ratio | 0.27 |
| Density (theoretical, g/cm$^3$) | 3.16 |

*Source*: Park, J.B. and Lakes, R.S. Ceramic implant materials, *Biomaterials: An Introduction*, 2nd ed., p. 133, Plenum Press, New York (1992). With permission.

compact bone ($E = 12{-}18$ GPa) contain comparatively less mineral. The properties of HA vary depending on the Ca/P ratio, the structure and the manufacturing process.

## 18.4 Other Ceramic Systems

### 18.4.1 Aluminum–Calcium–Phosphate (ALCAP) Ceramics

Initially calcium aluminate ceramic containing phosphorus pentoxide was fabricated which was later developed into aluminum–calcium–phosphorus oxide ceramic primarily by Bajpai et al. in 1980 (Billotte, 2000). ALCAP has insulating dielectric properties but no magnetic or piezoelectric properties. ALCAP is unique because they provide a multipurpose crystallographic system where one phase of the ceramic on implantation can be more rapidly resorbed than the others. The typical ratios of the various constituents are:

$Al_2O_3$:CaO:$P_2O_5 = 50{:}34{:}16$ which are mixed and calcined at a temperature of 1350°C for 12 h followed by sintering at 1400°C for 36 h. ALCAP materials exhibit good biocompatibility and gradual replacement of the ceramic with endogenous bone.

### 18.4.2 Coralline

Coral is a natural substance made by marine invertebrates which has a unique interconnected porous structure. Corals for use as bone implants were selected mainly on the basis of their structural similarity to bone. Coral provides an excellent structure for the ingrowth of bone, and the main component, $CaCO_3$ is gradually resorbed by the body (Khavari and Bajpai, 1993). Corals can also be converted to HA by a hydrothermal ion-exchange process. Interpore 200 is the commercial name for the coralline HA which resembles cancellous bone. Both pure coral (Biocoral) and coral transformed to HA are currently used to repair traumatized bone, to replace diseased bone and to correct a number of bone defects.

Biocoral comprises crystalline $CaCO_3$ or aragonite, the metastable form of $CaCO_3$. The compressive strength of Biocoral varies from 26 (50% porous) to 395 Mpa (dense) depending on the porosity. Similarly, the elastic modulus ranges from 8 (50% porous) to 100 Gpa (dense).

### 18.4.3 Zinc–Calcium–Phosphorus Oxide (ZCAP) Ceramics (Billotte, 2000)

Zinc is essential for human metabolism and is a component of at least 30 metalloenzymes. In addition, Zn may also be involved in the process of wound healing. Thus Zn–Ca–$P_2O_5$ polyphasic ceramics (ZCAP) were synthesized to repair bone defects and deliver drugs. ZCAP is prepared by thermal mixing of ZnO, CaO, and $P_2O_5$ in various ratios and calcining at 800°C for 24 h.

### 18.4.4 Zinc–Sulfate–Calcium–Phosphate (ZSCAP) Ceramics (Scheidler and Bajpai, 1992; Billotte, 2000)

Zn–sulfate–Ca–phosphate polyphasic ceramics (ZSCAP) are prepared from stock powders of $ZnSO_4$, ZnO, CaO, and $P_2O_5$ in a ratio of 15:30:30:25 and calcined in a crucible at 650°C for 24 h. ZSCAP sets and hardens upon the addition of water. These materials have been used to repair experimentally induced defects in bone.

### 18.4.5 Ferric–Calcium–Phosphorus–Oxide (FECAP) Ceramics (Stricker et al., 1992; Larrabee et al., 1993)

FECAP ceramics are prepared from powders of $Fe_2O_3$, CaO, and $P_2O_5$. The powders are combined in various ratios and calcined at 1100°C for 12 h. The composite when mixed with ketoglutaric acid and water sets and hardens. Studies apparently indicate that complete resorption occurs when implanted in bone within 60 days.

### 18.4.6 Bioactive or Surface-Reactive Ceramics (Billotte, 2000)

These are ceramics or inorganic materials that upon implantation in the host form strong bonds with the adjacent tissue. These materials include *dense nonporous glasses, Bioglass and Ceravital, and hydroxyapatite*. One of the uses is application of coatings on metal implants to form a bond with the adjacent tissue. However, delamination and spalling is a recurring problem due to the brittleness of the ceramic. There are a number of uses for surface reactive ceramics as listed below:

*Uses of surface reactive ceramics*

1. Coating of metal prostheses
2. In construction of dental defects
3. For filling space vacated by bone screws, donor bone, excised tumors, and diseased bone loss
4. As bone plates and screws
5. As replacements of middle ear ossicles
6. For lengthening of rami
7. For correcting periodontal defects
8. In replacing subperiosteal teeth

## 18.5 Glass-Ceramics

Several variations of Bioglass and Ceravital glass-ceramics have been used in the last decade. These glasses were first developed by Professor Larry Hench at the University of Florida in the early 1980s. Glass-ceramics for implantation are silicon oxide based systems with or without phosphorus pentoxide.

Glass-ceramics are crystalline materials nucleated within and from a glass developed by S.D. Stookey of Corning Glass in the early 1960s (Park, 1992). The formation of the glass-ceramic is initiated by the addition of nucleating agents that help nucleate and grow small crystals uniformly within the glass. These nucleating agents can be metals such as Cu, Ag, Au, Pt as well as $TiO_2$, $ZrO_2$, and $P_2O_5$. The nucleation is carried out at temperatures lower than the melting temperature and further annealing is conducted at appropriate temperatures to cause uniform growth of the crystallites. The nucleating agents and the heat treatment temperatures help to control the grain size to 0.1–1 $\mu$m. The typical thermal treatment can be illustrated by Figure 18.6.

Glass-ceramics developed for implantation are $SiO_2$–CaO–$Na_2O$–$P_2O_5$ and $Li_2O$–ZnO–$SiO_2$ systems. Although there are several glass forming systems, the best compositions are the ones which representatively contain $SiO_2$, CaO, and $P_2O_5$.

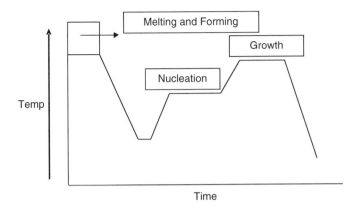

**FIGURE 18.6**
Temperature–time cycle for a typical glass-ceramic. (*Source*: Taken from Kingery, W.D., Bowen, H.K., and Uhlmann, D.R., *Introduction to Ceramics*, 2nd ed., John Wiley & Sons, New York, p. 368 (1976). With permission.)

The main reason is that the bonding to bone is related to the simultaneous formation of a calcium phosphate and $SiO_2$ rich film layer on the surface. If a silica rich layer forms first and a calcium phosphate film develops later or no phosphate film is formed for the case containing 60 mol% $SiO_2$ then direct bonding with the bone does not occur. The approximate region of the $SiO_2$–CaO–$Na_2O$ system for the tissue–glass–ceramic reaction is shown in Figure 18.7 (Hench and Ethridge, 1982). The optimum composition is given by the Bioglass (46S5.2) whose composition is

$SiO_2$:46.1
CaO:26.9
$Na_2O$:24.4
$P_2O_5$:2.6

### 18.5.1  Ceravital

Composition of Ceravital is similar to Bioglass in $SiO_2$ content except that they differ in other contents, see Table 18.6 (Park, 1992; Billotte, 2000). In order to control the resorption rate, $Al_2O_3$, $TiO_2$, and $Ta_2O_5$ are added to the Ceravital glass-ceramic. The mixtures are melted in a Pt-crucible at 1500°C for 3 h followed by annealing and cooling. The nucleation and crystallization temperatures are 680 and 750°C each for 24 h. The crystallite sizes are in the range of 4 Å and the crystals are unformly distributed to give a glass-ceramic that has a thermal expansion coefficient of $10^{-7}$ to $10^{-5}$/°C. Due to controlled crystallization,

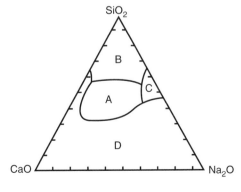

**FIGURE 18.7**
Approximate phase fields corresponding to the tissue–glass–ceramic bonding for the $SiO_2$–CaO–$Na_2O$ system. A: represents bonding within 30 days. B: Nonbonding; indicating reactivity is too low. C: Nonbonding; reactivity is too high. D: Bonding; does not form glass. (*Source*: Taken from Hench, L.L. and Ethridge, E.C., *Biomaterials: An Interfacial Approach*, Academic Press, New York, p. 147 (1982). With permission.)

**TABLE 18.6**

Typical Compositions of Bioglass and Ceravital Glass-Ceramics (Park, 1992)

| Type | Code | SiO$_2$ | CaO | Na$_2$O | P$_2$O$_5$ | MgO | K$_2$O |
|---|---|---|---|---|---|---|---|
| Bioglass | 42S5.6 | 42.1 | 29.0 | 26.3 | 2.6 | — | — |
| | (45S5) | 46.1 | 26.9 | 24.4 | 2.6 | — | — |
| | 46S5.2 | | | | | | |
| | 49S4.9 | 49.1 | 25.3 | 23.8 | 2.6 | — | — |
| | 52S4.6 | 52.1 | 23.8 | 21.5 | 2.6 | — | — |
| | 55S4.3 | 55.1 | 22.2 | 20.1 | 2.6 | — | — |
| | 60S3.8 | 60.1 | 19.6 | 17.7 | 2.6 | — | — |
| Ceravital | Bioactive[a] | 40–50 | 30–35 | 5–10 | 10–15 | 2.5–5 | 0.5–3 |
| | Nonbioactive[b] | 30–35 | 25–30 | 3.5–7.5 | 7.5–12 | 1–2.5 | 0.5–2 |

[a]  Ceravital composition is in wt% while Bioglass compositions are in mol%.

[b]  In addition Al$_2$O$_3$ (5–15), TiO$_2$ (1–5) and Ta$_2$O$_5$ (5–15) are added.

the grain size can be kept to a minimum to provide improved mechanical properties. The strength of these materials are in the range of 100–200 MPa (at least twice that of the glass). Figure 18.8 shows a TEM micrograph of a Bioglass glass-ceramic implanted in the femur of a rat for 6 weeks showing intimate contact between the mineralized bone and the Bioglass. The mechanical strength of the interfacial bond between bone and Bioglass ceramic is of the same order of magnitude as the strength of the bulk glass ceramic (850 kg/cm$^2$ or 83.3 MPa), which is about 3/4 that of the host bone strength (Beckham et al., 1971).

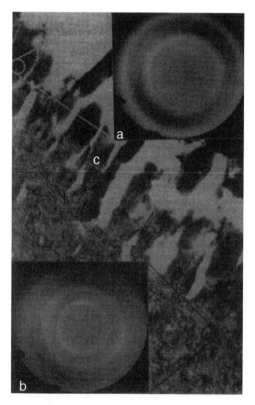

**FIGURE 18.8**

Transmission electron micrograph of well-mineralized bone (b) juxtaposed to the glass-ceramic (c), which was fractured during sectioning, × 51,500. Inset (a) is the selected area diffraction pattern from the ceramic area and (b) is the diffraction pattern from the bone area. (*Source*: Taken from Beckham, C.A., Greenlee, T.K., Jr., and Crebo, A.R., *Calcif. Tissue Res.*, **8**, 165–171 (1971). With permission.)

The major disadvantage of glass-ceramics is their brittleness. In addition, there are limitations on the compositions used for producing a biocompatible glass-ceramic which hinders the production of a glass-ceramic that has good mechanical properties. Thus they cannot be used for load-bearing applications although they can be used as fillers for bone cement, dental restorative composites, and coating material.

## 18.6 Deterioration of Ceramics

The performance of a ceramic similar to metal is paramount within the body or in vivo. Controlled degradation with time upon implantation is desirable when new tissue or bone has already formed. However, ceramics fail under static and dynamic stress, a condition known as fatigue which is accelerated in the presence of water. It is, therefore, essential to review some of the fundamental concepts of mechanical behavior needed to interpret the performance and response of degradation of ceramic materials.

### 18.6.1 Stress–Strain Behavior

For a material that undergoes mechanical deformation under the application of load, stress is defined as the force per unit area. The stress is usually expressed in newtons per square meter (Pa, Pascal) or pounds force per square inch (psi).

$$\text{Stress}(s) = \text{force/cross-sectional area, } (N/m^2) \text{ or } (lbf/in.^2)$$

Typically loads or forces can be applied upon a material in *tension, compression,* and *shear* or any combination of these *forces* (or stresses). Tensile stresses are generated in response to loads (forces) that relate to pulling an object apart (see Figure 18.9a) while compressive stresses tend to squeeze the object (see Figure 18.9b). Shear stresses resist loads that deform or separate by sliding layers of molecules past each other on one or more atomic planes (Figure 18.9c). Shear stresses can also be found in uniaxial tension or compression since the applied stress produces the maximum shear stress on planes at 45° to the direction of loading (Figure 18.9d).

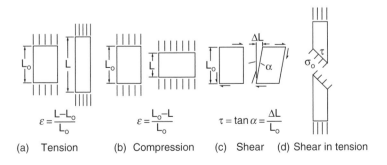

(a) Tension    (b) Compression    (c) Shear    (d) Shear in tension

**FIGURE 18.9**
Schematic representation of three modes of deformation in solids. The shear stresses can be produced by tension or compression as in (d). (*Source*: Park, J.B. and Lakes, R.S., Ceramic implant materials, *Biomaterials: An Introduction*, 2nd ed., Plenum Press, New York, p. 30. (1992). With permission.)

The deformation of an object in response to an applied load is called *strain*:

$$\text{Strain}(s) = \text{change in length/original length}$$
$$= \text{new length} - \text{original length (m/m) or (in./in.)}$$

The new length can arise due to deformation resulting in an extension of the object causing an increase in the length of the object. Similarly, compression could result in deformation causing the material to reduce its dimension in which case the strain would be negative in sign only. The deformations related to the different types of stresses are called tensile, compressive, and shear strain (see Figure 18.9).

If the stress–strain behavior is plotted on a graph, a curve that represents a continuous response of the material toward the imposed force can be obtained as shown in Figure 18.10. The stress–strain curve of a solid is usually characterized by a linear region where the stress increases linearly with strain until the point where the material displays nonlinear relation. This point is typically called the yield point which demarcates the material response into elastic and plastic deformation zones (Park, 1992).

In the elastic region, the strain ($\varepsilon$) increases in direct proportion to the applied stress ($\sigma$) given by Hooke's law:

$$\sigma = E\varepsilon; \quad \text{stress} = (\text{initial slope})(\text{strain}) \tag{18.2}$$

The slope ($E$) or the proportionality constant of the tensile/compressive stress–strain curve is called *Young's modulus* or the *modulus of elasticity*. It is the value of the increment of stress over the increment of strain. A stiff material normally provides a higher value of $E$ which reflects its stronger resistance to deformation. Similar analysis can be performed for the shear deformation, in which case the shear modulus, $G$, is defined as the initial slope of the plot of shear strain and shear stress. The unit for the modulus is the same as that of stress since strain is dimensionless.

The shear modulus of an isotropic material is given by Young's modulus: $E = 2G(1 + \nu)$; where $\nu$ is the Poisson ratio of the material. Poisson's ratio is defined as the negative ratio of the transverse strain to the longitudinal strain for tensile or compressive loading of a material. Poisson's ratio is close to 1/3 for common stiff materials, and is slightly less than 1/2 for rubbery materials and for soft biological tissues.

In the plastic region, strain changes are no longer proportional to the applied stress or load. In addition, when the applied load or stress is removed, the material will no longer return to its original shape but will remain permanently deformed. This deformation is

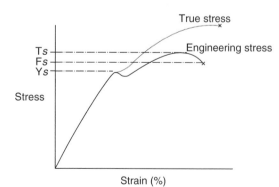

**FIGURE 18.10**
Stress–strain behavior of a representative ideal material depicting the engineering and true stress–strain response. (*Source*: Park, J.B., Lakes, R.S., Ceramic implant materials, *Biomaterials: An Introduction*, 2nd ed., p. 30, Plenum Press, New York (1992). With permission.)

called plastic deformation. When the load is released before atoms can slide over the other neighboring atoms, the atoms will go back to their respective original positions, thus resulting in an elastic deformation. When a material is deformed plastically, the atoms are moved past each other in such a manner that the atoms will now have a new environment of atoms and when the load is removed, they can no longer go back to their original positions.

Referring back to the stress–strain curve, a peak stress can be seen which is often followed by an apparent decrease until a point is reached where the material ruptures. The peak stress is known as the tensile or ultimate tensile strength (UTS); the stress where the material fails is called the failure or fracture strength (FS).

In solid materials such as metals and ceramics, the yield point is clear although in steels for example, the yield point undergoes further changes into upper and lower yield points related to specific atom movements resulting in a saw tooth like behavior. This point is typically characterized by a temporary increase in strain without a further increase in stress. Because of the difficulty in categorically identifying this change from linear to plastic deformation, an offset typically about 0.2% is called the yield point in lieu of the original yield point.

It must also be noted that the above definitions of stress and strain are called engineering stress and engineering strain which differ from true stress and true strain. The difference being that in the former case the stress relates to the force being applied to a material with constant cross-sectional area. As a result, the curve is obtained by assuming a constant cross-sectional area over which the load is applied from the initial loading to the point of failure. Hence a peak is seen in the plot (see Figure 18.10). Normally, when the material deforms, typically before failure there is rapid movement of atoms causing a sharp reduction in the area, a phenomenon known as *necking* occurs which actually causes an increase in stress rather than a decrease as seen when the original cross sectional area is considered. If more measurements are made of the changes in cross-sectional area that typically occur at this point and the true area is used in the calculations, then the stress is represented by the dotted curve as shown in Figure 18.10 above.

Another term that is often used to define the permanent strain that is realized before the test material fractures is called *ductility*. As is the case with strength, there is more than one way to define strain. Elongation is thus the linear plastic strain accompanying fracture (Van Vlack, 1989):

$El_{gage\ length} = (L_f - L_o)/L_o$, where $L_f$ is the final length and $L_o$ is the original length. It is important to note the gage length because plastic strain is almost invariably localized.

A second measure of ductility is the reduction of area, R of A, at the point of failure: R of A $(D) = (A_o - A_f)/A_o$, where $A_o$ is the original area and $A_f$ is the area at failure. Thus true stress at failure is defined as:

$$\sigma_f = F/A_f = [F/A_o][A_o/A_f] = \sigma[A_o/A_f]$$

$$= \sigma/[1 - D]; \text{ where } \sigma \text{ is the engineering stress} \qquad (18.3)$$

Similarly, true strain $\varepsilon$ can be represented as:

$$\varepsilon = \int_{l_o}^{l_f} \frac{dl}{l} = \ln(l_f/l_o) \qquad (18.4)$$

Assuming constant volume, $Al = A_o l_o$ then

$$\varepsilon = \ln(l/l_o) = \ln(A_o/A) \qquad (18.5)$$

The above equation gives a definition of true strain that holds for all strains and is independent of gage length.

## 18.6.2  Mechanical Failure

Mechanical failure is usually followed by fracture of the material. Fracture can be characterized by the amount of energy per unit volume required to produce failure. The quantity is called toughness and can be expressed in terms of stress and strain as follows:

$$\text{Toughness} = \int_{\varepsilon_o}^{\varepsilon_f} \sigma \, d\varepsilon = \int_{l_o}^{l_f} \sigma \frac{dl}{l} \tag{18.6}$$

Expressed in another way, toughness is essentially the summation of the product of stress and the normalized strain over which the strain acts taken over small increments. The area under the stress–strain curve thus provides a simple method of estimating the toughness as shown in Figure 18.11.

A material that can withstand high stresses and can undergo considerable plastic deformation (ductile–tough) material is tougher than one that resists high stresses but has no capacity for deformation (hard–brittle material) or one that has a high capacity for deformation but can only withstand relatively low stresses (ductile–soft or plastic material).

Brittle materials are known to exhibit fracture strengths far below the theoretical strengths predicted based on known atomic bond strengths. Moreover, there is much variation in strength from specimen to specimen, so that the practical strength is difficult to predict. These aspects, along with the comparative weakness of ceramics in tension, are the major reasons why ceramic and glassy materials are categorized as weak and brittle making them questionable for load bearing applications although they are excellent in terms of their compatibility with tissues. The brittleness of ceramics and glasses can be explained in terms of cracks and size of cracks explained below.

In the case of ceramic materials used for implants, reduction in strength occurs if water penetrates the ceramic. It is reasonable to assume that static failure occurs due to the presence of inherent cracks or cracks formed due to increased stress levels. The presence of impurities or any surface flaws contributes to this situation.

Studies of fatigue behavior of vapor-deposited pyrolitic carbon fibers (4000–5000 Å thick) onto a stainless steel substrate show that the film does not break unless the substrate undergoes plastic deformation at $1.3 \times 10^{-2}$ strain and up to one million cycles of loading. Fatigue is closely related to the substrate. Similarly, substrate–carbon adherence is responsible for the pyrolitic carbon deposited polymer arterial grafts.

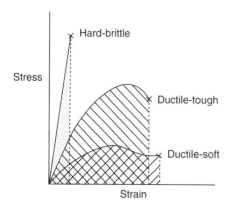

**FIGURE 18.11**
Stress–strain curves showing the characteristic response of different types of bioceramic materials. The areas underneath the curves are a measure of the toughness. (*Source*: Park, J.B. and Lakes, R.S., Ceramic implant materials, *Biomaterials: An Introduction*, 2nd ed., Plenum Press, New York, p. 133 (1992). With permission.)

The fatigue life of ceramics can be predicted by assuming that the fatigue fracture is due to the slow growth of preexisting flaws. Generally, the strength distribution, $s_i$, in an inert environment can be related to the probability of failure, $F$, given by the following equation:

$$\ln \ln(1/1 - F) = m \ln(s_i/s_o) \tag{18.7}$$

where $m$ and $s_o$ are constants. Figure 18.12 shows a good fit for Bioglass coated alumina (Ritter et al., 1979).

A minimum service life ($t_{min}$) of a specimen can be predicted by means of a proof test wherein it is subjected to stresses that are greater than those expected in service. Proof tests also eliminate the weaker pieces. This minimum life can be predicted from the following equation:

$$t_{min} = B\sigma_p^{N-2}\sigma_a^{-N}$$

where $\sigma_p$ is the proof test stress, $\sigma_a$, the applied stress, and $B$ and $N$ are constants (Ritter et al., 1979)

Rearrangement leads to

$$t_{min}\sigma_a^2 = B[\sigma_p/\sigma_a]^{N-2} \tag{18.8}$$

Figure 18.13 shows a plot of the above equation for alumina on a logarithmic scale (Ritter et al., 1979).

### 18.6.3 Brittle Crack Failure in a Ceramic (Kingery et al., 1976; Park, 1992)

The stress on a defect crack is not distributed uniformly over the entire cross-sectional area of the crack. If the crack is a narrow elliptical hole as shown in a specimen subjected to a tensile stress, the maximum stress ($\sigma_{max}$) acting at the ends of the hole is given by:

$$\sigma_{max} = \sigma_{app}(1 + 2a/b) \tag{18.9}$$

as shown in Figure 18.14.

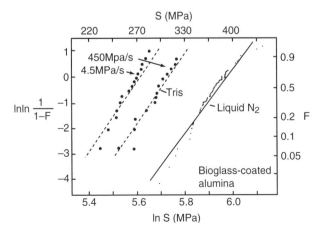

**FIGURE 18.12**
Plot of $\ln \ln[1/(1 - F)]$ vs. $\ln s$ for bioglass-coated alumina in a tris-hydroxyamino-methane buffer and liquid nitrogen. $F$ is the probability of failure and $S$ is the strength (*Source*: Ritter, J.E. Jr., Greenspan, D.C., Palmer, R.A., and Hench, L.L., *J. Biomed. Mater. Res.* **13**: 260 (1979). With permission.)

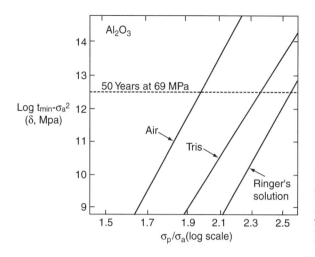

**FIGURE 18.13**
Plot showing the relation of equation 18.8 for alumina after proof testing. $N = 43.85$, $m = 13.21$, and $s_o = 55728$ psi (*Source*: Ritter, J.E., Jr., Greenspan, D.C., Palmer, R.A., and Hench L.L., *J. Biomed. Mater. Res.* **13**, 261 (1979). With permission.)

In Equation 18.9 above, $\sigma_{app}$ is the applied or nominal tensile stress experienced away from the crack. On rearranging:

$$\sigma_{max}/\sigma_{app} = (1 + 2a/b) \qquad (18.10)$$

The ratio $\sigma_{max}/\sigma_{app}$ is called the stress concentration factor (SCF) which can be substantial if the $a/b$ ratio is high, i.e., a sharp crack. If the crack tip has a radius of curvature ($r = b^2/a$) then we can rewrite:

$$\sigma_{max} = \sigma_{app}[1 + 2(a/r)^{0.5}] \qquad (18.11)$$

Since $a \gg r$ for a crack,

$$\sigma_{max} = 2\sigma_{app}(a/r)^{0.5} \qquad (18.12)$$

This indicates that the stress concentration becomes large for a sharp crack tip as well as for long cracks. Thus, the propagation of a sharp crack can be prevented if one increases the crack tip radius.

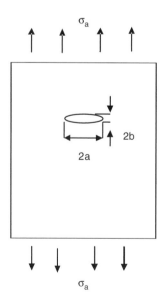

**FIGURE 18.14**
Schematic representation of an elliptic microcrack inclusion in a brittle ceramic material (Kingery et al., 1976; Park, 1992).

Griffith proposed an energy approach to failure. The elastic energy stored in a test specimen of unit thickness is:

$$\sigma \times \varepsilon = \pi a^2 \sigma(\sigma/E) = \pi(a\sigma)^2/E \tag{18.13}$$

One can observe that the elastic energy for a brittle material is twice the area under the stress–strain curve. The elastic energy is used to create two new surfaces as the crack propagates. The surface energy $4\gamma a$ ($\gamma$ is the surface energy) should be smaller than the elastic energy for the crack to grow. Thus the incremental changes of both energies for the crack to grow can be written as:

$$\frac{d}{da}\left(\frac{\pi(a\sigma)^2}{E}\right) = \frac{d}{da}(4\gamma a) \tag{18.14}$$

Hence,

$$\sigma = \sigma_f = \sqrt{\frac{2\gamma E}{\pi a}} \tag{18.15}$$

Since for a given material, $E$ and $g$ are constants,

$$\sigma_f = K/(\pi a)^{0.5} \tag{18.16}$$

$K$ has units of psi sq. root in. or $MPa(m)^{0.5}$ and is proportional to the energy required for failure; $K$ is also called the fracture toughness. Stress concentration also occurs in ductile materials, but their effect is not as serious as in the case of brittle materials since local yielding that occurs in the region of peak stress will effectively blunt the crack and alleviate the stress concentration.

## 18.7 Nanostructured Calcium Phosphates (NanoCaPs) — Emerging Materials

Calcium phosphates are considered as attractive biomedical materials owing to their excellent biocompatibility and nontoxicity of their chemical components. As discussed earlier, there are many phases of calcium phosphates exhibiting different crystal structures and Ca/P ratios which represent resorbable and nonresorbable ceramics and cements (Driessens, 1983; Aoki, 1991; Elliott, 1994). Several forms of these materials can be used as scaffolds for tissue engineering, as drug delivery agents, nonviral gene carriers, as prosthetic coatings and composites (Masaaki et al., 1998; Melde and Stein, 2002; Choi et al., 2004). All of these manifestations of calcium phosphates find applications for bone reconstruction and replacement as bone defect-filling drug carriers and as coatings for metal prostheses. The applicability of CaP materials for drug delivery and as carriers of plasmid DNA for nonviral gene delivery requires the synthesis of these structures under conditions in which the plasmid DNA is stable. Furthermore, the efficacy of these carriers for gene delivery is also dependent on their ability to bind and condense DNA effectively while also releasing the bound DNA after the complex is taken up by the cell. It is known that plasmid DNA is a negatively charged molecule (Billotte, 2000). Hence electrostatic interaction would necessitate the use of positively charged species to ensure adequate binding of plasmid DNA to the synthesized particles.

Thus CaP structures with varying Ca/P ratios could provide the desired balance of charge to favor optimum electrostatic interaction. Additionally, from the catalysis literature (Kumta et al., 2005) it is known that particles with smaller dimensions exhibit higher specific surface areas which in turn imply larger binding centers to enhance higher binding capacity of plasmid DNA. Thus nanostructured CaP particles with varying Ca/P ratios is a direction worth exploring for obtaining enhanced binding, release and delivery of plasmid DNA. Although the present article is not focused on outlining the effects of each of these individual aspects, the results of the studies presented do provide an indication of the validity and, moreover, the importance of the above-mentioned factors. Subsequent publications will provide more detailed descriptions of the results of ongoing research activities in the laboratory of the author validating the above important aspects for plasmid gene delivery.

In a recent publication by the author and his co-workers, they report a novel precipitation approach for synthesizing HA which can be represented by the following equation:

$$10CaCl_2 + 6Na_3PO_4 + xNaOH \rightarrow Ca_{9+(x/2)}(PO_4)_6(OH)_2 + (18+x)NaCl$$
$$+ (1-(x/2))CaCl_2 \qquad (x = 0,1,2)$$

This is a simple and easy approach under aqueous conditions for synthesizing thermally stable nanostructured HA powder. They also studied the effect of NaOH addition ($x = 0, 1, 2$) on the chemical reaction, the composition and thermal stability of the synthesized HA powder. Figure 18.15 is an SEM micrograph showing agglomerates (3–5 $\mu$m) of nanocrystallites ($\approx 10$ nm) of the synthesized HA powder. They also describe a new approach for synthesizing Mg-substituted brushite and Mg-substituted β-TCMP under physiological conditions. The synthesis of pure undoped brushite is based on the following reaction (Kumta et al., 2005).

$$Na_2HPO_4 + CaCl_2 + 2H_2O \rightarrow CaHPO_4 \cdot 2H_2O + 2NaCl \qquad (18.17)$$

After the solutions were prepared, the $CaCl_2 \cdot 2H_2O$ solution was added dropwise to $Na_2HPO_4$ solution while stirring. The precipitate was then centrifuged, washed with distilled water, and dried at 60°C overnight in a drying-oven.

The synthesis of 14% Mg substituted brushite is based on the following reaction:

$$Na_2HPO_4 + 0.86CaCl_2 + 0.14MgCl_2 + 2H_2O \rightarrow (Ca_{0.86}Mg_{0.14})HPO_4 \cdot 2H_2O + 2NaCl$$
$$(18.18)$$

Two separate aqueous solutions were prepared one containing the $Ca^{2+}$ and $Mg^{2+}$ ions and the other containing sodium phosphate. Both solutions were stirred until the salts were completely dissolved. 14% Mg/Ca solution was then added dropwise to the $Na_2HPO_4$ solution while stirring. The precipitate was then centrifuged, washed with distilled water, and dried overnight at 60°C in a drying oven. Figure 18.16 shows the SEM image of 14% Mg substituted brushite. The characteristic platelet morphology (10–20 $\mu$m, length and 1 $\mu$m thickness) is retained. In order to synthesize TCP, the authors report the

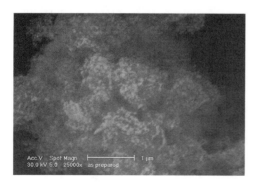

**FIGURE 18.15**
SEM micrograph of the as-prepared HA powder synthesized using a new simple aqueous approach. The synthesized powder consists of ($\sim 10$ nm) nanocrystallites of HA (Kumta et al., 2005).

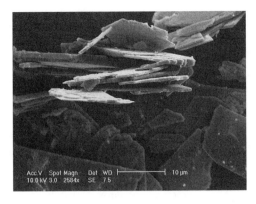

**FIGURE 18.16**
SEM image of the 14% Mg substituted brushite powder showing the characteristic platelet morphology (Kumta et al., 2005).

synthesis of Mg-substituted brushite phase containing 50% Mg. An interesting aspect is that with the incorporation of 50% Mg, the platelet morphology of brushite is lost resulting in nano-sized (100 nm) spherical particles (see Figure 18.17). The substituted brushite powder is then subjected to a slow in situ hydrolysis step to form Mg-substituted TCP, called TCMP. Figure 18.18 shows the ~80 nm nanostructured crystallites of TCP growing out of the initial spherical particles of the Mg-substituted brushite indicating a pseudomorphous transformation process. The synthesized CaP structures serve as potential carriers of plasmid DNA for nonviral gene delivery which have been discussed by the authors. Figure 18.19 shows the initial transfection efficiency results for the luciferase marker gene of the nanostructured CaP phase corresponding to hydroxyapatite (HA) with varying Ca/P ratios (Kumta et al., 2005).

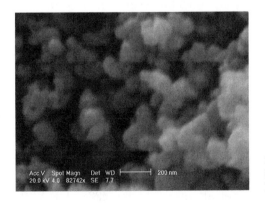

**FIGURE 18.17**
SEM image of 50% Mg substituted brushite showing the 100 nm size spherical particles (Kumta et al., 2005).

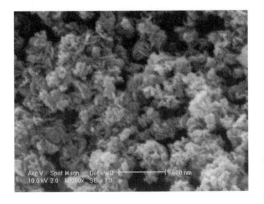

**FIGURE 18.18**
SEM image of 50% Mg TCMP showing 80 nm size TCP crystallites growing from spherical brushite crystals (Kumta et al., 2005).

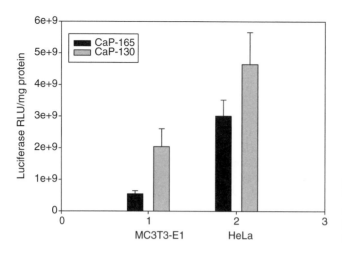

**FIGURE 18.19**
Transfection efficiency analysis of two different calcium to phosphate ratios of hydroxyapatite in MC3T3-e1 and HeLa cells (Kumta et al., 2005).

### 18.7.1   Enhanced Functions

The biocompatibility and osteo-response of nanostructured hydroxyapatite (HA) has also been recently studied. Webster et al. (Webster et al., 2000) have studied select functions of osteoblasts on nanophase (grain sizes less than 100 nm) alumina, titania and HA using in vitro cellular models. Compared to conventional ceramics, they observed that the surface occupancy of osteoblast colonies was significantly less on all nanophase ceramics that were tested by the group after 4 and 6 days of culture. They also report that the osteoblast proliferation was noticeably greater on nanophase alumina, titania and HA than on these ceramics fabricated using traditional ceramic processing methods namely of consolidation and prolonged sintering at high temperatures after 3 and 5 days. More significantly, compared to conventional large grained ceramics, synthesis of alkaline phosphatase and deposition of calcium containing mineral was apparently greater by osteoblasts cultured on nanophase than on conventional ceramics after 21 and 28 days. Their results appear to provide evidence of enhanced long-term (comprising days and weeks) functions of osteoblasts cultured on nanophase ceramics. They synthesized nanophase ceramics of alumina and titania using nanophase powders that were then compacted in a tool-steel die via a uniaxial pressing cycle (0.2–1 GPa over a 10 min period). The compacts were then sintered at 1000 and 600°C, respectively, to obtain final grains sizes less than 100 nm. In order to obtain larger grain sizes the compacts were sintered at temperatures of 1200°C to obtain grain sizes larger than 100 nm (Webster et al., 2000). In the case of HA, the nanophase materials were chemically synthesized and the cold pressed pellets were then sintered at 1100°C for 60 min. They report average grain sizes of 24 nm for nanophase alumina and 167 nm for conventionally fabricated alumina. In the case of titania, the grain sizes varied from 39 nm for nanophase and 4520 nm for the coarsened material. For HA, the nanophase material exhibited a grain size of 67 nm while the conventionally sintered ceramic displayed a grain size of 179 nm. They conducted osteoblast cell proliferation using rat calvarial osteoblasts in Dulbeco modified Eagle medium supplemented with 10% fetal bovine serum that were seeded with 2500 cells/cm$^2$ on the nanophase and large grained ceramic surfaces. They report that the proliferation of osteoblasts was significantly greater ($P < 0.01$) by almost 17% on nanophase than on conventional alumina and titania after 5 days of culture while showing almost 28% increase in nanophase HA after 5 days of culture. Their study also indicated evidence of decreased surface occupancy by osteoblasts cultured on nanophase ceramic formulations after 4 and 6 days of culture by almost 50%

compared to conventionally synthesized ceramic after 4 days in culture. Another interesting aspect of their research highlighting the influence of nanophase ceramics was seen on the alkaline phosphatase activity. They observed no detectable amounts of alkaline phosphatase activity by osteoblasts cultured on all substrates tested after 7 days and 14 days of culture. In contrast they observed that specifically after 28 days of culture, alkaline phosphatase activity on nanophase alumina, titania and HA was 36, 22, and 37% greater than on conventional ceramic formulations.

Normally, increased osteoblast adhesion coupled with decreased cell motility, as well as enhanced proliferation, synthesis of alkaline phosphatase and deposition of calcium-containing mineral has been observed on surfaces for example, borosilicate glass and titanium modified with immobilized peptide sequences such as arginine–glycine–aspartic acid–serine (RGDS) and lysine–arginine–serine–arginine (KRSR) contained in extracellular matrix proteins such as vitronectin and collagen (Dee et al., 1998). Their studies demonstrated for the first time that nanophase materials enhance these functions of osteoblasts without the need to modify the surface by immobilizing peptides. It is therefore believed that nanophase structures of biocompatible ceramics such as calcium phosphates will enhance bonding of orthopaedic/dental implants to juxtaposed bone and thus result in improved overall implant efficacy.

As a follow-on study, the research group of Webster et al. (2001) also studied the in vitro functions of osteoclasts which have been well documented on conventional orthopedic/dental materials including HA ceramics (Gomi et al., 1993; Matsunaga et al., 1999). They explored for the first time select functions particularly, synthesis of tartrate-resistant-acid phosphatase (TRAP) and the presence of resorption pits on nano-phase ceramics. It is known from Gomi et al. and Matsunaga et al. that compared to devitalized bone, these functions (such as decreased synthesis of TRAP) and smaller and fewer resorption pits) characteristic of osteoclast-like cells decrease on synthetic HA that exhibit grain sizes larger than 0.1 $\mu$m.

Their results show that compared to conventional ceramics exhibiting grain sizes larger than 100 nm, synthesis of TRAP was significantly greater (5-fold) in nanophase alumina while it was undetectable in large grained (167 nm) alumina after 10 and 13 days of culture of osteoclast-like cells. However, in the case of HA, they observed that TRAP synthesis was significantly greater by almost 83% (12-fold) in nanophase (67 nm) HA compared to large grained (179 nm) HA after 13 days. They also carried studies to investigate the enhanced resorption activity by osteoclast-like cells cultured on nanophase ceramics. In the presence of $10^{-8}$ M calcitonin in the cell culture media, the formation of resorption pits were apparently inhibited on all the substrates including devitalized bone for 13 days. However, in the absence of calcitonin, resorption pits were formed when osteoclast-like cells were cultured either on devitalized bone, alumina or on HA for 13 days (Webster et al., 2001). They observed that compared to conventional ceramics, formation of resorption pits was significantly greater when osteoclast-like cells were cultured on nanophase alumina and on nanophase HA. In particular, compared to conventional ceramics, after 13 days of culture, the numbers of resorption pits on nanophase alumina and on nanophase HA were three- and fourfold greater, respectively. In addition, they observed that compared to results obtained on nanophase alumina, formation of resorption pits was 25% greater when osteoclast-like cells were cultured on nanopase HA for 13 days. Their results on nanophase ceramics shed light on important aspects such as enhanced reactivity, surface wettability, and increased surface roughness that would mediate enhanced osteoclastic functions. These constitute parameters that could play an important role when designing and synthesizing the next generation of orthopaedic/dental implants. Since bone resorption by osteoclasts is accompanied by subsequent events leading to deposition of minerals containing calcium by osteoblasts *in vivo*, their results imply that enhanced coordinated functions of osteoclasts and osteoblasts could occur on nanophase ceramics. These events could form the basis of better osseointegration of orthopaedic and/or dental implants to the attached bone.

# References

Abrams, L.A.B. and Bajpai, P.K., Hydroxyapatite ceramics for continuous delivery of heparin, *Biomed. Sci. Instrum.*, **30**, 169–174 (1994).

Adams, D.A.W. and Williams, D.F., Carbon fiber-reinforced carbon as a potential implant materials, *J. Biomed. Mater. Res.*, **12**, 35–42 (1978).

Alexander, H.P., Parsons, J.R., Ricci, J.L., Bajpai, P.K., and Weiss, A.B., Calcium-based ceramics and composites in bone reconstruction, *Crit. Rev.*, **4**, 43–47 (1987).

Aoki, H., *Science and Medical Applications of Hydroxyapatite*, Takayama Press, Tokyo, Japan, p. 137 (1991).

Arrar, H.A.A.B. and Bajpai, P.K., Insulin delivery by zinc calcium phosphate (ZCAP) ceramics, *Biomed. Sci. Instrum.*, **28**, 172–178 (1992).

Beckham, C.A.G., Greenlee, T.K. Jr., and Crebo, A.R., Bone formation at a ceramic implant interface, *Calcif. Tissue Res.*, **8**, 165–171 (1971).

Billotte, W.G., Ceramic biomaterials, In: *The Biomedical Engineering Handbook*, Vol. 1. Bronzino, J.D., Ed., CRC Press, Boca Raton, FL, pp. 38-31–38-33, (2000).

Choi, D.M., Marra, K.G., and Kumta, P.N., Chemical synthesis of hydroxyapatite/poly($\varepsilon$-caprolactone) composites, *Mater. Res. Bull.*, **39**, 417–432 (2004).

Dee, K.C.A., Andersen, T.T., and Bizios, R., Design and function of novel osteoblast-adhesive peptides for chemical modification of biomaterials, *J. Biomed. Mater. Res.*, **40**, 371–377 (1998).

Drennen, J.A.S. and Steele, B.C.H., Zirconia and hafnia, In: *Concise Encyclopedia of Advanced Ceramic Materials*, Brook, R.J., Ed., Pergamon Press, Oxford, pp. 525–528 (1991).

Driessens, F.C.M., *Bioceramics of Calcium Phosphates*, de Groot, K., Ed., CRC Press, Boca Raton, FL, pp. 1–32 (1983).

Elliott, J.C., *Structure and Chemistry of the Apatites and Other Calcium Orthophosphates*, Elsevier, Amsterdam, pp. 1–62 (1994).

Gomi, K.L., Lowerberg, B., Shapiro, G., and Davies, J.E., Resorption of sintered synthetic hydroxyapatite by osteoclasts in vitro, *Biomaterials*, **14**, 91–96 (1993).

Guillemin, G.M., Meunier, A., Dallant, P., Christen, P., Pouliquen, J.C., and Sedel, L., Comparison of coral resorption and bone apposition with two natural corals of different porosities, *J. Biomed. Mater. Res.*, **23**, 765–779 (1989).

Hench, L.L., Bioceramics: from concept to clinic, *J. Am. Ceram. Soc.*, **74**, 1487–1510 (1991).

Hench, L.L.A.E. and Ethridge, E.C., *Biomaterials: An Interfacial Approach*, Academic Press, New York (1982).

Hulbert, S.F. and Young, F.A.S., *Artificial Bones, Use of Ceramics in Surgical Implants*. Gordon and Breach Science Publisher, New York (1969).

Kaae, J.L., Structure and mechanical properties of isotropic pyrolytic carbon deposited below 1600°C, *J. Nucl. Mater.*, **38**, 42–50 (1971).

Khavari, F.A.B. and Bajpai, P.K., Coralline-sulfate bone substitutes, *Biomed. Sci. Instrum.*, **29**, 65–69 (1993).

Kingery, W.D.B., Bowen, H.K., and Uhlmann, D.R., *Introduction to Ceramics*, John Wiley & Sons, New York, pp. 3–4 (1976).

Kumta, P.N., Introduction to Biomaterials, in *Class Notes*, Pittsburgh (2004).

Kumta, P.N.S., Speir, C., Lee, D.-H., Olton, D., and Choi, D., Nanostructured calcium phosphates for biomedical applications: novel synthesis and characterization, *Acta Biomater.*, **1**, 65–83 (2005).

Larrabee, R.A.F., Fuski, M.P., and Bajpai, P.K., A ferric-calcium-phosphorus-oxide ceramic for rebuilding bone, *Biomed. Sci. Instrum.*, **29**, 59–64 (1993).

LeGeros, R.Z., *Calcium Phosphates in Oral Biology and Medicine*, Karger, Basel, pp. 1–201 (1991).

Masaaki, T.Y., Youji, M., Kunio, I., Masaru, N., Masayuki, K., Kenzo, A., and Kazuomi, S., *J. Biomed. Mater. Res.*, **39**, 308 (1998).

Matsunaga, T.I., Inoue, H., Kojo, T., Hatano, K., Tsujisawa, T., Uchiyama, C., and Uchida, Y., Disaggregated osteoclasts increase in resorption activity in response to roughness of bone surface, *J. Biomed. Mater. Res.*, **48**, 417–423 (1999).

Mattie, D.R. and Bajpai, P.K., Analysis of the biocompatibility of ALCAP ceramics in rat femurs, *J. Biomed. Mater. Res.*, **22**, 1101–1126 (1988).

Melde, B.J.S. and Stein, A., *Chem. Mater.*, **14**, 3326 (2002).

Park, J.B., Aluminum oxides: biomedical applications, In: *Concise Encyclopedia of Advanced Ceramic Materials*, Brook, R.J., Ed., Pergamon Press, Oxford, pp. 13–16 (1991).

Park, J.B.A.L. and Lakes, R.S., *Biomaterials: An Introduction*, Kluwer Academic Press, Dordrecht, pp. 132–135 (1992).

Peltier, L.F., The use of plaster of Paris to fill defects in bone, *Clin. Orthop.*, **21**, 1–29 (1961).

Ravaglioli, A.A.K.A., *Bioceramics—Materials, Properties and Applications*, Chapman & Hall, London (1992).

Ritter, J.E. Jr., Greenspan, D.C., Palmer, R.A., and Hench, L.L., Use of fracture of an alumina and bioglass coated alumina, *J. Biomed. Mater. Res.*, **13**, 251–263 (1979).

Scheidler, P.A.A.B., and Bajpai, P.K., Zinc sulfate calcium phosphate (ZSCAP) composite for repairing traumatized bone, *Biomed. Sci. Instrum.*, **28**, 183–188 (1992).

Sharma, C.P., LTI carbons: blood compatibility, *J. Colloid Interface Sci.*, **97**, 585–586 (1984).

Stricker, N.J.L., Larrabee, R.A., and Bajpai, P.K., Biocompatibility of ferric calcium phosphorus oxide ceramics, *Biomed. Sci. Instrum.*, **28**, 123–128 (1992).

Van Vlack, L., *Elements of Materials Science and Engineering*, Addison-Wesley, Reading, MA, pp. 251–277 (1989).

Webster, T.J., Ergun, C., Doremus, R.H., Siegel, R.W., and Bizios, R., Enhanced functions of osteoblasts on nanophase ceramics, *Biomaterials*, **21**, 1803–1810 (2000).

Webster, T.J., Ergun, C., Doremus, R.H., Siegel, R.W., and Bizios, R., Enhanced osteoclast-like cell functions on nanophase ceramics, *Biomaterials*, **22**, 1327–1333 (2001).

# 19

---

## Biomaterials for Drug and Gene Delivery

---

**Yihua Loo and Kam W. Leong**

## CONTENTS

## 19.1  Introduction

The goal of drug delivery is to attain a controlled release of pharmaceutical compounds to specific target tissues. Precise delivery of the drug is necessary to maximize the therapeutic effect of the drug while simultaneously minimizing the undesirable side effects. Many excellent reviews cover the advanced aspects of polymeric controlled release (Kuo and Saltzman, 1996; Kuntz and Saltzman, 1997; Langer, 2000; Hoffman, 2002; Chen and Mooney, 2003; Langer and Tirrell, 2004; Peppas, 2004a, 2004b). In this chapter we will cover the fundamentals of drug delivery and methods of achieving controlled, sustained targeted drug release. This will be followed by a description of how biomaterials can be used to manipulate drug release profiles via different routes of drug administration and device designs.

The goal of gene delivery is to deliver a foreign gene to the nuclei of target cells (Nishikawa and Huang, 2001; Thomas and Klibanov, 2003; Williams and Baum, 2003; Cavazzana-Calvo et al., 2004). Gene delivery is more challenging than drug delivery as the intact DNA has to cross extra intracellular barriers to reach the nucleus. Viruses possess innate ability to penetrate these barriers. However, the immunogenicity and toxicity of viral gene vectors generate significant concerns over the long-term safety of the viral gene transfer approach. We will focus only on the nonviral approach in this chapter. Efficient delivery of the DNA to the nuclei of specific cell populations will lead to the production of peptides encoded by the gene. In most cases where the gene product is a soluble instead of membrane bound protein, gene delivery can be viewed as an advanced protein delivery system, where the transfected cell produces the protein in a sustained manner. The latter portion of the chapter will describe the potential of biomaterials in enhancing gene delivery, as well as emphasize the major barriers limiting effective nonviral gene delivery.

## 19.2  Fundamental Concepts of Drug Delivery

What happens after one swallows the pill? As the drug passes through the gastrointestinal (GI) tract, it gradually dissolves and gets absorbed into the blood capillaries lining the gut. The rate of absorption is dependent on multiple factors, such as the solubility of the pill and/or its coating, the surface area of the GI tract, the region of the GI tract, the presence of enzymes and the presence of any targeting ligands. In general, maximal absorption occurs in the intestines. As the blood travels from the intestinal veins to the liver (via the hepatic portal vein), first-pass metabolism occurs as the multitude of enzymes in the liver degrades or neutralizes a large percentage the pharmaceutical compound in the blood. The remainder of the drug is transported via the bloodstream to tissues where it exerts a biochemical effect.

If one is given an injection or an intravenous infusion, the drugs are administered directly into the systemic circulation and transported or partitioned to various tissues. Although first-pass metabolism is bypassed, a significant portion is excreted via glomerular filtration in the kidneys and eliminated via the reticuloendothelial system (RES) in the liver and spleen.

Within the systemic blood circulation, the drug continuously diffuses out of the bloodstream to distribute into surrounding tissues. Absorption by tissues and clearance from the bloodstream decrease the plasma drug level. Since the diffusion of the drug from the blood capillaries is indiscriminate, at different tissues, the drug can exert different biochemical effects. At the target tissues where the drug exerts a therapeutic effect, the disease can be cured or the symptoms of the disease can be alleviated. Uptake at target tissues can be further enhanced by using specific ligands that target cells expressing certain receptors. At nontarget tissues, the presence of the drug should ideally have no effect. Unfortunately, in many instances, undesirable systemic side effects of the drug occur, causing toxicity as the drug compromises physiological function in nontarget organs or affect other metabolic pathways.

In summary, the administration of drug leads to a certain concentration of plasma drug level. This concentration is decimated by uptake at different tissues, drug degradation at the liver, elimination by the RES and excretion by the kidneys. The concentration of drug in the plasma for a bolus administration is reflected in Figure 19.1.

In order for a drug to be effective, the level of drug in the plasma has to be above a critical minimum ($C_{min}$). However, when the drug concentration exceeds a critical level ($C_{max}$), adverse drug reactions may occur due to drug toxicity. There is a therapeutic window within which the plasma drug level should be maintained. The therapeutic index is defined as a ratio of the maximum tolerated drug concentration and the minimum drug concentration for a therapeutic effect. The larger the TI, the more effective the drug is.

$$\text{Therapeutic index, TI} = \frac{C_{max}}{C_{min}} \tag{19.1}$$

When the medication is first administered, for example via the oral route, the rate of drug absorption into the plasma exceeds the drug clearance. Thus, the plasma drug level initially rises to overshoot the critical maximum. This compensates for the gradual decrease in plasma drug level in the face of declining absorption rates at constant elimination rates. At its peak value, the rate of absorption and elimination are comparable. Following this, the level begins to fall as the body begins to clear the drug from the blood while the absorption rate is negligible as the drug is administered as a bolus. The cycle begins anew when a second bolus of drug is administered. If the second dosage is administered shortly after the first, the plasma drug level is more likely to exceed $C_{max}$, resulting in drug toxicity. Hence, it is important to monitor the duration between dosings.

For a continuous drug infusion, the shape of the curve may vary slightly. In addition, defining AUC as the area under the curve for a graph of plasma drug concentration

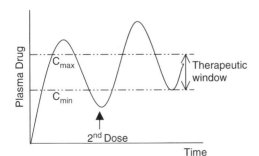

**FIGURE 19.1**
Changes in plasma drug concentration over time.

over time,

$$\text{Clearance} = \frac{\text{Dose}}{\text{AUC}} \tag{19.2}$$

The desired steady-state drug input rate for a continuous infusion may be calculated.

$$\text{Drug input rate} = \text{Target plasma concentration} \times \text{Clearance} \tag{19.3}$$

## 19.3   Ideal Drug Delivery System

An ideal drug delivery system is noninvasive, noncytotoxic, nonimmunogenic, and capable of delivering the pharmaceutical compound in a sustained and controlled fashion. Such a system will be able to release its medication in a manner appropriate to treating the disease, and for a prolonged time frame if necessary. If possible, localized delivery of the medication will also limit the concentration of drug to a specific region of the body and so minimize the systemic side effects. In short, an ideal drug delivery system has the following macroscopic properties.

### 19.3.1   Controlled Release

An ideal controlled release drug delivery system is one that can release the medication when appropriate. Thus, depending on the disease and drug properties, the kinetics of drug release is designed to maximize the beneficial pharmacological effects of the drug.

For a disease that requires a constant baseline level of medication, an ideal drug delivery system is one that demonstrates zero-order release kinetics over a long period of time. In other words, in the long run, the rate at which the drug is absorbed by the body is equivalent to the physiological drug clearance; the plasma drug concentration remains steady and within the therapeutic window over the duration of use (Figure 19.2).

For an illness that requires burst-phases of release in response to some external stimuli, drug delivery systems that exhibit bi- or multiphasic release profiles may be more appropriate (Figure 19.3). An example would be an insulin delivery system (Miyata et al., 2002) where the insulin release is responsive to the fluctuating glucose level as a result of food ingestion or exercise.

By means of an appropriate controlled release drug delivery system, the rate at which the drug is released from its carrier can be controlled for a definite period of use through

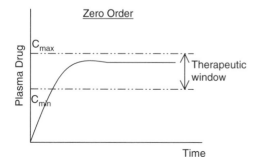

**FIGURE 19.2**
Changes in plasma drug concentration over time for a zero-order release system.

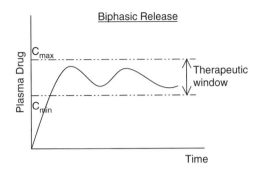

FIGURE 19.3

Changes in plasma drug concentration over time for a biphasic release system.

modifications to component design, initial drug concentration, drug solubility, drug diffusion characteristics, and physiological drug clearance rates.

Common controlled-release formulations include polymeric transdermal patches, polymeric implants, and drug pumps. Under optimal conditions, these drug delivery systems are capable of maintaining a constant plasma drug level within the therapeutic window, thereby limiting unfavorable side effects and maximizing drug performance. In addition, most controlled-release systems extend the apparent half-life of the drug by protecting the unreleased drug from degradation. Commercially, an innovative drug delivery system can extend the patent protection of a drug that is coming off a patent. In addition, it increases the pool of drug candidates that are previously rejected on the basis of poor solubility, high toxicity at moderate concentrations, or instability under physiological conditions.

## 19.3.2 Sustained Release

Sustained release formulations keep the patient's plasma drug level within the therapeutic window for a longer period of time compared to conventional drug release methods. As shown in Figure 19.4, a sustained-release drug delivery system stretches out the conventional release profile along the time axis. Since the plasma drug concentrations remain within the therapeutic window for a longer duration, less frequent dosages are required. This bodes well for patient compliance as it is much more convenient.

The common sustained-release formulations on the market include: drug complexes, coatings, suspensions, emulsions, and compressed tablets. Drug complexes have a slower rate of drug release as the conjugated pharmaceutical moieties are less soluble under physiological conditions. The rate of drug release can be correlated to the dissociation rate of the drug from the complexing agent. Similarly, the presence of slowly dissolving coatings around the drug limits the surface area exposed to extracellular fluid, thereby

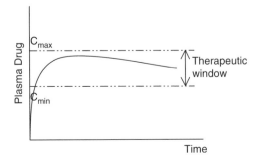

FIGURE 19.4

Changes in plasma drug concentration over time for a sustained-release system.

placing a cap on the rate at which drug can dissolve in plasma. Suspensions and emulsions delay the rate at which the drug diffuses into plasma.

### 19.3.3 Targeted Delivery

Targeted delivery selectively dispenses the pharmaceutical compound to the tissue or even cells of interest. It is advantageous as it increases drug concentration at target sites, while minimizing the (often adverse) effects on other organs. Three main methods (Park, 1997) are used, namely,

- Active targeting by means of specific ligands conjugated to therapeutic moieties or their carriers to "home-in" on the target cells.
- Passive targeting via physiological deposition processes.
- Local administration of drug delivery systems to the locality of diseased tissue.

The attachment of the ligand to the therapeutic moiety facilitates cell-specific uptake via receptor-mediated endocytosis, or in some cases simply improves accumulation in the target tissue. Lectin-decorated microparticles, for example, may bind to the surface carbohydrates on mucosal epithelial cells (Jepson et al., 2004). The ligand of interest is linked to the pharmaceutical compound in several different ways. For instance, the ligand can be conjugated with a "carrier" polymer which is used to complex the pharmaceutical component. The ligand can also be conjugated to or complexed with the pharmaceutical component. Lastly, the therapeutic moiety can be genetically engineered as a fusion protein with the ligand incorporated as part of its structure (Table 19.1).

Passive targeting is effective when the cells of interest preferentially uptake particulates in their surroundings. Examples include macrophages in different tissues, antigen-presenting cells of the immune system, and Kuffer cells in the liver. Restricted drug delivery to a general region of the body can also be achieved using administration routes and systems that keep the drug concentration high at the site of administration and low in other regions of the body. Embolization of arteries by drug-loaded particles, for example, has been applied to treat nonresectable tumors (Weisse et al., 2002).

**TABLE 19.1**

Ligands of Interest in Drug Delivery and Their Target Cells (Huang et al., 1999)

| Ligand | Target |
|---|---|
| Hormones | Hormone receptors. Can be used to target a wide variety of cells with ubiquitously expressed hormone receptors such as insulin receptors; or selectively expressed hormone receptors such as that for Steel factor and erythropoietin |
| Cell adhesion molecules (ICAMs, selectins and integrins) | Extracellular matrix. These ligands may also target highly metastatic cancer cells that express mutant forms of selectins |
| Transferrin | Actively metabolizing cells that uptake iron |
| Immunoglobulins | Highly specific cell surface epitopes, which include mutant or selectively expressed cell adhesion molecules |
| Asialoglycoproteins | Liver hepatocytes |

## 19.4   Routes of Drug Delivery

In addition to injections and implants, which directly deposit the therapeutic moiety within the body, there is a diversity of drug delivery routes corresponding to regions of the body that come into contact with the external environment. Table 19.2 outlines such routes and Table 19.3 highlights the salient features of these delivery routes.

## 19.5   Drug Delivery Systems and Their Mechanism of Action

Polymers, serving as drug carriers, are often used to achieve the desired drug delivery characteristics described above. Careful selection of material properties used in the manufacturing of components of drug delivery devices can optimize the rate and duration of controlled release. The three main mechanisms by which the rate of drug release from a delivery system hinge upon are diffusion, water penetration, and polymer degradation (Ratner et al., 1996) (Table 19.4).

**TABLE 19.2**

Drug Delivery Routes Corresponding to Regions of the Body that Come into Contact with the External Environment

| Physiological Barrier | Location in the Body | Mode of Delivery |
|---|---|---|
| Mucosal tissue | GI tract | Oral formulations, sublingual formulations, enemas |
| | Nasal passages | Nasal sprays, inhalants |
| | Lung | Pulmonary delivery systems |
| | Uterus | Intrauterine delivery systems |
| | Vagina | Intravaginal delivery systems |
| Epidermis | Skin | Topical creams, transdermal patches |
| | Eyes | Ocular delivery systems |

**TABLE 19.4**

Classification of Rate-Controlled Mechanisms

| Diffusion Controlled System | Water Penetration Controlled System | Polymer Degradation Controlled System |
|---|---|---|
| Diffusion through polymer | Osmotic pump | Surface erosion |
| Diffusion through membrane | Swelling controlled | Bulk degradation, Polymer sidechain cleavage |

**TABLE 19.3**

Brief Description of Different Routes of Drug Delivery

| Route of Delivery | Brief Description | Advantages | Disadvantages |
|---|---|---|---|
| Oral formulations | Pills, powders, capsules, suspensions and liquid mixtures that are swallowed | Convenient and noninvasive form of drug delivery<br>Easy to manufacture | Drug undergoes extensive first pass metabolism, hence dosage required is often high<br>Not suitable for drugs unstable in the gastrointestinal (GI) environment or poorly absorbed through the GI tract |
| Sublingual (Buccal) formulations | Device, tablet or patch placed under the tongue. Drug diffuses from the device through the skin and into the underlying blood vessels | Easy application and removal<br>Permeation of the drug through the buccal mucosa is very rapid, especially for low molecular weight drugs<br>Avoids first pass metabolism as drug enters systemic circulation directly | Patient may dislike the taste of the drug<br>Small surface area under the tongue limits the flux of the drug<br>Drug that gets dissolved in saliva and swallowed will undergo first pass metabolism<br>Dilution of the drug by saliva also decreases the flux of the drug<br>A sublingual patch has some risk of bacterial growth and occlusion of salivary glands |
| Enemas, suppositories | Rectal delivery systems which involve placing a tablet or applying cream in the rectum | Relatively high permeability of rectal mucosa<br>Capable of delivering peptide drugs due to low enzymatic activity<br>Localized treatment can be effected in the lower regions of the digestive tract | Still somewhat subjected to hepatic first pass metabolism<br>Distasteful and possibly uncomfortable |
| Pulmonary delivery systems (Edwards et al., 1997; Edwards and Dunbar, 2002) | Nasal sprays and inhalants deliver the drug in the form of fine particles or mist to the lung and the nasal passages via the nostrils or pharynx. Particles reach the deeper regions of the lung through the processes of impaction, sedimentation, Brownian motion and interception | Large surface area of the lung and nasal passages promotes absorption<br>Lack of enzymatic activity and mild pH facilitates the delivery of peptide drugs<br>Deep lung mucosa is highly permeable to proteins as the walls of the alveoli are very thin<br>Noninvasive and acts quickly<br>Avoids hepatic first pass metabolism<br>Capable of both local and systemic delivery | Ultra-fine particles present in sprays tend to aggregate<br>Particles that reach the deep lung are rapidly phagocytosed by the macrophages<br>Multiple branching of the airway tracts acts as a good filter for particles, which are then cleared by the cilia |

| Delivery system | Description | Advantages | Disadvantages |
|---|---|---|---|
| Intrauterine delivery systems | The device is inserted through the vagina and cervix to be implanted in the uterus. Commonly used for birth control and hormones | Avoids hepatic first pass metabolism; Localized treatment can be applied to the female reproductive system | Invasive, and so carries the risk of infection |
| Intravaginal delivery systems | Implants of monolith systems or creams are applied to the vagina. Commonly used for birth control drugs | Convenient for self-application; High permeability of the vaginal mucosa; Avoids hepatic first pass metabolism | Local microorganism population may interfere with drug metabolism |
| Topical creams | Drug is manufactured as a cream that is applied on the skin or lips. This is popularly used to deliver lipophilic compounds to epidermal tissue | Easy application and removal. Noninvasive; Localized treatment can be effected where the patch is placed on the skin above the targeted area. This reduces the systemic drug concentration, thus minimizing adverse systemic side effects | The strateum corneum of the skin is a very effective diffusion barrier, and the epidermis has a highly effective immune system. This prevents the entry of drugs that are not lipid soluble; Drugs may irritate the skin; Contact sensitization can be developed from long-term or repeated exposure, resulting in side effects such as rashes and eczema |
| Transdermal patches (Ranade, 1991) | Devices that are diffusion-controlled can be used to deliver drugs from an external flat reservoir, matrix or hydrogel to the epidermis, whereupon the drug diffuses through the different layers of the epidermis to the blood capillaries in the dermis for systemic circulation. Drug release by transdermal systems can be enhanced by ionotophoresis, electroporation, and ultrasound | Appropriate for lipid soluble drugs with short half-life; Avoids hepatic first pass metabolism; Zero-order release can be achieved for transdermal patches, where the plasma drug concentration is consistently within the therapeutic window | Easy removal implies that the cream may be inadvertently wiped off or the patch may accidentally peel off; Lag time before steady state release occurs |
| Ocular delivery systems | Eye drops or ointments which are applied to the lens or cornea directly. Hydrogel contact lens can be used to release drugs at a rate proportional to the square root of time elapsed | Localized treatment to the eye. Many of the drugs are active only in the eye and become inactivated upon entering systemic circulation; Convenient and permits self-application | Small surface area renders drug unsuitable for systemic drug delivery; Controlled release is challenging as drug retention in the eye is problematic; Viscous solutions have to be used to prevent the drug from being drained by lachrymal fluid |

*(continued)*

**TABLE 19.3** (Continued)

| Route of Delivery | Brief Description | Advantages | Disadvantages |
|---|---|---|---|
| Injections | Drug is injected directly into a vein The drug may be packaged as a micro- or nanoparticle, whereupon sustained and controlled delivery is possible | Rapid effect | Bolus administration Drug is rapidly cleared by the RES and excreted by the kidney Has to be administered by trained personnel Risk of infection increases if needles and syringes are reused |
| Continuous infusions | A catheter is inserted into a vein and the drug (in the form of solution, suspension or microspheres) is perfused into the systemic circulation | Rapid effect Continuous input of drug permits the plasma drug concentration to be maintained at a constant level (Zero-order release) Avoids hepatic first pass metabolism | Some degree of discomfort and inconvenience Catheter has to be inserted by trained personnel Risk of infection increases due to the presence of open needle hole |
| Implants | A hydrogel, reservoir or scaffold containing the therapeutic moiety is implanted Hydrogels and polymer microcapsules may be injected | Specific tissues can be targeted, thereby reducing systemic side effects Targeted regions can receive a consistently high level of drug within the therapeutic window. Controlled and sustained release kinetics can be attained Suitable for drugs with short half-life and easily degraded Avoids hepatic first pass metabolism | An immune response against the implant may be developed Injected polymer microcapsules and implanted polymer scaffolds may not be biodegradable Implantable devices (pumps, matrices, and scaffolds) have to be surgically implanted |

### 19.5.1 Diffusion Controlled Systems

#### 19.5.1.1 Monolithic Drug Delivery Systems

Monolithic drug delivery systems consist of the pharmaceutical compound being dissolved or dispersed in a polymer matrix. The rate at which the drug is released from the system is dependent on the rate at which it diffuses out of the polymer. Hence, the polymer chosen for such systems should have a degradation rate that is significantly slower than the diffusion rate of the drug from the matrix. Most often the polymer is nonbiodegradable, such as poly(ethylene vinyl acetate) used to control the release of contraceptive steroids for a period of several years. Other factors which determine the flux of the drug include solubility of drug in the matrix and in plasma, porosity of the polymer, and the geometry of the polymer matrix. There are three possible cases.

##### 19.5.1.1.1 Dissolved Drug That Diffuses through the Polymer

The rate-limiting step is diffusion through the polymer matrix and the driving force of drug release is the drug concentration gradient between the matrix and its environment. The drug is soluble in the polymer and the polymer is either nondegradable or the degradation rate is significantly slow such that the polymer matrix remains unchanged during the course of drug diffusion. The amount of drug loaded into the matrix is lower that its saturation concentration. The device can be fabricated by simply soaking the polymer "sponge" in a solution containing the drug. This system can be modeled as a nonsteady-state system with a dynamic drug concentration gradient (Park, 1997; Saltzman, 2001).

Assuming that the polymer matrix is a thin slab of thickness $L$, at a given time $t$,

$$\frac{M}{M_T} = 1 - \sum_{n=0}^{\infty} \frac{8 \exp[-D(2n+1)^2 \pi^2 t/L^2]}{(2n+1)^2 \pi^2} \tag{19.4}$$

where $M$ = mass of drug released at time $t$, $M_T$ = total mass of drug in the device, and $D$ = diffusion coefficient of the drug in the polymer matrix.

The amount of drug released can be simplified by early and late time approximations. At early time where $\leq 60\%$ of the drug is released.

$$\frac{M}{M_T} = 4\left[\frac{Dt}{\pi L^2}\right]^{1/2} \quad \text{for } 0 \leq \frac{M}{M_T} \leq 0.6; \quad \frac{dM}{dt} = 2M_T\left(\frac{D}{\pi L^2 t}\right)^{1/2} \tag{19.5}$$

At late time points,

$$\frac{M}{M_T} = 1 - \frac{8}{\pi^2}\exp\left[\frac{-D\pi^2 t}{L^2}\right] \quad \text{for } 0.4 \leq \frac{M}{M_T} \leq 1; \quad \frac{dM}{dt} = \frac{8DM_T}{L^2}\exp\left(-\frac{D\pi^2 t}{L^2}\right) \tag{19.6}$$

The release rate of a drug initially dissolved in a slab as a function of time, using both the early- and late-time approximations is shown in Figure 19.5 (Baker and Lonsdale, 1974). The full line shows the portion of the curve over which the approximations are valid $(D/L^2 = 1)$.

##### 19.5.1.1.2 Dispersed Drug That Diffuses through the Polymer

Like the dissolved drug, the rate-limiting step in this instance is diffusion through the polymer matrix and the driving force of drug release is the drug concentration

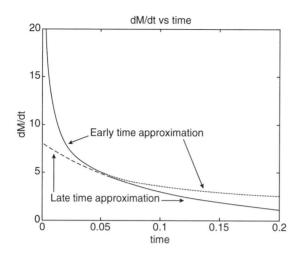

**FIGURE 19.5**
The release rate of a drug initially dissolved in a slab as a function of time, using both the early- and late-time approximations.

gradient between the matrix and its environment. However, the amount of drug loaded into the matrix exceeds its saturation concentration. The device can be fabricated via solvent casting or compression molding. It is modeled by the Higuchi equation (Higuchi, 1961; Park, 1997; Peppas and Siepmann, 2001).

$$M = [C_{sat}Dt(2C_{load} - C_{sat})]^{1/2} \quad \text{for } C_{load} \gg C_{sat} \quad (19.7)$$

where $C_{sat}$, $C_{load}$ = saturation and loading concentrations of the drug, respectively.

This model assumes that the drug is uniformly suspended as miniscule particles, there is no expansion or contraction of the device and the interface between the dispersed and the dissolved drug moves into the interior of the system as a continuous front.

### 19.5.1.1.3 *Dispersed Drug That Diffuses through the Channels*

This system is akin to that above, except that in the wake of drug particles that have already dissolved or diffused away, a channel within the solid polymer matrix is formed. The drug need not be soluble in the polymer, provided drug loading is high (>30%) to ensure the formation of channels to access drug in the interior of the matrix. The drug is diffusing through the fluid filled channel and so the diffusivity term changes. $D_{plasma}$ = diffusivity of the drug in plasma. The number of channels also affects diffusion and this is incorporated as a porosity term $\varepsilon$. Similarly, the tortuosity, $\tau$, of the channels is also incorporated (Park, 1997). The modified Higuchi equation is

$$M = C_{load}\left[\frac{D_{plasma}}{\tau}C_{sat}t(2C_{load} - \varepsilon C_{sat,plasma})\right]^{1/2} \quad (19.8)$$

### 19.5.1.2 *Membrane Controlled Drug Delivery Systems*

Monolithic drug delivery systems where the drug is uniformly dissolved or dispersed in a polymer matrix typically have release profiles that decline with time, due to the diminishing concentration gradient. To improve their release kinetics, monolithic polymer matrixes can be modified using rate-controlling membranes. Thus, the rate of drug release

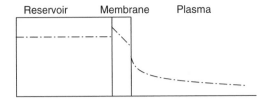

Reservoir    Membrane    Plasma

**FIGURE 19.6**
The concentration profile changes from reservoir, membrane to plasma, for a hydrophobic drug in a membrane-controlled release system.

depends on drug solubility and diffusivity in the membrane (Park, 1997).

$$\text{Fick's first law } J = -D\frac{dC}{dx} \tag{19.9}$$

can be used to predict the flux.

$$\text{Drug flux } J = DK\frac{C_{\text{reservoir}} - C_{\text{plasma}}}{L} \tag{19.10}$$

where $D$ = diffusivity of drug in membrane, $K$ = partition coefficient (calculated using thermodynamics), and $L$ = thickness of the membrane.

If the drug is equally soluble in the membrane, plasma and reservoir, $K = 1$ and $D/L$ can be viewed as the diffusional resistance. The drug concentration profile of the membrane can be further calculated using Fick's Second Law

$$\frac{\partial C}{\partial t} = D\nabla^2 C \tag{19.11}$$

Assuming steady-state and one-dimensional diffusion,

$$\frac{\partial C}{\partial t} = 0 \tag{19.12}$$

$$\text{Drug concentration at distance } x, \quad C_x = C_{\text{reservoir}} - \frac{x}{L}(C_{\text{reservoir}} - C_{\text{plasma}}) \tag{19.13}$$

If the drug is hydrophobic, it will preferentially partition into the membrane and so the concentration on either ends of the membrane is higher than the concentration in plasma and reservoir (Figure 19.6). The permeability coefficient is then defined as

$$P = \frac{DK}{L} \tag{19.14}$$

### 19.5.2 Water Penetration Controlled Systems

#### 19.5.2.1 Osmotic Pumps

Osmotic pumps (Figure 19.7) utilize semipermeable membranes that only permit the unidirectional movement of water into the osmotic agent compartment ($V_s$). This causes the compartment to expand, pushing the movable partition and forcing the drug ($V_d$) out of the delivery orifice. The system can be described as follows (Park, 1997)

$$\text{Volume of water entering the osmotic agent component} = \frac{dV_s}{dt} = \frac{A}{L}\lambda(\sigma\Delta\pi - \Delta P_H) \tag{19.15}$$

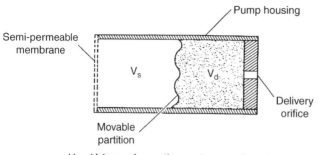

**FIGURE 19.7**
Schematic of an osmotic pump. (*Source:* From Theeuwes, F. and Yum, S.I., *Ann. Biomed. Eng.*, 4, 343–353, 1976. With permission.)

$V_s$   Volume of osmotic agent compartment
$V_d$   Volume of drug compartment

where $A$, $L$ = membrane area and thickness, respectively, $\lambda$ = membrane permeability coefficient, $\sigma$ = solute reflection coefficient (usually = 1) which reflects membrane selectivity, $\Delta\pi$ = osmotic pressure difference across semi-permeable membrane

$$\pi \approx C_{\text{osmotic agent}}RT \qquad (19.16)$$

($R$ = universal gas constant, $T$ = temperature), and $\Delta P_H$ = hydrostatic pressure difference across semi-permeable membrane.
    Assuming that efflux of drug = influx of water

$$\text{Drug release rate from pump,} \quad \frac{dM}{dt} = \frac{dV_s}{dt}C_D = \frac{A}{L}\lambda(\sigma\Delta\pi - \Delta P_H)C_D \qquad (19.17)$$

where $C_D$ = concentration of drug.
    An approximation can be made if the orifice is large, $\Delta\pi \gg \Delta P_H$.
    Thus,

$$\frac{dV_s}{dt} = \frac{A}{L}\lambda(\sigma\Delta\pi) \qquad (19.18)$$

and

$$\frac{dM}{dt} = \frac{A}{L}\lambda(\sigma\Delta\pi)C_D \qquad (19.19)$$

From the above equation, the rate of drug efflux can be achieved by increasing the membrane area, increasing the concentration of drug loaded, or use a more soluble salt as the osmotic agent. Osmotic pumps are usually implanted and can be refilled if necessary.

### 19.5.2.2  *Swelling Controlled Drug Delivery Systems*

Water penetration into a dehydrated hydrophilic crystalline polymer matrix containing the drug can cause the polymer to swell. As the polymer transitions from its crystalline phase into an amorphous phase, the diffusion of drug from the device is accelerated.
    Another swelling-controlled system is one that results in a single burst of drug release after a lag period (Yan Zhang and Wu, 2003). The drug and a dehydrated hydrophilic polymer are encapsulated in a semipermeable membrane. Water penetration causes the polymer to swell and rupture the membrane, thereby releasing the drug.

### 19.5.3 Polymer Degradation Controlled Systems

Biodegradable polymers are often used to deliver therapeutic moieties systemically and locally. They are desirable as they undergo hydrolysis into nontoxic molecules under physiological conditions. Hydrolysis can occur in three different ways, depicted in Figure 19.8.

Surface erosion controlled and bulk erosion controlled drug delivery systems consist of drug being dispersed within a polymer matrix or microsphere. Water penetration (shaded areas) into the polymer matrix or microsphere leads to the degradation of the bonds between the monomers by hydrolysis. Hence, the rate at which bond cleavage occurs is strongly correlated with rate of water penetration.

#### 19.5.3.1 Surface Erosion

In surface erosion controlled release systems, the rate of bond cleavage is significantly higher than the rate of water penetration. Consequently, only the polymer at/near the surface gets degraded. For example, a polyanhydride with a hydrophobic backbone might exhibit such behavior. The anhydride bond is highly hydrolytically labile while the hydrophobic and crystalline backbone would resist water penetration (Kumar et al., 2002). If drug release for these matrix-degradation-controlled systems is governed solely by the erosion of the matrix, a constant release rate may be obtained, provided the surface area of the device is maintained constant. However, that represents an idealized case that is rarely realized. In reality the drug molecules can also diffuse through the matrix. This is particularly true if the drug is hydrophilic, which presents a high driving force for diffusion. The release is often intermediate between zero-order and first-order kinetics. In an ideal case, doubling the thickness of the polymer matrix would double the duration of release but does not significantly the affect the rate of release. A constant release can sometimes be achieved if the diffusion is accompanied by a change in the matrix properties which boosts the diffusivity of the drug. For instance, the diffusivity may increase with time as a result of partial degradation or swelling of the matrix. Such an

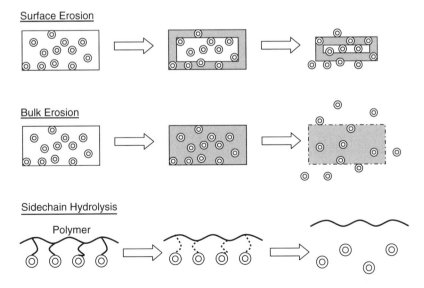

**FIGURE 19.8**
Schematic illustrating surface erosion, bulk erosion, and side chain hydrolysis.

increase may compensate for the decrease in the concentration gradient and lead to a constant release.

### 19.5.3.2  Bulk Erosion

In bulk degradation controlled release systems, the rate of bond cleavage is significantly lower than the rate of water penetration. Backbone cleavage of the polymer occurs uniformly throughout the interior of the device. Polyesters with an aliphatic backbone will exhibit such a behavior. Polylactide and polyglycolide are prime examples of bulk-degrading polymers. The mass loss of these polymers is biphasic. There is little detectable mass loss at initial time points because the degraded polymer chains are not yet water soluble. Only when the average molecular weight of the sample reaches a threshold and the oligomeric fragments of the polymer become water soluble will mass loss be apparent. The degradation behavior of these polyesters is also fueled by a feed-forward mechanism. Ester hydrolysis is acid catalyzed. The hydrolytic breakdown products of polyester are hydroxyl–carboxylic acids. The bulk-degrading situation creates a low pH microenvironment in the interior of the sample because of the trapped acidic breakdown products, which in turn accelerates the degradation. If the drug dispersed within the polymer is water soluble, water penetration will lead to the diffusion of the drug out of the matrix before complete degradation of the matrix occurs; drug release is therefore diffusion controlled. The biphasic degradation phenomenon of the polyesters can be exploited to produce pulsed release profile, for example, for vaccination applications (Jiang et al., 2005).

The mathematics of drug release from biodegradable matrices (Siepmann and Gopferich, 2001) will not be covered as the models are significantly more complex due to the presence of time-dependent factors such as permeability (increases with time), surface area, and volume (decrease with time).

### 19.5.3.3  Hydrolysis of Covalent Bond between Drug and Polymer Backbone

For drugs that are covalently attached to the backbone of a polymer chain, termed a pendant system, hydrolysis of the bond between the therapeutic moiety and the polymer backbone results in drug release. If the drug is attached to the polymer via a spacer, the hydrolysis of the polymer-spacer and the spacer–drug bonds are both relevant. The spacer approach provides an effective means of controlling the release rate. A spacer may also be necessary in some cases to render the conjugation bond accessible to hydrolysis. Although penetration of water into the matrix and outward diffusion of the cleaved drug molecules constitute part of the rate barrier, the cleavage of the polymer–drug bond as the rate-determining step is preferred for better control. Generally, the release rate drops with time as the drug concentration decreases.

The potential advantage of the pendant system is the high drug-loading level. While the drug-loading level of biodegradable matrix systems would be generally under 20 wt%, a higher drug-to-polymer ratio is possible in a pendant system (Yoo and Park, 2001). This may also be the only system that can provide a sustained release, for example a release period of weeks, for highly hydrophilic drugs. It might be possible to provide a sustained release for highly hydrophilic drugs using other release systems described above if the drug loading is small, for instance, less than 1 wt%. At high loading, sustained release will not be possible from a matrix system because the hydrophilic drug creates a high drive force for diffusion as well as swelling of the matrix. Conceptually, the pendant system affords the best chance to retard the release of hydrophilic drugs through the use of a relatively stable polymer–drug bond. The disadvantage of the pendant system is that extensive chemical development may be required for each drug, in conjugation, optimization of the release rate, and in ensuring that the integrity of the drug is restored after release.

### 19.5.3.4 Factors That Affect Degradation Rate (Siepmann and Gopferich, 2001)

a. Geometry of the matrix: Slabs and microspheres have different mass loss rates as the surface areas exposed to water differ.

b. Temperature: Although there would be little deviation from 37°C *in vivo*.

c. pH: The drug carrier may rarely encounter alkaline pH except in the GI tract, but would come across low pH environments such as the stomach, bladder, and tumor tissues.

d. Hydrophilicity of the polymer that determines the rate of water penetration.

e. Morphology of the polymer: The degree of crystallinity affects water penetration. The more crystalline the polymer structure, the slower water penetration occurs.

f. Presence of excipients: Typically these are water-soluble compounds that would enhance degradation.

g. Presence of enzymes: Cleavage of ester, amide, and phosphate bonds is enhanced in tissues abounding with these specific enzymes.

## 19.6  Pharmacokinetics

Pharmacokinetics is the study of processes that affect drug distribution and rate of change of drug concentrations within various tissues (compartments) of the body. It can be used as a tool to quantitatively model the absorption, accumulation, and elimination of drugs in different compartments (Figure 19.9).

### 19.6.1  Single-Compartment Model — Bolus Injection

A one-compartment model is the most straightforward model used to demonstrate the pharmacokinetics of drug distribution and elimination in a body (Saltzman, 2001). The single compartment represents the blood plasma volume of the body and its interaction with the surrounding tissues that take up the drug (Figure 19.10).

Assuming that

(1) the drug is administered as an intravenous injection (bolus)

(2) removal of drug from the plasma is purely attributed to physiological drug clearance

(3) physiological drug clearance is a first-order process with elimination rate constant $k$

A mass balance results in the equation

Rate of change of plasma drug concentration = Rate of drug elimination

$$\frac{dC}{dt} = -kC \qquad (19.20)$$

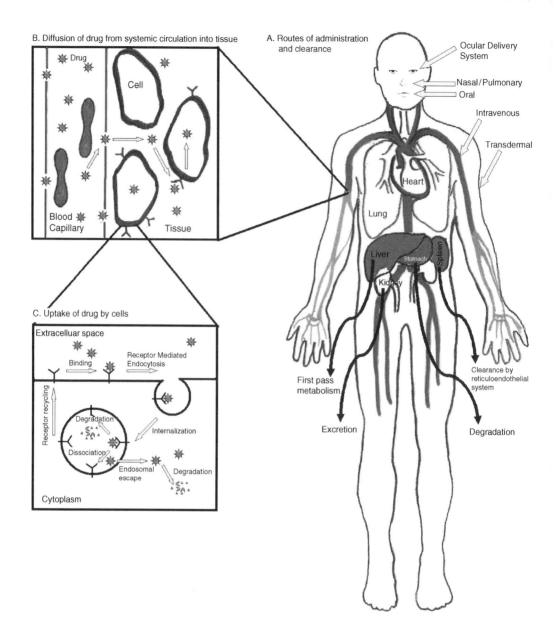

**FIGURE 19.9**
Schematic summarizing (a) routes of administration and clearance; (b) diffusion of drug from the systemic circulation into tissues; (c) uptake of drugs by cells (Stokes, 1995).

Hence,

$$\text{Plasma drug concentration at time } t, \quad C_t = C_0 e^{-kt} \qquad (19.21)$$

where $C_0$ = initial plasma drug concentration, $k$ = drug elimination rate constant (specific to drug used), and $t$ = time elapsed.

Thus, at $t = t_{1/2}$,

$$\frac{1}{2}C_0 = C_0 e^{-kt_{1/2}} \qquad (19.22)$$

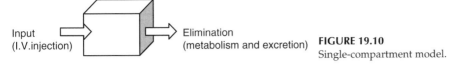

Input
(I.V.injection)

Elimination
(metabolism and excretion)

**FIGURE 19.10**
Single-compartment model.

$$t_{1/2} = \frac{\ln 2}{k} \quad (19.23)$$

Half-life of a drug, $t_{1/2}$ is the time taken for the body to reduce the plasma drug level to half the initial concentration following a bolus administration (such as an intravenous injection).

The single-compartment model can also be extended to drugs absorbed via various mucosal surfaces such as the GI tract and the lungs.
Additional assumptions include

(4) Absorption is a first-order process with absorption rate constant $k_a$.
   The mass balance yields the equation

Rate of change of plasma drug concentration
= Rate of absorption − Rate of elimination

$$\frac{dC}{dt} = (k_a C_d) - (kC) \quad (19.24)$$

where $k_a$ = rate constant of absorption and $C_d$ = concentration of drug remaining in the absorption compartment.
   For an initial drug concentration $C_{d,0}$,

$$\frac{dC}{dt} = (k_a C_{d,0} e^{-k_a t}) - (kC) \quad (19.25)$$

In the absence of any initial drug in the plasma compartment, i.e., $C_0 = 0$ at $t = 0$,

Plasma drug concentration at time $t$, $\quad C_t = C_{d,0}\left[\dfrac{k_a}{k - k_a}\right][e^{-k_a t} - e^{-kt}] \quad (19.26)$

### 19.6.2 Multiple-Compartment Models

In order to more realistically model the drug delivery system, more complicated multiple-compartment pharmacokinetic models can be applied. Such models are used to predict the distribution of drugs in various organs with different drug absorption and degradation rates. They can also be used to describe the uptake and partitioning of drug into various intracellular compartments.

## 19.7 Fundamental Concepts of Gene Delivery

The science of drug delivery has advanced to the point where it is possible to protect therapeutic moieties with very short half-lives and successfully deliver them to a targeted site. This sparked the advent of gene delivery using biomaterials. Instead of delivering a drug or a protein, the therapeutic moiety is an extraneous gene which subsequently stimulates the patient's cells to produce the specific functional therapeutic protein that relieves the disease symptoms or cures the disease. Such a system has multiple advantages of conventional drugs. First, by "turning-on" the cell to serve as a factory for the therapeutic protein; this produces sustained delivery that can last for days to weeks. Secondly, the expressed protein is bioactive, unlike other polymeric protein delivery systems where a certain degree of loss of bioactivity of the protein is often unavoidable. Thirdly, biological signals acting at the molecular level and cannot be delivered as a soluble factor can be achieved by gene delivery. Examples are membrane-bound proteins or transcription factors. Gene delivery renders administration of such biological signals possible. Lastly, the gene may code for a protein with a very short half-life, or one that is difficult to manufacture in large quantities synthetically.

Gene medicines typically consist of a gene expression system and a gene delivery system. The gene expression system encodes a therapeutic protein that is either not produced in the patient or produced in a nonfunctional manner. In addition, promoters and regulators could be added to enhance and regulate the production of the protein. The gene delivery system is responsible for transporting the gene to a specific cell population, as well as to augment successful gene expression in the nucleus. Occasionally, naked DNA can be injected into the target tissue to induce gene expression, the most successful being intramuscular injections. However, this is not feasible for many tissues due to rapid degradation of the DNA by endonucleases. Traditionally, gene delivery systems are broadly classified as either viral-mediated or nonviral-mediated. Viral vectors are significantly more efficient in delivering the gene as well as inducing gene expression as a result of their highly evolved and specialized components. Commonly used viral vectors are adenovirus, retrovirus, adeno-associated virus, and herpes-simplex virus (Stone et al., 2000). However, their use in the clinic is limited due to inherent drawbacks, such as immunogenicity, restricted targeting of specific cell types, size limitation on DNA, and potential for mutagenesis. Consequently, nonviral vectors are increasingly being proposed as alternatives as they have a better safety profile despite their low transfection efficiency. In addition, gene expression in nonviral delivery systems is usually transient, making it feasible for the treatment of nonchronic diseases. The more well-known nonviral vectors are the gene gun, cationic lipids, and cationic polymers. Hence, there is great promise for biomaterials to serve in the synthesis of nonviral vectors.

## 19.8   Delivery Obstacles in Nonviral Gene Delivery

Conventional routes of drug administration are used for gene delivery. However, such methods are only capable of delivering the gene/vector complex to the cell. Therein lies another difference between drug and gene therapy. Whereas a drug only needs to bind to a receptor on a cell surface or enter cytoplasm to have a therapeutic effect, a gene has to translocate into the nucleus in order to exploit the cell's transcriptional and translational machinery to synthesize the therapeutic protein. Hence, it is critical to examine the key hurdles that lie along the pathway from the extracellular space to protein expression (Leong) (Figure 19.11).

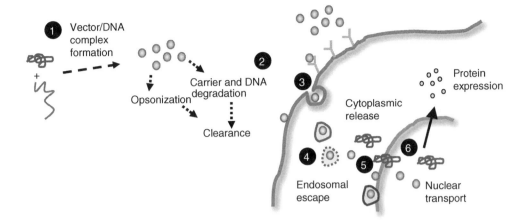

**FIGURE 19.11**
Barriers in nonviral gene delivery.

The key impediments to successful gene delivery are as follows

1. *Vector/DNA complex formation*: There are three major factors to consider during vector/DNA complex formation, namely, condensing the DNA, minimizing the size of the complex, and preventing the aggregation of complexes. First, DNA has to be condensed in order for efficient cellular uptake to occur and for efficient gene expression. The extent of DNA condensation is mediated by the charge density and ionicity of the polymer or lipid. Secondly, although there is no consensus regarding the optimal particle size, smaller particles below 150 nm are believed to be favorably uptaken by receptor-mediated endocytosis. Larger complexes ($>1\,\mu m$) will be favorably phagocytosed by cells of the immune system. Although this may be potentially useful in DNA vaccination, more often than not, it represents clearance. Particle size can in part be controlled by varying the intensity of agitation during complex formation, the molecular weight of the polymer, charge of the polymer, and by preventing aggregation. Thirdly, aggregation of complexes increases the likelihood of clearance. Aggregation may occur as a result of charge interactions with neighboring complexes, or with proteins in the plasma. Aggregation may be minimized by incorporating hydrophilic residues into the polymer (such as conjugating PEG to the polymer backbone). This will reduce nonspecific interactions with plasma proteins. In summary, an ideal vector/DNA complex contains highly condensed DNA, has a small and compact structure, but does not aggregate.

2. *Transport of the vector/DNA complex to the targeted cell*: After being administered to a patient, the vector/DNA complex must travel via the blood stream or other tissue compartments such as muscle or lung to its target tissue. Along the way, the gene carrier must protect the DNA from degradation by nucleases, in addition to avoiding clearance by the RES and the immune system. In order to avoid nuclease degradation, it is imperative that the vector/DNA complexes be stable in extracellular fluid so that they can be delivered to target cells in the body, as the electrostatic interaction between DNA and its vector may be compromised by high concentrations of polyelectrolytes present in plasma. Stability implies that the complexes will not dissociate into their vector and DNA components, and can

be enhanced by selecting cationic polymers which bind strongly to DNA. Such polymers are usually strongly charged, which may potentially compromise the transport of the complex to the targeted cell. This is because excessive positive surface charge increases the risk of aggregation and coating by negatively-charged serum proteins. In order to avoid clearance, stealth polymers such as PEG can be conjugated on to the polymer backbone to reduce nonspecific interactions with plasma proteins, as well as to elude complement system activation. Thus, the incorporation of PEG on to a strongly cationic polymer can facilitate DNA binding to produce a compact polyplex structure which will inhibit nuclease degradation while at the same time reduce aggregation and evade clearance by the immune system.

3. *Internalization of the vector/DNA complex by the cell*: The cell internalizes the vector/DNA complex via endocytosis. The mechanism of endocytosis can be either specific (via receptor-mediated endocytosis) or nonspecific (via pinocytosis and phagocytosis), clathrin-mediated or nonclathrin-mediated pathways. At this stage, receptor-mediated endocytosis can be exploited to enhance the uptake by specific target cells. When cell-specific targeting ligands (such as monoclonal antibodies, ICAMs, peptides, and substrates) are conjugated to the vector/DNA complex, cells which express the corresponding receptor will preferentially uptake the complex.

4. *Escape from the endosome*: Endocytosis usually results in the vector/DNA complex being sequestered into endosomes. The endosomes will eventually fuse with lysosomes. The potent lysozymes and low pH in these compartments will degrade the cationic polymer or cause it to swell, which results in DNA release. Once the vector/DNA complex dissociates, DNA is degraded by enzymes in the endosome. It is thus necessary for the DNA to escape from the endosome in order to reach the nucleus. Endosomal escape can be achieved in several ways. The endosomal membrane can be destabilized in the presence of endosomolytic reagents (such as chloroquine), lipophilic sidechains in the polymer and/or peptides which interact with the vesicular membrane. Another strategy is to use polymers with multiple amine groups that will bind the protons in the endosome. The build-up of positive charges then causes an influx of chloride ions to neutralize the charge gradient. Water follows the entry of chloride ions due to osmosis, which in turn causes the polymer to swell and the endosome to rupture. This mechanism is known as the proton-sponge effect. The destabilization of the endosomal membrane and the rupture of the endosomal vesicle results in the DNA being released into the cytoplasm. The lack of endosomal escape is a major barrier to efficient gene delivery as intracellular trafficking experiments show that most of the internalized particles are subsequently trapped in the endolysosomal pathway.

5. *Transport to the perinuclear space*: After escaping from the endosome, the DNA or the vector/DNA complex has to diffuse to the nuclear envelope. There is also some evidence that molecular motors drive the transport of vesicles containing vector/DNA complexes towards the nuclear envelope, though the polymeric property that causes this phenomenon is not known. As the complex traverses the cytoplasm, it is liable to unpack and release its DNA. From microinjection experiments, the apparent half-life of DNA in cytoplasm is determined to be 50 to 90 min, which is relatively fast compared to diffusional transport through the cytoplasm. Hence, during the course of transport to the perinuclear space, a large percentage of the dissociated DNA will be degraded. Complexes which escape the

endosome and do not dissociate are thus better able to protect against DNA degradation. Vectors that facilitate nuclear transport and remain complexed with the DNA at this stage are limited to synthetic polymers such as PEI. This demonstrates the need for mechanistic insight on the transport to the perinuclear space and the polymeric characteristics that enhance the process.

6. *Translocation into the nucleus*: Undissociated vector/DNA complexes can translocate into the nucleus during cell division, when the nuclear envelope is dispersed. Despite some evidence that intact complexes are present in the nuclei of nondividing cells, the mechanism remains a mystery. The more prevalent scenario would be the dissociated DNA translocating into the nucleus to be transcribed into mRNA. In other words, the complex has to unpack in the vicinity of the nuclear membrane to release the DNA. Transport into the nucleus is limited by the size and location of the nuclear pores. However, the translocation of plasmids into the nucleus can be facilitated by the inclusion of viral nuclear localization sequences (NLS). NLS are peptide sequences which are recognized by the cellular machinery, which then complexes with the DNA to promote nuclear accumulation.

It will be a challenge to design polymers that would incorporate features to overcome all the above-mentioned obstacles in gene delivery. More research into various transport mechanisms will undoubtedly shed light on polymeric characteristics that optimize the process of endocytosis, endosomal escape, transport through the cytoplasm to the perinuclear space, and translocation into the nucleus. Such knowledge will help determine the rate-limiting steps of gene delivery and from which optimal gene delivery systems can be rationally designed.

## 19.9   Nonviral Vectors for Gene Delivery

### 19.9.1   Microinjection of DNA into the Cell

DNA can be directly injected into a cell using microinjectors, when viewed under a microscope equipped with micromanipulators. This method has the advantage of introducing the gene of interest directly into the locality of the nucleus, circumventing the acidic endosomal/lysosomal pathway. However, specialized equipment such as micropipette pullers, microinjectors and microscopes equipped with micromanipulators have to be bought and special training is required in order to perform such a procedure. In addition, the procedure is tedious and difficult to scale-up, hence limited to research and not therapeutic purposes.

### 19.9.2   Gene Gun

The gene gun utilizes physical bombardment in order to get the DNA into the cell. Gold particles or rods are first coated with DNA, and then transferred to a Mylar carrier sheet. A high-voltage discharge then causes the DNA-coated particles to accelerate to high velocities, thereby facilitating the penetration of the particles into exposed tissues or a monolayer of cultured cells. The high-pressure bombardment needs to be optimized to minimize tissue damage. This method, though relatively efficient, is limited to exposed organs such as skin. It is especially attractive for DNA vaccination, where transfection of the dermal tissue can be easily achieved and the preponderance of immune cells such as Langerhans cells can lead to a strong immune response.

### 19.9.3 Electroporation

The cells are placed in a fluid medium containing the gene of interest. An electric field is then used to disrupt the cell membrane briefly, thereby increasing membrane permeability. Thus, the likelihood of extracellular material (including the gene of interest) entering the cell through the transient pores is increased. Although it has been mostly used for *in vitro* transfection in the past, recent instrument designs have made *in vivo* application of electroporation common. The indiscriminate nature of electroporation in admitting any compounds surrounding the tissue raises the concern of undesirable uptake. Cell toxicity and tissue damage remain an issue for electroporation.

### 19.9.4 Cationic Lipids

DNA is negatively charged and so is able to form complexes with cationic lipids (Zhang et al., 2004). Cationic lipids that have been developed for this purpose include quaternary ammonium salts (Dioctadecyldimethylammonium bromide (DODAB), and dioctadecyl-dimethylammonium chloride (DODAC)), cationic derivatives of cholesterol and diacyl glycerol and lipid derivatives of polyamines. Colipids such as dioleoyl phosphatidy-lethanolamine (DOPE) and dioleoyl phosphatidylcholine (DOPC) are frequently incorporated into the complex. The association of cationic lipid with DNA is a highly cooperative process. However, the interaction between the cationic lipids and DNA is poorly understood, and so difficult to manipulate to control-size distribution of the resulting complex (lipoplex). Electron microscopy of the lipoplex shows that DNA is condensed in the presence of cationic lipids (Gershon et al., 1993). Further experiments show that the shape of the lipoplex varied from spherical at low lipid/DNA ratios to smooth rod-like structures at high lipid/DNA ratios. The size of the lipoplex increases with lipid concentration. At extremely high lipid concentrations, a highly ordered multilamellar structure with DNA sandwiched between cationic lipid bilayers is formed (Safinya, 2001). Thus, by varying the lipid concentration and lipid/DNA ratio, the properties of the cationic lipid vector can be changed to influence transfection. Cationic lipids are probably the most highly effective nonviral vectors. However, some degree of cytotoxicity results in cell death.

### 19.9.5 Cationic Polymers

Like cationic lipids, cationic polymers such as polylysine and polyethylenimine, will form complexes with DNA. Cationic polymers are emerging as potential gene delivery vectors because of their versatility. Multiple parameters such as rigidity of the polymer backbone, hydrophobicity/hydrophilicity, charge density, adjustable molecular weight, and ionicity can be manipulated to achieve an optimal complexation with DNA. In addition, the biodegradability and ability to form nanoparticles and matrices will enable the control of DNA-release kinetics and sustained release. Consequently, the design of new polymeric gene carriers is an area of research that is intensively pursued in the recent years. Polyethyleneimine (PEI) is the most potent synthetic gene carrier and the most widely studied. It can mediate gene delivery in a variety of cells *in vitro* and tissues *in vivo*. However, PEI is extremely cytotoxic and methods to decrease toxicity (such as incorporating PEG) are being studied. Polylysine is one of the first gene carriers to be studied as it is able to condense DNA very well and so protect DNA from nuclease degradation. However, it is also extremely cytotoxic and has low transfection efficiencies.

Polyamidoamine dendrimers with either ammonia or ethylenediamine as core molecules are used to form starburst dendrimers which can then be used to condense DNA. High-generation dendrimers are very effective at disrupting anionic vesicle membranes, resulting in high transfection efficiencies close that of PEI. Cytotoxicity is also a main concern. The advantages of using synthetic polymers include: ability to study the effect of charge groups on cytotoxicity and DNA condensation, ease of forming copolymers to enhance the effects of gene delivery, ease of conjugating targeting ligands and excipients to the polymer backbone. Natural polymers can also be used as gene carriers due to their biocompatibility. Chitosan is extensively studied as a potential vector for mucosal gene delivery. Collagen and gelatin have also been investigated as potential gene carriers, though their transfection efficiencies are limited by instability under physiological conditions and poor DNA binding efficiency, respectively.

## 19.10 Conclusion

The use of biomaterials in drug delivery has enabled the achievement of controlled and sustained release of drugs to targeted tissues. This is mostly attributed to matching the desired drug release kinetics to the parameters of the biopolymer, such as its kinetics of degradation, drug solubility, and diffusion in the polymer. By manipulating the drug release profile, the therapeutic effect of the drug can be maximized while at the same time minimizing the adverse systemic reactions. This is monitored by studying the biodistribution of the drug after administration.

Nonviral gene delivery systems harbor great potential in the treatment of a diversity of inherited and acquired diseases. However, in order to improve nonviral gene expression to therapeutic levels, significant challenges of low transfection efficiencies, DNA condensation, and biocompatibility have to be overcome. A deeper insight into the barriers underscoring in nonviral gene delivery will facilitate the design of biomaterials to address these obstacles. The diversity of polymeric gene carriers available bodes well for tackling different gene therapy applications. For instance, cell types with different metabolic and surface characteristics can be targeted using polyplexes with different properties for optimal transfection. Likewise, different routes of administration will require polyplexes of different surface and dissociation characteristics. It is likely that continuing research in gene carrier synthesis and intracellular trafficking studies will lead to the successful development of efficient gene delivery systems for clinical applications.

## References

Baker, R.W. and Lonsdale, H.S., Controlled release: Mechanisms and rates. In A.C. Tanquary and R.E. Lacey (eds)., *Controlled Release of Biologically Active Agents*, Plenum Press, New York, (1974).

Cavazzana-Calvo, M., Thrasher, A. et al., The future of gene therapy, *Nature*, **427** (6977), 779–781 (2004).

Chen, R.R. and Mooney, D.J., Polymeric growth factor delivery strategies for tissue engineering, *Pharm. Res.*, **20** (8), 1103–1112 (2003).

Edwards, D.A. and Dunbar, C., Bioengineering of therapeutic aerosols, *Annu. Rev. Biomed. Eng.*, **4**, 93–107 (2002).

Edwards, D.A., Hanes, J., Caponetti, G., Hrkach, J., Ben-Jebria, A., Eskew, M.L., Mintzes, J., Deaver, D., Lotan, N., and Langer, R., Large porous particles for pulmonary drug delivery, *Science*, **276** (5320), 1868–1871 (1997).

Gershon, H., Ghirlando, R., Guttman, S.B., and Minsky, A., Mode of formation and structural features of DNA-cationic liposome complexes used for transfection, *Biochemistry*, **32** (28), 7143–7151 (1993).

Higuchi, T., Rate of release of medicaments from ointment bases containing drugs in suspension, *J. Pharm. Sci.*, **50**, 874–875 (1961).

Hoffman, A.S., Hydrogels for biomedical applications, *Adv. Drug Deliv. Rev.*, **54** (1), 3–12 (2002).

Huang, L., Hung, M.-C., and Wagner, E., Eds. *Nonviral Vectors for Gene Therapy*, Academic Press, New York (1999).

Jepson, M.A., Clark, M.A. et al., M cell targeting by lectins: a strategy for mucosal vaccination and drug delivery, *Adv. Drug Deliv. Rev.*, **56** (4), 511–525 (2004).

Jiang, W., Gupta, R.K., Deshpande, M.C., and Schwendeman, S.P., Biodegradable poly(lactic-*co*-glycolic acid) microparticles for injectable delivery of vaccine antigens, *Adv. Drug Deliv. Rev.*, **57** (3), 391–410 (2005).

Kumar, N., Langer, R.S. et al., Polyanhydrides: an overview, *Adv. Drug Deliv. Rev.*, **54** (7), 889–910 (2002).

Kuntz, R.M. and Saltzman, W.M., Polymeric controlled delivery for immunization, *Trends Biotechnol.*, **15** (9), 364–369 (1997).

Kuo, P.Y. and Saltzman, W.M., Novel systems for controlled delivery of macromolecules, *Crit. Rev. Eukaryot. Gene Expr.*, **6** (1), 59–73 (1996).

Langer, R., Biomaterials in drug delivery and tissue engineering: one laboratory's experience, *Acc. Chem. Res.*, **33** (2), 94–101 (2000).

Langer, R. and Tirrell, D.A., Designing materials for biology and medicine, *Nature*, **428** (6982), 487–492 (2004).

Leong, K.W., Polymeric Controlled Nucleic Acid Delivery, MRS Bulletin, **30** (9), 640–647 (2005).

Miyata, T., Uragami, T., and Nakamae, K., Biomolecule-sensitive hydrogels, *Adv. Drug Deliv. Rev.*, **54** (1), 79–98 (2002).

Nishikawa, M. and Huang, L., Nonviral vectors in the new millennium: delivery barriers in gene transfer, *Hum. Gene Ther.*, **12** (8), 861–870 (2001).

Park, K., Ed., *Controlled Drug Delivery: Challenges and Strategies*, American Chemical Society, Washington (1997).

Peppas, N.A., Devices based on intelligent biopolymers for oral protein delivery, *Int. J. Pharm.*, **277** (1–2), 11–17 (2004a).

Peppas, N.A., Intelligent therapeutics: biomimetic systems and nanotechnology in drug delivery, *Adv. Drug Deliv. Rev.*, **56** (11), 1529–1531 (2004b).

Peppas, N.A. and Siepmann, J., Modeling of drug release from delivery systems based on hydroxypropyl methylcellulose (HPMC), *Adv. Drug Deliv. Rev.*, **48** (2–3), 139–157 (2001).

Ranade, V., Drug delivery systems. 6. Transdermal drug delivery, *J. Clin. Pharmacol.*, **31** (5), 401–418 (1991).

Ratner, B.D., Hoffman, A.S., Schoen, F.J., and Lemons, J.E., Eds. *Biomaterials Science*, Academic Press, New York (1996).

Safinya, C., Structures of lipid–DNA complexes: supramolecular assembly and gene delivery, *Curr. Opin. Struct. Biol.*, **11** (4), 440–448 (2001).

Saltzman, W.M., *Drug Delivery: Engineering Principles for Drug Delivery*, Oxford University Press, Oxford (2001).

Siepmann, J. and Gopferich, A., Mathematical modeling of bioerodible, polymeric drug delivery systems, *Adv. Drug Deliv. Rev.*, **48** (2–3), 229–247 (2001).

Stokes, C.L., The pros and cons of drug 'trafficking', *Nat. Med.*, **1** (11), 1135–1136 (1995).

Stone, D., David, A., Bolognani, F., Lowenstein, P.R., and Castro, M.G., Viral vectors for gene delivery and gene therapy within the endocrine system, *J. Endocrinol.*, **164** (2), 103–118 (2000).

Theeuwes, F. and Yum, S.I., Principles of the design and operation of generic osmotic pumps for the delivery of semisolid or liquid drug formulations, *Ann Biomed Eng.*, **4** (4), 343–354 (1976).

Thomas, F. and Klibanov, A.M., Non-viral gene therapy: polycation-mediated DNA delivery, *Appl. Microbiol. Biotechnol.*, **62** (1), 27–34 (2003).

Weisse, C., Clifford, C.A. et al., Percutaneous arterial embolization and chemoembolization for treatment of benign and malignant tumors in three dogs and a goat, *J. Am. Vet. Med. Assoc.*, **221** (10), 1430–1436 (2002).

Williams, D.A. and Baum, C., Medicine. Gene therapy — new challenges ahead, *Science*, **302** (5644), 400–401 (2003).

Zhang, Y., Zhang, Z., and Wu, F., A novel pulsed-release system based on swelling and osmotic pumping mechanism, *J. Controlled Release*, **89** (1), 47–55 (2003).

Yoo, H.S. and Park, T.G., Biodegradable polymeric micelles composed of doxorubicin conjugated PLGA–PEG block copolymer, *J. Controlled Release*, **70** (1–2), 63–70 (2001).

Zhang, S., Xu, Y., Wang, B., Qiao, W., Liu, D., and Li, Z., Cationic compounds used in lipoplexes and polyplexes for gene delivery, *J. Controlled Release*, **100** (2), 165–180 (2004).

# 20

## Orthopedic Prostheses and Joint Implants

Shanfeng Wang, Lichun Lu, Bradford L. Currier, and Michael J. Yaszemski

## CONTENTS

## 20.1  Introduction

The clinical needs for orthopedic implants come from a variety of conditions that include fractures and soft-tissue injuries resulting from trauma, *arthritis*, and degenerative disk disease. *Osteoarthritis, rheumatoid arthritis,* and *post-traumatic arthritis* are the most common forms of arthritis to cause joint pain and stiffness. Osteoarthritis is a disease in which the articular cartilage cushioning the bones wears away and the bones themselves become the articulating bearing surfaces. Rheumatoid arthritis is a disease in which the synovial membrane becomes inflamed, and the end result of this inflammatory process is destruction of the articular cartilage. Post-traumatic arthritis is joint destruction that results from sports injuries or other accidents. *Osteonecrosis* can also cause osteoarthritis. Intervertebral disk degeneration is a normal aging process in which the gelatin-like center of the disk degenerates and the space between the vertebrae narrows. Thereafter, the disk and facet joints of the spine experience increased stress that results in further wear and degenerative changes.

Orthopedic devices are used to relieve pain, improve function, and address deformity caused by the above defects and diseases. They include implants such as joint replacement prostheses, fracture fixation devices (nails, pins, screws, and plates), and spinal implants for both trauma and reconstruction applications. Orthopedics ranks behind cardio-vascular as the second most important sector in the U.S. medical implant market. It accounts for 24% of the U.S. medical device industry and is projected to experience a growth rate of 7 to 9% (Kouidri, 2004). The most dominant products within the orthopedic sector are devices that are implanted for reconstruction in hip, knee, and spine applications.

## 20.2  Considerations for Materials in Orthopedic Implants

The aim of biomaterials usage in orthopedic implants is to restore the structural integrity and functionality of the damaged bones and joints, and to minimize complications such as implant structural failure, loosening, or articulating surface wear. To attain these objectives, the materials selection process must incorporate the chemical and mechanical demands of the biologic environment to achieve the desired functional outcome. In addition to *in vivo* performance, a material must also satisfy practical manufacturing, marketing, and clinical requirements, including reasonable cost, the ability to be fabricated into intricate shapes and sizes, and the provision of desired design properties to the implant. The requirements fall into three interrelated major categories: mechanical properties, biocompatibility, and manufacturing (Williams, 1980; Smith, 1985; Hoeppner and Chandrasekaran, 1994; Kohn, 1995; Long and Rack, 1998). These categories are depicted in Figure 20.1.

### 20.2.1  Mechanical Properties

Materials undergo mechanical testing in tension, compression, bending, shear, and torsion. The measurement of toughness and ductility provide information to mitigate against catastrophic failure as a result of unanticipated overload or localized strain. In addition, these properties facilitate plate "contouring" for fracture fixation without severely jeopardizing plate strength. The mechanical property of hardness refers to

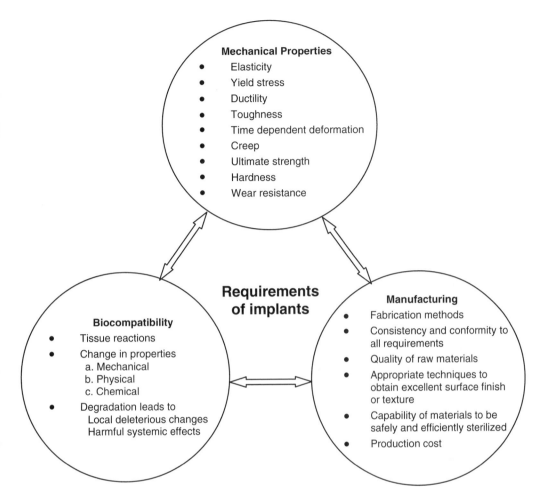

**FIGURE 20.1**
Implant material requirements for orthopedic applications. (*Source*: Adapted from Hoeppner, D.W. and Chandrasekaran, V., *Wear*, **173**, 189 (1994). With permission.)

a material's resistance to indentation, which is important, particularly when combining various materials for bearing or wear conditions.

Implant materials are required to have both high static (as above) and cycle-dependent mechanical properties. A fracture-fixation device typically remains in service for a period of months or years and must endure repeated loading under corrosive conditions. The mechanical properties of "fatigue," "creep," and "stress relaxation" reflect time-dependent materials' behavior and are important parameters in the selection process.

*Fatigue* refers to a mode of failure from repeated stress at magnitudes lower than that required to cause failure in a single application. Implant materials necessarily must have a high degree of fatigue resistance to perform over the long term. Certain materials may undergo progressive deformation with time under constant stress. This mode of deformation and failure is called *creep* and relates to the viscoelastic characteristics of a material. Noncrystalline materials such as polymers, consisting of long-chain molecules having weak van der Waals forces between chains, are particularly prone to this time-dependent form of deformation. The process in polymers is also more temperature-sensitive than in metals and deformations may occur rapidly on exposure to quite low stresses. Creep phenomena may be minimized in the implant design process by using metal alloys having a high melting point and a face-centered cubic crystalline structure to inhibit dislocation movement. Plastics can be made more resistant to creep by adding fillers or other reinforcing materials that raise the viscosity and restrict the movement of dislocations. *Stress relaxation* is a time-dependent, viscoelastic process similar to creep, but it refers to the decay of internal stress under constant strain. Musculoskeletal tissues including muscle, tendons, and bone all exhibit viscoelastic properties. An excellent biologic example of stress relaxation is the time-dependent reduction in applied interfragmentary compression at a fracture site that is fixed and compressed with a dynamic compression plate. Creep and stress relaxation are usually, but not always, undesirable properties of orthopedic biomaterials because they dissipate forces necessary to maintain rigid internal fixation (Smith, 1985).

## 20.2.2 Biocompatibility

Material choices also must take into account *biocompatibility* with surrounding tissues, the environment and corrosion issues, friction and wear of the articulating surfaces, and implant fixation either through osseous integration (the degree to which bone will grow next to or integrate into the implant) or bone cement. First of all, the materials must be nontoxic and noncarcinogenic, causing little or no foreign-body reaction. Additionally, the material must not degrade in response to the corrosive conditions of the biologic environment, thereby impairing mechanical properties or releasing potentially harmful degradation by-products locally and systemically. However, such a state, that is, complete inertness, is unachievable, and therefore a relative degree of implant interaction with the host is considered acceptable for permanent implants. Indeed, in the area of tissue-engineered medical products (TEMPS), specific interactions between the host and the typically degradable implant are desirable. The *degradation* process must not impair significantly the mechanical strength of the device nor allow the release locally or systemically of by-products that might evoke a deleterious biologic response.

The *corrosion* of metals in biologic fluids is an electrochemical reaction that results in the release of metal ions into the surrounding aqueous electrolyte. This dissolution reaction is coupled with a corresponding reduction reaction of constituents in the aqueous environment to maintain charge neutrality. The alloys currently used as orthopedic biomaterials have a corrosion rate typical for the specific material decreased by a passivating oxide layer that acts like an electrical resistor to retard the anodic dissolution of metal cations. Plasma coating can also enhance the fatigue strength, the corrosion and wear resistance as well as the loadbearing capacity. Under optimum passivation conditions, all implant alloys have a finite, albeit slow, uniform corrosion rate *in vivo*. However, damage to this passivating layer, such as by fretting or wear, may produce conditions conducive to accelerated focal corrosion and failure.

Degradation of nonmetallic implant materials is more difficult to assess than that of metals. Of importance in the degradation process of polymers are the types of chemical bonds present, steric hindrance and electronegativity effects produced by atoms in close proximity with these chemical bonds, and supramolecular structure (e.g., a crystalline structure is generally more inert than an amorphous one). Also important is a knowledge of the low-molecular weight mobile moieties and their cytotoxicity, since such molecules constitute a diffusible fraction consisting of polymeric chain degradation by-products or stabilizing additives or plasticizers. Failures that have been observed in surgically-implanted polymers appear to relate to the susceptibility of nonmetallic materials to various forms of mechanochemical deterioration, such as stress-solvent crazing, friction, wear, and fatigue (Smith, 1985).

Note that the definition of biocompatibility refers to the specific application. Many materials may be biocompatible under one or more conditions but cannot be assumed to display biocompatibility under all the conditions. Biocompatibility is the situation that exists when an implanted material interacts with the host such that the desired functional outcome occurs for the expected period of time in the absence of unwanted adverse effects on the host caused by the presence of the material.

### 20.2.3  Manufacturing Requirements

Manufacturing requirements dictate that the material has properties that permit fabrication in the optimum design configuration. Sterilization and cleanliness are essential for all implantable devices. Each sterilization method must accomplish the same goal: remove or destroy living organisms and viruses from the biomaterial. Three methods commonly employed are steam sterilization, ethylene oxide (EtO) gas sterilization, and gamma radiation sterilization. Recently some other sterilization techniques have been developed using low-temperature gas plasma, ionized gases, and supercritical carbon dioxide. Selection of a specific sterilization method is based on economic considerations and implant material properties, for example, heat resistance, solubility, and radiation sensitivity. Furthermore, the packaging of medical devices such as ultra-high molecular weight polyethylene (UHMWPE) components influences the susceptibility of those implants to oxidative degradation. Since the 1990s, air-permeable UHMWPE packaging has been replaced by sterilization under a nitrogen atmosphere and barrier packaging to minimize oxidative degradation during long-term shelf storage (Davis, 2003).

Cleanliness is a concept that differs from sterility, and is just as important with respect to implant performance. Cleanliness defines specified levels of nonbiologic contaminants (for example, oils that may remain on the implant from a prior processing step), which are the maximum levels of those contaminants that may remain on the implant prior to its distribution. An implant can be sterile but not clean, just as it may be clean but not sterile.

## 20.3  Materials in Orthopedic Devices

The term "orthopedic materials" is a general term for biomaterials used in orthopedic surgery applications, and includes devices that are as diverse as bone graft substitutes and total joint prostheses. The bone graft substitutes (Laurencin et al., 1999; Lu et al., 2000) based on autograft, allograft, metals, ceramics, polymers, cells, and growth factors will be discussed in Chapter 22. Here, materials used in fracture fixation devices, total joint prostheses, and musculoskeletal repair and reconstruction implants are described in the following categories: metals, ceramics, and polymers (Smith, 1985; Agrawal, 1998; Donachie, 1998; Hallab et al., 2002; Katti, 2004). The mechanical properties of those most common orthopedic biomaterials are tabulated in Table 20.1, and compared with those of cortical bone.

### 20.3.1  Metals

Metals are attractive for structural implant purposes owing to their high strength. With advances in refining technology, many metals and alloy systems have been

**TABLE 20.1**

Mechanical Properties of Common Orthopedic Biomaterials Compared with Cortical Bone

| Orthopedic Biomaterial | Elastic Modulus (Young's Modulus) (GPa) | Yield Strength (Elastic Limit) (MPa) | Ultimate Strength (MPa) | Fatigue Strength (Endurance Limit) (MPa) | Hardness HVN | Elongation at Fracture (%) | Primary Use(s) |
|---|---|---|---|---|---|---|---|
| *Cortical bone*[a] | | | | | | | |
| Low strain rate | 15.2 | 114[e] | 150[c]/90[e] | 30–45 | — | — | — |
| High strain rate | 40.8 | — | 400[c]–270[e] | — | — | — | — |
| *Metals* | | | | | | | |
| Stainless steels | | | | | | | |
| ASTM F138[b] | 190 | 792 | 930[e] | 241–820 | 130–180 | 43–45 | TJA[d] components, screws, plates, cabling |
| Co–Cr alloys | | | | | | | |
| ASTM F75[b] | 210–253 | 448–841 | 655–1277[e] | 207–950 | 300–400 | 4–14 | TJA[d] components |
| ASTM F90[b] | 210 | 448–1606 | 1896[e] | 586–1220 | 300–400 | 10–22 | |
| ASTM F562[b] | 200–230 | 300–2000 | 800–2068[e] | 340–520 | 8–50 (RC) | 10–40 | |
| ASTM F1537[b] | 200–300 | 960 | 1300[e] | 200–300 | 41 (RC) | 20 | |
| Ti alloys | | | | | | | |
| CPTi ASTM F67[b] | 110 | 485 | 760[e] | 300 | 120–200 | 14–18 | Plates, screws, TJA[d] |
| Ti-6Al-4V ASTM 136[b] | 116 | 897–1034 | 965–1103[e] | 620–689 | 310 | 8 | Components (nonbearing surface) |
| *Ceramics* | | | | | | | |
| Al$_2$O$_3$ (Alumina) | 366 | — | 3790[c], 310[e] | — | 20–30 (GPa) | — | Bearing-surface TJA[d] components |
| ZrO$_2$ (Zirconia) | 201 | — | 7500[c], 420[e] | — | 12 (GPa) | — | TJA[d] components |

| Polymers | | | | | | |
|---|---|---|---|---|---|---|
| UHMWPE | 0.5–1.3 | 20–30 | 30–40[e] | 13–20 | 60–90 (MPa) | 130–500 | Low-friction inserts for bearing surfaces in TJA[d] |
| PMMA | 1.8–3.3 | 35–70 | 38–80[e] | 19–39 | 100–200 (MPa) | 2.5–6 | Bone cement |
| Silicone rubber | 0.008 | — | 7.6 | — | — | 350 | Finger joint |

*Source:* Adapted from Hallab, N.J., Jacobs, J.J., and Katz, J.L., In: *Biomaterials Science: An Introduction to Materials in Medicine*, Ratner, B.D., Hoffman, A.S., Schoen, F.J., and Lemons, J.E., Eds., Elsevier Academic Press, Amsterdam, 526–555, (2002). With permisssion.

RC, Rockwell Hardness Scale; HVN, Vickers Hardness Number, kg/mm.

[a] Cortical bone is both anisotropic and viscoelastic. Thus, properties listed are representative, and reflect testing conditions used to generate them with respect to both specimen orientation and rate of loading.

[b] Designation by American Society for Testing and Materials (ASTM).

[c] Compression.

[d] Total joint arthroplasty.

[e] Tension.

developed with a high degree of corrosion resistance. Seven alloy systems have been selected for review here based on a combination of properties that makes them desirable for musculoskeletal applications. These properties include biocompatibility, low cost, high elastic modulus and ultimate strength, high ductility for loads exceeding the yield stress (thus reducing the risk of catastrophic brittle failure), ease of manufacturing for their intended application, and corrosion resistance. The seven alloys shown in Table 20.1 may be grouped according to composition into three alloy systems: the austenitic stainless steels (iron, chromium, molybdenum), the cobalt-based alloys, and the titanium-based alloys.

### 20.3.1.1   Stainless Steels

The primary stainless steel alloy presently recommended for device manufacture is the American Iron and Steel Institute (AISI) type 316LV (ASTM F138 in Table 20.1). The exact composition may vary slightly relative to the casting or forging variant. However, both forms are derived from the very common 18-8 stainless steel alloy (18% chromium, 8% nickel) used in tableware and other commercial applications. The composition differences between the 18-8 and 316LV alloy are necessitated by the superior corrosion resistance required of implant devices. The addition of molybdenum (3%) to the 18-8 alloy and the reduction of carbon content (0.03% max) confers improved corrosion resistance on the alloy, particularly to pitting and intergranular attack. Such compositional changes, however, necessitate the addition of nickel (12%) to maintain the stability of the desired austenitic microstructure (Smith, 1985).

Of the alloys currently specified for device manufacture, stainless steel is the cheapest and most easily fabricated. To obtain high quality devices, careful attention must be given to the melting process, the carbon and impurity content, and the various thermal treatments necessary for shaping and developing desirable mechanical properties. Surface preparation is typically accomplished by mechanical polishing or electropolishing to remove draw marks, pits, burrs, and surface contamination. The final step in processing stainless steel implants is that of surface passivation in nitric acid to remove surface iron particles and to artificially thicken the surface oxide layer.

### 20.3.1.2   Cobalt-Based Alloys

The two Co–Cr alloys predominantly used as implant alloys are cobalt–chromium–molybdenum (Co–Cr–Mo) (ASTM F-75 and F-76), and cobalt–nickel–chromium–molybdenum (Co–Ni–Cr–Mo) (ASTM F-562) in Table 20.1. Other Co-based alloys approved for implant use include one that incorporates tungsten (Co–Cr–Ni–W, ASTM F-90) and another with iron (Co–Ni–Cr–Mo–W–Fe, ASTM F-563). These four Co-based alloys can be divided in to two main types by the manufacturing condition: cast alloy or wrought alloy. Co–Cr–Mo is a cast alloy and the other three are wrought alloys. The Co-based alloys display a useful balance between mechanical properties and biocompatibility, both forms being somewhat superior to stainless steel in strength and corrosion resistance, but more expensive to manufacture.

Co–Cr–Mo alloy cannot be contoured at the time of surgery because of its high rate of work hardening. Accordingly, this alloy is typically reserved for implantable devices having a fixed configuration (e.g., total hip prosthesis). In addition, because of its high abrasion resistance, it is sometimes used for bearing applications such as metal-on-metal total joint devices. The wrought Co–Cr alloys mechanically exhibit a lower rate of work hardening than the cast alloy. In the fully annealed state, the wrought alloy displays a yield stress similar to the more brittle cast variant. However, it has a much-improved ductility (60% strain at fracture), and an ultimate tensile strength approaching that of a heavily cold-worked stainless steel. Moreover, with appropriate working and annealing treatments, the wrought alloy can be made to span a useful range of strengths and ductilities, giving it much versatility as an implant alloy. The wrought alloy, however, is somewhat less resistant to crevice corrosion than the cast Co–Cr–Mo alloy. Its use for fracture fixation devices is not as yet commonplace, probably as a result of its increased cost compared with that of stainless steel.

### 20.3.1.3 *Titanium-Based Alloys*

This third alloy system used in manufacturing structural implants includes two titanium-based alloys: commercially pure titanium (CPTi) and Ti-6Al-4V, containing a nominal 6% aluminum and 4% vanadium. CPTi must adhere to specified impurity maxima, particularly with respect to oxygen, since mechanical properties vary markedly with impurity content. The higher the impurity content, the stronger but less ductile the metal. Mechanically, the disadvantages of pure titanium include its relatively low elastic modulus (approximately half that of stainless steel and Co–Cr), low shear strength, and its poor abrasion resistance. The low abrasion resistance causes it to gall or seize when it is in sliding contact with another metal surface. In addition, it is more difficult and expensive to fabricate than stainless steel. Beyond light weight, the major advantage of titanium lies in its inherent corrosion resistance, particularly in saline solutions. This inertness results primarily from the spontaneous formation of a strong passivating oxide layer (Smith, 1985).

The addition of 6% aluminum and 4% vanadium to commercially pure titanium results in an alloy having mechanical properties similar to cold-worked stainless steel (including superior fatigue resistance) yet retaining excellent corrosion resistance. In addition, the Ti-6Al-4V alloy is more easily weldable and machinable than the pure form. The greatest drawback to Ti-based alloys is their relative softness compared to Co–Cr–Mo alloys. Thus, titanium alloys are seldom used as materials where hardness or resistance to wear is an important design criterion. However, titanium alloys are the material of choice for patients having known hypersensitivity reactions to any of the constituents of stainless steel or Co–Cr alloys.

### 20.3.1.4 *New Metals and Surface Coatings*

Novel alloys for orthopedic applications have often been designed by adding small quantities of new elements to the above three major alloys to provide specific new properties to those alloys. In addition, some metals, such as zirconium (Zr) and tantalum (Ta) have also been used in special circumstances because of their chemical stability, high strength, and outstanding resistance to wear. Oxidized zirconium femoral components haven been commercialized as Oxinium because of enhanced mechanical and biocompatibility properties. However, they are costly to manufacture.

Currently, surface coatings are used to improve the performance of implants by encouraging bone growth and providing enhanced fixation. The coated surfaces include roughened Ti, porous coatings made of Co–Cr or Ti beads, Ti wire (or fiber) mesh, plasma-spayed Ti, and bioactive nonmetallic materials such as hydroxyapatite or other calcium phosphate compositions. Osteoconductive and osteoinductive growth factors are also being developed in coatings for enhancing fixation (Hallab et al., 2002).

## 20.3.2 Ceramics

Ceramic materials often reduce osteolysis and are regarded as favorable materials for joints or joint-surface materials due to their excellent wear resistance, high compressive strength, good biocompatibility, and stability in physiological environments. However, they have not as yet been applied to fracture fixation applications largely because of their poor ductility, i.e., susceptibility to brittle fracture. Commercially, alumina ($Al_2O_3$) and zirconia ($ZrO_2$) ceramics have been used in total hip replacements (THR) for the last 30 years. In February 2003, the FDA approved two newly-designed hip implants made of durable ceramics.

Certain glasses, ceramics, and glass-ceramics that contain oxides of silicon, sodium, calcium, and phosphorus ($SiO_2$, $Na_2O$, $CaO$, and $P_2O_5$) are the only materials known currently that form a chemical bond with bone, resulting in a strong mechanical implant/bone interface (Blanchard, 1995). These materials are referred to as *bioactive* because they bond to bone (and in some cases to soft tissue) through a time-dependent, kinetic modification of the surface triggered by their implantation. In particular, an ion-exchange reaction between the bioactive implant and surrounding body fluids results in the formation of a biologically active hydrocarbonate apatite (calcium phosphate) layer on the implant that is chemically and crystallographically equivalent to the mineral phase of bone. This equivalence is responsible for the relatively strong interfacial bonding between the implant and the host bone.

### 20.3.3   Polymers

#### 20.3.3.1   *Ultrahigh-Molecular Weight Polyethylene (UHMWPE)*

Because of its low coefficient of friction with metal, UHMWPE has been widely used since the early 1960s by Charnley as a load-bearing articulating surface in several multi-component total joint devices after polytetrafluoroethylene (PTFE) failed due to its accelerated creep and poor stress corrosion. The wear of UHMWPE is a major problem in orthopedics (Hallab et al., 2002). Any use of the joint, such as walking in the case of total hip arthroplasty, results in cyclic loading of the polymeric cup against the metal or ceramic ball. Due to significant localized contact stresses at the ball/socket interface, small regions of UHMWPE tend to adhere to the metal or ceramic ball. During the reciprocating motion of normal joint use, fibrils will be drawn from the adherent regions on the polymer surface and break off to form submicrometer-sized wear debris. This adhesive wear mechanism, coupled with fatigue-related delamination of the UHMWPE, results in tiny polymer particles being shed into the surrounding synovial fluid and tissues. The biological interaction with small particles in the body then becomes critical. The body's immune system attempts, unsuccessfully, to digest the wear particles. Enzymes are released that eventually result in the death of adjacent bone cells and resorption of the local bone extracellular matrix, a process termed osteolysis. Over time, sufficient bone is resorbed around the implant to cause mechanical loosening, which necessitates implant removal and insertion of a new, revision prosthesis. Wear tests have shown that the wear resistance of UHMWPE can be improved by cross-linking with gamma irradiation. However, this can negatively affect some physical properties such as tensile strength. In addition, the history of total joint replacement is replete with examples of novel implants that have worked well in preclinical studies, and then demonstrated unanticipated problems after a period of widespread clinical use has occurred. Indeed, early reports are appearing in the literature that demonstrate wear of explanted highly cross-linked polyethylene cup liners after a time period much shorter than would have been expected from the preclinical studies.

#### 20.3.3.2   *Poly(methylmethacrylate) (PMMA)*

PMMA is used widely as a bone cement in orthopedics, particularly for femoral stem fixation to bone in total hip arthroplasty, femoral and tibial prosthesis fixation to bone in total knee arthroplasty, and as a permanent bone substitute in the treatment of pathologic fractures of the vertebrae and appendicular skeleton. The development of current bone cement techniques has significantly reduced the rates of loosening associated with total joint replacement. PMMA manufactured for orthopedic purposes is stored in sterile packaging and subsequently polymerized *in situ* by thoroughly mixing powdered, prepolymerized methyl methacrylate with liquid methylmethacrylate monomer. Manufacturers have added the appropriate "opacifiers," "initiators," and "activators" to the components to begin the polymerization process, which normally occurs over a time period of about 15 min. Barium sulfate is usually added as an opacifier, which allows the PMMA to be visible on a standard radiograph. The initiator, benzoyl peroxide, is a solid at room temperature, and is included as a powder with the prepolymerized PMMA. It is the source of free radicals that will initiate the polymerization process. The rate of benzoyl peroxide's spontaneous decomposition into peroxide radicals at room temperature is too low to initiate the polymerization, and this rate is increased to an appropriate value by the presence of *N,N*-dimethyl-*p*-toluidine, an accelerator that is a liquid at room temperature. It is included and stored with the liquid methylmethacrylate monomer, and reacts with the benzoyl peroxide upon mixing the liquid and solid components of the cement to produce the free radicals that initiate the reaction. The polymerization proceeds through phases that may be separated by time points called "dough time" and "working time." The time interval that begins with mixing the cement components and ends when the cement has gained enough viscosity to be handled as a cohesive mass is called the "dough time," and typically lasts about 2 to 4 min. The time period from this point, until the cement is too hard to mold any more, is the "working time," and lasts about 8 to 11 min. These times vary somewhat depending upon the initial temperature of the cement and the ambient room temperature. The reaction is exothermic with attainment of temperatures as high as 122°C in the center of the material and 92°C at the surface. It is advisable to control heat production as much as possible, such as by using the minimum amount of PMMA to accomplish a given task, or by adding fillers. Another issue in the use of *in situ* PMMA polymerization is the release of the monomer, MMA, into the circulation, with the potential to cause direct toxic effects such as a precipitous fall in blood pressure and death.

Mechanically, PMMA is strong but brittle when fully hardened. Compared with other common thermoplastics, it demonstrates excellent properties, including its tensile modulus, tensile strength, flexural rigidity, and resistance to creep. However, it is mechanically inferior to the metal alloys, having low ductility (<5% strain to failure) and a high susceptibility to stress solvent crazing. It should also be recognized that PMMA has poor adhesive properties. In fact, the term "bone cement" is a misnomer, since the PMMA does not adhere to the bone. Fixation to the bone occurs by intrusion of the cement, while early in the polymerization process and in a low viscosity state, into the interstices of the host's trabecular bone.

### 20.3.3.3 *Poly(dimethyl siloxane) (PDMS)*

Silicone (PDMS) is an odorless, tasteless material, which does not support bacteria growth and will not stain or corrode other materials. Silicones also resist water and many chemicals, such as acids, oxidizing chemicals, ammonia, and isopropyl alcohol. They are used in many applications because of their stability, low surface tension (20.4 mN/m), lack of toxicity, and superior compatibility with human tissue and body fluids. Silicones can be easily cross-linked to elastomers with varying physical properties for making artificial finger joints as well as other soft-tissue implants. However, due to its low strength and modulus, silicone has limited use in other orthopedic implants.

## 20.4   Applications

Orthopedic implants far exceed any other biomaterial applications by weight or volume. They are used both as fracture fixation devices (which may or may not be removed after fracture healing) (Figure 20.2) and as joint replacement devices or prostheses designed to remain in the body for a life time (Figure 20.3). Prosthetic devices serve as joint replacements (replacing either the total joint or only one of the two articulating surfaces) or as bone replacements (replacing larger sections of bone, for example, after tumor resection) (Williams, 1980; Park, 1984; Hallab et al., 2002; Davis, 2003; López et al., 2003).

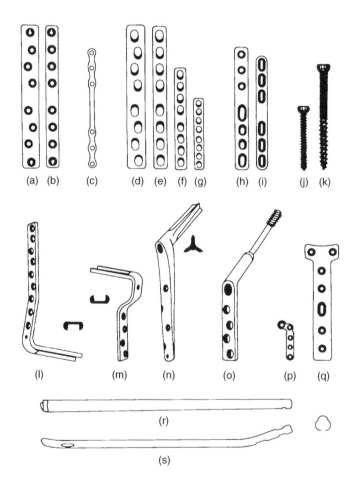

**FIGURE 20.2**

Typical examples for orthopedic internal fixation devices (schematic). (a) and (b) Round hole plates (can be used with compression devices). (c) Sherman bone plate (historical, not in current use). (d) to (g) Dynamic compression plates of various sizes. (h) Compression bone plate with glide holes. (i) Bagby compression bone plate (historical, not in current use). (j) Cortical bone screw. (k) Cancellous bone screw (with smooth shank to allow compression of fracture fragments). (l) Condylar angle blade plate. (m) Hip blade plate for osteotomies. (n) Jewett nail plate with three-flanged nail (historical, not in current use). (o) Two-component dynamic hip screw plate. (p) Miniature L-plate used for hand surgery applications. (q) T-plate for proximal humeral fractures and tibial plateau fractures. (r) Intramedullary femoral nail. (s) Intramedullary tibia nail. (*Source*: Davis, J.R., *Handbook of Materials for Medical Devices*, ASM International, Cleveland, OH (2003). With permission.)

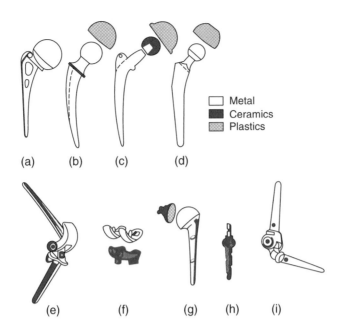

**FIGURE 20.3**
Historical examples of joint prostheses. (a) Moore hip endoprosthesis. (b) Müller total hip prosthesis (metal against polyethylene acetabular cup). (c) Weber total hip prosthesis with modular head and metal, ceramic, and polyethylene components. (d) Müller total hip prosthesis with straight stem. (e) Hingelike knee joint prosthesis; metal against metal (G.E.U.P.A.R.). (f) Sliding knee joint prosthesis; metal against plastic (Geomedic). (g) Total shoulder joint prosthesis; metal against plastic (St. Georg). (h) Total finger joint prosthesis with metal and plastic components (St. Georg). (i) Total elbow joint prosthesis; metal-to-metal (McKee). (*Source*: Davis, J.R., *Handbook of Materials for Medical Devices*, ASM International, Cleveland, OH (2003). With permission.)

## 20.4.1 Fracture Fixation Devices

Fracture fixation devices include external and internal fracture fixation devices. External fixation may be used to immobilize the fracture site by casts or by devices fixed to adjacent bone, to provide temporary fixation, and to protect soft tissues during major extremity trauma.

Internal fixation uses a device placed directly across the fracture site, such as a plate, wire, screw, pin, or nail (Figure 20.2). Often, various combinations of these devices are employed and the instrumentation is inserted after open reduction. Alternatively, fixation devices may be inserted percutaneously after closed-fracture reduction.

Almost all of these devices are made from metal alloys. The simplest but most versatile implants are metal wires, which can be used in a variety of situations for diverse applications that include bone fixation and soft tissue reattachment to bone. Bone plates, introduced in the early 1900s to assist in the healing of skeletal fractures, were among the earliest successful biomedical implants. The bone plate's job is done once the bone has healed and can support the loads encountered during the activities of daily living without refracturing. However, unlike a cast, which can be easily removed after fracture healing, an internal fixation device requires a second operation for its removal. Thus, these devices are usually left in place unless a specific reason exists for their removal that justifies the anesthetic and surgical risks. Such reasons include the treatment of infection at the site of the fracture, and pain from pressure caused by overlying objects such as shoes. Intramedullary devices are used to fix fractures of the long bones by inserting the devices into the intramedullary cavity. Spinal fixation devices are used for the treatment of spinal deformities, degenerative spinal conditions, or fractures.

### 20.4.2  Joint Replacements

#### 20.4.2.1  *Hip*

Total hip replacement (THR) was the first and is most frequently performed of all the total joint replacements. The early methods of treating diseased or fractured hip joints that were not amenable to repair involved only the acetabular cup or the femoral head. One technique of restoring hip joint function is to place an interpositional device over the femoral head while the surface of the acetabulum is sculpted to fit the device. The implant serves as a mold interposing the two surfaces, which eventually adapt according to the loads and motions experienced by the joint. Most femoral head replacements are performed in conjunction with the installation of an acetabular cup (total hip arthroplasty). The insertion of a femoral component alone, which articulates with the person's native acetabulum, is called a hemiarthroplasty. As indicated in Table 20.2, the choice of the articulating materials for the femoral component and socket component is rather crucial in wear behavior. Currently, the most frequent choice in the U.S. for artificial hips is a plastic cup made of UHMWPE, articulating with a metal (Co–Cr alloy) or ceramic (alumina or zirconia) ball affixed to a metal stem (Figure 20.4a).

The most difficult short-term problem in hip joint replacement, as well as other joint replacements, is initial fixation of the implants to the bone. As depicted in Figure 20.5, a cemented prosthesis is fixed in the femoral canal by PMMA bone cement that attaches the metal to the bone, while an uncemented prosthesis is held in place by the tight press fit of the uncemented prosthesis into the femoral canal. Also, the stress concentration experienced by the bone-implant structure at points of changing construct rigidity, such as at the distal end of the femoral stem, makes the bone in such areas more susceptible to fracture during use. The femoral prosthesis depicted in Figure 20.5 is a monoblock design. That is, the femoral stem and the head are a single unit. This implies that the choice of head diameter and neck length must be made prior to cementing the femoral prosthesis in place. Modular femoral designs, such as the prosthesis shown in Figure 20.4a, allow the

**TABLE 20.2**

Materials Combinations in Total Hip Replacement (THR) Prostheses

| Femoral Component | Socket Component | Results |
| --- | --- | --- |
| Co–Cr–Mo | Co–Cr–Mo | Metal-on-metal total hip bearing couple in clinical use in Europe. Preclinical studies demonstrate lowest wear rate of any bearing surface combination to date |
| Co–Cr–Mo | UHMWPE | Currently the most widely employed total hip bearing couple in use in the U.S. |
| Alumina/zirconia | UHMWPE | Very low wear rate compared to metal on UHMWPE. Zirconia is more impact resistant than alumina |
| Ti-6Al-4V | UHMWPE | High rate of UHMWPE wear and particle induced osteolysis. Not in clinical use |
| Surface-coated Ti-6Al-4V | UHMWPE | Enhanced wear resistance to abrasion compared to Ti-6Al-4V on UHMWPE |

*Source*: Adapted from Davis, J.R., *Handbook of Materials for Medical Devices*, ASM International, Cleveland, OH (2003). With permission.

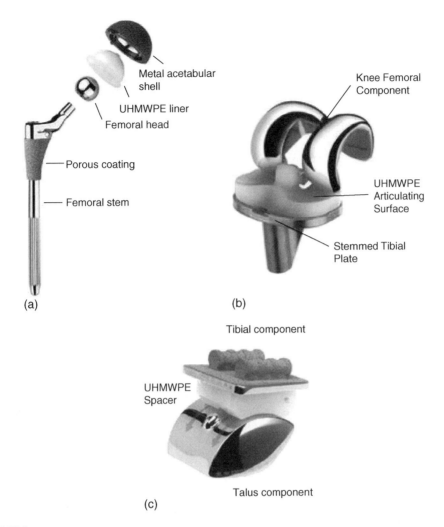

**FIGURE 20.4**
Components and examples of lower extremity joint arthroplasty prostheses: (a) hip, (b) knee, and (c) ankle (Scandinavian).

decision regarding stem size to be made independently of the decision regarding neck length and head diameter. The head can undergo a trial fitting after the cement hardens from the stem insertion. This allows fine-tuning of both the leg length and the stability of the hip prosthesis against dislocation. It is the preferred implant choice and insertion technique in current clinical practice.

### 20.4.2.2 Knee

Total knee replacement (TKR) is a surgical procedure in which arthritic or damaged surfaces of the knee joint are removed and replaced by synthetic biomaterials. The knee is not just a hinge joint, but has a complex gliding and rotational motion. The knee joint implants can be classified into hinged and nonhinged types. Historical design examples that led to the currently used total knee prostheses appear in Figure 20.3e,f. The nonhinged types are further divided into unicompartmental and tricompartmental devices, based on the articulating knee surfaces that are replaced. The tricompartmental designs, which are

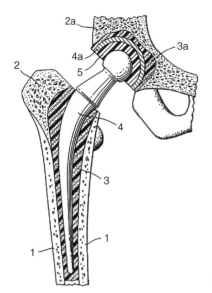

**FIGURE 20.5**
Schematic of the components of a cemented total joint replacement: (1) cortical bone, (2, 2a) trabecular bone, (3, 3a) bone cement, (4) metallic femoral prosthesis, (4a) metal backing of acetabular cup, (5) polyethylene acetabular cup. (*Source*: Courtesy of Topoleski, L.D.T., PhD thesis, University of Pennsylvania, (1990). With permission.)

the most frequently implanted knee replacements, are classified as either posterior cruciate ligament retaining or posterior cruciate ligament removing designs. The selection of a particular implant depends on the functional and geometric status of the knee, the nature of the disease that caused the need for knee replacement, and the range of activities required by the individual patient. The most frequently used method of fixation to bone is cementation of all three components (femoral, tibial, and patellar) to the bone. The most frequently used combination of materials for these components is a metal femoral component, a metal tibial component to which is affixed an UHMWPE component for articulation with the femoral component, and an all polyethylene patellar component for articulation with the metal femoral component (Figure 20.4b). Porous-coated knee replacement implants are available, and are designed to induce bone tissue in-growth to the implant. These devices are used less frequently in the U.S. than are the cemented knee replacement devices.

### 20.4.2.3 Ankle

The ankle joint is made up of the two bones of the leg (the tibia and the fibula), and the most proximal bone in the foot, the talus. It has three articulating surfaces: the distal tibia and the superior surface of the talus, the medial malleolus of the tibia and the medial side of the talus, and the distal fibula (lateral malleolus of the ankle), and the lateral side of the talus. The ankle joint moves in dorsiflexion, plantar flexion, inversion, and eversion. Its range of inversion–eversion is approximately 14° in normal walking. Ankle joint kinematics are not accurately modeled by the hinge plus rotational motion system as in the knee. The ankle has more complex kinematics throughout the six possible degrees of freedom in three dimensions, which makes it more difficult to duplicate in an implant.

Though there are a variety of ankle implants available in the U.S., there are currently two prostheses that are most frequently used in current practice. The first resurfaces the ankle joint medially, laterally, and superiorly. This prosthesis requires the conversion of a three-bone ankle into a two-bone ankle through fusion of the distal tibia and fibula to each other. The second design resurfaces the superior talus, and requires a mobile-bearing polyethylene component to enhance mobility of the ankle while limiting bone resection.

The FDA has extended the clinical trials of the Scandinavian Total Ankle Replacement (STAR) device (Figure 20.4c), which is approved in Europe and has been used there for more than ten years.

### 20.4.2.4  Shoulder

Shoulder arthroplasty may be recommended for patients with glenohumaral arthritis or for proximal humeral fractures that are better treated, for a variety of clinical reasons, with replacement rather than repair. The hemispherical, incongruent glenohumeral joint is the least constrained and provides the largest motion of any joint in the body. As had occurred in hip-joint replacements, the first shoulder-joint replacement prosthesis, introduced by Neer, was designed as a hemiarthroplasty to replace only the humeral head. Current designs offer a glenoid replacement component that allows the surgeon and patient to choose total shoulder arthroplasty as a reconstruction option (Figure 20.6a). A more challenging task in shoulder replacements occurs when the rotator cuff does not function normally. The Neer prosthesis was designed to function with an intact, functioning rotator cuff. There are more constrained designs that are indicated for patients who have a nonfunctioning rotator cuff either through injury or degeneration.

The most common total shoulder arthroplasty configuration consists of a humeral component made of a metal (usually a cobalt/chromium-based alloy), and a glenoid component made of UHMWPE. The articulation usually occurs between the metal ball on the humeral component, and the UHMWPE cup, which constitutes the glenoid component. There have been recent designs that have been classified as "reverse total shoulder arthroplasty implants," which have the ball component attached to the glenoid, and the cup component attached to the humerus.

### 20.4.2.5  Elbow

The elbow is a hinge-type joint allowing flexion and extension, and, in addition, supination and pronation of the forearm. The goal of elbow replacement as a treatment for elbow arthritis is to restore the functional mechanics of the joint by removing scar tissue, balancing muscles, and inserting a replacement for the articulating surfaces. One stem of the artificial joint is fixed to the distal humerus and another stem to the proximal ulna. As shown in Figure 20.6b, there are two types of elbow implants: linked (semi-constrained) or unlinked (unconstrained) differentiated by the presence or absence of a physical connection between the humeral and ulnar components. Linked implants are chosen when the surrounding joint structures are unable to provide stability to the joint. Unlinked implants more closely reproduce the natural kinematics of the joint, and are an appropriate choice when the joint capsule, ligaments, and muscles can provide stability throughout the elbow's range of motion.

The metal stems inserted into the humerus and ulna are precision-engineered and are available in various sizes to allow for optimum fit. Depending on the type of elbow implant, the bearing components can vary. Typically, a linked elbow implant is more common in the U.S. In a linked elbow, the bearing components include a linked metal piece and a linked screw that is placed on the ulna, and a high-grade plastic "yoke" that is attached to the humeral stem. The plastic "yoke" is commonly used on the humerus to serve as a cushion to prevent metal-on-metal contact. A pin assembly is then attached to link the bearing components to the humeral and ulnar stems. These elbow bearing components form the linked hinge for the two stems. Alternatively, an unlinked elbow has a pin assembly and a metal piece called a bobbin that are placed on the humeral stem and a high-grade plastic component that is attached to the ulnar stem.

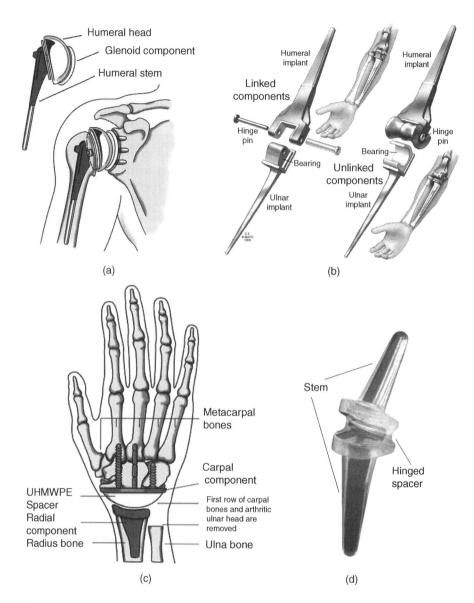

**FIGURE 20.6**
Components and examples of upper extremity joint replacement prostheses: (a) shoulder, (b) elbow, (c) wrist, (d) finger (Graphs (a) and (c) courtesy of American Academy of Orthopaedic Surgeons. With permission.)

### 20.4.2.6 *Wrist*

The wrist joint has complicated kinematics, allowing flexion and extension, supination (palm up) and pronation (palm down), and deviation (radial and ulnar). Shown in Figure 20.6c, the eight carpal bones are arranged in two rows of four bones in each row. The long metacarpal bones radiate out from the second row of carpal bones, and the bones of the fingers and thumb attach to their respective metacarpals. The two bones of the forearm (radius and ulna) participate with the proximal row of carpal bones in the formation of the wrist joint.

A total wrist replacement implant consists of several components. First, it has an ellipsoid head, which simulates the curvature of the patient's natural radiocarpal joint to allow for a functional range of motion. This allows the patient to flex and extend the wrist and move it side-to-side. Second, it has an offset trapezoidal-shaped radial stem. This stem anchors the implant in the radius and adds stability, as well as eliminating rotation of the implant within the bone. Third, it has an elongated radial tray with a molded bearing made of UHMWPE. This component is crucial to "load sharing," distributing forces over the entire surface of the implant. Fourth, it has a curved metacarpal stem. This component is shaped to accommodate the natural curvature of the metacarpal medullary canal, and secures the wrist implant to the hand.

### 20.4.2.7  Finger

Many small joints of the hand and foot can be replaced. The natural finger joints include a metacarpophalangeal (MCP) joint, and proximal and distal interphalangeal joints. Stability is provided by ligaments and tendons so that fingers do not collapse under load. Current treatment options include replacement arthroplasty, resection or fusion of the arthritic joint. Resection usually relieves pain and corrects deformity but lacks stability and strength. Fusion relieves pain and provides strength, but takes away motion. The replacement options include hinged prostheses, polycentric prostheses, and space-filler prostheses. Some artificial finger joints (Figure 20.6d) are made of silicone, and others are metal on plastic bearing surfaces. The implants are inserted into the gap created when the arthritic surfaces of the MCP joint are removed. The artificial finger joint has a stem on each side that is inserted into the canals created in the bone of the finger and the metacarpal joint.

### 20.4.2.8  Spine and Intervertebral Disk Replacement

The anatomic components that comprise the intervertebral disk, and their attachment into bone, contribute significantly to spinal stability by absorbing pressure and permitting spinal range of motion within a physiologic range. At the same time, these structures, the nucleus pulposus and the annulus fibrosus, limit motions in excess of the physiologic range that might otherwise risk injury to the neurologic tissues that are contained within the bony spine. Disk arthroplasty must also take into consideration the presence of the paired posterior facet joints. These synovial joints participate in transmitting spinal loads and determining spinal range of motion, and may, in conjunction with the anterior disk, contribute to pain and abnormal spinal motion because of degenerative changes. The biomaterials for total disk replacement must satisfy the high demands of a lifetime of repetitive, cyclic loads imparted to the implant. The anticipated age of a person who is a candidate for this implant is decades younger than the typical age of a person who is a candidate for total hip or knee arthroplasty. Thus, the projected life span of a total disk arthroplasty implant is 30 to 50 years. During this time the device will undergo between 10 and 30 million loading cycles (Le et al., 2004; Oskonian et al., 2004; Smith et al., 2004).

Link SB Charité III became commercially available in 1987. The Charité artificial disk is a three-piece articulating medical device consisting of a minimally constrained polyethylene core sandwiched between two metal endplates as shown in Figure 20.7. In 1989, another disk replacement device, the ProDisc, was introduced. It is a metal-on-metal design and has yielded favorable long-term outcomes. So far, of all the spinal arthroplasty devices in use, only the SB Charité and the ProDisc have more than 5 years of clinical follow-up, and both have been used in Europe for more than a decade. There are not yet data from long-term prospective randomized clinical trials available for these devices. In the U.S., these clinical trials were initiated in 2000 for the SB Charité and in 2001 for the ProDisc. The SB Charité was approved for use in the U.S. by the FDA in 2004.

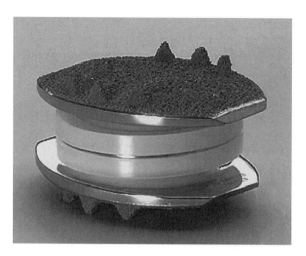

**FIGURE 20.7**
The LINK SB Charité III artificial disk.

Complications and implant failures occur with orthopedic implants (Anderson et al., 2002). Therefore, implant retrieval and evaluation plays a critical role in the evolution of medical devices from development to clinical use. The clinical utility of orthopedic implant retrieval and evaluation is summarized in Table 20.3.

## 20.5   Perspectives

Novel technologies are being applied to the development of new orthopedic implants, and will likely change aspects of clinical practice in the near future (Kouidri, 2004). These changes may include the elimination of certain procedures, the introduction of new procedures, a reduction in the length of hospital inpatient stay for some existing procedures, and an increase in the expected service life of implants. Technology developments are in the area of implant composition and manufacture (i.e., direct manufacturing of shape specific degradable tissue engineering products via solid freeform fabrication), and novel materials, including combination products that contain various mixtures of metals, natural and synthetic polymers, bioactive molecules, and cells. Novel therapies to augment existing treatment options are being made possible by the introduction of existing technology to new applications. For example, *lithotripsy* machines, already in use for the treatment of kidney stones, have now been approved by the FDA for the treatment of plantar fasciitis. The use of these shock wave instruments to break up plantar scar tissue, help increase local blood flow, and ultimately provide an environment for local tissue repair have been available in the U.S. since 2000. However, the effectiveness of such therapies has been questioned. *Knee Navigation Systems* help surgeons identify the appropriate landmarks during total knee arthroplasty to accurately position the implants. These navigation systems, based on either preoperative axial imaging datalinked to intraoperative skeletal landmark registration, or on intraoperative x-ray fluoroscopic data, have also been developed for use in other joints and in the spine. *Minimally Invasive Surgery* (MIS) technology may allow certain orthopedic operations to be done with less trauma to structures that would otherwise need to be manipulated and retracted during the procedure. MIS techniques could bring about improvements that include less postoperative pain, shorter hospital stays, faster rehabilitation times, and an overall lower

## TABLE 20.3
Clinical Utility of Retrieval Studies Involving Orthopedic Implants

| Implant Type | Knowledge Gained/Lessons Learned |
|---|---|
| Plates, screws, and rods used for fracture fixation | Do not mix metal alloys in same device |
| | Match the hardness and stiffness with the application |
| | Metallic implant wear and corrosion may lead to problems associated with allergic reactions |
| Femoral stems of THR (fracture analysis) | Cobalt alloys require high-quality casting |
| | High-strength superalloys may be advantageous |
| | Welded regions may fail in tensile-loaded locations |
| | Part numbers should not be etched in tensile-loaded locations |
| Femoral stem, modular interface | Corrosion at an interface is dependent on metallurgical and mechanical design factors |
| Polymeric components of total joint replacements (excluding one-piece flex hinge joints like finger) | Teflon performs poorly in wear applications |
| | Reinforcement of UHMWPE with chopped fiber is ineffective, and accelerates wear |
| | Laboratory wear simulation should be done using clinically realistic implant motion, fluid environment, and loading patterns |
| | Mechanical designs that produce high localized stresses may cause delamination of the polymer, and the subsequent generation of wear debris |
| | Radiation sterilization to produce cross-linking is useful, but can lead to molecular chain scission, oxidation, and aging |
| Analysis of tissue surrounding total joint replacements. | Wear particles derived from breakdown of the implant-bone interface or wear of the articulation (bearing) materials cause inflammation, osteolysis, and implant loosening |
| Titanium and titanium-alloy implants | A good material for one implant application may not necessarily be good in another application |
| | Commercially pure titanium is appropriate for fracture fixation devices |
| | Titanium alloys may yield severe wear in some total joint applications |

*Source*: Adapted from Anderson, J.M., Schoen, F.J., Brown, S.A., and Merritt, K., In: *Biomaterials Science: An Introduction to Materials in Medicine*, Ratner, B.D., Hoffman, A.S., Schoen, F.J., and Lemons, J.E., Eds., Elsevier Academic Press, Amsterdam, 771–782 (2002). With permission.

cost of care. Tissue engineering strategies that take advantage of bone's ability to repair and remodel itself have already resulted in bone graft substitute devices for some applications. These strategies, as they continue to develop and be refined, may lead to an ability to discontinue using autograft bone for grafting needs, and eliminate the potential complications that can occur at the iliac crest and other bone graft harvest sites.

Biomaterials and implant research will continue to concentrate on serving the needs of patients by leading to devices that physicians consider to be appropriate for the care of those patients, and that industry can produce at a reasonable cost (Piehler, 2000; Medlin, 2004). Examples of novel designs include increasingly smaller implants, modular implants, and the use of shape-memory alloys. Smaller implants may have more stringent material property requirements to meet strength, fatigue, and functional performance goals in smaller and smaller device volumes. Examples include the class of implantable microelectromechanical devices (MEMS) that have been developed for both diagnostic and therapeutic functions. Modular implant devices have multiple components, each of which is selected during the procedure to optimize a given function, and which are then assembled during the operation. This design approach results in a better ability to adapt to changing situations intraoperatively, but has the disadvantage of producing a junction in the implant, which may produce fretting and crevice corrosion. Shape-memory alloys can be malleable at room temperature (or in a water–ice bath) and then assume their memory shape at body temperature as the austenitic–martensitic transition occurs. This ability to assume a predetermined shape can be exploited in a number of surgical situations, such as the spinal deformity reduction in scoliosis.

Novel medical applications are being explored in the field of nanotechnology. For example, self-assembling DNA nanotubes could find use in TEMPS that seek to mimic natural extracellular matrix. In addition, nanotube-coated titanium implants provide surfaces to which osteoblasts attach and express their phenotypic functions (Webster and Ejiofor, 2004). Recently, the graft polymerization of a biocompatible phospholipid polymer on to a polyethylene surface has been investigated (Moro et al., 2004), and a total hip arthroplasy bearing surface has been made from the resulting material. Hip-joint simulator studies using this material revealed that the grafting markedly decreased the wear-related production of the polyethylene particles that are responsible for osteolysis.

## 20.6   Conclusions

In summary, total joint arthroplasty is a good solution for many arthritic problems. New alloy chemistries, creative thermal–mechanical processing, novel coating technologies, and advanced surface treatments will be expected to fulfill higher mechanical property requirements. TEMPS and bioactive implants also represent a promising addition to the clinical armamentarium.

## Problems

1. Why are orthopedic prostheses and joint implants important, and what are the major goals that joint arthroplasty should achieve?
2. What are three categories of design requirements for orthopedic biomaterials to be used in joint arthroplasty applications?
3. What are three major time- or cycle-dependent properties and why are they important for orthopedic materials?
4. Name five primary orthopedic implant biomaterials. List their advantages and disadvantages.
5. What is the major issue associated with the longevity of total joint replacement implants? Suggest a strategy to solve this problem by improving biomaterial properties.
6. What is the chemical composition of bone cement? Name one clinical application that uses bone cement and the process for implanting the cement.

7. What are two major types of orthopedic devices?

8. What are the two most frequently performed total joint replacements?

9. Name two new technologies that are under development in the field of orthopedic implants.

10. Search for a new biomaterial or surface treatment in the recent literature. List and explain its advantages and disadvantages, and give your suggestions for possible clinical applications in which it might be used.

## Answers

1. The importance stems from the burden of joint arthritis and intervertebral disk degeneration on our population. These diseases account for almost 25% of the medical devices implanted in the U.S. The goals of joint arthroplasty are to relieve pain, improve function, and correct deformity (see Introduction).

2. Three design requirement categories for joint implant biomaterials are mechanical properties, biocompatibility, and manufacturing (see Section 20.2).

3. Three properties that are time or cycle dependent include creep, stress relaxation, and fatigue fracture. See the discussion of these properties in Section 20.2.1 for a discussion of their importance in the selection of biomaterials for orthopedic devices.

4. Five general classes of materials in use for orthopedic applications include the stainless steels, the cobalt-based alloys, the titanium-based alloys, the ceramics, and the polymers. Each of these categories includes several specific biomaterials. For example, the polymer class includes UHMWPE, PMMA, and PDMS (silicone). See Section 20.3 and Table 20.1 for further discussion of the advantages and disadvantages of each of these materials.

5. The most important issue affecting joint arthroplasty longevity is the bearing couple, i.e., the chemical and physical nature of the articulating surfaces. The wear that occurs at this interface, and the resulting particulate debris, is the basis for the osteolysis whose end result is often implant loosening and the need for revision surgery. See Section 20.3.3.1 and Table 20.3 for further information on this issue.

6. Bone cement is poly(methylmethacrylate). Formulations from different companies vary slightly. Most include barium sulfate as an opacifier, so that the cement can be seen on an x-ray image. The ingredients are packaged as a powder and a liquid, which are mixed during surgery, and produce a mixture that is at first a low viscosity liquid. This mixture increases in viscosity over about 15 min, and passes through stages during which it is injectable, then moldable, and finally becomes a hard solid. The liquid component contains the accelerator, *N,N*-dimethyl-*p*-toluidine, to increase the rate of free radical formation by the initiator, and an inhibitor, hydroxyquinone, to prevent premature polymerization of the liquid methylmethacrylate (MMA) monomer. The MMA monomer makes up the balance of the liquid component. The powder component contains previously polymerized and powdered poly(methylmethacrylate), the barium sulfate, and the initiator, benzoyl peroxide. See Section 20.3.3.2 for further details.

7. The two major classes are fracture fixation devices and joint replacement devices. The fixation devices include spinal instrumentation devices, both for anterior and posterior spinal applications. See Section 20.4 for additional details.

8. The two most frequently performed joint replacements are total hip arthroplasty and total knee arthroplasty.

9. There are some novel technologies on the horizon in the field of orthopedic implants, for example, Minimally Invasive Surgery (MIS) and Knee Navigation Systems. See Section 20.5 for additional discussion of this topic.

10. Refer to the references listed in this chapter or other recent publications in the biomaterials literature to select a material for evaluation. Then, choose an implant issue, such as bearing surface wear and its effect on joint implant longevity, and discuss how the novel material might be used to address that issue.

# References

Agrawal, C.M., Reconstructing the human body using biomaterials, *JOM*, **50**, 1 (1998).

Anderson, J.M., Schoen, F.J., Brown, S.A., and Merritt, K., Implant retrieval and evaluation, In: *Biomaterials Science: An Introduction to Materials in Medicine*, Ratner, B.D., Hoffman, A.S., Schoen, F.J., and Lemons, J.E., Eds., Elsevier Academic Press, Amsterdam, pp. 771–782 (2002).

Blanchard, C.R., *Body Parts of the Future*, *Technology Today*, Southwest Research Institute, San Antanio, TX (1995).

Davis, J.R., *Handbook of Materials for Medical Devices*, ASM International, Cleveland, OH (2003).

Donachie, M., Biomaterials, In: *Metals Handbook Desk*, 2nd ed., Davis, J.R., Ed., ASM Internatuional, Cleveland, OH, pp. 702–709 (1998).

Hallab, N.J., Jacobs, J.J., and Katz, J.L., Orthopedic applications, In: *Biomaterials Science: An Introduction to Materials in Medicine*, Ratner, B.D., Hoffman, A.S., Schoen, F.J., and Lemons, J.E., Eds., Elsevier Academic Press, Amsterdam, pp. 526–555 (2002).

Hoeppner, D.W. and Chandrasekaran, V., Fretting in orthopaedic implants: a review, *Wear*, **173**, 189 (1994).

Katti, K.S., Biomaterials in total joint replacement, *Colloid. Surf. B: Biointerfaces*, **39**, 133 (2004).

Kohn, D.H., Structure-property relations of biomaterials for hard tissue replacement, In: *Encyclopedic Handbook of Biomaterials and Bioengineering*, Part B, Vol. 1, Wise, D.L., Trantolo, D.J., Altobelli, D.E., Yaszemski, M.J., Gresser, J.D., and Schwartz, E.R., Eds., Marcel Dekker, New York (1995).

Kouidri, D., Orthopedics, Chapter 5, In: *The U.S. Market for Medical Devices — Opportunities and Challenges for Swiss Companies*, von Walterskirchen, M., Ed. Swiss Business Hub USA, Chicago, pp. 37–45 (2004).

Laurencin, C.T., Ambrosio, A.M.A., Borden, M.D., and Cooper, J.A. Jr., Tissue engineering: orthopedic applications, *Annu. Rev. Biomed. Eng.*, **1**, 19 (1999).

Le, H., Thongtrangan, I., and Kim, D.H., Historical review of cervical arthoplasty, *Neurosurg. Focus*, **17**, E1 (2004).

Long, M. and Rack, H.J., Titanium alloys in total joint replacement — a materials science perspective, *Biomaterials*, **19**, 1621 (1998).

López, R.A. Jr., Miro, L.A., Cancel, L.M., and Cardona, C.J., Biomechanics of joint replacement: finger to shoulder, In: *Proceedings of Applications of Engineering Mechanics in Medicine*, 8 December 2003, University of Puerto Rico—Mayaguez, pp. C1–C19.

Lu, L., Currier, B.L., and Yaszemski, M.J., Synthetic bone substitutes, *Curr. Opin. Orthopedics*, **11**, 383 (2000).

Medlin, D.J., Future challenges for metals in orthopedic implant devices, *Adv. Mater. Processes*, **November**, 81 (2004).

Moro, T., Takatori, Y., Ishihara, K., Konno, T., Takigawa, Y., Matsushita, T., Chung, U.-I., Nakamura, K., and Kawaguchi, H., Surface grafting of artificial joints with a biocompatible polymer for preventing periprosthetic osteolysis, *Nat. Mater.*, **3**, 829 (2004).

Oskouian, R.J., Whitehill, R., Samii, A., Shaffery, M.E., Johnson, J.P., and Shaffery, C.I., The future of spinal arthroplasty: a biomaterial perspective, *Neurosurg. Focus*, **17**, E2 (2004).

Park, J.B., *Biomaterials Science and Engineering*, Plenum Press, New York (1984).

Piehler, H.R., The future of medicine: biomaterials, *MRS Bull.*, **August**, 67 (2000).

Smith, G.K., Orthopaedic biomaterials, Chapter 13, In: *Textbook of Small Animal Orthopaedics*, Newton, C.D. and Nunamaker, D.M., Eds., International Veterinary Information Service, Ithaca (1985).

Smith, H.E., Wimberley, D.W., and Vaccaro, A.R., Cervical Arthroplasty: material properties, *Neurosurg. Focus*, **17**, E3 (2004).

Topoleski, L.D.T., Failure mechanisms of poly(methyl methacrylate) bone cement and fracture characteristics of titanium fiber reinforced bone cement, Ph.D thesis, University of Pennsylvania (1990).

Webster, T.J. and Ejiofor, J.U., Increased osteoblast adhesion on nanophase metals: Ti, Ti6Al4V, and CoCrMo, *Biomaterials*, **25**, 4731 (2004).

Williams, D.F., Implantable prostheses, *Phys. Med. Biol.*, **25**, 611 (1980).

# 21

## Dental Implants

Bruce A. Doll, Ash Kukreja, Ali Seyedain, and Thomas W. Braun

## CONTENTS

## 21.1 Introduction

Current applications for dental implants have developed from a long history of attempts to restore edentulous areas. Over the past decades the increase in the elderly population has been characterized by a rise in the incidence of tooth loss. Therapies for tooth loss encompass numerous attempts to restore the form and function of the dentition utilizing biocompatible material. To gain perspective, the first section of the chapter will discuss the historical events culminating in the present therapies. Present therapy indications and complications will be presented. Discussion of the implant design and the use of intraoral/extraoral implants will be followed by future directions for implants in craniofacial therapy.

### 21.1.1   History of Dental Implants

Tooth loss has been apparent in skulls dating back several thousand years. Whether for function, adornment, religious connotations, or other reasons, efforts to engineer adequate replacements for the lost tooth have developed. Logically, designs for implantation into the oral tissues were loosely based upon the shape or function of a tooth as guideline for the material and shapes tested. *Implantation* was first defined by Congdon in 1915 as a term used to "designate the operation of introducing either a natural or an artificial root into an artificial socket cut into the alveolar process" (Congdon, 1915; Hoek et al., 1959).

According to Cranin, in prehistoric Egyptian dynasties, intraosseous implantation of animal teeth and artificial teeth carved of ivory was performed prior to mummification in the corpse's jaw to ensure suitable preparation for the afterlife. Furthermore, Cranin stated that the earliest recorded dental implant was placed during the pre-Columbian era. Depicting a global problem, Galliardot in 1862 excavated a site in the Middle East, where he uncovered an appliance dating to 400 BC. The appliance contained four lower teeth holding two carved ivory teeth held by a gold wire to replace two missing incisors (Weinberger, 1948; Ring, 1985). In 1931, while in Honduras, Popenoe discovered a skull with an artificial tooth carved from a dark stone. This skull, dated to 600 AD, had three tooth-shaped pieces of shell which had been implanted in the alveolar sockets of missing lower incisors (Saville, 1913).

Attempts to replace missing teeth in ancient times were not solely confined to creating artificial alternatives. Transplantation of teeth was described by an Arab surgeon named Abul Kasim. Though transplantation seemed to be a widespread procedure in Europe in the 1500s, popularity waned by the 19th century as an understanding of disease transfer became apparent (Ring, 1985).

As a result, considerations given to the type of material used to construct the root form dental implant became the focus of many scientists and clinicians. In 1809, the use of a gold implant inserted into a fresh extraction site was performed by Maggilio (Driskell, 1987). In 1887, lead became the material of choice when Harris successfully cemented a crown on to a leaded root implant. Support for Harris's choice of material was provided when a publication by Berry in 1888 considered the use of wood, tin or silver as root substitutes. However, he concluded that lead was the material of choice since it was well tolerated. The 20th century brought about the implantation of silver capsules and artificial roots (Ring, 1985). In 1909, Greenfield, introduced the first lattice cage root form design made of iridioplatinum noteworthy for lacking close resemblance to the shape of a tooth root as had been the prevailing practice. Interestingly the design incorporated the concept of tissue in-growth into the implant framework (Figure 21.1) (Greenfield, 1915).

Subsequently, the foundation of today's biomaterials are prefaced by the works of Venable, who in 1937, developed the cast cobalt–chromium–molybdenum alloy known as vitallium (Ring, 1985). In 1939, using Venable's vitallium, Strock developed the first true endosteal root form implant. Using their new "screw" implant, they utilized animal models followed by evaluations in humans and provided the first histological evidence of bone apposition and osseointegration (Strock, 1939). In addition to providing histological success, they provided clinical success. After replacing a maxillary left incisor tooth, it was documented that the root-form implant was in function for over 15 years (Figure 21.2) (Strock and Strock, 1949).

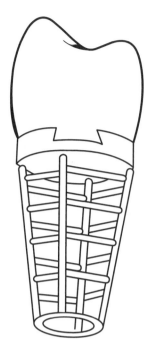

**FIGURE 21.1**
The iridioplatinum artificial root design. The design incorporated an appreciation for the tooth conical root form, biocompatible material and anticipated bone growth into the retentive mesh. Difficulties with implant stability, fixed length and alignment of the crown with the existing dentition were significant disadvantages.

The Strocks' success, though limited, prompted a period of innovation, and experimentation. Consequently, the implant root form design has undergone various morphogenic changes. Corkscrew-shaped implants, screw-shaped implants, trombone-shaped implants, vented implants, nonvented implants, threaded implants, nonthreaded implants, coiled implants, double-helical-spiraled implants, cylindrical implants, and an assortment of others have all made an appearance.

While the development of the root-form implant was taking place, other implant devices were attempted with varying success. Gershkoff and Goldberg introduced the concept of the subperiosteal implant to the United States in the late 1940s. The implant

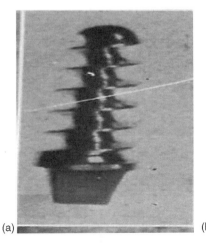
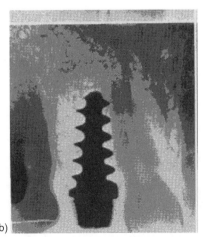

(a)        (b)

**FIGURE 21.2**
Strock implanted a vitallium root form implant (a) that functioned successfully for over 15 years. (b) Conical, tapered root-form thread design with a modifiable retentive core represents concepts applicable to present implant design.

represented a response to improve stability and retention for a mandibular denture. Though the idea was patented by Dahl in 1941, Gershkoff and Goldberg modified the design to improve predictability (Dahl, 1957). The implant had a novel design including a portion placed between the periosteum and the cortical bone (Figure 21.3). Successful therapy with the subperiosteal implant can be attributed to Lew and Berman who, in 1951, introduced the protocol of taking direct bone impressions which significantly enhanced the fit of the metal casting. They also provided long term clinical follow-ups demonstrating stability with their technique (Lew, 1952). However, the subperiosteal implant had limited application for narrow edentulous ridges. The design was used successfully for several decades before other designs superseded its utility.

Concurrently, Linkow introduced another form of an endosteal implant known as the blade-vent implant or plate-form implant that deviated from normal root form anatomy (Linkow, 1984). This implant system provided a solution for treating a narrow and constricted edentulous alveolar ridge. Thus the system design used the bone for support by surgical placement of the blade within the bone utilizing a vertical interface for stability. In addition the implant had openings (i.e., vents, slots, holes) that allowed bone in-growths thus providing resistance to vertical forces (Figure 21.4). One initial objection of the plate-form implant was the frequent result of a fibrous tissue interface as opposed to the more desirable bony interface. However, over time, techniques were developed to overcome this pitfall.

Clinicians have sought an acceptable tooth replacement working with available material, logic, and when available, a knowledge of previous attempts. Present-day root-form implant design and protocol can be largely attributed to Per-Invar Bränemark who developed a landmark implant study in Sweden which started in 1951 (Figure 21.5). He and his colleagues provided the long-term successful human clinical trials as well as the irrefutable histological evidence of true osseointegration that launched the dental community into the present era of implantology (Bränemark et al., 1983).

Unfortunately, today's implant systems remain insufficient to fulfil all expectations. Certain systemic conditions, oral habits, time restrictions, dental and skeletal anatomy are some of the factors that may contraindicate implant placement in edentulous areas. However, new material and knowledge of the biology of osseointegration offer encouragement for expanded, more predictable implant therapies.

### 21.1.1.1 Dental Implant Biomaterial

The biocompatibility profiles of biomaterials use for the replacement or augmentation of biological tissues have been a critical concern. Special circumstances are associated with dental implant prosthetic reconstruction of the oral-maxillofacial region because the

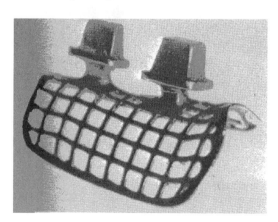

**FIGURE 21.3**
Modified subperiosteal implant accommodated anatomical limitations imposed by endosteal implant. The meshwork rested upon the mandible. Union of the two abutments increased stability relative to two single implants. However, failure of integration of bone within the supporting mesh prevented widespread application.

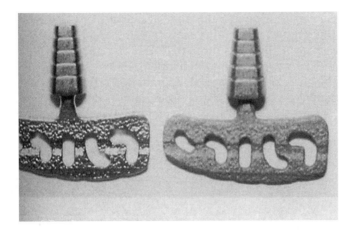

**FIGURE 21.4**
Blade implant. Note the openings which were designed to allow bony in-growth through the base grid and prosthetic cementation over the customized post. Unlike the supraperiosteal implant (Figure 21.3), the blade placement endosteally improved retention. The adjustable abutment height broadened clinical application.

implant extends from the bone, across the epithelial layers and into the oral cavity. The functional aspects of use include the transfer of force from the occlusal surfaces of teeth through the crown and neck connective region of the implant and into the implant for interfacial transfer to the supporting soft and hard tissues — a complex series of chemical, biochemical, mechanical and biomechanical challenges to design. Ultimately, a lost tooth would be replaced by another tooth. Previous efforts to transplant teeth have been successful on a case basis; however, donor tooth availability, tooth size and shape, and edentulous anatomy limit the application of the procedure. Presently, efforts are underway to "grow" teeth but the accompanying discoveries will not yield clinical therapies for another decade or more. Therefore, concurrent emphasis has been focused on improving available dental implants with respect to design and function. The disciplines of biomaterials and biomechanics are complementary to the understanding of device-based function. The physical, mechanical, and chemical properties of the basic material components must be fully evaluated for a biomedical application. The roles of macroscopic implant shape and microscopic transfer of stress and strain along biomaterial-to-tissue interfaces. The shape and form of the implant predominantly

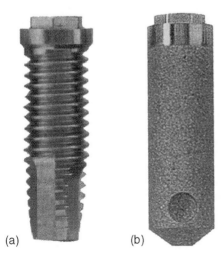

(a)    (b)

**FIGURE 21.5**
Threaded root-form (a) and cylindrical HA-coated (b) implant designs (Nobelpharma) are representative of present endosteal implant systems employing mechanical and/or chemical surface properties to improve retention.

control the mechanical stress and strain. The basic properties of the biomaterial (surface chemistry, microtopography and modulus of elasticity) and the nature of the union of the surface with the adjacent tissue control the localized microscopic strain distribution. Engineering analysis of implant systems include optimizing design and biomaterial. The favorable control of tissue response and biodegradation often places restrictions on which materials can be safely used within the oral environment. Designs are often evolved for specific biomaterials because of the imposed biological or restorative conditions.

## 21.1.2 Biology of Alveolar Bone Implantation

Principles of bone biology underlying the integration of implants has been thoroughly covered in several fine reviews (Steigenga et al., 2003; Triplett et al., 2003). Therefore, relevant concepts will be reviewed as they relate to implant design and function. Traditional therapy with dental implants requires extended periods of time for integration. Enhanced tissue compatability of implants have expanded the therapeutic applications of implant dentistry. Recent designs of endosseous implants were initially proposed with a two-stage surgical protocol for load-free and submerged healing to ensure predictable osseointegration. Discomfort, inconvenience, and anxiety associated with the interim healing period remains a challenge to both patients and clinicians. Long-term stability depends on the integration between osseous tissue and the implant. Integrity of the osseous tissue requires the contribution of mesenchymal stem cells and their continuous differentiation into an osteoblastic phenotype. Compromised healing responses in elderly patients further confound successful, prolonged integration of implants. Improvement of the implant/bone interface remains an open problem. However, the prospect of integration has been marked by significant therapeutic advances due to case selection, surgical and restorative protocols, implant design, construction, and enhanced biocompatability.

The predominant biological consideration in endosseous implant placement and retention has been the bone/implant interface. Predictable anchorage of the implant requires it to closely contact the bone tissue. Through initial studies in dogs, Bränemark recommended a submerged approach to placing implants, thereby minimizing initial contact with the gingival tissues. The concern emphasized decreased exposure to the oral environment, encouraging bone apposition against the implant surface, impeding the extension of gingival epithelium to encapsulate the implant and minimizing bacterial colonization (O'Sullivan et al., 2004).

Integration of the dental implant involves both the gingival and osseous tissue adaptation to the implant surface. With the two-stage approach, implant placement initially positions the surface adjacent to the cortical and cancellous components of craniofacial bone. A one-stage approach where the implant remains exposed to the oral environment, introduces additional contact with the gingival and mucosal tissues concurrent with the osseous tissue contact. Several conditions must be present to obtain implant integration and long-term clinical success when using the one-stage implant placement procedure with immediate loading (Astrand et al., 2002). These conditions include (1) primary stability, (2) sufficient bone quality, and (3) elimination of micromovement of the implant before osseous integration is complete.

Professor Per-Ingvar Bränemark demonstrated the capacity for osseous tissue to integrate with titanium. He proposed the term osseointegration to describe the direct structural and functional connection between living bone and the surface of a load carrying implant (Bränemark et al., 1983; Smith, 1985; Meffert, 1986). Several fine reviews of the subject of osseointegration are available to amplify chapter content (Pjetursson et al., 2004; Wood and Vermilyea, 2004). A brief summary of the events culminating in approximation of the hard tissue against the implant are provided with emphasis on recent advances.

The quality of the tissue-implant interface was evaluated using light and scanning electron microscopy with morphometric analysis. Nine dogs were implanted with three types of dental implants (titanium, zirconia, or alumina). Dubruille and coworkers proposed the division of osseointegration into two phases: (1) osseocoaptation involving a physical contact between the implants and the bone without an interpenetration process, and (2) osseocoalescence to describe the infiltration of the bioactive material, ultimately substituted by newly formed bone. There was no significant statistical difference between the three types of material used for implants (Dubruille et al., 1999).

The interaction between implant materials and bone and oral epithelial cells contributes to the clinical success of dental implants. Comparison of the attachment and behavior of osteoblastic cells on titanium and hydroxyapatite revealed more cells attached on hydroxyapatite and the cells spread more rapidly than on titanium. Cells on titanium possessed well-defined and polarized stress fibers; in contrast cells did not form good stress fibers or vinculin-positive focal adhesions on hydroxyapatite (Goto et al., 2004). The functional activity of cells in contact with an implant is determined by surface properties. Before cells attach, the extracellular matrix in the serum deposits on the implant; rounded cells then attach and spread upon it. Cells may form focal adhesions and polarize, and either migrate or proliferate and form colonies.

Adaptation of the soft tissue to the implant surface involves epithelial cell migration and adhesion. Laminin-5 (Ln-5), a component of the basement membrane (BM), regulates epithelial cell migration and adhesion. The distribution of Ln-5 during the formation of peri-implant epithelium (PIE) in rats was investigated and compared to the distribution of Ln-5 during oral mucosa formation after tooth extraction. One day after extraction, the junctional epithelium had disappeared. Two weeks post extraction, the new epithelium became the PIE and spread further apically along the implant surface. Ln-5 was expressed at the PIE-connective tissue interface, but not at the implant/PIE interface until 4 weeks post surgery. The PIE originated from oral sulcular epithelium and remained nonkeratinized epithelium. Ln-5 may induce cell migration during PIE formation and contribute to the attachment of PIE to Ti, regardless of the delay in the synthesis and deposition of Ln-5 at the Ti-PIE interface (Atsuta et al., 2005).

## 21.1.3 Dental Implants: Geometry and Biomaterials

The variety of dental implants presently exceeds 200 and they are manufactured by approximately 80 companies. Different materials, dimensions, and surface modifications offer the clinician a variety of options with clinical applications. However the scientific literature does not provide any clear recommendations concerning physical characteristics of dental implants and their clinical specifications (Jokstad et al., 2003; Triplett et al., 2003). Characteristcs shared by the more commonly employed dental implants include: form, geometry, surface, and composition.

### 21.1.3.1 Dental Implant Form

The engineering design of implants is based on many interrelated factors, including the geometry of the implant, mechanical properties, and the initial and long-term stability of the implant/tissue interface. The external contour of an implant and the magnitude of occlusal loading can have significant effects on the load transfer characteristics and may result in different bone failure rates for different implant systems. There is no one optimal design criterion. However, implants can be engineered to maximize strength, interfacial stability, and load transfer by using different materials, surfaces, and thread designs.

### 21.1.3.1.1   Implant Thread Geometry

Dental implant thread geometry has been proposed as a potential factor affecting implant stability and the percentage of osseointegration. Recently, Steigenga and coworkers evaluated thread design in a prospective, randomized, parallel arm study to consider quality and percentage of implant osseointegration and resistance to reverse torque in the tibia of rabbits. Data showed that the square thread design implants had significantly more bone-to-implant contact and greater reverse-torque measurements compared to the V-shaped and reverse-buttress thread designs. No differences were found in radiographic bone density assessments, suggesting square thread design may be more retentive for endosseous dental implant systems (Figure 21.6) (Steigenga et al., 2004).

### 21.1.3.1.2   Implant Surface

The rate and degree of osseointegration at turned and sand blasted and acid etched implant surfaces during early phases of healing were evaluated in a canine model by Abrahamsson and coworkers. While healing showed similar characteristics with resorptive and appositional events for both acid-etched and turned surfaces, the rate and degree of osseointegration were superior for the sand blasted surfaces (Abrahamsson et al., 2004).

The surface of the implant may also be modified through retention of biomolecules. Osteogenic proteins, bone morphogenetic proteins (BMP), may be retained on Ti surfaces whereas a possible chemical union is evident on hydroxyapatite surfaces (Ong and Chan, 2000; Talib and Toff, 2004). The osteoinductive and regenerative potential of recombinant human (rh) BMP-2 is of clinical benefit in cases where bone augmentation is indicated and improved levels of osseointegration are expected. Alternatively, the biomolecules may be delivered to the implant sites coincident with implant placement. The effect of rhBMP-2 on implant osseointegration was determined using histomorphometric and radiographic imaging analyses. Hollow-cylinder implants filled with an absorbable collagen sponge soaked with rhBMP-2 exhibited the same mean histologic bone-implant contact on the outer surface of the implant as controls (Sykaras et al., 2004). No additional benefit to integration was available with rhBMP-2.

### 21.1.3.2   Dental Implant Materials

Biomaterial implantation depends upon full integration of the implant with living bone. Titanium and bioceramic materials, such as hydroxyapatite are extensively used as fabrication materials for dental implants due to their high compatibility with hard tissue and living bone, despite artificial implants' lack of biomechanical properties equivalent to

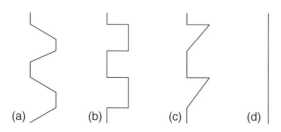

**FIGURE 21.6**
Implant thread design: (a) V-shaped, (b) square, (c) reverse buttress, (d) nonthreaded (modified from Steigenga et al., 2004).

**TABLE 21.1**

Engineering Properties of Metals and Alloys Used for Dental Implants

| Material | Nominal Analysis (w/o) | Modulus of Elasticity GN/m$^2$ (psi × 10$^6$) | Ultimate Tensile Strength MN/m$^2$ (ksi) | Elongation to Fracture (%) | Surface |
|---|---|---|---|---|---|
| Titanium (Ti) | 99$^+$Ti | 97 (14) | 240–550 (25–70) | >15 | Ti oxide |
| Titanium–aluminum–vanadium (Ti–Al–V) | 90Ti–6Al–4V | 117 (17) | 860–896 (125–130) | >12 | Ti oxide |
| Zirconium (Zr) | 99$^+$Zr | 97 (14) | 207–310 (30–45) | >30 | Zr oxide |

Minimum values for the American Society for Testing and Materials Committee F4 documents are provided. Selected products provide a range of properties. GN/m$^2$ = giganewton per meter squared. MN/m$^2$ = meganewton per meter squared; ksi = thousand pounds per inch squared; psi = pounds per inch squared; w/o = weight percent. (Reprinted with permission; Lemmons and Phillips, 1993.)

the original tissue. Hydroxyapatite has low stiffness, and low strength, whereas Ti has reasonable stiffness and strength (Table 21.1). Both materials possess predictable capacity for integration with living bone. Minimum stresses in the implant and the bone must be achieved to enhance the retention of the implant and prevent bone resorption (Hedia and Mahmoud, 2004). The force applied to the bone implant interface is nearly proportional to the magnitude of the force applied to a prosthesis. The range of forces applied to the bone/ implant interface are dependent upon the location and magnitude of the applied force. Present implant design best accommodates compressive forces to coincide with tolerances established for properties cortical bone (Table 21.2). Like cortical bone, tension and shear are less tolerated by the implant components and the implant bone interface.

*21.1.3.2.1 Titanium*

Currently, Ti is favored for endosseous root-form implants. A Ti implant may have several configurations, but screw-type or cylindrical predominate. The implant surface is most often machined Ti or Ti alloy, or a rough surface usually composed of Ti, Ti alloy or hydroxyapatite. Compatible with the proximal hard and soft tissues, durable, modifiable, relatively inexpensive, and resistant to corrosion, Ti is a preeminent material utilized in the

**TABLE 21.2**

Cortical Bone Strengths in Human Femur Specimens (Reprinted with permission) (Reilly and Burstein, 1975)

| Type of Force Applied | Strength (MPa)[a] | Load Direction/Comments |
|---|---|---|
| Tensile | 133.0 (11.7) | Longitudinal |
| | 100.0 (8.6) | 30° off-axis |
| | 60.5 (4.8) | 60° off-axis |
| | 51.0 (4.4) | Transverse |
| Compressive | 193.0 (13.9) | Longitudinal |
| | 173.0 (13.8) | 30° off-axis |
| | 133.0 (15.0) | 60° off-axis |
| | 133.0 (10.0) | Transverse |
| Shear | 68.0 (3.7) | Torsion |

[a] Standard Deviation given in parentheses.

present generation of implants. However, bioactivity, a modulus unlike bone, probable microparticulate and ion accumulation at the implant site and clinical limitations mandate continued efforts to improve upon present designs.

There may be a risk of greater ion release for surface-enlarged implants than conventionally turned components. The possible relationship between ion release and a surface roughness was investigated by Wennerberg and coworkers. For the *in vivo* investigation, synchrotron radiation x-ray fluorescence spectroscopy and secondary ion mass spectroscopy (SIMS) were performed 12 weeks and 1 year after implantation in rabbit tibiae. No correlation was found between increasing roughness and ion release, neither *in vitro* nor *in vivo*. *In vivo*, slightly higher values for the roughest surface up to a distance of 400 $\mu$ from the implant surface; thereafter no difference was found. SIMS demonstrated no difference in ion release for the roughest and smoothest surfaces, but slightly more Ti in bone tissue after 1 year than after 12 weeks. Titanium particulate concentration rapidly decreased with distance from the implant surface (Wennerberg et al., 2004).

Titanium endosseous dental screws with different surfaces: smooth titanium, titanium plasma-sprayed (TPS), alumina oxide sandblasted and acid-etched (Al-SLA), zirconium oxide sandblasted and acid-etched were evaluated for the presence of Ti debris adjacent to the implant. Implants were placed in sheep femura and tibiae and evaluated immediately after surgery and after 14 days. The biological evolution of the peri-implant tissues and detachment of Ti debris from the implant surfaces during the first 14 days post healing were investigated. All samples showed new bone trabeculae and vascularized medullary spaces in those areas where gaps between the implants and host bone were visible. However, no osteogenesis was induced in the areas where the implants were initially positioned in close contact with the host bone. Chips of the preexisting bone inducing new peri-implant neoosteogenesis were surrounded by new bone trabeculae. The threads of some screws appeared to be deformed where the host bone showed fractures. Ti granules of 3 to 60 $\mu$ were detectable only in the peri-implant tissues of TPS implants both, thus suggesting the presence of debris may be related to the friction of the TPS coating during surgical insertion (Franchi et al., 2004). To enhance tissue compatability, Ti has been coated with HA and bioactive glass composites obtained via sol-gel process.

### 21.1.3.2.2 *Bioceramics*

Metal implants such as Ti, stainless steel and Co–Cr–Mo have been used for load bearing purposes such as hip-joint prostheses, fixing plates and dental root implants. For practical application, plasma-sprayed coatings of hydroxyapatite on metal implants are applied to promote early formation of strong bonds between metal implant and osseous tissue. Plasma spray coating involves heating of hydroxyapatite material to a semimolten or molten state and then propelling it on to a metal substrate. The plasma flame temperature is in the range of 6000 to 16,000°C, but the surface temperature of the substrate rarely exceeds 150°C. The hydroxyapatite materials are fed into the spray gun in the form of powders (Talib and Toff, 2004). Better osseointegration of hydroxyapatite and Ti/bioactive glass sol–gel coated dental implants with respect to uncoated Ti. *In vitro*, the hydroxyapatite coating stimulates osteoblastic cells in producing higher level of alkaline phosphatase and collagen, whereas *in vivo* this surface modification resulted in a higher torque for implant removal and an increased bone-implant contact area (Ramires et al., 2003). The coating/substrate interface of commercially available dental implants coated with plasma-sprayed hydroxyapatite have been analyzed by EPMA spectrometry and XPS. A thin Ti oxide film containing calcium (Ca) and phosporus (P) was found at the interface. Under mechanical stress, a mixed mode of cohesive and interfacial fractures occurred in the implant. The cohesive fracture was due to separation of the oxide film from the substrate, while the interfacial fracture was due to exfoliation of the coating from the oxide film bonded to the substrate. The interfacial bond was the result of both mechanical and chemical forces. Calcium diffused into the metal substrate. A chemical bond appeared to exist at the interface (Mimura et al., 2004).

### 21.1.3.2.3  *Nanostructured Ceramics*

Promising new implant designs will depend upon recent advances in the synthesis, characterization, and biological compatibility of nanostructured ceramics for implants. In an attempt to simulate the mechanical properties of natural bone, novel nanoceramic/polymer composite formulations have been fabricated and characterized with respect to their cytocompatibility and mechanical properties. The development of three nanostructured implant coatings: diamond, hydroxyapatite, and functionally graded metalloceramics based on the Cr–Ti–N ternary system, will enhance mechanical properties such as hardness, toughness, friction coefficient, and the bioactivity. Given the present evidence for interfacial fracture of conventional metal ceramic interactions (Persson et al., 1996; Suansuwan and Swain, 2003), nanostructured diamond produced by chemical vapor deposition (CVD) techniques and composed of nanosize diamond grains provide a combination of ultrahigh hardness, improved toughness over conventional microcrystalline diamond, low friction, and satisfactory adhesion to Ti alloys. Nanostructured processing applied to hydroxyapatite coatings is used to achieve the desired mechanical characteristics and enhanced surface reactivity and has been found to increase osteoblast adhesion, proliferation, and mineralization (Huang et al., 2004; McManus et al., 2005; Sato et al., 2005). Finally, nanostructured metalloceramic coatings provide continuous variation from a nanocrystalline metallic bond at the interface to the hard ceramic bond on the surface and have the ability to overcome adhesion problems associated with ceramic hard coatings on metallic substrates (Catledge et al., 2002).

Through the decomposition of oxygenated compounds (single-source precursors) or the reaction of oxygen-free metal compounds with oxygenating agents, metal–organic chemical vapour deposition (MOCVD) has recently been proposed as a technique to coat dental prostheses with metal nanostructured oxide films. Gaivaresi and coworkers compared the histomorphometric, biocompatibility, ultrastructural and microhardness properties of commercially pure Ti implants, Ti/MA, (psi 2 mm × 5 mm length) coated with nanostructured $TiO_2$ films by MOCVD (Ti/MOCVD) in rabbit cortical and cancellous sites. Four and 12 weeks after surgery, significant increases in AI of Ti/MOCVD implants were observed as compared to Ti/MA implants. Bone microhardness results showed significant increases for the Ti/MOCVD versus Ti/MA implants in both the cancellous and cortical sites at 12 weeks. Nanostructured $TiO_2$ coating positively affected the osseointegration rate of commercially pure Ti implants and the bone mineralization at the bone/biomaterial interface (Franchi et al., 2004).

Carbon nanofibers possess nanoscale fiber dimensions similar to crystalline hydroxyapatite found in bone. Their mechanical properties (such as low weight-to-strength ratios) that and may facilitate their use as a dental implant material. Compared to conventional carbon fibers, nanometer dimension carbon fibers promoted selective osteoblast adhesion. In contrast, adhesion of other cells was not influenced by carbon fiber dimensions. In fact, smooth muscle cell, fibroblast, and chondrocyte adhesion decreased with an increase in either carbon nanofiber surface energy or simultaneous change in carbon nanofiber chemistry. Furthermore, carbon fibers with nanometer dimensions may be optimal materials to selectively increase osteoblast adhesion necessary for successful dental implant applications due to a high degree of nanometer surface roughness (Price et al., 2003).

### 21.1.3.2.4  *Zirconia*

To further improve the esthetic aspect of dental implants, efforts have been undertaken to develop implant systems derived from durable, biocompatible, tooth-colored materials. Zirconium is a material possessing these properties. Kohal demonstrated the utility of an all-ceramic custom-made zirconia implant-crown system for the replacement of a single tooth (Kohal and Klaus, 2004).

Zirconium can be deposited on Ti to enhance cell and bone apposition. In a recent study, $ZrO_2$ (4% $CeO_2$), and $ZrO_2$ (3% $Y_2O_3$) coatings were deposited on Ti and CoCrMo implants using plasma spraying. Diffraction patterns showed that both the coatings appeared to be primitive tetragonal phase. Scanning electron microscopy (SEM) observations demonstrated both the $ZrO_2$ coatings appeared to be rough, porous and melted. The average surface roughness of $ZrO_2$ (3% $Y_2O_3$ and $ZrO_2$ 4% $CeO_2$) coatings was correlated to the starting powder size and substrates. No significant difference between the hardness of all coatings and substrates was observed. The adhesive strengths of $ZrO_2$ (4% $CeO_2$) coating to Ti and CoCrMo substrates were higher than 68MPa and significantly greater than that of $ZrO_2$ (3% $Y_2O_3$) coatings (Yang et al., 2003).

Zirconia ceramic implants also possess biocompatible and osteoconductive properties (Scarano, 2003; Knabe et al., 2004). After 4 weeks of implantation in rabbit's tibias, significant quantities of newly formed bone were observed in close contact with zirconia ceramic surfaces. Osteoblasts were noted in close association with the implant surface. Mature bone, characterized by small marrow spaces with detectable areas of osteoblastic activity, was detected (Scarano, 2003).

Zirconia may become an alternative to Ti for dental implant fabrication. During a 14-month study, Kohal and coworkers investigated the osseointegration of loaded zirconia implants compared with Ti implants in monkeys. Titanium implant surfaces were sandblasted with $Al_2O_3$ and subsequently acid etched. The zirconia implants were sandblasted. Five months after insertion of the crowns, the implants with the surrounding hard and soft tissues were harvested, and evaluated for the peri-implant soft-tissue dimensions and mineralized bone-to-implant contact. No statistically significant differences were found in the extent of the different soft-tissue compartments. Custom-made zirconia implants osseointegrated to the same extent as custom-made Ti control implants and demonstrated similar peri-implant soft tissue dimensions (Kohal and Klaus, 2004).

The effects of Ti and zirconium on mesenchymal stem cell osteoblastic-like activity was investigated. *In vitro*, human mesenchymal stem cells (hMSCs) isolated from femoral head bone marrow are capable of osteogenic differentiation, expressing alkaline phosphatase, osteocalcin, collagen type I, and bone sialoprotein, accompanied by extracellular matrix mineralization. Exposure of OS-treated hMSCs to submicron commercially pure Ti particles suppressed BSP gene expression, reduced collagen type I and bone sialoprotein production, decreased cellular proliferation and viability, and inhibited matrix mineralization. In comparison, exposure to zirconium oxide ($ZrO_2$) particles of similar size did not alter osteoblastic gene expression and resulted in only a moderate decrease in cellular proliferation and mineralization. Confocal imaging of cpTi-treated hMSC cultures displayed disorganized cytoskeletal architecture and low levels of extracellular bone sialoprotein. Chronic exposure of marrow cells to Ti wear debris *in vivo* may contribute to decreased bone formation at the bone/implant interface by reducing the population of viable hMSCs and compromising their differentiation into functional osteoblasts (Wang et al., 2002).

### 21.1.4   Dental Implant Treatment Planning Criteria

To appreciate the challenge to tissue engineering to propose restoration of the dentition requires a brief introduction to the demands of restoring functionality. The treatment with implants entails the placement of a biomaterial into an osseous tissue site. Implant treatment-planning criteria are available to evaluate each clinical presentation for the appropriateness of implants. Conversely, understanding the clinical utility of implants further establishes the criteria for selecting a suitable biomaterial.

#### 21.1.4.1   Treatment Planning

Dental implants replace teeth. This consideration dictates the majority of protocols and steps in the surgical placement of dental implants. The location, angulation, separation, size, design, and other characteristics of these implants are directly related to the anticipated suprastructure (crown) attached to the implant. The selection and placement of implants within an "anatomical range" that allows a clinically acceptable suprastructure is most important. The placement of dental implants would be contraindicated if the available anatomy in the maxilla and the mandible does not permit the placement of implants that would support clinically acceptable prostheses. Osseous regeneration procedures such as alveolar ridge augmentation and maxillary sinus augmentation can improve the deficient surgical sites to allow acceptable implant supported dental treatment planning.

An acceptable dental implant treatment plan should address all or most of the following:

(1) Clinically stable occlusion
(2) Improved esthetics and function
(3) Mechanical stability and longevity of parts
(4) Phonetics
(5) Pathology prevention or resistance
(6) Patient comfort

In addition to the mechanical and geometric considerations, prevention of pathology around implants requires careful consideration and assessment. Infection prevention and treatment around dental implants depends on many factors such as

(1) Patient's health status (compromised by immune status, diabetes, history of smoking)
(2) Patient's periodontal status
(3) Patient's level of oral hygiene and compliance with home dental care
(4) Sources of infection such as retained root tips or existing endodontic lesions
(5) Prosthetic design
(6) Surface characteristics of a dental implant

With the use of computer-assisted surgery and other modern imaging technologies, the surgeon's procedures have been improved. With an acrylic template and computed tomographic images, a treatment plan is established with appropriate software. The first osteotomy can be achieved through the template of the pilot drill. Implant placement with standard clinical procedures is then completed. This new technology improves the treatment outcome and optimizes the surgical procedure (Blanchet et al., 2004).

### 21.1.4.2  Complications

The inflammatory process affecting the soft and hard tissues resulting in rapid loss of supporting bone associated with bleeding and suppuration has been termed peri-implantitis. The causes of early and late peri-implantitis is less well understood and seems to be related to the peri-implant environment and to the soft tissues/implant interface, to patient-related factors (e.g., smoking, systemic diseases, plaque control) and to host-parasite equilibrium. However, there is wide scientific evidence that demonstrates the direct correlation between oral microbiota and peri-implant mucositis or peri-implantitis. In particular, adherence and colonization of microbiota on plaque-exposed biomaterials, like Ti, are discriminant factors for the development of infection.

Tooth loss may be a predictor for susceptibility to peri-implantitis (Karoussis et al., 2003). Implants replacing teeth lost due to periodontitis are more susceptible to peri-implantitis when compared to implants replacing teeth lost due to other reasons. Patients with peri-implantitis have been shown to harbor high levels of periodontal pathogens, *Actinobacillus actinomycetemcomitans*, *Porphyromonas gingivalis*, *Prevotella intermedia*, *Bacteroides forsythus* and *Treponema denticola*. The successful treatment and stabilization of a patient's periodontal condition or maintenance of periodontal health is vital to the long term stability of an implant implant. The treatment of peri-implantitis can be challenging and difficult. There are to date no data available to support specific treatment protocols in the treatment of peri-implantitis. Prevention of peri-implantitis by addressing all potential causes would be an easier solution than the repair of infected implants. Consultation with a patient's physician to verify health status may predict susceptibility to infections including peri-implantitis (Klinge et al., 2002). This along with the periodontal status of a patient may have an affect on the recommended treatment plans or course of treatment for the patient.

Bone loss around dental implants due to peri-implantitis could have significant effects on the mechanical stability of the implant and its superstructure. Regardless of the magnitude, infected implants may represent a threat to the longevity of the associated prosthetic replacement (Fartash et al., 1997; Hultin et al., 2000; Klinge et al., 2002). Implants are susceptible to occlusal trauma and prone to plaque accumulation. The patient's oral health status systemic health will contribute to susceptibility (Quirynen et al., 2002).

Regenerative or resective surgical approaches are proposed for the treatment of peri-implantitis depending on the morphology and the shape of bone defects. The therapeutical approach to peri-implantitis surrounding dental implants comprises several aspects such as the removal of supragingival bacterial plaque, an appropriate surgical approach, the removal of granulation tissue and detoxification of the exposed implant surface, the elimination of the anaerobic ecosystem by the removal of peri-implant pocket (gingivectomy or apically repositioned flap) or by the regeneration of the peri-implant hard tissues and, finally, the establishment of an efficient plaque control regimen (Garg, 2004; Romeo et al., 2004).

### 21.1.5  Loading of Dental Implants

To minimize the risk of implant failure, osseointegrated oral implants are conventionally kept load-free during the healing period. During healing, removable prostheses are used, however; many patients find these temporary prostheses inconvenient. It would be beneficial if the healing period could be abbreviated. Dental implants have been loaded either following a period of subgingival, intraosseous retention (two-stage), immediately (one-stage) or as a delayed immediate experience (Ericsson and Nilner, 2002). As clinicians' understanding of the biological and mechanical factors involved in immediate occlusal loading has evolved, the success of these procedures has increased, particularly as a treatment option for the restoration of the edentulous mandible (Lazzara et al., 2004). Early loading of dental implants has been defined as restoration of implants in or out of occlusion at least 48 h after implant placement, but at a shorter time interval than conventional healing (3 months for mandible, 5 to 6 months for maxilla) (Krug and Mounajjed, 2003). Immediate loading or restoration has been defined as attachment of a restoration in or out of direct occlusal function within 48 h of surgical placement (Ganeles and Wismeijer, 2004). Animal studies have demonstrated that successful osseointegration of implants can occur when implants are placed and loaded immediately. The histological findings involving implants that were placed in humans and immediately loaded showed no fibrous tissue formation (encapsulation). The bone-to-implant contact was found to be excellent between the immediately-loaded implants and the surrounding alveolar bone (Romanos, 2004). Following an evaluation of seven random controlled trials and six case studies, 124 patients in total were considered for evaluation of immediate loading of implants. Implants had been either immediately loaded after insertion (2 to 3 days), early loaded (6 weeks) or conventionally loaded (3 to 8 months) in edentulous mandibles of adequate bone quality and shape. On a patient basis, there were no statistically significant differences for prosthesis failures, implant failures and marginal bone loss on intra-oral radiographs (Esposito et al., 2004). As a result, loading implant immediately after placement gained popularity among clinicians. Concerns related to this approach remain open. More marginal bone loss has been noted with immediate loaded implants (Lorenzoni et al., 2003). Factors that may influence the success of immediate implant loading, including patient selection, type of bone quality, required implant length, micro- and macrostructure of the implant, surgical skill, need for achieving primary stability/ control of occlusal force, and prosthesis guidelines, must be considered prior to therapy. Various studies have demonstrated the feasibility and predictability of this technique. Anatomic locations, implant designs, and restricted prosthetic guidelines are the key to ensure successful outcomes.

To reasonably evaluate the success of immediate-loaded implants several factors must be considered: single- or multiple-tooth conditions, immediate or delayed placement in extraction sockets, effect of implant surface and geometry, bone quality, implant stability, surgical technique, occlusal design, effect of cigarette smoking, and stability of results. No single study comprehensively considered all these factors, yet case-study formats have indicated success with rapid loading of implants compared with the two-stage process. Due to statistically inconclusive numbers of implants and patients, conclusions concerning the success of immediate-loaded implants must be considered carefully. Random-controlled studies will improve our understanding of the predictability of immediate and early loading. Priority should be given to trials assessing the effectiveness of immediately-loaded implants rather than early-loaded ones. Future studies, preferably randomized, prospective longitudinal studies, are needed before this approach can be widely used (Esposito et al., 2004).

### 21.1.6 Extraoral Applications of Endosseous Implants

The advent of osseointegrated implants brings with it extraoral as well as intraoral applications. The uses essentially parallel each other with the intent being restoration of missing or otherwise inadequate tissue. Intraoral use permits the restoration of dentition in areas where it is otherwise lost. The utility is far reaching and has dramatically changed the nature of intraoral restoration and reconstruction. Extraoral uses have permitted wide-ranging applications such as prosthetic restoration of virtually all facial structures. As early as the 1960s, animal and human studies indicated the possibility of epidermal and mucosal penetration of implants for bone anchoring (Jansen et al., 1994; Paquay et al., 1996). Implants used in this role have achieved demonstrable and predictable long-term utility using Ti implants.

Sites of extraoral use, often referred to as craniofacial, have most commonly included the mastoid process and periorbital and perinasal regions for auricular, orbital, and nasal prostheses. It appears that, by and large, one of the most commonly used extraoral implant is the Nobelbiocare extraoral craniofacial implant system (Figure 21.7). These implants have specific design characteristics which are believed to enhance immobilization and prevent undue migration. Both one-stage and two-stage placements have been described. While traditional two-stage placement is the norm, results with one-stage placement in some studies have been encouraging. The lack of heavy loading and repetitive motion may contribute to success. Implant maintenance and hygiene are necessary as intraoral uses to ensure longevity.

Not unlike the intraoral counterpart, peri-implant management is a frequent determinant to success and failure. Skin infections and tissue breakdown are complications which follow exposure of subcutaneous implants and which may lead to implant loss. Motion and instability, as in oral applications, contribute to loss of osseoadegration. This factor is determined, in part, by the amount and quality of cortical bone available to anchor the implant and the time permitted for integration.

Patient related factors, such as nutritional status, metabolic diseases, immunosuppression, and radiation therapy with subsequent tissue alteration may contribute significantly to implant failures. Operator-related factors may also determine failure. Bacterial and fungal infection may be related to inadequate hygiene which, in turn, can also be related to prosthesis or device placement on the implant. Typical means of topical infections are useful, including culture and sensitivity of potential organisms involved, and maintenance of a regular program of hygiene with the intention of biofilm elimination (Eliades, 1997; Ueda et al., 1998; Montanaro et al., 2004).

Extraoral implants have proven to be a valuable way to secure prosthetic eyes, noses, ears, cheeks, hearing aids, and other contour-deficient areas.

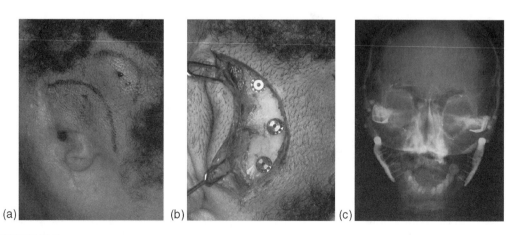

(a)                                   (b)                                   (c)

**FIGURE 21.7**
Extraoral implantation for prosthetic ear retention. (a) Post-auricular incision site, (b) implant placement in post-auricular area, (c) frontal radiograph assessing bilateral implant placement. (Photographs by Dr. M. Buckley.)

### 21.1.7  Maintenance

Osseointegration is becoming increasingly routine in the rehabilitation of partially or fully edentulous patients. However, the surrounding tissues may be subject to inflammatory conditions similar to periodontal disease and so require maintenance.

Little is known about the mechanisms of bacterial interaction with implant materials in the oral cavity. A correlation between plaque accumulation and progressive bone loss around implants has been reported (Scarano et al., 2004). Bacterial adhesion shows a direct positive correlation with surface roughness. Other surface characteristics also seem to be extremely important with regard to plaque formation. Different adhesion affinities of bacteria have been reported for different materials (Gatewood et al., 1993; Groessner-Schreiber et al., 2004; Kuula et al., 2004; Lange et al., 2004). To facilitate elimination of bacterial plaque, different surfaces have been evaluated for bacterial adherence. In Ti discs, zirconium oxide had a relatively lower bacterial colonization potential (Scarano et al., 2004). The use of metals with lower disposition to plaque accumulation will improve implant retention.

Professional maintenance is as important for patients with dental implants as it is for patients with natural teeth. However, ideal maintenance instruments do not exist. Sato and coworkers compared the effects of a new ultrasonic scaler (VR), a conventional ultrasonic scaler (SP), and a plastic scaler (PS) on Ti surfaces. Artificial debris was removed with the VR, SP, or PS scaler for 60 sec under standardized conditions. No significant differences in the surface roughness or SEM observations were found among the VR, SP, or PS scalers, suggesting ultrasonic scalers with nonmetal tips would be suitable for implant maintenance (Cheng et al., 2002; Sato et al., 2004).

### 21.1.8  Craniofacial Maintenance

To ensure the long-term success of a facial rehabilitation, hygienic homecare maintenance for patients who have received a maxillofacial prosthesis is very important. Craniofacial implant therapy requires a specific protocol to care for the peri-implant tissues and material used for the prosthesis. Proper follow-up management of a maxillofacial ear prosthesis includes instruction in home care methods emphasizing the insertion and the disconnection of the ear prosthesis, hygiene of the bar abutments before and after postdefinitive connection to the craniofacial implants, washing of the device, and periodic professional evaluation (Ciocca et al., 2004).

## 21.2  Conclusion

Patients with virtually every clinical indication have been treated with endosseous dental implants. Tissue integration of the implant can occur if certain conditions are satisfied: minimal damage to the surrounding bone during placement and stable placement. Loading may be delayed or immediate, both situations have resulted in stable implant function, though controversy persists as to which approach may be more appropriate. Implant placement in craniofacial areas can be further expanded as the biocompatibility of the metals is improved. Given an historical perspective, craniofacial implants and specifically, dental implant design, have improved as a predictable therapy yet more remains to be accomplished. New biomaterials, an expanding knowledge of the biology of osseointegration, and refined surgical techniques, offer encouragement for expanded, more predictable implant therapies.

## Problems

1. What are the advantages for the selection of zirconium as a dental implant material?
   **Answer:** Tooth colored (esthetics), biocompatible.

2. What are the advantages for the selection of titanium as a dental implant material?
   **Answer:** Biocompatible, inexpensive, amenable to various surface preparations.

3. What are the criteria for case selection for implants?
   **Answer:** Clinically stable occlusion, improved esthetics and function, mechanical stability and longevity of parts, phonetics, pathology prevention or resistance, patient comfort.

4. What is the definition of osseointegration?
   **Answer:** The direct structural and functional connection between living bone and the surface of a load-carrying implant.

5. What tissues are adjacent to an implant?
   **Answer:** Alveolar bone, gingival epithelium, gingival connective tissue.

6. What are possible options for loading the implant?
   **Answer:** Delayed, early and immediate.

7. What is the intent of covering the implant for several months?
   **Answer:** To enhance bone apposition against the implant.

8. What criteria are important for a decision as to when the implant will be loaded?
   **Answer:** Implant stability, bone quality, opposing occlusion, esthetics.

9. How is bacterial plaque removed from the implant?
   **Answer:** Homecare includes brushing, flossing and an antimicrobial rinse. Professional care may include the use of plastic instrumentation around the implant.

10. What are the possible complications with implant placement?
    **Answer:** Infection, pain, mobility of the implant, alveolar bone fracture, and nerve damage represent possible complications.

## References

Abrahamsson, I., Berglundh, T., Linder, E., Lang, N.P., and Lindhe, J., Early bone formation adjacent to rough and turned endosseous implant surfaces, An experimental study in the dog, *Clin Oral Implants Res.*, **15** (4), 381–392 (2004).

Astrand, P., Engquist, B., Anzen, B., Bergendal, T., Hallman, M., Karlsson, U., Kvint, S., Lysell, L., and Rundcrantz, T., Nonsubmerged and submerged implants in the treatment of the partially edentulous maxilla, *Clin. Implant Dent. Relat. Res.*, **4** (3), 115–127 (2002).

Atsuta, I., Yamaza, T., Yoshinari, M., Mino, S., Goto, T., Kido, M.A., Terada, Y., and Tanaka, T., Changes in the distribution of laminin-5 during peri-implant epithelium formation after immediate titanium implantation in rats, *Biomaterials*, **26** (14), 1751–1760 (2005).

Blanchet, E., Lucchini, J.P., Jenny, R., and Fortin, T., An image-guided system based on custom templates: case reports, *Clin. Implant Dent. Relat. Res.*, **6** (1), 40–47 (2004).

Bränemark, P.I., Adell, R., Albrektsson, T., Lekholm, U., Lundkvist, S., and Rockler, B., Osseointegrated titanium fixtures in the treatment of edentulousness, *Biomaterials*, **4** (1), 25–28 (1983).

Catledge, S.A., Fries, M.D., Vohra, Y.K., Lacefield, W.R., Lemons, J.E., Woodard, S., and Venugopalan, R., Nanostructured ceramics for biomedical implants, *J. Nanosci. Nanotechnol.*, **2** (3–4), 293–312 (2002).

Cheng, A.C., Wee, A.G., Li, J.T., and Archibald, D., A new prosthodontic approach for craniofacial implant-retained maxillofacial prostheses, *J. Prosthet. Dent.*, **88** (2), 224–228 (2002).

Ciocca, L., Gassino, G., and Scotti, R., Home care maintenance protocol for ear prostheses, *Minerva Stomatol.*, **53** (10), 611–617 (2004).

Congdon, M., The plantation of teeth, *Panama-Pacific Dent. Congress Trans.*, **2**, 295–305 (1915).

Dahl, G., Subperiosteal implants and superplants, *Dent. Abstr.*, **2**, 685 (1957).

Driskell, T., History of implants, *J. Calif. Dent. Assoc.*, **15**, 16–25 (1987).

Dubruille, J.H., Viguier, E., Le Naour, G., Dubruille, M.T., Auriol, M., and Le Charpentier, Y., Evaluation of combinations of titanium, zirconia, and alumina implants with 2 bone fillers in the dog, *Int. J. Oral Maxillofac. Implants*, **14** (2), 271–277 (1999).

Eliades, T., Passive film growth on titanium alloys: physicochemical and biologic considerations, *Int. J. Oral Maxillofac. Implants*, **12** (5), 621–627 (1997).

Ericsson, I. and Nilner, K., Early functional loading using Bränemark dental implants, *Int. J. Periodontics Restorative Dent.*, **22** (1), 9–19 (2002).

Esposito, M., Worthington, H.V., Thomsen, P., and Coulthard, P., Interventions for replacing missing teeth: different times for loading dental implants, *Cochrane Database Syst. Rev.*, (3), CD003878 (2004).

Fartash, B., Hultin, M., Gustafsson, A., Asman, B., and Arvidson, K., Markers of inflammation in crevicular fluid from peri-implant mucosa surrounding single crystal sapphire implants, *Clin. Oral Implants Res.*, **8** (1), 32–38 (1997).

Franchi, M., Bacchelli, B., Martini, D., Pasquale, V.D., Orsini, E., Ottani, V., Fini, M., Giavaresi, G., Giardino, R., and Ruggeri, A., Early detachment of titanium particles from various different surfaces of endosseous dental implants, *Biomaterials*, **25** (12), 2239–2246 (2004).

Ganeles, J. and Wismeijer, D., Early and immediately restored and loaded dental implants for single-tooth and partial-arch applications, *Int. J. Oral Maxillofac. Implants*, **19 (Suppl.)**, 92–102 (2004).

Garg, A.K., Complications associated with implant surgical procedures part 1: prevention, *Dent. Implantol. Update*, **15** (4), 25–32 (2004).

Gatewood, R.R., Cobb, C.M., and Killoy, W.J., Microbial colonization on natural tooth structure compared with smooth and plasma-sprayed dental implant surfaces, *Clin. Oral Implants Res.*, **4** (2), 53–64 (1993).

Goto, T., Yoshinari, M., Kobayashi, S., and Tanaka, T., The initial attachment and subsequent behavior of osteoblastic cells and oral epithelial cells on titanium, *Biomed. Mater. Eng.*, **14** (4), 537–544 (2004).

Greenfield, E., Implanted artificial roots, *Panama -Pacific Dent. Congress Trans.*, **2**, 538–539 (1915).

Groessner-Schreiber, B., Hannig, M., Duck, A., Griepentrog, M., and Wenderoth, D.F., Do different implant surfaces exposed in the oral cavity of humans show different biofilm compositions and activities?, *Eur. J. Oral Sci.*, **112** (6), 516–522 (2004).

Hedia, H.S. and Mahmoud, N.A., Design optimization of functionally graded dental implant, *Biomed. Mater. Eng.*, **14** (2), 133–143 (2004).

Hoek, R.B., Costich, E.R., and Avery, J.K., Terminology in the field of tooth plantation, *J. Oral. Surg. Anesth. Hosp. Dent. Serv.*, **17** (4), 46–47 (1959).

Huang, J., Best, S.M., Bonfield, W., Brooks, R.A., Rushton, N., Jayasinghe, S.N., and Edirisinghe, M.J., In vitro assessment of the biological response to nano-sized hydroxyapatite, *J. Mater. Sci. Mater. Med.*, **15** (4), 441–445 (2004).

Hultin, M., Fischer, J., Gustafsson, A., Kallus, T., and Klinge, B., Factors affecting late fixture loss and marginal bone loss around teeth and dental implants, *Clin. Implant Dent. Relat. Res.*, **2** (4), 203–208 (2000).

Jansen, J.A., Paquay, Y.G., and van der Waerden, J.P., Tissue reaction to soft-tissue anchored percutaneous implants in rabbits, *J. Biomed. Mater. Res.*, **28** (9), 1047–1054 (1994).

Jokstad, A., Braegger, U., Brunski, J.B., Carr, A.B., Naert, I., and Wennerberg, A., Quality of dental implants, *Int. Dent. J.*, **53** (6 Suppl. 2), 409–443 (2003).

Karoussis, I.K., Salvi, G.E., Heitz-Mayfield, L.J., Bragger, U., Hammerle, C.H., and Lang, N.P., Long-term implant prognosis in patients with and without a history of chronic periodontitis: a 10-year prospective cohort study of the ITI Dental Implant System, *Clin. Oral Implants Res.*, **14** (3), 329–339 (2003).

Klinge, B., Gustafsson, A., and Berglundh, T., A systematic review of the effect of anti-infective therapy in the treatment of peri-implantitis, *J. Clin. Periodontol.*, **29** (Suppl. 3), 213–225 (2002).

Knabe, C., Berger, G., Gildenhaar, R., Klar, F., and Zreiqat, H., The modulation of osteogenesis in vitro by calcium titanium phosphate coatings, *Biomaterials*, **25** (20), 4911–4919 (2004).

Kohal, R.J. and Klaus, G., A zirconia implant-crown system: a case report, *Int. J. Periodontics. Restorative Dent.*, **24** (2), 147–153 (2004).

Krug, J. and Mounajjed, R., Two ways of immediate rehabilitation of edentulous mandible with dental implants and prostheses–critical view on Bränemark System Novum, *Acta Medica (Hradec Kralove)*, **46** (4), 205–212 (2003).

Kuula, H., Kononen, E., Lounatmaa, K., Konttinen, Y.T., and Kononen, M., Attachment of oral gram-negative anaerobic rods to a smooth titanium surface: an electron microscopy study, *Int. J. Oral Maxillofac. Implants*, **19** (6), 803–809 (2004).

Lange, K., Herold, M., Scheideler, L., Geis-Gerstorfer, J., Wendel, H.P., and Gauglitz, G., Investigation of initial pellicle formation on modified titanium dioxide (TiO2) surfaces by reflectometric interference spectroscopy (RIfS) in a model system, *Dent. Mater.*, **20** (9), 814–822 (2004).

Lazzara, R.J., Testori, T., Meltzer, A., Misch, C., Porter, S., del Castillo, R., and Goene, R.J., Immediate Occlusal Loading (IOL) of dental implants: predictable results through DIEM guidelines, *Pract. Proc. Aesthet. Dent.*, **16** (4), 3–15 (2004).

Lemmons, J.E. and Phillips, R.W., Biomaterials for dental implants, In: *Contemporary Implant Dentistry*, Misch, C.E., Ed., Mosby-Year Book, Inc., St Louis, 259–278 (1993).

Lew, I., Full upper and lower dentures implant, *Dent. Concepts*, **4**, 17 (1952).

Linkow, L.I., Evolutionary design trends in the mandibular subperiosteal implant, *J. Oral. Implantol.*, **11** (3), 402–438 (1984).

Lorenzoni, M., Pertl, C., Zhang, K., Wimmer, G., and Wegscheider, W.A., Immediate loading of single-tooth implants in the anterior maxilla. Preliminary results after one year, *Clin. Oral Implants Res.*, **14** (2), 180–187 (2003).

McManus, A.J., Doremus, R.H., Siegel, R.W., and Bizios, R., Evaluation of cytocompatibility and bending modulus of nanoceramic/polymer composites, *J. Biomed. Mater. Res. A*, **72A** (1), 98–106 (2005).

Meffert, R.M., Endosseous dental implantology from the periodontist's viewpoint, *J. Periodontol.*, **57** (9), 531–536 (1986).

Mimura, K., Watanabe, K., Okawa, S., Kobayashi, M., and Miyakawa, O., Morphological and chemical characterizations of the interface of a hydroxyapatite-coated implant, *Dent. Mater. J.*, **23** (3), 353–360 (2004).

Montanaro, L., Campoccia, D., Rizzi, S., Donati, M.E., Breschi, L., Prati, C., and Arciola, C.R., Evaluation of bacterial adhesion of streptococcus mutans on dental restorative materials, *Biomaterials*, **25** (18), 4457–4463 (2004).

Ong, J.L. and Chan, D.C., Hydroxyapatite and their use as coatings in dental implants: a review, *Crit. Rev. Biomed. Eng.*, **28** (5–6), 667–707 (2000).

O'Sullivan, D., Sennerby, L., Jagger, D., and Meredith, N., A comparison of two methods of enhancing implant primary stability, *Clin. Implant Dent. Relat. Res.*, **6** (1), 48–57 (2004).

Paquay, Y.C., De Ruijter, A.E., van der Waerden, J.P., and Jansen, J.A., A one stage versus two stage surgical technique. Tissue reaction to a percutaneous device provided with titanium fiber mesh applicable for peritoneal dialysis, *Asaio J*, **42** (6), 961–967 (1996).

Persson, P., Nilsson, N., and Sjoberg, S., Structure and bonding of orthophosphate ions at the iron oxide-aqueous interface, *J. Colloid. Interface Sci.*, **177** (1), 263–275 (1996).

Pjetursson, B.E., Tan, K., Lang, N.P., Bragger, U., Egger, M., and Zwahlen, M., A systematic review of the survival and complication rates of fixed partial dentures (FPDs) after an observation period of at least 5 years, *Clin. Oral Implants Res.*, **15** (6), 625–642 (2004).

Price, R.L., Haberstroh, K.M., and Webster, T.J., Enhanced functions of osteoblasts on nanostructured surfaces of carbon and alumina, *Med. Biol. Eng. Comput.*, **41** (3), 372–375 (2003).

Quirynen, M., De Soete, M., and van Steenberghe, D., Infectious risks for oral implants: a review of the literature, *Clin. Oral Implants Res.*, **13** (1), 1–19 (2002).

Ramires, P.A., Wennerberg, A., Johansson, C.B., Cosentino, F., Tundo, S., and Milella, E., Biological behavior of sol-gel coated dental implants, *J. Mater. Sci. Mater. Med.*, **14** (6), 539–545 (2003).

Reilly, D.T. and Burstein, A.H., The elastic and ultimate properties of compact bone tissue, *J. Biomech.*, **8** (6), 393–405 (1975).

Ring, M., *Dentistry: An Illustrated History*, CV Mosby Co, St. Louis (1985).

Romanos, G.E., Present status of immediate loading of oral implants, *J. Oral Implantol.*, **30** (3), 189–197 (2004).

Romeo, E., Ghisolfi, M., and Carmagnola, D., Peri-implant diseases. A systematic review of the literature, *Minerva Stomatol.*, **53** (5), 215–230 (2004).

Sato, S., Kishida, M., and Ito, K., The comparative effect of ultrasonic scalers on titanium surfaces: an in vitro study, *J. Periodontol.*, **75** (9), 1269–1273 (2004).

Sato, M., Slamovich, E.B., and Webster, T.J., Enhanced osteoblast adhesion on hydrothermally treated hydroxyapatite/titania/poly(lactide-co-glycolide) sol-gel titanium coatings, *Biomaterials*, **26** (12), 1349–1357 (2005).

Saville, M., Pre Columbian decoration of teeth in Ecuador, *Am. J. Anthropol.*, **15**, 380 (1913).

Scarano, A., Di Carlo, F., Quaranta, M., and Piattelli, A., Bone response to zirconia ceramic implants: an experimental study in rabbits, *J. Oral Implantol.*, **29** (1), 8–12 (2003).

Scarano, A., Piattelli, M., Caputi, S., Favero, G.A., and Piattelli, A., Bacterial adhesion on commercially pure titanium and zirconium oxide disks: an *in vivo* human study, *J. Periodontol.*, **75** (2), 292–296 (2004).

Smith, G.C., Surgical principles of the Bränemark osseointegration implant system, *Aust. Prosthodont. Soc. Bull.*, **15**, 37–40 (1985).

Steigenga, J.T., al-Shammari, K.F., Nociti, F.H., Misch, C.E., and Wang, H.L., Dental implant design and its relationship to long-term implant success, *Implant Dent.*, **12** (4), 306–317 (2003).

Steigenga, J., Al-Shammari, K., Misch, C., Nociti, F.H. Jr, and Wang, H.L., Effects of implant thread geometry on percentage of osseointegration and resistance to reverse torque in the tibia of rabbits, *J. Periodontol.*, **75** (9), 1233–1241 (2004).

Strock, A., Experimental work on a method for the replacement of missing teeth by a direct implantation of a metal support into the alveolus, *Am. J. Orthodont. Oral Surg.*, **25**, 467–472 (1939).

Strock, A. and Strock, M., Further studies on inert metal implantation for replacement, *Alpha Omega*, (1949).

Suansuwan, N. and Swain, M.V., Adhesion of porcelain to titanium and a titanium alloy, *J. Dent.*, **31** (7), 509–518 (2003).

Sykaras, N., Woody, R.D., Lacopino, A.M., Triplett, R.G., and Nunn, M.E., Osseointegration of dental implants complexed with rhBMP-2: a comparative histomorphometric and radiographic evaluation, *Int. J. Oral Maxillofac. Implants*, **19** (5), 667–678 (2004).

Talib, R.J. and Toff, M.R., Plasma-sprayed coating of hydroxyapatite on metal implants–a review, *Med. J. Malaysia*, **59**, 153–154 (2004).

Triplett, R.G., Frohberg, U., Sykaras, N., and Woody, R.D., Implant materials, design, and surface topographies: their influence on osseointegration of dental implants, *J. Long Term Eff Med Implants*, **13** (6), 485–501 (2003).

Ueda, M., Hata, K.I., Sumi, Y., Mizuno, H., and Niimi, A., Peri-implant soft tissue management through use of cultured mucosal epithelium, *Oral Surg. Oral Med. Oral Pathol. Oral Radiol. Endod.*, **86** (4), 393–400 (1998).

Wang, M.L., Nesti, L.J., Tuli, R., Lazatin, J., Danielson, K.G., Sharkey, P.F., and Tuan, R.S., Titanium particles suppress expression of osteoblastic phenotype in human mesenchymal stem cells, *J. Orthop. Res.*, **20** (6), 1175–1184 (2002).

Weinberger, B., *An Introduction to the History of Dentistry*, CV Mosby Co, St. Louis (1948).

Wennerberg, A., Ide-Ektessabi, A., Hatkamata, S., Sawase, T., Johansson, C., Albrektsson, T., Martinelli, A., Sodervall, U., and Odelius, H., Titanium release from implants prepared with different surface roughness, *Clin. Oral Implants Res.*, **15** (5), 505–512 (2004).

Wood, M.R. and Vermilyea, S.G., A review of selected dental literature on evidence-based treatment planning for dental implants: report of the Committee on Research in Fixed Prosthodontics of the Academy of Fixed Prosthodontics, *J. Prosthet. Dent.*, **92** (5), 447–462 (2004).

Yang, Y., Ong, J.L., and Tian, J., Deposition of highly adhesive ZrO(2) coating on Ti and CoCrMo implant materials using plasma spraying, *Biomaterials*, **24** (4), 619–627 (2003).

# 22

---

## *Tissue Engineering of Bone*

---

Sanjeev Kakar and Thomas A. Einhorn

## CONTENTS

## 22.1   Introduction

Autogenous bone grafting is considered the standard of treatment for the management of bone defects. By 2004, over 1.5 million of these procedures will be performed each year to treat various craniofacial disorders such as missing alveolar bone in cleft palates and orthopedic conditions such as fractures and nonunions (Deutche Banc, 2001). Shortcomings from autografting include numerous procedures, lengthy recovery times, donor site morbidity and difficulties in shaping the graft to fill the defect (Banwart et al., 1995; Fowler et al., 1995; Goulet et al., 1997). These limitations have led to alternate graft materials such as allogeneic bone. However, despite allogeneic bone being readily available, the risk of disease transmission, loss of biologic and mechanical properties, and increased cost have limited its use (Parikh, 2002).

With these difficulties, researchers have sought alternatives to current treatment modalities. Tissue engineering represents a field of biological research where promising progress has been made to develop new clinical options. Tissue engineering in orthopedics emphasizes the restoration of function by replacing damaged or diseased tissues through the application of biological and engineering principles (Alsberg et al., 2001). In terms of its applicability to bone, the goal is to create a bone healing response in a precise anatomic area so that the tissue formed is integrated structurally with the surrounding skeleton and has the biomechanical properties necessary to be durable and effective (Fleming et al., 2000a).

The repair and regeneration of bone by tissue engineering occurs through an ordered sequence of cellular events that are affected by several biological and mechanical factors. In terms of biological factors, the first principle is that all newly formed tissue requires the presence of osteoprogenitor cells (Fleming et al., 2000a). These cells can be harvested from the patient and delivered into skeletal defects to ensure bone healing. The osteoprogenitor cells can be grown on to naturally derived or synthetic scaffolds, which act as passive three-dimensional mechanical matrices supporting attachment, proliferation and differentiation. The cells form their own matrix, which is integrated with the host tissue as the implant degrades over time. These properties are considered to be *osteoconductive* as they promote the bone healing response to progress throughout the defect (Fleming et al., 2000a).

The osteoprogenitor cells are derived from a pluripotent population and are capable of differentiating along several tissue lines. It is desirable to control cell migration, differentiation and subsequent tissue formation with growth factors and adhesion molecules either contained in or on the surface of the implanted matrix, or secreted by cells incorporated in the matrix. The stimuli from these growth factors and adhesion molecules are termed *osteoinductive* as they are capable of determining cell differentiation and consequently the osseous tissue produced at the graft recipient site (Fleming et al., 2000a; Alsberg et al., 2001).

Bone formation can be affected by the mechanical environment. Distraction osteogenesis (DO) is the process by which application of a tensile force at an optimal rate and frequency controls new bone formation (McCarthy et al., 2001). Initially popularized by Ilizarov in the 1950s for the management of leg-length discrepancies, it has recently become a useful technique for the treatment of numerous traumatic, congenital, and acquired conditions of the extremities and craniofacial region (Swennen et al., 2001).

Based on the biological and mechanical principles involved in tissue engineering of bone, this chapter focuses on a detailed description of these factors from their evolution to current-day practice.

## 22.2 Biological Components Involved in Tissue Engineering of Bone

### 22.2.1 Cells

#### 22.2.1.1 Bone Marrow Cells

Bone marrow contains osteoprogenitor and mesencyhmal stem cells (MSC) (Beresford, 1989; Connolly et al., 1989; Connolly et al., 1991; Grundel et al., 1991). MSC are pluripotent and have the ability to differentiate along several different lineages to form bone, cartilage, muscle, or adipose tissue (Beresford, 1989; Connolly et al., 1989; Connolly et al., 1991; Grundel et al., 1991). In contrast, osteoprogenitor cells are a step further along their differentiation and are committed to producing only bone (Beresford, 1989; Connolly et al., 1989; Connolly et al., 1991; Grundel et al., 1991). Connolly and Shindell (1986) first reported on bone marrow osteogenic precursor cells for the management of tibial nonunions by injecting bone marrow into these defects. Clinical and radiographic studies demonstrated union by 6 months. Others have described similar successes (Healey et al., 1990; Garg et al., 1993). In a study of delayed unions in eight osteosarcoma patients, Healey et al. (1990) reported bone formation and union in seven cases following percutaneous bone marrow grafting.

The ability of bone marrow cells to heal bony defects can be potentiated by adding osteoinductive agents. Lane and co-workers (1999) demonstrated that combining recombinant human bone morphogenetic protein (BMP)-2 to bone marrow cells resulted in higher union rates with superior mechanical properties compared to treatments using autogenous bone graft or bone marrow.

Despite the success of these procedures, the number of osteoprogenitor stem cells within bone marrow is limited. For example in young individuals, one stem cell per 50,000 nucleated cells have osteogenic capacity and this number falls dramatically to one per 2 million in the elderly (Werntz et al., 1996). As the success of bone marrow grafting is dependent upon the transfer of sufficient osteoprogenitor cells, several investigators have tried numerous techniques to increase their concentrations. Connolly (1995) described a method involving the injection of marrow concentrate into scaphoid nonunions. Out of the five patients treated, four experienced healing as a result of this application. Bruder et al. (1998a) expanded the number of osteoprogenitor cells by growing them under special culture conditions. These cells, when added to a composite mixture of ceramics and collagens, were able to bridge critical osseous femoral defects in adult rats.

#### 22.2.1.2 Mesenchymal Stem Cells

Mesenchymal stem cells (MSCs) comprise a population of resting, undifferentiated cells that have the ability to regenerate throughout life. They have a number of advantages over fully differentiated cells including ease of expansion, maintenance of their phenotype and lack of senescence.

MSCs are capable of dividing into clones or differentiating into multiple connective tissue lineages such as muscle, cartilage, and bone (Bruder et al., 1998a). Consequently, techniques have been developed to isolate and expand MSC numbers, while ensuring that their phenotype is maintained and there is no loss in osteogenic or chondrogenic potential (Bruder et al., 1997). These properties make MSCs a useful source of osteoprogenitor cells for bone tissue engineering.

Several investigators have reported on the clinical applicability of using MSCs in tissue regeneration. Bruder et al. (1998a) studied the use of MSCs to heal segmental bone defects in the femora of adult athymic rats. MSCs isolated from human bone marrow were grown in culture, loaded on to a ceramic carrier and implanted into critical-sized segmental defects. Controls comprised of cell-free ceramics implanted into the contralateral limb. The femurs were harvested and analyzed by high-resolution radiography, immuno-histochemistry, quantitative histomorphometry, and biomechanical testing. Mesenchymal stem-cell-treated defects had evidence of new bone formation by 8 weeks. Biomechanical evaluation confirmed treated femurs were significantly stronger than the controls. These findings demonstrate that human MSCs can regenerate bone in clinically significant osseous defects and may therefore provide an alternative to autogenous bone grafts.

The repair of cranial bone defects is a major challenge for craniofacial surgeons owing to the limited availability of autologous bone graft. Consequently, surgeons have experimented with other materials to find a suitable alternative. Shang et al. (2001) used autologous MSCs isolated from eight adult sheep to treat parietal bone defects. The cells were expanded in culture and added to a calcium–alginate composite. The bony defects were treated by either calcium alginate/MSC composites or calcium alginate alone. New bone formation was observed within the experimental group only, with CT scans revealing almost complete repair of these defects. Importantly, this tissue-engineered bone had the same biomechanical properties as native parietal bone.

In an attempt to enhance the osteogenic potential of MSCs, investigators have studied ways of pretreating these cells (Yoshikawa et al., 1996). Yoshikawa et al. described a technique where hydroxyapatite/MSC composites were cultured in mediums with or without dexamethasone, a known osteogenic agent, for 2 weeks. After being implanted subcutaneously in rats, the composites were harvested and analyzed for alkaline phosphatase activity and bone gamma carboxy glutamic acid (Gla) protein. Results showed that dexamethasone-treated bone marrow cells exhibited an enhanced osteogenic response immediately after transplantation. In contrast, the untreated composite did not show any bone formation. These results indicate that the inherent osteogenic ability of marrow stromal stem cells can be stimulated using tissue culture technology.

### 22.2.1.3 Muscle Cells

In 1965, Urist first noted that when demineralized bone matrix is implanted into skeletal muscle, a new ossicle of bone is formed. In subsequent reports, this phenomenon of osteoinduction was attributed to the mitogenic effects of BMP on cells in muscle and muscle planes (Urist, 1965). This was further reported by Katagiri et al. (1994), who incubated myoblasts with BMP2 and demonstrated a down-regulation of myogenic markers such as troponin T, but an increase in alkaline phosphatase and osteocalcin expression. This suggests that muscle cells had been transformed into osteoblast-like cells in the presence of this osteoinductive stimulus. Research by Khouri et al. (1996) demonstrated that these cells are functionally active by comparing the ability of BMP3, a muscle flap and a combination of the two to heal a rat calvarial defect. Results showed that a muscle flap injected with BMP3 was capable of healing the defect completely. In contrast, defects treated with either the muscle flap or BMP3 alone demonstrated only 37 and 64% healing, respectively. These findings support the concept that muscle-based osteopro-genitor cells are functionally effective and lay the foundation for future investigations regarding the use of skeletal muscle as a source of inducible osteoprogenitor cells for bone healing.

Muscle derived stem cells have been genetically engineered to express human BMP-4, vascular endothelial growth factor (VEGF) or VEGF specific antagonist (soluble Flt1) to study the interaction between angiogenic and osteogenic factors in bone healing (Peng et al., 2002). Using a mouse model, Peng et al. intramuscularly implanted a designated number of transduced cells into the lateral aspect of each femur. Ectopic bone formation was monitored radiographically and histologically for up to 4 weeks postoperatively. Results showed that VEGF acted synergistically with BMP-4 to increase the recruitment of MSCs, enhance cell survival and promote cartilage formation in the early stages of endochondral ossification. In contrast, Flt1 inhibited this bone healing response elicited by BMP-4. From these studies, the authors concluded that VEGF had an important role in enhancing BMP-4 elicited bone formation and regeneration.

### 22.2.1.4   Embryonic Stem Cells

Recent reports have described the use of human embryonic stem cells in tissue engineering. Thomson et al. (1998) demonstrated that these cells can be grown *in vitro* from human blastocysts and maintain their developmental potential to form all three germ layers. As a result, cartilage, bone and muscle may be derived from the mesoderm. This development of human embryo technology represents a new therapeutic approach that may be used in the future for regeneration of skeletal tissues. Nevertheless, major challenges exist, including the ethical issues.

## 22.2.2   Role of Scaffolds

Scaffolds act as a conduit for the delivery of cells, genetic material and growth factors to the site of interest (Doll et al., 2001). In addition, they support vascular invasion, maintain uniform distribution and retention of cells throughout its three-dimensional lattice, facilitate efficient diffusion of molecules, and undergo resorption and replacement by new bone as it is formed (Bruder and Fox, 1999).

Several materials have been used in bone–tissue engineering and can be divided into acellular and cellular systems (Burg et al., 2000). The former is comprised of an absorbable filler material, which encourages bony in-growth without any additional cellular component. In contrast, cellular scaffolds include cells embedded in the implanted scaffold.

### 22.2.2.1   Acellular Systems

#### 22.2.2.1.1   Natural Matrices

Demineralized bone matrix (DBM) is produced from the acid extraction of human cortical bone. Since the earlier observations of Urist and co-workers on its ability to induce ectopic bone formation (Van de Putte and Urist, 1965; Van de Putte and Urist, 1966), interest has developed within the orthopedic community as to its role in treating bony defects. Tuli and Singh (1978) demonstrated that DBM has osteoinductive and osteoconductive properties in the healing of rabbit bony defects. After 12 weeks of treatment with DBM, 13 out of the 16 animal defects had been bridged by new bone formation with no local foreign body or immunogenic reaction to the graft.

Tiedeman et al. (1995) reported on the efficacy of DBM used in conjunction with bone marrow in the treatment of patients with bony disorders such as comminuted fractures with associated bone loss. After a follow-up period averaging 19 months, 30 out of 39 patients demonstrated successful bone formation with the patients grafted with DBM demonstrating healing comparable to those who were treated with autogenous bone graft.

The osteoinductive properties of DBM vary depending on its source. This was highlighted by Rabie and co-workers (Rabie et al., 2000) during a study examining the healing of rabbit parietal bone defects in the presence of DBM extracted from intramembranous bone (imDBM) or endochondral bone (ecDBM). In the experimental animals, defects were grafted with endochondral bone, endochondral bone mixed with imDBM, intramembranous bone mixed with imDBM, or with endochondral bone mixed with ecDBM. Controls comprised of defects that were either left untreated (passive control) or grafted with rabbit skin collagen (active control). Results showed a total of 41.4, 70.8 and 85% more new bone formation in defects grafted with composite endochondral bone with imDBM, intramembranous bone mixed with imDBM and endochondral bone mixed with ecDBM, respectively, than those grafted with endochondral bone alone ($P < .001$). No bone was formed in either passive or active controls. The authors concluded that DBM, particularly those derived from intramembranous bone, have extremely high osteoinductive properties.

### 22.2.2.1.2 Ceramics

Ceramics are biomaterials produced from the heating of natural mineral salts to high temperatures (Ladd and Pliam, 1999). Of the various types, calcium phosphate ceramics have been extensively used in the treatment of bony defects owing to their similar architectural properties and surface chemistry to bone. The most widely used include tricalcium phosphate (TCP) and hydroxyapatite (HA) (Hollinger and Battistone, 1986). They display excellent biocompatibility, osteoconductivity, and osseointegration (Ohgushi et al., 1989; Goshima et al., 1991; Ripamonti, 1996).

From a functional perspective, calcium phosphate ceramics can be divided into slow and rapid resorbing ceramics (Fleming et al., 2000b). HA is a slow resorbing compound that may be derived from marine coral (Chiroff et al., 1975) by a simple hydrothermal treatment process. Holmes et al. (Holmes et al., 1984; Holmes et al., 1987) conducted a series of experiments to determine the capabilities of HA in treating osseous defects. In the radial diaphyses of dogs, bilateral cortical windows were created and filled with either HA or an iliac autograft (Holmes et al., 1987). Specimens were harvested at 3, 6, 12, 24, and 48 months. Results showed that the HA implants encouraged significant bony in-growth compared to the grafts.

In light of these findings, HA has been used to treat a number of orthopedic conditions. Thalgott et al. (2002) first reported HA for spinal reconstruction. Twenty patients underwent circumferential lumbar fusion with HA blocks placed anteriorly and autografted with transpedicular or translaminar facet screw fixation posteriorly. Radiographs demonstrated solid arthrodesis rates of over 90%. Clinical follow-up reflected these positive findings with over 80% of patients reporting good or excellent pain relief. From these observations, coralline HA is a practical alternative to autograft or allograft in anterior lumbar interbody fusions.

One of the major drawbacks associated with HA use is its poor handling properties. To overcome this, Friedman et al. (1998) developed an HA-based cement paste for craniofacial reconstruction. The material can be used to treat defects that were previously not amenable to ceramic fixation. It is rapidly adherent and directly converted to bone without loss of implant volume. In their study of over 100 patients undergoing craniofacial reconstructive procedures using this cement, success rates were reported to be 97% at 2 years.

A further disadvantage of HA is related to its slow resorption. In order to overcome this, manipulating the thermal conversion process of calcium carbonate may produce faster resorbing HA. The resulting compound is of calcium carbonate with a thin coating of HA. Once this coating is resorbed, however, after a few months, the remaining calcium carbonate is absorbed much more rapidly.

By contrast to HA, TCP is a more rapidly resorbing ceramic and has been used in formulations to enhance fracture repair. It undergoes the same remodeling process and forms tissue with the same structural characteristics to bone (Parikh, 2002). The mechanism by which TCP encourages new bone formation, however, remains unclear. Frost (1991) hypothesized that it may be related to the calcium phosphate crystals that are produced as a consequence of TCP dissolution. These particles stimulate osteoclast proliferation which has an indirect stimulatory effect on osteoblast function.

TCP has been studied as a potential bone filler in traumatic bone injuries. This was reported by Hinz et al. (2002), who used the material to treat calcaneal fractures. Biopsy results demonstrated active bone formation within the scaffold.

Despite these relative successes in achieving osteoinduction, TCP is limited as a bone-graft substitute owing to its porosity which is too small to allow complete bony in-growth before the matrix is resorbed. In order to enhance its osteoinductive properties, Laffargue et al. (1999) described a technique of adding rhBMP-2 to TCP cylinders to treat femoral condyle defects in rabbits. They observed increased trabecular bone formation prior to implant resorption.

### 22.2.2.1.3 Synthetic Polymers

Synthetic matrices have been increasingly used in bone–tissue engineering. These scaffolds have the advantage of being bioresorbable, biocompatible, osteoconductive, and can be easily molded to fit the individual defect (Oreffo and Triffitt, 1999). Meinig et al. (1996) demonstrated this by treating 1-cm mid-diaphyseal radial bone defects with poly-L-lactide (PLLA) in New Zealand White rabbits. Untreated defects of a similar size on the contralateral limb served as controls. Results showed cortical bone formation spanning the defects in the experimental animals compared to radial-ulnar synostosis with no new bone formation in the controls.

Defect size limits the ability of these synthetic polymers to promote bone formation. This was highlighted by Gugala and Gogolewski (1999), when they attempted to treat 4-cm tibial defects in sheep with PLLA. In the cases where membranes were used alone, no osseous repair was noted. In contrast, defects treated with both cancellous bone graft and synthetic membrane demonstrated significant bony repair.

### 22.2.2.2 Cellular Systems

### 22.2.2.2.1 Natural Matrices

Type I collagen is the most abundant extracellular matrix protein in bone and promotes mineral deposition by providing binding sites for matrix proteins such as osteonectin. Nevertheless, collagen is a poor bone graft material when used alone. This was demonstrated by Werntz et al. (1986), who noticed collagen scaffolds were unable to promote healing of diaphyseal defects. In contrast, collagen and bone marrow cell composites stimulated bony repair and were more effective than those seen using cancellous bone graft.

The addition of rhBMP-2 to collagen has similar osteoinductive effects. This was demonstrated by Boyne et al. (1997), when they examined the combination of rhBMP-2 with an absorbable collagen sponge (ACS) (rhBMP-2/ACS) in human maxillary floor reconstruction. Significant bone growth was documented by computer tomography in all patients. There were no serious or unexpected immunologic or adverse effects. Histologic examinations of core bone biopsies confirmed the quality of the bone induced by rhBMP-2/ACS. These results suggest that rhBMP-2/ACS may provide an acceptable alternative to traditional bone grafts for maxillary floor reconstruction procedures.

Collagraft®, a composite of fibrillar collagen and porous calcium phosphate ceramic, has been compared in a multicenter prospective randomized trial with iliac crest autografts for the treatment of long bone fractures (Cornell et al., 1991). Initial results suggest no significant differences between the two groups, thereby lending support to the use of Collagraft® as a substitute for autogenous bone grafts. Further work by Alvis et al. (2003) examining the role of Collagraft® showed that its osteoconductive properties can be enhanced by adding bone marrow cells. Implants of Collagraft®, Collagraft® plus bone marrow, and bone marrow alone were placed subcutaneously in a rat model and results showed that by 3 weeks, new bone formation was only seen within the Collagraft®/bone marrow composites.

### 22.2.2.2.2 Ceramics

Osteoprogenitor cells have been added to ceramic materials to improve their osteogenic properties. This was described by Okamura et al. (1997), where they subcutaneously implanted porous HA impregnated with rat marrow cells. Results suggested that HA may facilitate osteogenic differentiation of MSCs, as analysis of the composite revealed the appearance of osteoblast-like cells and mineralized bone on the HA surface.

This observation of ceramics supporting MSC differentiation along osteogenic lines led Bruder et al. (1998b) to study the effects of implants loaded with MSCs on the healing of large segmental femoral defects in a canine model. Animals were treated with either MSC-laden ceramic cylinders (HA and TCP) or empty ceramic cylinders. A third control group comprised of untreated defects. After 4 months, the femora were harvested and processed for histological examination. Atrophic nonunion was seen within the control group. In contrast, woven and lamellar bony in-growth was seen in the implants loaded with MSCs.

Quarto et al. (2001) reported on a series of three patients in which bone marrow osteoprogenitor cells were placed on macroporous HA scaffolds to treat large bone defects. In all subjects, radiographic analysis revealed abundant callus formation along the implants and good integration at the interfaces with the host bone by 2 months postoperatively.

The problems associated with the use of synthetic ceramics for MSC delivery is their brittle nature and lack of interconnecting pores (Doll et al., 2001). Natural ceramic composites, on the other hand, combine favorable mechanical properties with an open porous structure. An example is the natural coral exoskeleton, which has been used in several clinical applications (Roux et al., 1988). Petite et al. (2000) explored its use as a delivery vehicle for MSCs in the treatment of large bony defects in sheep. The authors compared its efficacy to coral scaffold alone to achieve osseous union. Results showed significant increases in clinical union rates in the experimental group compared to controls.

### 22.2.2.2.3 Synthetic Polymers

Creating osteoconductive scaffolds from nonbiological materials offers many advantages, including excellent biocompatibility, ease of assembly, unlimited supply, and a lack of disease transmission. The ideal material would serve as a scaffold for the in-growth of new tissue and as a source of growth factors to support cell differentiation. It should initially provide the mechanical stability required for a healing process to begin, and with time, be able to transfer these properties to developing skeletal tissues (Laurencin, 1996).

Polyglycolic acid (PGA) is already used in many areas of modern medicine (e.g., suture material). More recently, proponents have investigated its use in bone–tissue engineering and in particular its effects on fracture healing (Puelacher et al., 1996). Standardized 9-mm defects were created in athymic rat femurs and bridged with titanium miniplates. Half the defects were treated with PGA constructs containing bovine periosteum-derived cells, whereas the remaining defects were either left untreated or filled with polymer templates alone. After 12 weeks, new bone formation was seen primarily bridging the defects in the experimental groups. Histologic evaluation revealed new bone formation in all experimental animals with islands of cartilage indicative of endochondral bone formation.

In addition to stimulating bone repair, synthetic polymers have been used to create artificial joints. Isogai et al. (1999) described a technique in which they were able to create a finger joint from a composite of bovine periosteum, chondrocytes and tenocytes seeded on to a polyglycolic and poly-L-lactic acid copolymer. The composite was implanted subcutaneously into athymic mice. After 20 weeks, the new tissue that was formed had the shape and dimensions of human phalanges. Histological examination revealed mature articular cartilage and subchondral bone with a tenocapsule that had a structure similar to that of a human finger.

### 22.2.3 Role of Growth Factors

Growth factors are proteins secreted by cells and function as signaling molecules. They comprise a family of molecules that have autocrine, paracrine or endocrine effects on appropriate target cells. In addition to promoting cell differentiation, they have direct effects on cell adhesion, proliferation, and migration by modulating the synthesis of proteins, other growth factors, and receptors (Johnson et al., 1988).

#### *22.2.3.1 Bone Morphogenetic Proteins*

Since the discovery of the osteoinductive properties of DBM (Urist, 1965), attention has focused on the role of bone morphogenetic proteins (BMP) in embryological bone formation and bone repair of the postnatal skeleton (Johnson et al., 1988; Ripamonti and Duneas, 1998; Cho et al., 2002). BMPs are a group of noncollagenous glycoproteins that belong to the transforming growth factor beta (TGFβ) superfamily. They are synthesized locally and predominantly exert their effects by autocrine and paracrine mechanisms. Over 15 different BMPs have been identified and their genes cloned (Croteau et al., 1999). The best studied examples are BMP-2, BMP-3, and BMP-7 (Osteogenic Protein 1), as these are known to play important roles in bone repair by stimulating MSC differentiation along osteogenic lines.

The importance of BMPs in bone repair has been the subject of much investigation. Cho et al. (2002) defined and characterized their temporal expression during murine fracture healing. BMP-2 showed maximal expression on day 1 after fracture, suggesting its role as an early response gene in the cascade of healing events. BMP-3, 4, 7, and 8 exhibited a restricted period of expression from day 14 through day 21, when the resorption of calcified cartilage and osteoblastic recruitment were most active. BMP-5 and 6 were constitutively expressed from day 3 to day 21. These findings suggest that several members of the BMP family are actively involved in fracture healing, with each having a distinct temporal expression pattern and potentially unique role in the repair process.

Gerhart et al. (1993) studied the effects of rhBMP-2 on the healing of segmental femoral bone defects in sheep. Fractures were stabilized by plate fixation and treated with bone matrix devoid of bone inductive proteins (inactive), rhBMP-2 mixed with this inactive bone matrix, or autogenous bone graft. A control group with no intervention was also included. Radiographs showed bony union in all defects treated with rhBMP-2 and bone graft. No bone formation was detected in the control and inactive bone-matrix groups. Biomechanical testing revealed that the new bone formed in the rhBMP-2-treated group was stronger than that seen in the animals receiving autogenous graft. Long-term analyses of the bone formed by rhBMP-2 revealed that it had undergone a normal sequence of ossification, modeling and remodeling (Kirker-Head et al., 1995). Results from these and other studies support investigations on the use of BMP-2 in clinical settings as an alternative to autograft for traumatic and reconstructive procedures.

Govender et al. (2002) conducted a prospective, randomized, controlled multicenter trial evaluating the effects of rhBMP-2 on the treatment of open tibial fractures. Four hundred and fifty patients were randomized to receive either intramedullary (IM) nail fixation alone or IM fixation plus an implant containing either 0.75 or 1.5 mg/ml of rhBMP-2 at the time of definitive treatment. The implant was placed over the fracture site during closure. Routine soft-tissue management was used in all patients. Results showed that the 1.5 mg/ml rhBMP-2 group had accelerated times to union, improved wound healing, reduced infection rates and fewer secondary invasive interventions.

In addition to its use in fracture healing, BMPs have been used in spine surgery. Sandhu et al. (1995) conducted a study analyzing the efficacy of rhBMP-2 in comparison to autograft in sheep anterior spinal fusion. Comparisons were made using radiographic, mechanical, and histological analyses after 6 months of treatment. Radiographs revealed complete fusion in all of the rhBMP-2-treated animals compared to only 40% in the autograft group. Biomechanical testing demonstrated that segments treated with rhBMP-2 were 20% stiffer in flexion than were those treated with autograft. The authors concluded that treatment with rhBMP-2 improves fusion rates and strength of repair compared to using autograft in anterior spinal fusions.

With similar positive results seen in a rhesus monkey model (Boden et al., 1998), Boden et al. (2002) conducted a prospective, randomized controlled clinical study evaluating the use of rhBMP2 in posterolateral lumbar spine fusion in patients who had single-level disc degeneration, grade 1 or less spondylolisthesis, mechanical low back pain with or without leg pain and at least 6 months failure of nonoperative treatment. Patients were randomized into groups receiving autograft/Texas Scottish Rite Hospital (TSRH) pedicle screw instrumentation (controls), rhBMP-2/TSRH or rhBMP-2 alone without internal fixation. Results showed a significantly improved radiographic fusion rate between those receiving rhBMP-2 (100%) compared to those in which an autograft had been used (40%). Clinical symptoms improved at a faster rate in the rhBMP-2 group with successful posterolateral spine fusion being present after 1 year follow-up.

As with BMP-2, BMP-7 (OP-1) has proved to be efficacious in animal models. Cook et al. (1995) studied the effects of rhBMP-7 on the healing of ulnar and tibial fractures in a monkey model. Ulnar and tibial defects were treated with a composite of rhBMP-7 and bovine type 1 collagen. Controls were comprised of defects treated with collagen carrier alone or autogenous cancellous bone graft. Radiographs demonstrated that five of the six ulnae and four of the five tibiae treated with rhBMP-7 had completely healed by 6 to 8 weeks postoperatively. In contrast, none of the defects treated with the collagen carrier or bone graft had demonstrated bony union. Histological evaluation revealed the formation of new cortices with areas of woven and lamellar bone and normal appearing bone marrow elements. Mechanical testing of the defects treated with BMP showed higher torsional strengths to failure than those treated with autogenous bone graft.

The osteogenic effect of BMP-7 has been used in a prospective, randomized double-blind trial to evaluate its ability to heal fibular defects in patients who have undergone high tibial osteotomy (Geesink et al., 1999). Results showed significant new bone formation in the patients treated with BMP compared to controls. In a larger study, Friedlaender et al. (2001) assessed the efficacy of rhBMP-7 over iliac crest bone graft to treat patients with tibial nonunions. Nine months after surgery, 81% of the BMP-7-treated nonunions and 85% of those treated with bone graft had achieved clinical union. The authors concluded that whilst no statistical difference was noted between the two groups, BMP-7 was a safe and effective alternative to bone graft in the treatment of tibial nonunions.

### 22.2.3.2 *Fibroblast Growth Factors*

Fibroblast growth factors (FGF) are a group of structurally related compounds that share between 30 and 50% sequence homology. Acidic FGF (aFGF, FGF1) and basic FGF (bFGF, FGF2) are the most well-studied members of this family, with bFGF considered to be the more potent. It stimulates angiogenesis, endothelial cell migration and is mitogenic for fibroblasts, chondrocytes and osteoblasts (Ingber and Folkman, 1989; Hurley et al., 1993).

During fracture repair, FGFs differ in their temporal and spatial expression (Rundle et al., 2002). In the early stages, FGF 1 and 2 are localized to the proliferating periosteum. This expression is then limited to osteoblasts during intramembranous bone formation and in the chondrocytes and osteoblasts during endochondral bone formation.

In light of their active involvement during fracture repair, investigators have studied the potential therapeutic roles of FGF in bone formation. Nakamura et al. (1998) injected bFGF into mid-diaphyseal transverse tibial fractures in dogs and compared bone healing rates to controls that were injected with carrier molecules. Specimens were harvested at 2, 4, 8, 16, and 32 weeks and assessed in terms of callus formation, morphology, and strength. Results showed that bFGF had positive effects on callus formation, remodeling rates, maximum load, bending stress, and energy absorption.

Radomsky et al. (1999) demonstrated combining FGF with hyaluronic acid resulted in superior bone forming potential. Bilateral fibula fractures were created in a primate model and the experimental side was injected with a basic FGF/hyaluronic acid composite gel. The contralateral fibula was left untreated and acted as a control. Increased callus formation and mechanical strength were noted in the treated defects. Radiographic and histologic analyses demonstrated that the callus size, periosteal reaction, vascularity, and cellularity were consistently greater in the treated osteotomies than in the controls. Similar findings were reported by Lisignoli et al. (2002). Segmental radial fractures were produced in rats and treated with either a biodegradable hyaluronic acid scaffold or a hyaluronic acid polymer/MSC composite that had been grown in medium with or without supplemental bFGF. Enhanced mineralization of the bone defects was noted in the presence of the composites grown in bFGF. These results suggest that FGF has the potential to promote skeletal repair.

### 22.2.3.3 *Transforming Growth Factor β*

Transforming Growth Factor β (TGFβ) influences a number of cell processes. These include stimulating MSC growth and differentiation, acting as a chemotactic factor for fibroblast and macrophage recruitment, and enhancing collagen and other extracellular matrix (ECM) product secretion (Khan et al., 2000).

TGFβ has been used to stimulate bone regeneration. This was demonstrated by Lind et al. (1993), where they continuously administered TGFβ for 6 weeks to rabbits in whom unilateral plated tibial defects had been created. The control group comprised of defects treated with solvent without the growth factor. Results showed that TGFβ had a positive effect on fracture repair with increased bending strengths and callus formation seen in the experimental group.

Critchlow et al. (1995) performed a study to test the hypothesis that the anabolic effects of TGFβ on bony repair are dependent on the mechanical stability at the fracture site. Unilateral tibial fractures were produced in a rabbit model and held in either an unstable or stable configuration using plastic or steel plates, respectively. TGFβ-2 was injected into the calluses 4 days after fracture. In animals with unstable mechanical fixation, TGFβ-2 did not have an anabolic effect on callus formation. In contrast, those with stable mechanical constructs developed enlarged calluses. Histological analyses revealed that the calluses comprised almost entirely of bone compared to those seen within the unstable group, which were predominantly comprised of cartilage. These findings demonstrate that stable fracture fixation is important for TGFβ-2 mediated skeletal repair.

From the above studies, it can be seen that TGFβ augments fracture healing in experimental models. It is difficult however, to draw definitive conclusions regarding these effects, as reported studies testing several isoforms of TGFβ at different dosages in numerous animal models have yielded inconsistent results. Consequently, some believe that the anabolic effects of TGFβ may be due to its potentiation of BMPs (Centrella et al., 1994). Ripamonti and co-workers (Ripamonti et al., 1997) reported enhanced BMP-7 effects on bone differentiation when low doses of TGFβ-1 were added. Combinations of BMP-7 and TGFβ-1 yielded a two- to three-fold increase in cross-sectional area of newly generated ossicles compared to BMP-7 alone. The tissue had distinct morphological differences with larger amounts of endochondral bone formation compared to BMP-7 generated specimens.

### 22.2.3.4 *Insulin-Like Growth Factor*

Insulin-like growth factors (IGF) 1 and 2 are the two main types in this class to have an anabolic effect on bone metabolism by stimulating osteoblast and osteoclast cell proliferation and matrix synthesis (Khan et al., 2000). Reductions in their levels have been linked to age related declines in bone mineral density (Bennett et al., 1984). Jehle and co-workers (Jehle et al., 2003) conducted a cross sectional study of the relationship between serum IGF levels and bone metabolism in patients with osteoporosis. Serum parameters including IGF-1 and IGF binding proteins (IGFBP) 1 through 6 were measured. Dual-energy x-ray absorptiometry was used to determine lumbar spine bone mineral density. Compared to age- and sex-matched controls, patients with osteoporosis had a 73% decrease in free IGF-1, a 29% decrease in total IGF-1, a 10% decrease in IGFBP-3, and a 52% decrease in IGFBP-5 levels. These reductions were most evident in the patients who had sustained vertebral fractures. The authors concluded that derangements in IGF system components reflect alterations in bone metabolism and a subsequent increase in susceptibility to fractures in these patients.

For tissue engineering purposes, researchers have tended to favor IGF-1 over IGF-2 due to its greater stimulatory effects on osteoblast function and its expression during fracture healing (Bak et al., 1990; Andrew et al., 1993). Thaller et al. (1993) first examined its ability to promote healing of critical-size calvarial defects in rats. Animals received either subcutaneous administration of IGF-1 or were left untreated to act as controls. Within the experimental group, repair commenced after 1 week of treatment with complete bone formation seen by 6 weeks. Delayed osseous repair was detected in the control animals by 8 weeks.

Shen et al. (2002) demonstrated similar positive findings using MSCs transfected with an IGF-1 gene. The cells were systemically injected into mice, which had earlier sustained closed, mid-diaphyseal femoral fractures. Their findings demonstrated that the cells preferentially localized to the fracture site and exerted a positive effect on the repair process. This resulted in enhanced callus formation and ossification in the experimental group compared to controls.

This positive effect on bone formation has been used to promote spinal fusion. Kandziora et al. (2002) compared the efficacy of IGF-1 with TGFβ-1 to autologous bone grafts in cervical fusion. After C3-4 discectomy, stabilization was achieved using a titanium cage, a titanium cage with autologous bone graft, or a titanium cage with IGF-1 and TGFβ-1. After 12 weeks, animals treated with IGF-1/TGFβ-1 had significantly higher fusion rates than the bone-grafted animals. This could be attributed to the increased callus mineral density seen in the IGF-1 group.

### 22.2.3.5 *Platelet Derived Growth Factor*

Platelet derived growth factor (PDGF) is synthesized by numerous cell types including platelets, macrophages, and endothelial cells. It consists of two polypeptide A and B chains that share 60% amino acid sequence homology (Solheim, 1998). PDGFs possess strong mitogenic properties and stimulate the proliferation of osteoblasts (Canalis, 1981; Canalis et al., 1989). This is particularly important in fracture healing where they exhibit differential spatial and temporal expression (Andrew et al., 1995). Nash et al. (1994) examined the efficacy of PDGF on bone formation using a rabbit tibial osteotomy model. Each osteotomy was injected with either collagen or collagen containing PDGF. An increase in callus formation and a more advanced stage of endosteal and periosteal osteogenic differentiation was seen in the experimental group compared to the controls after 28 days. Osteotomies treated with PDGF were not statistically different in strength from the nonoperated contralateral bones. In the control group, however, the osteotomies were statistically weaker than their intact contralateral bones. From these observations, it appears that exogenous PDGF has a stimulatory effect on fracture healing.

PDGF has been used clinically to stimulate periodontal regeneration (Howell et al., 1997). Patients with periodontal osseous defects underwent reconstructive flap surgery and received either PDGF-BB and IGF-1 (50 $\mu$g/ml or 150 $\mu$g/ml) or underwent no further intervention. Results showed that those receiving low-dose PDGF had no increase in bone regeneration compared to controls. In contrast, patients treated with the higher doses developed statistically significant increases in alveolar bone formation.

Based on these promising findings, Giannobile et al. (2001) examined the use of adenoviral vectors encoding for PDGF-A gene on root lining cells. Results showed that this genetic delivery vehicle stimulated root lining cell proliferation and may provide beneficial results in periodontal tissue engineering.

### 22.2.4 Gene Therapy

Gene therapy is an emerging technology in the field of bone tissue engineering. It involves the transfer of genetic material into a cell's genome, thereby altering its synthetic function. For this process, the selected gene's messenger ribonucleic acid (mRNA) is reversely transcribed into complementary deoxyribonucleic acid (cDNA). It is then inserted into a plasmid and placed into a vector (viral or nonviral) carrier that facilitates gene transfer into the targeted cell lines. Successful gene transfer using nonviral vectors is termed *transfection* whereas with viral carriers it is known as *transduction*.

Viruses are efficient vectors owing to their increased ability to infect host cells. They can be divided into *integrating* or *nonintegrating* subtypes depending upon their effects on the host cell's genome (Table 22.1). The former group is designed to integrate its genetic material into the cell's DNA without causing the replication of the virus or inducing an immunological response (Evans and Robbins, 1995; Robbins and Ghivizzani, 1998; Salypongse et al., 1999). Examples include adeno-associated viruses and retroviruses. Adeno-associated viruses are small DNA viruses originating from the parvovirus family. They have the advantages of being able to infect nondividing cells and of stable integration of its DNA into the host cell's genome at a precise location on chromosome 19 (Samulski et al., 1991). Disadvantages include difficulty in generating high titers of the recombinant viruses, their small size limiting the amount of exogenous DNA and their inability to insert DNA at specific sites in the host cell's genome.

Retroviruses are the best developed viral vectors for gene therapy and are being used in many clinical trials (Miller, 1992). They are small RNA viruses that, once inside the cell, have their RNA transcribed into double-stranded DNA by the cell's reverse

**TABLE 22.1**

Properties of Present Vectors

| Vector[a] | Advantages | Disadvantages |
|---|---|---|
| Integrating viral | | |
| Retrovirus | | |
| MMLV-based | Straightforward production | Require target cell division |
| | No viral proteins made | Possible insertional mutagenesis |
| | Extensive use in human trials | |
| Lentivirus-based | Transduce nondividing cells | More development required |
| AAV | Site-specific integration[b] | Difficult to produce |
| | Nonpathogenic | Small packaging capacity (4 Kb) |
| | Transduce nondividing cells | |
| | No viral proteins made | |
| Viral nonintegrating | Straightforward production | Inflammatory |
| Adenovirus | High titers | Immunogenecity of transduced cells |
| | Transduce nondividing cells | |
| HSV | Large packing capacity | Difficult to produce |
| | High titers | Cytotoxicity |
| | Transduce nondividing cells | |
| Nonviral | | |
| Naked DNA | Simple | Few cells transfect well |
| | Nonimmunogenic | |
| | Inexpensive | |
| | Safe | |
| Liposomes | As above | Gene expression usually transient and low |
| Particle bombardment (gene gun) | Used in conjunction with plasmid DNA | Cumbersome; requires specialized equipment |
| DNA–ligand complexes | May be targetable | Possible antigenicity |
| | Receptor-mediated uptake often efficient | Low expression |

Reprinted with permission from Evans, C.H. et al. Gene therapy for rheumatic diseases. *Arthritis Rheum.*, 42, 1 (1999).

[a]  All types of vectors are the subject of considerable research. This table summarizes the present state of development. MMLV = Moloney murine leukaemia virus; AAV = adeno-associated virus; HSV = herpes simplex virus.

[b]  Wild-type AAV integrates in a site-specific manner. Recombinant virus appears as if it does not.

transcriptase. The DNA is integrated into the cell's genome and is expressed throughout the duration of the cell's lifecycle. The main drawbacks to these vectors are that they only infect and transduce actively replicating cells and randomly integrate into the host cell's DNA. Concerns about possible mutagenesis resulting from placement of retroviral sequences could result in activation of an oncogene leading to the development of a malignant tumor.

Nonintegrating viruses do not insert their genetic material into the host cell's DNA but instead maintain it within the nucleus as an unintegrated, episomal form (Evans and Robbins, 1995). The adenovirus (Table 22.1) is the more-studied virus of this type and has the advantage of being able to infect both dividing and some nondividing cells, thereby achieving a high level of transient gene expression. However, it induces the formation of adenoviral antigens which results in an immune response against infected cells, thereby resulting in a loss of gene expression after a short period of time.

Herpes simplex viruses (HSV) are capable of infecting both dividing and nondividing cells, carry large amounts of DNA and infect many different cell types. The demonstration of HSV vector-associated toxicity has led to the development of a second generation of vector to minimize these effects.

Nonviral vectors possess limited immunogenecity and are safer than viral vectors. They are much cheaper and easier to produce in large quantities than viral carriers. The most commonly used nonviral vectors are liposomes, which are phospholipid vesicles that fuse with the cell membrane and deliver its contents into the cell (Musgrave et al., 2002). Their main disadvantage, however, is their poor rate of genetic transfer (Salypongse et al., 1999). Consequently, modern-day gene therapy applications employ transduction methods owing to greater efficiency over transfection techniques (Robbins and Ghivizzani, 1998).

The two main approaches to gene therapy involve *in vivo* and *ex vivo* gene transfer (Robbins and Ghivizzani, 1998). The *in vivo* technique involves the direct transfer of genetic material into the host. It is a technically easier method to perform but is limited by an inability to perform *in vitro* safety testing on transfected cells.

*In vivo* gene therapy has been used to promote fracture repair through the expression of BMP-2 (Baltzer et al., 2000). Segmental defects were created in the femora of New Zealand White rabbits and animals divided into three groups: a positive control with no intervention, a negative control receiving adenoviral vectors infected with a luciferase gene, and an experimental group receiving viral vectors encoding for BMP-2. Results demonstrated that BMP-2 exerted an anabolic effect with evidence of fracture healing in the treated animals. In contrast, the repair tissue in the control animals consisted of a fibrotic response with minimal osseous union. These observations add support to the use of local adenoviral delivery of an osteoinductive gene to promote fracture repair in defects that would have otherwise proceeded to nonunion.

Lumbar interbody fusions have been used to treat a number of conditions including spinal instability, tumors, and disc disruptions (Goldstein, 2000; Patil et al., 2000). Reports vary, but between 4 and 40% of these procedures are unsuccessful (Zoma et al., 1987; Steinmann and Herkowitz, 1992). Gene therapy has been investigated as a potential mechanism to enhance spinal fusion in these cases. Alden et al. (1999a, 1999b) reported on the use of an adenoviral construct containing the BMP-2 gene to achieve spinal fusion. Athymic rats were divided into three groups and the spinous process-lamina junction injected with either BMP-2 gene viral constructs, beta galactosidase gene viral vectors or both. Results showed enhanced bone formation in the BMP-2 group compared to the controls. Additionally, well-developed vasculature, cartilage, and cancellous bone were found within the paraspinal muscles where BMP-2 vectors were injected. There was no evidence of neural compromise in the BMP-2 treated animals, suggesting this direct *in vivo* model may be a safe method to achieve spinal fusion.

Gene therapy has been described for treating craniofacial disorders (Lindsey, 2001). Using an athymic rat model, Lindsey investigated whether nasal bone reconstruction could be enhanced using recombinant adenoviral vectors encoding for BMP-2 gene. Results showed significant osseous repair in the BMP-2 treated animals compared to the controls.

The use of direct *in vivo* techniques is not without problems. Generation of adenoviral vectors induces a florid immune response. Not only is this deleterious to the immunocompetent host (Brody et al., 1994), but it also limits the effectiveness of gene expression. This was demonstrated by Alden et al. (1999a, 1999b), when they investigated the endochondral response to BMP-2 adenoviral vector injections in immunocompetent and deficient animals. The former group showed evidence of acute inflammation without ectopic bone formation at the injection sites. In the athymic nude rats, BMP-2 gene therapy induced mesenchymal stem cell chemotaxis and proliferation, with subsequent differentiation into chondrocytes. The chondrocytes secreted a cartilaginous matrix, which underwent mineralization and subsequent replacement by bone. The study demonstrated that within immunocompetent animals, the endochondral response is limited by the immune response to adenoviral constructs.

The indirect *ex vivo* approach to gene therapy is technically more demanding than the *in vivo* method. It involves the removal of cells from a tissue biopsy and genetically modifying them *in vitro* before transfer back into the host. This offers the advantage of selecting the cells with the greatest gene expression and testing them for any abnormal behavior before reimplantation (Chen, 2001).

Using the principles of *ex vivo* gene transfer, Lieberman et al. (1999) generated BMP-2 producing bone marrow cells and investigated their ability to heal segmental femoral fractures in syngeneic rats. A group treated with rhBMP-2 served as a positive control. Negative controls included uninfected rat bone marrow cells, DBM and beta galactosidase-transduced cells. Results showed that the BMP-2-transduced cells induced greater trabecular bone formation in the fracture site compared to any of the control groups. Others have reported similar results using the *ex vivo* method of gene therapy to promote this repair process (Breitbart et al., 1999).

## 22.3   Mechanical Factors

Limb lengthening was first described by Codivilla in 1905 (Codivilla, 1905) for the treatment of limb length discrepancies. It was not until the work of Ilizarov (Ilizarov, 1978a; Ilizarov et al., 1978b) 50 years later that the technique of distraction osteogenesis (DO) gained popularity as a method for enhancing bone regeneration. Currently, the concept of DO is applied for the correction of a variety of orthopedic deformities and malformations with predictable results (Ilizarov, 1990). This was highlighted by Rozbruch (Rozbruch et al., 2002), where patients with leg-length discrepancy, malalignment, and nonunion following high tibial osteotomy were treated with distraction. Bone union was achieved with correction of the deformities and limb-length inequalities.

DO has been used as a method for correcting craniofacial defects (Davies et al., 1998). McCarthy et al. (1992) reported its use in mandibular reconstruction and achieved bone lengthening from 18 to 24 mm. Successful follow-up of the patients demonstrated that this technique may be used for early reconstruction of maxillofacial deformities without the need for bone grafts, blood transfusion, or intermaxillary fixation.

### 22.3.1   Biology of Distraction Osteogenesis

Distraction osteogenesis generates new tissue through the application of tensile forces to developing callus in a controlled osteotomy (Lewinson et al., 2001; Meyer et al., 2001). It is characterized by three separate stages: (1) the latency phase that immediately follows osteotomy; (2) the active or distraction phase, which permits active separation of bony segments; and (3) the consolidation phase, where active distraction has ended and healing of the callus begins (Tay et al., 1998; Sato et al., 1999; Isefuko et al., 2000). The period of time for each stage varies depending upon the anatomic site and the size of the osseous defect needing repair.

Bone formation is formed primarily by intramembranous ossification (Einhorn and Lee, 2001). The early events after the latency period closely resemble fracture healing with a localized inflammatory response and haematoma formation (Tajana et al., 1989). The callus within the distraction gap comprises of a number of different cell types with mesenchymal-like cells at the center, surrounded by fibroblast-like cells secreting a collagen-rich matrix (Lewinson et al., 2001). Chondrocyte-like cells can also be seen at the interface between trabecular bone and osteoblasts, secreting a mineralized matrix (Sato et al., 1999).

## 22.3.2 Physiological Factors Governing Distraction Osteogenesis

### 22.3.2.1 Latency Period

The latency period relates to the time between an osteotomy and the distraction of bone ends. Fluctuations in its length affect the tissue formed within the regenerate. This was demonstrated by the work of White and Kenwright (1990). Tibial osteotomies were created in New Zealand White rabbits and divided into groups receiving distraction immediately or after a latency of 7 days. Results showed that a delay in distraction influenced the osteogenic response. Immediate distraction resulted in the formation of fibrous tissue within the osteotomy defect. In contrast, those within the delayed distraction group produced a large volume of callus with areas of proliferating cartilage. This difference may be related to the well-developed capillary network found within the latter animals. The authors hypothesized that during the latency period, damaged blood vessels have the necessary time to repair and can better withstand the tensile forces of distraction.

Warren et al. (2000) further investigated the effects of gradual distraction vs. acute lengthening in rat mandibular DO. Animals either underwent immediate lengthening of 3 mm or gradual distraction of 0.25 mm twice a day after a 3-day latency period. Results showed a marked elevation of critical extracellular matrix molecules (osteocalcin and collagen Type I) during the consolidation phase of the gradually distracted groups compared with acute lengthening. These findings suggest that gradual distraction osteogenesis promotes successful osseous bone repair by regulating the expression of bone-specific extracellular matrix molecules. In contrast, decreased production or increased turnover of proteins like collagen and osteocalcin may lead to fibrous union during acute lengthening.

### 22.3.2.2 Distraction Rates

The rate and rhythm of distraction appears to determine the success of osseous repair. This was highlighted by the work of Ilizarov (Ilizarov, 1989) in which he investigated the effects of different distraction rates (0.5 mm, 1.0 mm, or 2.0 mm per day) and frequencies (1 step per day, 4 steps per day, 60 steps per day) on limb lengthening in canine tibiae. Results showed that a distraction rate of 1.0 mm per day led to the best results with optimum preservation of periosseous tissues, bone marrow and blood. Distraction of 0.5 mm per day led to premature consolidation of the regenerate, whereas rates of 2.0 mm adversely affected the surrounding tissues.

Farhadieh and co-workers (Farhadieh et al., 2000) examined the effects of several distraction rates on the biomechanical, mineralization, and histologic properties of regenerate tissue. A uniaxial distractor was applied to the angle of the mandible and varying rates of distraction applied (1, 2, 3, and 4 mm/day). After 5 weeks of distraction, results showed that the biomechanical, mineralization and histologic properties were significantly superior in the 1-mm group compared to the 4-mm group.

From these studies it can be seen that the biological nature of the regenerate is related to the stress/strain forces generated within the distraction gap. Meyer et al. (2001) demonstrated that the magnitude of these forces directly influences the phenotypic differentiation of the cells within the distraction gap. Li et al. (2000) reported similar findings using an experimental model of tibial leg lengthening. The authors' aims were to determine the morphology of the collagenous proteins present and the genes expressed within the regenerate at four different rates. At distraction rates of 0.3 mm per day, remodeled bone ends were separated by central areas of intramembranous bone and fibrocartilage. In the osteotomies distracted at 0.7 mm or 1.3 mm per day, new bone formation was seen at the corticotomy ends and was separated by central areas of fibrous tissue and cartilage. Fibrous tissue with sparse bone formation was seen within the animals distracted at 2.7 mm per day. Type I collagen was mainly expressed by the fibroblasts in the fibrous tissue, the bone surface cells and to a limited extent by the osteocytes. Type II collagen was produced by the chondrocytes. These results suggest that osteoblasts and chondrocytes within the regenerate originate from the same pool of osteoprogenitor cells, and their differentiation and expression of Types I and II collagen genes is affected by different rates of distraction.

### 22.3.2.3  *Blood Supply*

Studies of distraction have demonstrated the importance of blood vessel formation during this process. Rowe and co-workers (Rowe et al., 1999) analyzed this angiogenic process during mandibular DO. Osteotomies were created in the right hemimandible of rats and a distraction device applied. Distraction commenced after a 3-day latency period for 6 days. Results demonstrated that mandibular DO was associated with an intense vascular response during the early stages of distraction. Similar findings were reported by Choi et al. (2000). Using scanning electron microscopy, they studied the spatial and temporal expressions of new blood vessels during DO. They showed that proliferations of periosteal and medullary blood vessels occurred primarily during the latency and distraction periods.

Li et al. (1999) demonstrated that the angiogenic response is directly related to the distraction rate. Intense proliferations of capillary precursor cells were noticed within the fibrous interzone of the distracted gap, with maximum values occurring between 0.7 and 1.3 mm per day.

## 22.4   Conclusion

The field of tissue engineering to repair or regenerate the musculoskeletal system is developing rapidly and expanding in its applications. To date, strategies have met with limited success within the clinical setting. With ongoing research to enhance the osteogenic potential of cell concentrates, develop better delivery systems and gene therapy applications for growth factors and osteoinductive substances, tissue engineering will add to current treatment modalities and greatly enhance the management of musculoskeletal injuries and diseases in the future.

# References

Alden, T.D., et al., Percutaneous spinal fusion using bone morphogenetic protein-2 gene therapy, *J. Neurosurg.*, **90**, 109 (1999a).

Alden, T.D., et al., *In vivo* endochondral bone formation using a bone morphogenetic protein 2 adenoviral vector, *Hum. Gene Ther.*, **10**, 2245 (1999b).

Alsberg, E., Hill, E.E., and Mooney, D.J., Craniofacial tissue engineering, *Crit. Rev. Oral Biol. Med.*, **12**, 64 (2001).

Alvis, M., et al., Osteoinduction by a collagen mineral composite combined with autologous bone marrow in a subcutaneous rat model, *Orthopaedics*, **26**, 77 (2003).

Andrew, J.G., et al., Insulin-like growth factor gene expression in human fracture callus, *Calcif. Tissue Int.*, **53**, 97 (1993).

Andrew, J.G., et al., Platelet-derived growth factor expression in normally healing human fractures, *Bone*, **16**, 455 (1995).

Bak, B., Jorgensen, P.H., and Andreassen, T.T., Dose response of growth hormone on fracture healing in the rat, *Acta Orthop. Scand.*, **61**, 54 (1990).

Baltzer, A.W., et al., Genetic enhancement of fracture repair: healing of an experimental segmental defect by adenoviral transfer of the BMP-2 gene, *Gene Ther.*, **7**, 734 (2000).

Banwart, J.C., Asher, M.A., and Hassanein, R.S., Iliac crest bone graft harvest donor site morbidity: a statistical evaluation, *Spine*, **20**, 1055 (1995).

Bennett, A.E., et al., Insulin-like growth factors I and II: aging and bone density in women, *J. Clin. Endocrinol. Metab.*, **59**, 701 (1984).

Beresford, J.N., Osteogenic stem cells and the stromal system of bone and marrow, *Clin. Orthop.*, **240**, 270 (1989).

Boden, S.D., et al., Laparoscopic anterior spinal arthrodesis with rhBMP2 in a titanium interbody threaded cage, *J. Spinal Disord.*, **11**, 95 (1998).

Boden, S.D., et al., Use of recombinant human bone morphogenetic protein-2 to achieve posterolateral lumbar spine fusion in humans: a prospective, randomized clinical pilot trial: Volvo Award in clinical studies, *Spine*, **27**, 2662 (2002).

Boyne, P.J., et al., A feasibility study evaluating rhBMP-2/absorbable collagen sponge for maxillary sinus floor augmentation, *Int. J. Periodont. Restor. Dent.*, **17**, 11 (1997).

Breitbart, A.S., et al., Gene enhanced tissue engineering: applications for bone healing using cultured periosteal cells transduced retrovirally with the BMP7 gene, *Ann. Plast. Surg.*, **42**, 488 (1999).

Brody, S.L., et al., Acute responses of non human primates to airway delivery of an adenovirus vector containing the human cystic fibrosis transmembrane conductance regulator cDNA, *Hum. Gene Ther.*, **5**, 821 (1994).

Bruder, S.P. and Fox, B.S., Tissue engineering of bone, *Clin. Orthop.*, **S367**, S68 (1999).

Bruder, S.P., Jaiswal, N., and Haynesworth, S.E., Growth kinetics, self renewal and the osteogenic potential of purified human mesenchymal stem cells during extensive subcultivation and following cryopreservation, *J. Cell Biochem.*, **64**, 278 (1997).

Bruder, S.P., et al., Bone regeneration by implantation of purified, culture-expanded human mesenchymal stem cells, *J. Orthop. Res.*, **16**, 155 (1998a).

Bruder, S.P., et al., The effect of implants loaded with autologous mesenchymal stem cells on the healing of canine segmental bone defects, *J. Bone Joint Surg. Am.*, **80**, 985 (1998b).

Burg, K.J.L., Porter, S., and Kellam, J.F., Biomaterial developments for bone tissue engineering, *Biomaterials*, **21**, 2347 (2000).

Canalis, E., Effect of platelet-derived growth factor on DNA and protein synthesis in cultured rat calvaria, *Metabolism*, **30**, 970 (1981).

Canalis, E., McCarthy, T.L., and Centrella, M., Effects of platelet derived growth factor on bone formation *in vitro*, *J. Cell Physiol.*, **140**, 530 (1989).

Centrella, M., et al., Transforming growth factor beta gene family members and bone, *Endocr. Rev.*, **15**, 27 (1994).

Chen, Y., Orthopaedic applications of gene therapy, *J. Orthop. Sci.*, **6**, 199 (2001).

Chiroff, R.T., et al., Tissue ingrowth of replamineform implants, *J. Biomed. Mater. Res.*, **6**, 29 (1975).

Cho, T.J., Gerstenfeld, L.C., and Einhorn, T.A., Differential temporal expression of members of the transforming growth factor β superfamily during murine fracture healing, *J. Bone Miner. Res.*, **17**, 513 (2002).

Choi, I.H., et al., Vascular proliferation and blood supply during distraction osteogenesis: a scanning electron microscopic observation, *J. Orthop. Res.*, **18**, 698 (2000).

Codivilla, A., On the means of lengthening in the lower limbs, the muscles and tissues which are shortened through deformity, *Am. J. Orthop. Surg.*, **2**, 353 (1905).

Connolly, J., Injectable bone marrow preparations to stimulate osteogenic repair, *Clin. Orthop.*, **313**, 8 (1995).

Connolly, J.F. and Shindell, R., Percutaneous marrow injection for an ununited tibia, *Nebr. Med. J.*, **71**, 105 (1986).

Connolly, J.F., et al., Development of an osteogenic bone marrow preparation, *J. Bone Joint Surg.*, **71A**, 684 (1989).

Connolly, J.F., et al., Autologous marrow injection as a substitute for operative grafting of tibial nonunions, *Clin. Orthop.*, **266**, 259 (1991).

Cook, S.D., et al., Effect of recombinant human osteogenic protein-1 on healing of segmental defects in non-human primates, *J. Bone Joint Surg. Am.*, **77**, 734 (1995).

Cornell, C.N., et al., Multicenter trial of Collagraft as bone graft substitute, *J. Orthop. Trauma*, **5**, 1 (1991).

Critchlow, M.A., Bland, Y.S., and Ashhurst, D.E., The effect of exogenous transforming growth factor β2 on healing fractures in the rabbit, *Bone*, **16**, 521 (1995).

Croteau, S., et al., Bone morphogenetic proteins in orthopaedics: from basic science to clinical practice, *Orthopaedics*, **22**, 686 (1999).

Davies, J., Turner, S., and Sandy, J.R., Distraction osteogenesis — a review, *Br. Dent. J.*, **185**, 462 (1998).

Deutche Banc. Alex Brown. Estimates and Company Information (2001).

Doll, B., et al., Critical aspects of tissue engineered therapy for bone regeneration, *Crit. Rev. Eukaryot Gene Expr.*, **11**, 173 (2001).

Einhorn, T.A. and Lee, C.A., Bone regeneration. New findings and potential clinical applications, *J. Am. Acad. Orthop. Surg.*, **9**, 157 (2001).

Evans, C.H. and Robbins, P.D., Possible orthopaedic applications of gene therapy, *J. Bone Joint Surg.*, **77A**, 1103 (1995).

Farhadieh, R.D., et al., Effect of distraction rate on biomechanical, mineralization, and histologic properties of an ovine mandible model, *Plast. Reconstr. Surg.*, **105**, 889 (2000).

Fleming, J.E., Cornell, C.N., and Muschler, G.F., Bone cells and matrices in orthopedic tissue engineering, *Orthop. Clin.*, **31**, 357 (2000a).

Fleming, J.E., Cornell, C.N., and Muschler, G.F., Bone cells and matrices in orthopaedic tissue engineering, *Orthop. Clin.*, **31**, 357 (2000b).

Fowler, B.L., Dall, B.E., and Rowe, D.E., Complications associated with harvesting autogenous iliac bone graft, *Am. J. Orthop.*, **24**, 895 (1995).

Friedlaender, G.E., et al., Osteogenic protein 1 (bone morphogenetic protein 7) in the treatment of tibial nonunions, *J. Bone Joint Surg. Am.*, **83**, S1–S151 (2001).

Friedman, C.D., et al., BoneSource hydroxyapatite cement: a novel biomaterial for craniofacial skeletal tissue engineering and reconstruction, *J. Biomed. Mater. Res.*, **43**, 428 (1998).

Frost, H., A new direction for osteoporosis research, *Bone*, **12**, 249 (1991).

Garg, N.J., Gaur, S., and Sharma, S., Percutaneous autogenous bone marrow grafting in 20 cases of ununited fracture, *Acta Orthop. Scand.*, **64**, 671 (1993).

Geesink, R.G.T., Hoefnagels, N.H.M., and Bulstra, S.K., Osteogenic activity of OP1 bone morphogenetic protein (BMP7) in a human fibular defect, *J. Bone. Joint Surg. Br.*, **81**, 710 (1999).

Gerhart, T.N., et al., Healing segmental femoral defects in sheep using recombinant human bone morphogenetic protein, *Clin. Orthop.*, **293**, 317 (1993).

Giannobile, W.V., et al., Platelet-derived growth factor (PDGF) gene delivery for application in periodontal tissue engineering, *J. Periodontol.*, **72**, 815 (2001).

Goldstein, S.A., *In vivo* nonviral delivery factors to enhance bone repair, *Clin. Orthop.*, **S379**, S113 (2000).

Goshima, J., Goldberg, V.M., and Caplan, A.I., The osteogenic potential of culture expanded rat marrow mesenchymal cells assayed *in vivo* in calcium phosphate ceramic blocks, *Clin. Orthop.*, **262**, 298 (1991).

Goulet, J.A., et al., Autogenous iliac crest bone graft: complications and functional assessment, *Clin. Orthop.*, **339**, 76 (1997).

Govender, S., et al., Recombinant human bone morphogenetic protein 2 for treatment of open tibial fractures. A prospective, controlled, randomized study of four hundred and fifty patients, *J. Bone Joint Surg. Am.*, **84**, 2123 (2002).

Grundel, R.E., et al., Autogeneic bone marrow and porous biphasic calcium phosphate ceramic for segmental bone defects in canine ulna, *Clin. Orthop.*, **266**, 244 (1991).

Gugala, Z. and Gogolewski, S., Regeneration of segmental diaphyseal defects in sheep tibiae using resorbable polymeric membranes: a preliminary study, *J. Orthop. Trauma*, **13**, 187 (1999).

Healey, J.H., et al., Percutaneous bone marrow grafting of delayed union and nonunion in cancer patients, *Clin. Orthop.*, **256**, 280 (1990).

Hinz, P., et al., A new resorbable bone void filler in trauma: early clinical experience and histologic evaluation, *Orthopedics*, **25**, S597 (2002).

Hollinger, J.O. and Battistone, G.C., Biodegradable bone repair materials, *Clin. Orthop.*, **207**, 290 (1986).

Holmes, R.E., et al., A coralline hydroxyapatite bone graft substitute. Preliminary report, *Clin. Orthop.*, **188**, 252 (1984).

Holmes, R.E., Bucholz, R.W., and Mooney, V., Porous hydroxyapatite as a bone graft substitute in diaphyseal defects: a histometric study, *J. Orthop. Res.*, **5**, 114 (1987).

Howell, T.H., et al., A phase I/II clinical trial to evaluate a combination of recombinant human platelet-derived growth factor-BB and recombinant human insulin-like growth factor-I in patients with periodontal disease, *J. Periodontol.*, **68**, 1186 (1997).

Hurley, M.M., et al., Basic fibroblast growth factor inhibits type 1 collagen gene expression in osteoblastic MC3T3E1 cells, *J. Biol. Chem.*, **268**, 5588 (1993).

Ilizarov, G.A., The tension–stress effect on the genesis and growth of tissues: Pt II. The influence of the rate and frequency of distraction, *Clin. Orthop.*, **239**, 263 (1989).

Ilizarov, G.A., Clinical applications for a tension stress effect for limb lengthening, *Clin. Orthop.*, **250**, 34 (1990).

Ilizarov, G.A., et al., Characteristics of systemic growth regulation of the limbs under the effects of various factors influencing their growth and length, *Ortop. Travmatol. Protez.*, **8**, 37 (1978a), in Russian.

Ilizarov, G.A., Pereslitskikh, P.F., and Barabash, A.P., Closed directed longitudino-oblique or spinal osteoclasia of the long tubular bones (experimental study), *Ortop. Travmatol. Protez.*, **11**, 20 (1978b), in Russian.

Ingber, D.E. and Folkman, J., Mechanochemical switching between growth and differentiation during fibroblast growth factor stimulated angiogenesis *in vitro*: role of extracellular matrix, *J. Cell Biol.*, **109**, 317 (1989).

Isefuko, S., Joyner, C.J., and Simpson, H.R.W., A murine model of distraction osteogenesis, *Bone*, **27**, 661 (2000).

Isogai, N., et al., Formation of phalanges and small joints by tissue-engineering, *J. Bone Joint Surg. Am.*, **81**, 306 (1999).

Jehle, P.M., et al., Serum levels of insulin-like growth factor (IGF)-I and IGF binding protein (IGFBP)-1 to -6 and their relationship to bone metabolism in osteoporosis patients, *Eur. J. Intern. Med.*, **14**, 32 (2003).

Johnson, E.E., Urist, M.R., and Finerman, G.A., Repair of segmental defects of the tibia with cancellous bone grafts augmented with human bone morphogenetic protein. A preliminary report, *Clin. Orthop.*, 249 (1988).

Kandziora, F., et al., Comparison of BMP-2 and combined IGF-I/TGFβ1 application in a sheep cervical spine fusion model, *Eur. Spine J.*, **11**, 482 (2002).

Katagiri, T., et al., Bone morphogenetic protein-2 converts the differentiation pathway of C2C12 myoblasts into the osteoblast lineage, *J. Cell Biol.*, **127**, 1755 (1994).

Khan, S.N., et al., Bone growth factors, *Orthop. Clin.*, **31**, 375 (2000).

Khouri, R.K., et al., Repair of calvarial defects with flap tissue: role of bone morphogenetic proteins and competent responding tissues, *Plast. Reconstr. Surg.*, **98**, 103 (1996).

Kirker-Head, C.A., et al., Long-term healing of bone using recombinant human bone morphogenetic protein 2, *Clin. Orthop.*, **318**, 222 (1995).

Ladd, A.L. and Pliam, N.B., Use of bone graft substitutes in distal radius fractures, *J. Am. Acad. Orthop. Surg.*, **7**, 279 (1999).

Laffargue, P., et al., Evaluation of human recombinant bone morphogenetic protein-2-loaded tricalcium phosphate implants in rabbits' bone defects, *Bone*, **25**, S55 (1999).

Lane, J.M., et al., Bone marrow and recombinant human bone morphogenetic protein-2 in osseous repair, *Clin. Orthop.*, **361**, 216 (1999).

Laurencin, C.T., et al., Tissue engineered bone-regeneration using degradable polymers: the formation of mineralized matrices, *Bone*, **19**, 93S (1996).

Lewinson, D., et al., Expression of vascular antigens by bone cells during bone regeneration in a membranous bone distraction system, *Histochem. Cell Biol.*, **116**, 381 (2001).

Li, G., et al., Effect of lengthening rate on angiogenesis during distraction osteogenesis, *J. Orthop. Res.*, **17**, 362 (1999).

Li, G., et al., Tissues formed during distraction osteogenesis in the rabbit are determined by the distraction rate: localization of the cells that express the mRNAs and the distribution of types I and II collagens, *Cell Biol. Int.*, **24**, 25 (2000).

Lieberman, J.R., et al., The effect of regional gene therapy with bone morphogenetic protein-2-producing bone-marrow cells on the repair of segmental femoral defects in rats, *J. Bone Joint Surg. Am.*, **81**, 905 (1999).

Lind, M., et al., Transforming growth factor β enhances fracture healing in rabbit tibiae, *Acta Orthop. Scand.*, **64**, 553 (1993).

Lindsey, W.H., Osseous tissue engineering with gene therapy for facial bone reconstruction, *Laryngoscope*, **111**, 1128 (2001).

Lisignoli, G., et al., Osteogenesis of large segmental radius defects enhanced by basic fibroblast growth factor activated bone marrow stromal cells grown on non-woven hyaluronic acid-based polymer scaffold, *Biomaterials*, **23**, 1043 (2002).

McCarthy, J.G., et al., Lengthening the human mandible by gradual distraction, *Plast. Reconstr. Surg.*, **89**, 1 (1992).

McCarthy, J.G., et al., Distraction osteogenesis of the craniofacial skeleton, *Plast. Reconstr. Surg.*, **107**, 1812 (2001).

Meinig, R.P., et al., Bone regeneration with resorbable polymeric membranes: treatment of diaphyseal bone defects in the rabbit radius with poly(L-lactide) membrane. A pilot study, *J. Orthop. Trauma*, **10**, 178 (1996).

Meyer, U., et al., Mechanical tension in distraction osteogenesis regulates chondrocyte differentiation, *Int. J. Oral Maxillofac. Surg.*, **30**, 522 (2001).

Miller, A.D., Human gene therapy comes of age, *Nature*, **357**, 455 (1992).

Musgrave, D.S., Fu, F.H., and Huard, J., Gene therapy and tissue engineering in orthopaedic surgery, *J. Am. Acad. Orthop. Surg.*, **10**, 6 (2002).

Nakamura, T., et al., Recombinant human basic fibroblast growth factor accelerates fracture healing by enhancing callus remodeling in experimental dog tibial fracture, *J. Bone Miner. Res.*, **13**, 942 (1998).

Nash, T.J., et al., Effect of platelet-derived growth factor on tibial osteotomies in rabbits, *Bone*, **15**, 203 (1994).

Ohgushi, H., Goldberg, V.M., and Caplan, A.I., Heterotopic osteogenesis in porous ceramics induced by marrow cells, *J. Orthop. Res.*, **7**, 568 (1989).

Okamura, M., et al., Osteoblastic phenotype expression on the surface of hydroxyapatite ceramics, *J. Biomed. Mater. Res.*, **37**, 122 (1997).

Oreffo, O.C. and Triffitt, J.T., Future potentials for using osteogenic stem cells and biomaterials in orthopedics, *Bone*, **25**, 5S (1999).

Parikh, S.N., Bone graft substitutes: past, present and future, *J. Postgrad. Med.*, **48**, 142 (2002).

Patil, P.V., et al., Interbody fusion augmentation using localized gene delivery, *Trans. Orthop. Res. Soc.*, **25**, 360 (2000).

Peng, H., et al., Synergistic enhancement of bone formation and healing by stem cell-expressed VEGF and bone morphogenetic protein-4, *J. Clin. Invest.*, **110**, 751 (2002).

Petite, et al., Tissue engineered bone regeneration, *Nat. Biotechnol.*, **18**, 959 (2000).

Puelacher, W.C., et al., Femoral shaft reconstruction using tissue-engineered growth of bone, *Int. J. Oral Maxillofac. Surg.*, **25**, 223 (1996).

Quarto, R., Mastrogiacomo, M., and Cancedda, R., Repair of large bone defects with the use of autologous bone marrow stromal cells, *N. Engl. J. Med.*, 344 (2001).

Rabie, A.B., Wong, R.W., and Hagg, U., Composite autogenous bone and demineralized bone matrices used to repair defects in the parietal bone of rabbits, *Br. J. Oral Maxillofac. Surg.*, **38**, 565 (2000).

Radomsky, M.L., et al., Novel formulation of fibroblast growth factor 2 in a hyaluronan gel accelerates fracture healing in nonhuman primates, *J. Orthop. Res.*, **17**, 607 (1999).

Ripamonti, U., Osteoinduction in porous hydroxyapatite implanted in heterotopic sites of different animal models, *Biomaterials*, **17**, 31 (1996).

Ripamonti, U. and Duneas, N., Tissue morphogenesis and regeneration by bone morphogenetic proteins, *Plast. Reconstr. Surg.*, **101**, 227 (1998).

Ripamonti, U., et al., Recombinant transforming growth factor-beta1 induces endochondral bone in the baboon and synergizes with recombinant osteogenic protein-1 (bone morphogenetic protein-7) to initiate rapid bone formation, *J. Bone Miner. Res.*, **12**, 1584 (1997).

Robbins, P.D. and Ghivizzani, S.C., Viral vectors for gene therapy, *Pharmacol. Ther.*, **80**, 35 (1998).

Roux, F.X., et al., Madreporic coral: a new bone graft substitute for cranial surgery, *J. Neurosurg.*, **69**, 510 (1988).

Rowe, N.M., et al., Angiogenesis during mandibular distraction osteogenesis, *Ann. Plast. Surg.*, **42**, 470 (1999).

Rozbruch, S.R., et al., Distraction osteogenesis for nonunion after high tibial osteotomy, *Clin. Orthop.*, **394**, 227 (2002).

Rundle, C.H., et al., Expression of the fibroblast growth factor receptor genes in fracture repair, *Clin. Orthop.*, **403**, 253 (2002).

Salypongse, A.N., Billiar, T.R., and Edington, H., Gene therapy and tissue engineering, *Clin. Plast. Surg.*, **26**, 663 (1999).

Samulski, R.J., et al., Targeted integration of adeno-associated virus (AAV) into human chromosome 19, *EMBO J.*, **10**, 3941 (1991).

Sandhu, H.S., et al., Histologic evaluation of the efficacy of rhBMP-2 compared with autograft bone in sheep spinal anterior interbody fusion, *Spine*, **20**, 2669 (1995).

Sato, M., et al., Mechanical tension stress induces expression of bone morphogenetic protein(BMP) 2 and BMP 4, but not BMP6, BMP7 and GDF5 mRNA during distraction osteogenesis, *J. Bone Miner. Res.*, **14**, 1084 (1999).

Shang, Q., et al., Tissue engineered bone repair of sheep cranial defects with autologous bone marrow stromal cells, *J. Craniofac. Surg.*, **12**, 586 (2001).

Shen, F.H., et al., Systemically administered mesenchymal stromal cells transduced with insulin-like growth factor-I localize to a fracture site and potentiate healing, *J. Orthop. Trauma*, **16**, 651 (2002).

Solheim, E., Growth factors in bone, *Int. Orthop.*, **22**, 410 (1998).

Steinmann, J.C. and Herkowitz, H.N., Pseudoarthrosis of the spine, *Clin. Orthop.*, **284**, 80 (1992).

Swennen, et al., Craniofacial distraction osteogenesis: a review of the literature. Pt 1: clinical studies, *Int. J. Oral. Maxillofac. Surg.*, **30**, 89 (2001).

Tajana, G.F., Morandi, M., and Zembo, M., The structure and development of osteogenic repair tissue according to Ilizarov technique in man: characterization of the extracellular matrix, *Orthopedics*, **12**, 515 (1989).

Tay, B.K.-B., et al., Histochemical and molecular analysis of distraction osteogenesis in a mouse model, *J. Orthop. Res.*, **16**, 636 (1998).

Thalgott, J.S., et al., Anterior lumbar interbody fusion with processed sea coral (coralline hydroxyapatite) as part of a circumferential fusion, *Spine*, **27**, E518 (2002).

Thaller, S.R., Dart, A., and Tesluk, H., The effects of insulin like growth factor 1 on critical size calvarial defects in Sprague–Dawley rats, *Ann. Plast. Surg.*, **31**, 430 (1993).

Thomson, J.A., et al., Embryonic stem cell lines derived from human blastocysts, *Science*, **282**, 1145 (1998).

Tiedeman, J.J., et al., The role of a composite, demineralized bone matrix and bone marrow in the treatment of osseous defects, *Orthopaedics*, **18**, 1153 (1995).

Tuli, S.M. and Singh, A.D., The osteoinductive property of decalcified bone matrix. An experimental study, *J. Bone Joint Surg.*, **60**, 116 (1978).

Urist, M.R., Bone: formation by autoinduction, *Science*, **150**, 893 (1965).

Van de Putte, K.A. and Urist, M.R., Experimental mineralization of collagen sponge and decalcified bone, *Clin. Orthop.*, **40**, 48 (1965).

Van de Putte, K.A. and Urist, M.R., Osteogenesis in the interior of intramuscular implants of decalcified bone matrix, *Clin. Orthop.*, **43**, 257 (1966).

Warren, S.M., et al., Rat mandibular distraction osteogenesis: Pt III. Gradual distraction versus acute lengthening, *Plast. Reconstr. Surg.*, **107**, 441 (2000).

Werntz, J.R., Lane, J.M., and Piez, C., The repair of segmental bone defects with collagen and marrow, *Orthop. Trans.*, **10**, 262 (1986).

Werntz, J.R., et al., Qualitative and quantitative analysis of orthotopic bone regeneration by marrow, *J. Orthop. Res.*, **14**, 85 (1996).

White, S.H. and Kenwright, J., The timing of distraction of an osteotomy, *J. Bone Joint Surg. Br.*, **72**, 356 (1990).

Yoshikawa, T., Ohgushi, H., and Tamai, S., Immediate bone forming capability of prefabricated osteogenic hydroxyapatite, *J. Biomed. Mater. Res.*, **32**, 481 (1996).

Zoma, A., et al., Surgical stabilization of the rheumatoid cervical spine: a review of indications and results, *J. Bone Joint Surg.*, **49B**, 8 (1987).

# 23

## Tissue Engineering — Nervous System

**Lizzie Y. Santiago and Kacey G. Marra**

## CONTENTS

23.1  Overview of the Nervous System ............................................................................................ 442
23.2  Peripheral Nerve Repair ........................................................................................................... 443
    23.2.1  Injuries and Treatments ................................................................................................ 443
    23.2.2  Biomaterials in Peripheral Nerve Repair ................................................................... 444
        23.2.2.1  Biodegradable Materials ............................................................................... 444
        23.2.2.2  Nondegradable Biomaterials ........................................................................ 445
        23.2.2.3  Native Biomaterials ....................................................................................... 445
        23.2.2.4  Commercially Available Nerve Guides ...................................................... 446
    23.2.3  Cellular Nerve Guides ................................................................................................... 446
    23.2.4  Guides Containing Growth Factors ............................................................................. 447
    23.2.5  Summary .......................................................................................................................... 448
23.3  Spinal Cord Repair .................................................................................................................... 448
    23.3.1  Injuries and Treatments ................................................................................................ 448
    23.3.2  Pathophysiology of a Spinal Cord Injury .................................................................. 448
    23.3.3  Nonpermissive Environment for Nerve Regeneration ............................................. 449
    23.3.4  Models of Spinal Cord Injury Used in Animal Research ......................................... 449
        23.3.4.1  Contusion Model ............................................................................................ 449
        23.3.4.2  Transection Model .......................................................................................... 449
    23.3.5  Biomaterials in SCI Research ........................................................................................ 450
        23.3.5.1  Native Materials ............................................................................................. 450
        23.3.5.2  Synthetic and Biodegradable Polymers ..................................................... 450
            23.3.5.2.1  Poly(ethylene) Glycol ................................................................. 450
            23.3.5.2.2  Poly($\alpha$-hydroxy acids) (PLGA, PLA) .......................................... 450
            23.3.5.2.3  Synthetic Nondegradable Polymers ......................................... 451
    23.3.6  Neurotrophic Factors ..................................................................................................... 451
    23.3.7  Cellular Therapies in Spinal Cord Repair .................................................................. 451
        23.3.7.1  Olfactory Ensheathing Cells (OEC) ............................................................ 452
        23.3.7.2  Schwann Cells (SCs) ...................................................................................... 452
        23.3.7.3  Stem Cells ........................................................................................................ 452
        23.3.7.4  Genetically Engineered Cells ....................................................................... 453
    23.3.8  Summary .......................................................................................................................... 453
23.4  Challenges in Neural Tissue Engineering ............................................................................. 453
References .............................................................................................................................................. 453

## 23.1  Overview of the Nervous System

Anatomically, the human nervous system is subdivided into the central (CNS) and the peripheral nervous system (PNS). The central nervous system contains the brain and the spinal cord. The peripheral nervous system consists of several sets of nerve fibers that extend from the CNS.

The neuron, also called a nerve cell, is the structural and functional unit of the nervous system. Each neuron usually contains a cell body or soma from which a long nerve process, called axon, and a number of small branching processes, called dendrites, extends. The neuron is specialized to react to stimuli and to conduct the resulting stimuli to other parts of the cell or to other neurons or effector cells. The nervous system contains a network of neurons that communicate with each other by means of the synapse.

Another important cellular component of the nervous system is the glial or neuroglial cell. In the mammalian CNS the glial cells are more numerous than the neurons. The CNS contains four types of glial cells: astrocytes, oligodendrocytes, ependyma, and microglial cells. Each cell has different functions (Table 23.1). Schwann cells are the glial components of the PNS.

The spinal cord is a cylinder of gray and white matter located in the upper two-thirds of the vertebral canal (Figure 23.1). The gray matter, located in the center of the cylinder, contains cell bodies, dendrites, axons, and glial cells, whereas the white matter contains axons and glial cells. The spinal cord receives incoming signals from the body and sends signals to the body via the peripheral nerves.

The cross-sectional anatomy of the peripheral nerve is illustrated in Figure 23.2. Myelinated and unmyelinated axons are arranged in bundles or fascicles. Three layers of connective tissue known as the epineurium, perineurium, and endoneurium encircle and run between bundles. The innermost layer, the endoneurium, consists of a collagenous matrix that provides protection and nourishes the axons. Groups of fascicles are surrounded by a thin layer of connective tissue, the perineurium, which provides the tensile strength of the nerve. The outer layer, epineurium, protects and nourishes the bundles and maintains the structural continuity of the nerve.

**TABLE 23.1**

Major Functions of the Glial Cells of the Central (CNS) and Peripheral Nervous System (PNS)

| Glial Component | Location | Function |
| --- | --- | --- |
| Schwann cell | PNS | Myelinate PNS neurons |
| Astrocyte | CNS | Provide a structural and supporting framework for neuronal cells and capillaries |
| | | Capture, release, and store chemical neurotransmitters |
| | | Participate in neuronal guidance after CNS injury |
| Oligodendrocyte | CNS | Myelinate CNS neurons |
| Microglial cell | CNS | Show phagocytic properties |
| Ependyma | CNS | Interact with astrocytes to form a barrier separating the ventricles of the brain and cerebrospinal fluid (CSF) from the CNS neurons |

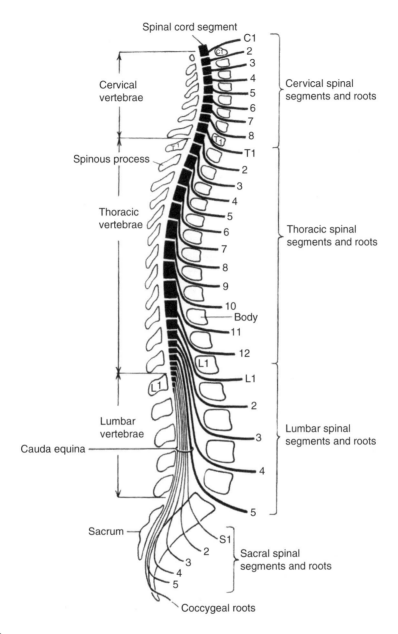

**FIGURE 23.1**
Segments of the spinal cord illustrating their corresponding nerve fibers. (*Source*: From Noback, N.L., Strominger, R.J., and Demarest, R.J., *Human Nervous System: Structure and Function*, 5th ed., Williams and Wilkins, p. 104 (1996). With permission.)

## 23.2 Peripheral Nerve Repair

### 23.2.1 Injuries and Treatments

Peripheral nerve injuries can occur due to trauma and disease. Current treatments for peripheral nerve regeneration include either surgical realignment of the severed ends or

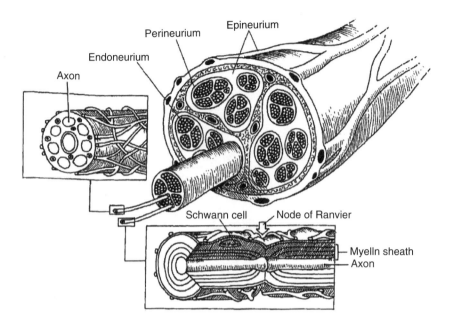

**FIGURE 23.2**
Cross-sectional view of a peripheral nerve. Myelinated and unmyelinated nerve fibers are arranged in bundles surrounded by three layers of connective tissue: endoneurium, perineurium, and epineurium. (*Source*: From Lee, S.K. and Wolfe, S.W., J. *Am. Acad. Orthop. Surg.*, **8** (4), 244 (2000). With permission.)

an autograft as a replacement. Results of nerve repair to date have been fair, with only 50% of patients regaining useful function (Lee and Wolfe, 2000). Muscle and vein grafts have also been examined as nerve conduits, with promising results (Glasby et al., 1986a, 1986b; Fansa et al., 2001; Meek et al., 2002). However, the comorbidity of harvesting donor grafts is a major deterrent. Furthermore, none of these approaches has resulted in robust axonal connections. Potential for regeneration decreases with multiple anastamoses and regeneration is currently limited by gap length. The development of a successful nerve guide from a biomaterial must result in a conduit that has the desired permeability, degradation rate, surface topography, diameter, and mechanical properties. Moreover, the biomaterial must be biocompatible, exhibit a low inflammatory response, and promote axonal elongation. All of these requirements have rendered the clinically successful peripheral nerve substitute for gaps >3 cm thus far elusive.

### 23.2.2  Biomaterials in Peripheral Nerve Repair

Both degradable and nondegradable materials have been examined as nerve conduits. Degradable biomaterials also include native as well as synthetic polymers. The following section is an overview of different biomaterials that have been examined as acellular nerve guides.

#### 23.2.2.1  *Biodegradable Materials*

Biodegradable nerve guides have consisted of FDA-approved polymers, such as poly(lactic acid), (PLA); poly(glycolic acid), (PGA); poly(caprolactone), (PCL), and copolymers (Hadlock et al., 1999; Rodriguez et al., 1999; Maquet et al., 2000). Maquet et al.

have prepared porous PLA conduits coated with poly(vinyl alcohol) and implanted into a 5-mm rat sciatic nerve defect model with fair results (Maquet et al., 2000). Similarly, Rutkowski and Heath have fabricated synthetic conduits of PLA following den Dunnen's method of fabrication (den Dunnen et al., 1996; Heath and Rutkowski, 1998; Rutkowski and Heath, 2002a, 2002b). Axon regeneration based on varying parameters of the conduit such as porosity, wall thickness, and Schwann cell seeding density have been examined (Rutkowski and Heath, 2002a, 2002b). To improve the flexibility of the nerve guides, plasticizers have been incorporated into PLA tubes (Luciano, 2000). However, implantation typically results in a rapid loss of plasticizer, which in turn quickly decreases the mechanical properties. PLA has been also modified with PCL by several groups, including Rodriguez et al., to improve the maintenance of mechanical properties during degradation and decrease the inflammatory response (e.g., by decreasing the PLA content) (Rodriguez et al., 1999). PCL/PLA copolymers are highly permeable, which permits the necessary exchange of nutrients and molecules in the wound site (den Dunnen and Meek, 2001). Caprolactone has been copolymerized with trimethylene carbonate to produce nerve guides with interesting properties, such as flexibility and tailored degradation rates (Pego et al., 2001). Both the mechanical properties and degradation rate can be modified by altering the monomer ratio during the synthesis of these copolymers.

### 23.2.2.2  *Nondegradable Biomaterials*

Nondegradable polymers such as polyethylene (Madison et al., 1987) and poly-urethanes (Robinson et al., 1991) have also been examined. Silicone has been studied as a clinical alternative to nerve autografts (Lundborg et al., 1982; Madison et al., 1988; Kakinoki et al., 1995). Madison et al. compared polyethylene vs. PLA tubes in a 4-mm mouse sciatic nerve defect model (Madison et al., 1987). The tubes were further modified by the inclusion of a laminin gel within the conduits, which enhanced axonal outgrowth. Teflon and polysulfone have been examined as nerve guides, with satisfactory results (Navarro et al., 1996). Conducting polymers such as poly(pyrrole) and poly(pyrrole)/hyaluronic acid composites have shown promise (Schmidt et al., 1997; Collier et al., 2000).

### 23.2.2.3  *Native Biomaterials*

Collagen is the major component of nerve tissue and has been widely studied as a biological conduit material (Valentini et al., 1987; Archibald et al., 1991; Li et al., 1992; Stocum, 1998; Ceballos et al., 1999; Hutmacher, 2001; Verdu et al., 2002). Gibby et al. (1983) demonstrated the potential of collagen as a nerve guide in cat radial and sural nerve defect models. Archibald et al. examined collagen-based nerve guides in both rat and nonhuman primate models and demonstrated that the collagen nerve guides were as efficient as autografts in the rat 4-mm sciatic nerve defect model (Archibald et al., 1991). More recently, collagen within silicone tubes has been shown to improve nerve regeneration in a mouse sciatic defect model (Verdu et al., 2002), although a previous study by Valentini et al. (1987) demonstrated that collagen gel-filled tubes impeded nerve regeneration in a mouse sciatic nerve model. Magnetic alignment of the collagen fibers within the tube has been explored (Ceballos et al., 1999), as has the alignment of fibrin fibers (Dubey et al., 2001). The combination of collagenous beads with PCL is also being examined (Waddell et al., 2003; Bender et al., 2004).

Agarose hydrogels have also been explored and the results are promising (Balgude et al., 2001). Small intestinal submucosa, (SIS), is another native polymeric material that has been examined as a tissue-engineered substrate for a variety of applications, including nerve regeneration (Voytik-Harbin et al., 1997; Badylak et al., 1998; Hadlock et al., 2001; Lindberg and Badylak, 2001).

### 23.2.2.4  *Commercially Available Nerve Guides*

Currently, one biodegradable, synthetic polymeric peripheral nerve guide on the market is NeuroTube™, manufactured by Synovis Micro Companies Alliance. This tube consists of poly(glycolic acid). A highly complex fabrication technique produces a flexible, spring-like tube. Weber et al. reported the use of these polyglycolic acid (PGA) tubes in 46 clinical cases (Weber et al., 2000). Compared to nerve graft, the PGA conduits outperformed the autograft in defects less than 3 cm. This is promising; however, improved outcomes in larger defects are needed prior to general clinical use.

A biodegradable native polymeric nerve guide that is commercially available is NeuroGen™, marketed by Integra Neurosciences. This commercial guide consists of bovine collagen and is available in lengths up to 2 cm.

### 23.2.3  Cellular Nerve Guides

Although synthetic tubular nerve guides can promote axonal elongation over relatively short gaps, the inclusion of cells within a guide can significantly improve nerve regeneration. Several groups have demonstrated enhanced peripheral nerve regeneration using Schwann cell-seeded nerve guides in sciatic nerve defects. The important role of Schwann cells in nerve regeneration has been well-documented (Porter et al., 1986; Levi and Bunger, 1994; Woerly et al., 1996; Ansselin et al., 1997, 1998; Jesson and Mirsky, 1999; Bryan et al., 2000; Hadlock et al., 2000; Rodriguez et al., 2000; Fansa et al., 2001; Hadlock et al., 2001; Chen and Strickland, 2003; Timmer et al., 2003; Fansa and Keilhoff, 2004; Galla et al., 2004). An interesting study by Hadlock et al. (2001) involved seeding SIS with Schwann cells, subsequently rolling the seeded construct into tubes, and implanting into a 7-mm rat sciatic nerve defect model. Results were near the performance of autografts. Fansa et al. described the inclusion of Schwann cells within acellular autologous matrices, such as veins, muscles and nerves (Fansa and Keilhoff, 2004). After 6 weeks in a 2-cm rat sciatic nerve defect, the muscle grafts demonstrated improved regeneration compared to unseeded muscle grafts. Galla et al. (2004) seeded poly(caprolactone) nerve guides with Schwann cells in a fibrin matrix and examined nerve regeneration in a rat 10-mm sciatic nerve gap. Although they did not compare nerve regeneration to unseeded PCL guides, they did compare nerve regeneration to seeded guides + LIF (leukemia inhibitory factor). Myelination rate was comparable to autograft. An earlier paper by Hadlock et al. (2000) demonstrated comparable nerve regeneration in PLGA guides seeded with Schwann cells as compared to autograft in a 7-mm sciatic nerve gap in rats. Finally, Ansselin's group has demonstrated that collagen tubes seeded with Schwann cells result in improved recovery in an 18-mm rat sciatic nerve gap after 7 months (Ansselin et al., 1997, 1998). Indeed, they report that "Supplementing guides with Schwann cells enhances regeneration of peripheral axons over a distance normally prohibitive. This effect is greatest in the early stages of regeneration (1 to 3 months) and is dependent on the number of cells implanted."

Although many of these cellular approaches are promising for long-gap nerve repair, a challenge for using autologous Schwann cells is the donor site morbidity. Currently, it is not clinically feasible to utilize a patient's own nerves to obtain a significant number of pure Schwann cells.

### 23.2.4  Guides Containing Growth Factors

Modifications to polymer nerve guides such as growth factor incorporation is an alternative approach. Growth factors are natural hormones, usually proteins, present in the body that can attract useful cells and proteins to the wound, stimulate and increase production of connective tissue, promote remodeling, and create a new supply of blood vessels to nourish the site. A tissue-engineered delivery system that results in the slow, controlled release of factors such as nerve growth factor (NGF), and insulin-like growth factor-I (IGF-I), could stimulate and guide axon growth. Such an approach could involve polymer microspheres. Drugs and other growth factors have been incorporated into polymer microspheres, such as human growth hormone (Cleland et al., 1997), Japanese encephalitis virus vaccine (Khang et al., 1999), vascular endothelial growth factor (King and Patrick, 2000), transforming growth factor $\beta_1$ (Lu et al., 2000; Peter et al., 2000), fibroblast growth factor (Nugent et al., 1992), and cisplatin (Verrijk et al., 1991). Additionally, microspheres containing growth factors have been injected into a porous scaffold post-fabrication (Mooney et al., 1996). Babensee et al. (2000) have written a comprehensive review on growth factor delivery. Recently, Richardson et al. (2001) described the fabrication and evaluation of a polymer scaffold that delivers two growth factors for bone regeneration.

The use of growth factors in nerve regeneration includes examination of the incorporation of glial growth factor (GGF) within a polymer conduit (Bryan et al., 2000). GGF is produced by neurons and stimulates proliferation of Schwann cells (Terenghi, 1999). The role of NGF in nerve regeneration has been more widely studied. The neurotrophin NGF promotes the differentiation of several classes of neurons, is a survival factor in both neuronal cell culture and *in vivo* (Yakovchenko et al., 1996), and has been encapsulated and delivered from polymer microspheres (Camarata et al., 1992; Krewson et al., 1996; Pean et al., 1998; Cao and Shoichet, 1999; Gouhier et al., 2000; Pean et al., 2000). Tranquillo's group has had promising results with the addition of NGF within guides (Rosner et al., 2003), and Shoichet's group has examined both the delivery of surface-immobilized NGF (Kapur and Shoichet, 2004) and the microsphere encapsulation of NGF (Cao and Shoichet, 1999).

Recently, Arsenijevic et al. (2001) reported that IGF-I is a key factor in the regulation of neural stem cell activity. The effects of IGF-I on cell types such as the widely studied rat pheochromocytoma cell line PC12 (Greene and Tischler, 1976; Monnier et al., 1994; Zachor et al., 1994), Schwann cells (Cheng and Feldman, 1997; Russell et al., 2000), dorsal root ganglia (Russell et al., 2000; Kimpinski and Mearow, 2001), as well as the expression of IGF-I from PC12 cells (Yakovchenko et al., 1996; Bach et al., 1997) have been reported. Lam et al. (2000) and Meinel et al. (2001) have recently published optimized procedures for IGF-I encapsulation.

Other growth factors that are being examined for their potential for peripheral nerve regeneration include the neurotrophin-3 (NT-3) and brain-derived neurotrophic factor (BDNF), which both show a beneficial effect on the survival and phenotypic expression of primary sensory neurons in the dorsal root ganglia and of motor neurons in the spinal cord (Terenghi, 1999). Other neurotrophic factors such as ciliary neurotrophic factor (CNTF), glial cell line-derived neurotrophic factor (GDNF), and leukemia inhibitory factor (LIF) also exert a variety of actions on neuronal cells, which appear to overlap and complement those of the neurotrophins, and hence are being investigated in neuronal tissue engineering applications (Tan et al., 1996; Yaginuma et al., 1996; Terenghi, 1999; Loh et al., 2001; Fine et al., 2002; Galla et al., 2004).

### 23.2.5 Summary

The elusive goal in peripheral nerve regeneration is a suitable nerve guide that will promote axonal regeneration over gaps of greater than 3 cm in humans. Many groups are studying the traditional tissue-engineering paradigm: scaffolds, cells, and growth factors. It is hopeful that a biodegradable nerve guide attaining the best mechanical properties which concurrently promotes nerve regeneration will be developed in the near future.

## 23.3   Spinal Cord Repair

### 23.3.1   Injuries and Treatments

The incidence of spinal cord injuries (SCI) in the United States has reached 11,000 new cases per year (Center, N.S.C.I.S., 2004); approximately 450,000 individuals already live with a spinal cord injury in the United States (Anonymous, http://www.spinalinjury. net/html/_spinal_cord_101.html). Motor vehicle accidents are the main cause of SCI (41%), followed by knife and gunshot injuries (22%), falls (21%), and recreational activities (8%) (Becker et al., 2003). Eighty percent of the cases occur in males (Becker et al., 2003; Talac et al., 2004), and 55% of the cases occur at ages between 16 and 30 years old (Center, N.S.C.I.S., 2004).

   Multiple health problems, such as recurrent kidney stones, urinary tract infection, pressure sores, and cardiac and respiratory dysfunction, arise as a result of the loss of sensory and motor functions in regions below the level of the injury (Talac et al., 2004). Pneumonia, pulmonary emboli, and septicemia are the leading causes of death in individuals that survive the initial spinal cord injury (Becker et al., 2003).

### 23.3.2   Pathophysiology of a Spinal Cord Injury

A spinal cord injury is characterized by the progressive destruction of spinal cord tissue (Norenberg et al., 2004; Talac et al., 2004). In the initial impact, which most commonly occurs in the form of a compression or contusion of the spinal cord tissue, fragments of bone, vertebral disc, or ligament affect axons, neurons, glial cells and blood vessels (Becker et al., 2003). The initial damage triggers focal hemorrhage, local edema, vasospasm, and the loss of microcirculation (Becker et al., 2003; Norenberg et al., 2004). The ischemia expands to the surrounding tissue, leading to additional neuronal death (Becker et al., 2003). Cytotoxic extracellular levels of excitatory amino acids such as glutamate and free radicals are reached after the impact (Norenberg et al., 2004; Talac et al., 2004). An inflammatory response that includes the infiltration of neutrophils, monocytes and lymphocytes to the site of the injury is observed 24 h after the initial insult (Norenberg et al., 2004; Talac et al., 2004). Cells far beyond the original lesion are affected in both antegrade and retrograde directions. Large cystic regions are formed surrounded by scar tissue (Profyris et al., 2004).

### 23.3.3  Nonpermissive Environment for Nerve Regeneration

Unlike the peripheral nervous system, the central nervous system has a limited capacity of regeneration following injury. As regenerating axons reach the proximity of the injury, the axons cease to grow. The inability for axons to regenerate in the site of injury have been attributed to the presence of chemical inhibitors and to the formation of a glial scar (Fawcett and Asher, 1999; Hermanns et al., 2001; McKerracher, 2001; Jacobs and Fehlings, 2003; Lee et al., 2003). Myelin associated inhibitors such as Nogo-A, myelin-associated glycoprotein (MAG), and oligodendrocyte myelin glycoprotein (OMgp) cause the collapse of the growth cones (McKerracher, 2001; Jacobs and Fehlings, 2003; Lee et al., 2003). However, using an *in vitro* system of adult dorsal root ganglion (DRG) in a gradient of agreccan, Tom and colleagues (2004) found that the induced dystrophic endings are dynamic and could possibly be "reawakened into a regenerative state".

Many different types of cells such as reactive astrocytes, meningeal cells, oligodendrocyte precursor cells, and inflammatory cells, contribute to the formation of the glial scar (Fawcett and Asher, 1999; McKerracher, 2001; Jacobs and Fehlings, 2003). The inability of axons to regenerate through the glial scar (composed mainly of reactive astrocytes and proteoglycans) was attributed for many years to the physical barrier presented by the scar (Fitch and Silver, 1997; Stichel et al., 1998; Silver and Miller, 2004). However, it appears that proteoglycans present in the scar (e.g., chondroitin sulfate proteoglycans: CSPGs) actually inhibit axonal regrowth (Fitch and Silver, 1997; Jacobs and Fehlings, 2003; Talac et al., 2004). Astrocytes in the glial scar produce four types of proteoglycans: heparan sulfate proteoglycan (HSPG), dermatan sulfate proteoglycan (DSPG), keratan sulfate proteoglycan (KSPG), and chondroitin sulfate proteoglycan (CSPG) (Silver and Miller, 2004). CSPGs are produced within 24 h after injury and remain in the injury site for months (Silver and Miller, 2004).

### 23.3.4  Models of Spinal Cord Injury Used in Animal Research

Animal models of spinal cord injury have been used to understand the pathology of spinal cord injury and to devise strategies for spinal cord repair. Contusion and transection are two widely used models in spinal cord injury research. Another model not discussed in this chapter involves the partial transection (i.e., hemisection) of the spinal cord (Bunge, 2001).

#### 23.3.4.1  Contusion Model

A contusion or compression is the most common type of spinal cord injury observed in humans (Talac et al., 2004). Different methods have been devised to reproducibly create this type of injury in animal models and include a "surgical spring-loaded clip" and a computer-controlled impactor (Talac et al., 2004).

#### 23.3.4.2  Transection Model

In this model of spinal cord injury, the spinal cord is completely transected and, if necessary, a small section (1 to 3 mm) of the spinal cord may be removed (Talac et al., 2004). A common transection model was introduced by Bunge and involves a transection of the rat spinal cord at the T8 level and the removal of T9-11 levels (Talac et al., 2004).

### 23.3.5 Biomaterials in SCI Research

Among other uses, biodegradable and nonbiodegradable polymeric materials have been examined in spinal cord injury research in the form of a sealant for injured membranes, as tubular conduits aimed to guide regeneration across the transected spinal cord, and as sponges or gels that could potentially reduce glial scar formation. Neurotrophic factors have been incorporated into some of these biomaterials to further improve axonal regrowth.

#### 23.3.5.1 Native Materials

Collagen (Liu et al., 1997, 2001; Taylor et al., 2004), alginate (Kataoka et al., 2004), fibrin (Taylor et al., 2004), and poly-β-hydroxybutyrate (Hazari et al., 1999) are examples of natural materials that have been tested in spinal cord research. Liu and colleagues (1997, 2001) observed axonal regrowth through a collagen guidance channel used to bridge the rat spinal cord and the nerve root (1997, 2001). Alginate sponges demonstrated a reduction in connective tissue scar formation in a completely transected rat spinal cord injury model (Kataoka et al., 2004). Alginate has also been used to encapsulate fibroblasts modified to produce brain-derived neurotrophic factor (BDNF) in the site of injury (Tobias et al., 2001). A heparin-based delivery system was designed for the cell-mediated delivery of NT-3 from fibrin gel (Taylor et al., 2004). Fibers of poly-β-hydroxybutyrate (PHB) (a biodegradable polymer of bacterial and algae origin; Hazari et al., 1999) coated with an alginate hydrogel containing fibronectin were implanted in a cervical spinal cord injury in adult rats (Novikov et al., 2002). PHB fibers demonstrated improved neuronal survival in comparison with the implantation of only alginate hydrogel or fibronectin.

#### 23.3.5.2 Synthetic and Biodegradable Polymers

##### 23.3.5.2.1 Poly(ethylene) Glycol

Polyethylene glycol (PEG) is a membrane fusogen (Luo et al., 2002). Donaldson and Borgens studied the topical application of PEG to seal the physically damaged cell membrane and to reverse the permeabilization produced by the injury to the spinal cord (Shi and Borgens, 1999; Borgens and Shi, 2000; Borgens et al., 2002; Donaldson et al., 2002). Both *in vitro* and *in vivo* studies using adult guinea pig spinal cords demonstrated an increase in nerve impulse conduction after treating the injured spinal cord membranes for 2 min with a 50% PEG solution prepared in distilled water (Shi and Borgens, 2000).

##### 23.3.5.2.2 Poly(α-hydroxy acids) (PLGA, PLA)

Gautier and colleagues studied the *in vitro* and *in vivo* degradation of guidance channels prepared from poly(D,L-lactic-co-glycolic acid) and poly(D,L-lactic acid) (Gautier et al., 1998). Guidance channels are thought to minimize scar tissue formation and contribute to the accumulation of growth promoting molecules in the injury site (Oudega et al., 2001). Channels that mimic spinal cord tracts could also be incorporated into these tubular structures (Friedman et al., 2002). The authors concluded that PLGA is not suitable for spinal cord applications due to the fast resorption of this polymer and the high degree of swelling that could potentially lead to the compression of the spinal cord stumps (Gautier et al., 1998). During the 10 weeks of observation, a slower degradation rate and less water absorption was obtained in guidance channels made of poly(D,L-lactic acid) (Gautier et al., 1998). In another study, guidance channels prepared using poly(D,L-lactic acid) and a mixture of poly(L-lactic acid) and 10% poly(L-lactic acid) oligomers were implanted into a 3- to 4-mm gap created at the T8–T9 level of a rat spinal cord (Oudega et al., 2001).

Although axons were observed to grow into the channel during the first 2 months of implantation, later time points show that the axons either retracted or died (Oudega et al., 2001). The collapse of the tube walls may have contributed to the loss of axons at the latest time points (Oudega et al., 2001). Patist and colleagues studied the suitability of a freeze-dried poly(D,L-lactic acid) foam containing BDNF in promoting regeneration in the transected adult rat thoracic spinal cord (Patist et al., 2004).

### 23.3.5.2.3  *Synthetic Nondegradable Polymers*

Poly(2-hydroxyethyl methacrylate) (pHEMA) hydrogels containing longitudinally oriented channels have been designed for entubulation strategies (Flynn et al., 2003). Nerve growth factor (NGF) has been bound to the pHEMA gels and the bioactivity of the hydrogel has been tested *in vitro* using PC-12 cells (Kapur and Shoichet, 2003). A poly(2-hydroxyethyl methacrylate-co-methyl methacrylate) (pHEMA-MMA) hydrogel guidance channel was implanted into a T8 transected spinal cord in adult Sprague–Dawley rats; the hydrogel supported the regeneration of brainstem motor axons (Tsai et al., 2004). In another study, a biocompatible hydrogel prepared from poly[N-(2-hydroxy-propyl)methacrylamide] (pHPMA) (NeuroGel™) and containing RGD peptides when implanted into a completely transected spinal cord reduced the necrosis and cavitation in the site of lesion (Woerly and Pinet, 2001). The same hydrogel (NeuroGel™) when implanted into the completely transected cat spinal cord, reduced cavitation and allowed angiogenesis (Woerly et al., 2004).

### 23.3.6  Neurotrophic Factors

Neurotrophic factors are growth factors that promote the growth and survival of neurons during development (Jones et al., 2001). Treatment with neutrophic factors reduced axonal degeneration and further promotes regeneration in spinal cord injury models (Oudega and Hagg, 1999; Sayer et al., 2002). In a spinal cord injury, neurotrophins can direct the growth of axons into the site of injury, which contains high concentrations of one or more growth factors delivered by continuous infusion (Oudega and Hagg, 1999; Novikov et al., 2002), direct injection (Sayer et al., 2002), and incorporation into a gel or scaffold (Oudega and Hagg, 1999; Patist et al., 2004; Taylor et al., 2004). NGF (Oudega and Hagg, 1999; Sayer et al., 2002), NT-3 (Oudega and Hagg, 1999; Sayer et al., 2002), and BDNF (Oudega and Hagg, 1999; Sayer et al., 2002), among others, have been tested in animal models of spinal cord injury. Each neurotrophic factor appears to stimulate the growth of specific axonal populations. For instance, the infusion of NGF for 2 weeks into a spinal cord injury promoted sensory axon growth (Oudega and Hagg, 1999). NT-3 elicited the growth of corticospinal axons after injection into a rat spinal cord injury (Oudega and Hagg, 1999). A localized and sustained delivery of high concentrations of neurotrophic factors have been achieved using *ex vivo* gene therapy which involves the removal of cells from a host, the genetic modification of these cells, and the transplantation of these genetically modified cells back into the host (Jones et al., 2001). In addition, NGF has been successfully encapsulated in biodegradable micro-spheres for CNS applications (Cao and Shoichet, 1999).

### 23.3.7  Cellular Therapies in Spinal Cord Repair

Cellular grafts have been transplanted into the site of injury to replace the spinal nervous tissue lost. The transplantation strategy should promote the survival and migration of the implanted cells, and in the case of stem cells, also their differentiation. Cell transplantation therapies tested for spinal cord injury repair include the use of olfactory ensheathing cells, Schwann cells, neural, and embryonic stem cells. *Ex vivo* gene therapy provides an alternative for the localized delivery of neurotrophic factors using genetically engineered cells.

### 23.3.7.1 *Olfactory Ensheathing Cells (OEC)*

OEC, originally described as Schwann cells, can be obtained from the nasal olfactory bulb or from the olfactory mucosa (Franklin, 2003; Jones et al., 2003; Barnett, 2004; Barnett and Riddell, 2004). OEC have been shown to myelinate peripheral nerves especially in the presence of meningeal cells (Franklin, 2003). In order to monitor the migratory ability of olfactory ensheathing cells, Lee and colleagues labeled OEC with superparamagnetic nanoparticles (Lee et al., 2004). After implanting the OEC in a completely transected spinal cord of female Sprague–Dawley rats, they concluded that the OEC were not able to cross the host/graft interface (Lee et al., 2004). OEC is seen as a substitute for Schwann cells in cell transplantation therapies for areas in which Schwann cell migration and remyelination is inhibited by the presence of astrocytes (Franklin, 2003; Barnett, 2004; Barnett and Riddell, 2004). For a review of OEC and OEC in the treatment of CNS injury, please refer to Barnett (2004), and Barnett and Riddell (2004).

### 23.3.7.2 *Schwann Cells (SCs)*

The implantation of peripheral nerves into a transected spinal cord and the growth of axons into the implanted nerve led to the theory that a suitable environment is essential for axonal growth in an injured spinal cord (Bunge, 2001). Schwann cells (SCs), known to contribute to the supportive environment present in peripheral nerves, became a substitute for the peripheral nerve bridge. SCs contribute to the regeneration by producing growth factors, cell adhesion molecules, and extracellular matrix components (Jones et al., 2003). SCs, when implanted into the injured rat spinal cord, can produce axon regeneration and myelination within the region of implantation (Jones et al., 2003). Schwann cells have been incorporated in poly($\alpha$-hydroxyacid) guidance channels in the transected adult rat spinal cord (Gautier et al., 1998; Oudega et al., 2001). Although axons were observed to grow into the channel, the collapse of the tube impeded further regeneration.

Combined strategies have been devised to overcome the failure of axons to grow beyond the SCs graft (Bunge, 2001). Combined strategies that involve demyelination of areas around the injury and Schwann cell transplantation increased the migration of implanted Schwann cells and improved axonal regeneration (Azanchi et al., 2004). In another study, the administration of cyclic adenosine monophosphate combined with Schwann cell transplantation promoted the growth of supraspinal axons and improved function after a thoracic (T8) contusion injury in adult rats (Pearse et al., 2004).

### 23.3.7.3 *Stem Cells*

Neural stem cells and embryonic stem cells have been proposed and examined as a possible cellular therapy for SCI. Embryonic stem cells are pluripotent cells able to differentiate into the various cell types of the body. McDonald and colleagues transplanted embryonic stem cells nine days after producing a contusion in a rat spinal cord and demonstrated that the implanted cells differentiated into astrocytes, oligodendrocytes, and neurons (McDonald et al., 2004). In another study, embryonic stem cells implanted into the spinal cord of adult rat 3 days after chemical demyelination differentiated mainly into oligodendrocytes (Liu et al., 2000).

Neural stem cells isolated from embryonic and adult rats when implanted into the injured rat spinal cord differentiated into the glial lineage (Cao et al., 2001). In another study, neural progenitor cells injected intravenously migrated to the injured spinal cord and differentiated into neurons, astrocytes, and oligodendrocytes (Fujiwara et al., 2004).

### 23.3.7.4 Genetically Engineered Cells

*Ex vivo* gene therapy has been employed for the localized delivery of high concentrations of neurotrophins into the site of injury. Fibroblasts and immortalized neural stem cells have been genetically engineered to produce BDNF, NGF, and NT-3. In the absence of immune suppression, BDNF-producing fibroblasts encapsulated in alginate-poly-L-ornithine survived for at least 4 weeks after transplantation into a rat cervical spinal cord injury (Tobias et al., 2001).

Fibroblasts and immortalized neural stem cells genetically engineered to produce NGF and NT-3 when implanted in adult rats with a T8 hemisection injury demonstrated improved neuronal survival (Himes et al., 2001). In another study, fibroblasts were genetically modified to produce NGF (Grill et al., 1997). All of these studies demonstrated the potential of gene therapy in spinal cord injury repair.

### 23.3.8 Summary

The successful repair of the injured spinal cord will likely require a combinatorial strategy that involves the use of agents that promote axonal growth and the elimination or neutralization of the inhibitory cues. In cases of extensive neural tissue loss, the implantation of stem cells or neural progenitor cells offers a strategy to replenish the glia and/or neurons lost. An important issue that needs to be resolved is the inability of the regenerating axons to emerge from the graft.

## 23.4 Challenges in Neural Tissue Engineering

The field of tissue engineering is a rapidly growing and exciting field. Neural tissue engineering is a relatively newcomer to the field of tissue engineering, but extensive research is being conducted in this area. Both PNS and CNS repair are challenging to tissue engineering. Long gaps are still unable to be bridged with synthetic nerve guides. The future trend of PNS repair is towards cell therapy, gene therapy, and drug delivery. Novel biomaterials with tailored mechanical properties and degradation rates are needed. For spinal cord injury, the challenges are even more daunting. The design of novel hydrogels that can encapsulate cells or deliver drugs to the injury are among the most promising treatments. Further elucidation of spinal cord repair, however, is needed in order to design a tissue-engineered system for SCI repair.

## References

Anonymous, Spinal cord 101, last accessed November 1, 2005 at http://www.spinalinjury.net/html/_spinal_cord_101.html

Ansselin, A.D., Fink, T., and Davey, D.F., Peripheral nerve regeneration through nerve guides seeded with adult Schwann cells, *Neuropathol. Appl. Neurobiol.*, **23** (5), 387–398 (1997).

Ansselin, A.D., Fink, T., and Davey, D.F., An alternative to nerve grafts in peripheral nerve repair: nerve guides seeded with adult Schwann cells, *Acta Chir. Aust.*, **30** (S147), 19–24 (1998).

Archibald, S.J., Krarup, C., Shefner, J., Li, S.T., and Madison, R.D., A collagen-based nerve guide conduit for peripheral nerve repair: an electrophysiological study of nerve regeneration in rodents and nonhuman primates, *J. Comp. Neurol.*, **306** (4), 685–696 (1991).

Arsenijevic, Y., Weiss, S., Schneider, B., and Aebischer, P., Insulin-like growth factor-I is necessary for neural stem cell proliferation and demonstrates distinct actions of epidermal growth factor and fibroblast growth factor-2, *J. Neurosci.*, **21** (18), 7194–7202 (2001).

Azanchi, R., Bernal, G., Gupta, R., and Keirstead, H.S., Combined demyelination plus Schwann cell transplantation therapy increases spread of cells and axonal regeneration following contusion injury, *J. Neurotrauma*, **21** (6), 775–788 (2004).

Babensee, J.E., McIntire, L.V., and Mikos, A.G., Growth factor delivery for tissue engineering, *Pharm. Res.*, **17** (5), 497–504 (2000).

Bach, L.A., Leeding, K.S., and Leng, S.L., Regulation of IGF-binding protein-6 by dexamethasone and IGFs in PC12 rat phaechromocytoma cells, *J. Endocrinol.*, **155** (2), 225–232 (1997).

Badylak, S.F., Record, R., Lindberg, K., Hodde, J., and Park, K., Small intestinal submucosa: a substrate for in vitro cell growth, *J. Biomater. Sci. Polym. Ed.*, **9** (8), 863–878 (1998).

Balgude, A.P., Yu, X., Szymanski, A., and Bellamkonda, R.V., Agarose gel stiffness determines rate of DRG neurite extension in 3D cultures, *Biomaterials*, **22** (10), 1077–1084 (2001).

Barnett, S.C., Olfactor ensheathing cells: unique glial cell types?, *J. Neurotrauma*, **21** (4), 375–382 (2004).

Barnett, S.C. and Riddell, J.S., Olfactory ensheathing cells (OECs) and the treatment of CNS injury: advantages and possible caveats, *J. Anat.*, **204**, 57–67 (2004).

Becker, D., Sadowsky, C.L., and McDonald, J.W., Restoring function after spinal cord injury, *The Neurologist*, **9**, 1–15 (2003).

Bender, M., Bennett, J.M., Waddell, R., Doctor, J.S., and Marra, K.G., Multi-channeled biodegradable polymer/cultispher composite nerve guides, *Biomaterials*, **25** (7–8), 1269–1278 (2004).

Borgens, R.B. and Shi, R., Immediate recovery from spinal cord injury through molecular repair of nerve membranes with polyethylene glycol, *FASEB*, **14**, 27–35 (2000).

Borgens, R., Shi, R., and Bohnert, D., Behavioral recovery from spinal cord injury following delayed application of polyethylene glycol, *J. Exp. Biol.*, **205**, 1–12 (2002).

Bryan, D.J., Holway, A.H., Wang, K.K., Silva, A.E., Trantolo, D.J., Wise, D., and Summerhayes, I.C., Influence of glial growth factor and Schwann cells in a bioresorbable guidance channel on peripheral nerve regeneration, *Tissue Eng.*, **6** (2), 129–138 (2000).

Bunge, M.B., Bridging areas of injury in the spinal cord, *The Neuroscientist*, **7** (4), 325–339 (2001).

Camarata, P.J., Suryanarayanan, R., Turner, D.A., Parker, R.G., and Ebner, T.J., Sustained release of nerve growth factor from biodegradable polymer microspheres, *Neurosurgery*, **30** (3), 313–319 (1992).

Cao, X. and Shoichet, M.S., Delivering neuroactive molecules from biodegradable microspheres for application in central nervous system disorders, *Biomaterials*, **20**, 329–339 (1999).

Cao, Q.-l., Zhang, Y.P., Howard, R.M., Walters, W.M., Tsoulfas, P., and Whittemore, S.R., Pluripotent stem cells engrafted into the normal or lesioned adult rat spinal cord are restricted to a glial lineage, *Exp. Neurol.*, **167**, 48–58 (2001).

Ceballos, D., Navarro, X., Dubey, N., Wendelschafer-Crabb, G., Kennedy, W.R., and Tranquillo, R.T., Magnetically aligned collagen gel filling a collagen nerve guide improves peripheral nerve regeneration, *Exp. Neurol.*, **158** (2), 290–300 (1999).

Center, N.S.C.I.S., Spinal cord injury: fact and figures at a glance, *J. Spinal Cord Med.*, **27** (2) (2004).

Chen, Z.L. and Strickland, S., Laminin gamma1 is critical for Schwann cell differentiation, axon myelination, and regeneration in peripheral nerve, *J. Cell Biol.*, **163**, 889–899 (2003).

Cheng, H.-L. and Feldman, E.L., Insulin-like growth factor-I (IGF-I) and IGF binding protein-5 in Schwann cell differentiation, *J. Cell. Physiol.*, **171**, 161–167 (1997).

Cleland, J.L. et al., The stability of recombinant human growth hormone in poly(lactic-co-glycolic) (PLGA) microspheres, *Pharm. Res.*, **14** (4), 420–425 (1997).

Collier, J.H., Camp, J.P., Hudson, T.W., and Schmidt, C.E., Synthesis and characterization of polypyrrole–hyaluronic acid composite biomaterials for tissue engineering applications, *J. Biomed. Mater. Res.*, **50** (4), 574–584 (2000).

den Dunnen, W.F. and Meek, M.F., Sensory nerve function and auto-mutilation after reconstruction of various gap lengths with nerve guides and autologous nerve grafts, *Biomaterials*, **22** (10), 1171–1176 (2001).

den Dunnen, W.F., Stokroos, I., Blaauw, E.H., Holwerda, A., Pennings, A.J., Robinson, P.H., and Schakenraad, J.M., Light-microscopic and electron-microscopic evaluation of short-term nerve regeneration using a biodegradable poly(DL-lactide-epsilon-caprolacton) nerve guide, *J. Biomed. Mater. Res.*, **31** (1), 105–115 (1996).

Donaldson, J., Shi, R., and Borgens, R., Polyethylene glycol rapidly restores physiological functions in damaged sciatic nerves of guinea pigs, *Neurosurgery*, **50**, 147–157 (2002).

Dubey, N., Letourneau, P.C., and Tranquillo, R.T., Neuronal contact guidance in magnetically aligned fibrin gels: effect of variation in gel mechano-structural properties, *Biomaterials*, **22** (10), 1065–1075 (2001).

Fansa, H. and Keilhoff, G., Comparison of different biogenic matrices seeded with cultured Schwann cells for bridging peripheral nerve defects, *Neurol. Res.*, **26** (2), 167–173 (2004).

Fansa, H., Keilhoff, G., Wolf, G., and Schneider, W., Tissue engineering of peripheral nerves: a comparison of venous and acellular muscle grafts with cultured Schwann cells, *Plast. Reconstr. Surg.*, **107** (2), 485–494 (2001).

Fawcett, J.W. and Asher, R.A., The glial scar and central nervous system repair, *Brain Res. Bull.*, **49** (6), 377–391 (1999).

Fine, E.G., Decosterd, I., Papaloizos, M., Zurn, A.D., and Aebischer, P., GDNF and NGF released by synthetic guidance channels support sciatic nerve regeneration across a long gap, *Eur. J. Neurosci.*, **15** (4), 589–601 (2002).

Fitch, M.T. and Silver, J., Glial cell extracellular matrix: boundaries for axon growth in development and regeneration, *Cell Tissue Res.*, **290**, 379–384 (1997).

Flynn, L., Dalton, P.D., and Shoichet, M.S., Fiber templating of poly(2-hydroxyethyl methacrylate) for neural tissue engineering, *Biomaterials*, **24**, 4265–4272 (2003).

Franklin, R.J.M., Remyelination by transplanted olfactory ensheathing cells, *Anat. Rec.*, **271B**, 71–76 (2003).

Friedman, J.A., Windebank, A.J., Moore, M.J., Spinner, R.J., Currier, B.L., and Yaszemski, M.J., Biodegradable polymer grafts for surgical repair of the injured spinal cord, *Neurosurgery*, **51**, 742–752 (2002).

Fujiwara, Y., et al., Intravenously injected neural progenitor cells of transgenic rats can migrate to the injured spinal cord and differentiate into neurons, astrocytes and oligodendrocytes, *Neurosci. Lett.*, **366**, 287–291 (2004).

Galla, T.J., Vedecnik, S.V., Halbgewachs, J., Steinmann, S., Friedrich, C., and Stark, G.B., Fibrin/Schwann cell matrix in poly-epsilon-caprolactone conduits enhancing guided nerve regeneration, *Int. J. Artif. Organs*, **27**, 127–136 (2004).

Gautier, S.E., Oudega, M., Fragoso, M., Chapon, P., Plant, G.W., Bunge, M.B., and Parel, J.-M., Poly(alpha-hydroxyacids) for application in the spinal cord: resorbability and biocompatibility with adult rat Schwann cells and spinal cord, *J. Biomed. Mater. Res.*, **42**, 642–654 (1998).

Gibby, W.A., Koerber, H.R., and Horch, K.W., A quantitative evaluation of suture and tubulization nerve repair techniques, *J. Neurosurg.*, **58** (4), 574–579 (1983).

Glasby, M.A., Gschmeissner, S., Hitchcock, R.J., and Huang, C.L., Regeneration of the sciatic nerve in rats. The effect of muscle basement membrane, *J. Bone Joint Surg. Br.*, **68** (5), 829–833 (1986a).

Glasby, M.A., Gschmeissner, S.E., Huang, C.L., and De Souza, B.A., Degenerated muscle grafts used for peripheral nerve repair in primates, *J. Hand Surg. [Br]*, **11** (3), 347–351 (1986b).

Gouhier, C., Chalon, S., Venier-Julienne, M.C., Bodard, S., Benoit, J., Besnard, J., and Guilloteau, D., Neuroprotection of nerve growth factor-loaded microspheres on the D2 dopaminergic receptor positive-striatal neurones in quinolinic acid-lesioned rats: a quantitative autoradiographic assessment with iodobenzamide, *Neurosci. Lett.*, **288** (1), 71–75 (2000).

Greene, L.A. and Tischler, A.S., Establishment of a noradrenergic clonal line of rat adrenal pheochromocytoma cells which respond to nerve growth factor, *Cell Biol.*, **73** (7), 2424–2428 (1976).

Grill, R.J., Blesch, A., and Tuszynski, M.H., Robust growth of chronically injured spinal cord axons induced by grafts of genetically modified NGF-secreting cells, *Exp. Neurol.*, **148**, 444–452 (1997).

Hadlock, T., Sundback, C., Hunter, D., Cheney, M., and Vacanti, J.P., A polymer foam conduit seeded with Schwann cells promotes guided peripheral nerve regeneration, *Tissue Eng.*, **6** (2), 119–127 (2000).

Hadlock, T.A., Sundback, C.A., Hunter, D.A., Vacanti, J.P., and Cheney, M.L., A new artificial nerve graft containing rolled Schwann cell monolayers, *Microsurgery*, **21** (3), 96–101 (2001).

Hadlock, T., Sundback, C., Koka, R., Hunter, D., Cheney, M., and Vacanti, J.P., A novel, biodegradable polymer conduit delivers neurotrophins and promotes nerve regeneration, *Laryngoscope*, **109** (9), 1412–1416 (1999).

Hazari, A., Johansson-Ruden, G., Junemo-Bostrom, K., Ljungberg, C., Terenghi, G., Green, C., and Wiberg, M., A new resorbable wrap-around implant as an alternative nerve repair technique, *J. Hand Surg.*, **24B** (3), 291–295 (1999), British and European Volume.

Heath, C.A. and Rutkowski, G.E., The development of bioartificial nerve grafts for peripheral-nerve regeneration, *Trends Biotechnol.*, **16** (4), 163–168 (1998).

Hermanns, S., Klapka, N., and Muller, H.W., The collagenous lesion scar — an obstacle for axonal regeneration in brain and spinal cord injury, *Restor. Neurol. Neurosci.*, **19**, 139–148 (2001).

Himes, B.T., Liu, Y., Solowska, J.M., Snyder, E.Y., Fischer, I., and Tessler, A., Transplants of cells genetically modified to express Neurotrophin-3 rescue axotomized Clarke's nucleus neurons after spinal cord hemisection in adult rats, *J. Neurosci. Res.*, **65**, 549–564 (2001).

Hutmacher, D.W., Scaffold design and fabrication technologies for engineering tissues-state of the art and future perspectives, *J. Biomater. Sci. Polym. Ed.*, **12** (1), 107–124 (2001).

Jacobs, W.B. and Fehlings, M.G., The molecular basis of neural regeneration, *Neurosurgery*, **53**, 943–949 (2003).

Jesson, K.R. and Mirsky, R., Schwann cells and their precursors emerge as major regulators of nerve development, *Trends Neurosci.*, **22** (9), 402–410 (1999).

Jones, D.G., Anderson, E.R., and Galvin, K.A., Spinal cord regeneration: moving tentatively towards new perspectives, *NeuroRehabilitation*, **18**, 339–351 (2003).

Jones, L.L., Oudega, M., Bunge, M.B., and Tuszynski, M.H., Neurotrophic factors, cellular bridges and gene therapy for spinal cord injury, *J. Physiol.*, **533**, 83–89 (2001).

Kakinoki, R., Nishijima, N., Ueba, Y., Oka, M., and Yamamuro, T., Relationship between axonal regeneration and vascularity in tubulation — an experimental study in rats, *Neurosci. Res.*, **23** (1), 35–45 (1995).

Kapur, T. and Shoichet, M.S., Chemically-bound nerve growth factor for neural tissue engineering applications, *J. Biomater. Sci., Polym. Ed.*, **14** (4), 383–394 (2003).

Kapur, T.A. and Shoichet, M.S., Immobilized concentration gradients of nerve growth factor guide neurite outgrowth, *J. Biomed. Mater. Res.*, **68A** (2), 235–243 (2004).

Kataoka, K. et al., Alginate enhances elongation of early regenerating axons in spinal cord of young rats, *Tissue Eng.*, **10** (3/4), 493–504 (2004).

Khang, G., Cho, J.C., Lee, J.W., Rhee, J.M., and Lee, H.B., Preparation and characterization of Japanese encephalitis virus vaccine loaded poly(L-lactide-co-glycolide) microspheres for oral immunization, *Biomed. Mater. Eng.*, **9** (1), 49–59 (1999).

Kimpinski, K. and Mearow, K., Neurite growth promotion by nerve growth factor and insulin-like growth factor-1 in cultured adult sensory neurons: role of phosphoinositide 3-kinase and nitrogen activated protein kinase, *J. Neurosci. Res.*, **63**, 486–499 (2001).

King, T.W. and Patrick, C.W. Jr., Development and in vitro characterization of vascular endothelial growth factor (VEGF)-loaded poly(D,L-lactic-co-glycolic acid)/poly(ethylene glycol) microspheres using a solid encapsulation/single emulsion/solvent extraction technique, *J. Biomed. Mater. Res.*, **51**, 383–390 (2000).

Krewson, C.E., Dause, R., Mak, M., and Saltzman, W.M., Stabilization of nerve growth factor in controlled release polymers and in tissue, *J. Biomater. Sci. Polym. Ed.*, **8** (2), 103–117 (1996).

Lam, X.M., Duenas, E.T., Daugherty, A.L., Levin, N., and Cleland, J.L., Sustained release of recombinant human insulin-like growth factor-I for treatment of diabetes, *J. Controlled Rel.*, **67** (2–3), 281–292 (2000).

Lee, I.-H. et al., In vivo magnetic resonance tracking of olfactory ensheathing glia grafted into the rat spinal cord, *Exp. Neurol.*, **187**, 509–516 (2004).

Lee, D.H.S., Strittmatter, S.M., and Sah, D.W.Y., Targeting the nogo receptor to treat central nervous system injuries, *Nature*, **2**, 1–7 (2003).

Lee, S.K. and Wolfe, S.W., Peripheral nerve injury and repair, *J. Am. Acad. Orthop. Surg.*, **8** (4), 243–252 (2000).

Levi, A.D. and Bunger, R.P., Studies of myelin formation after transplantation of human Schwann cells into the severe combined immunodeficient mouse, *Exp. Neurol.*, **130** (1), 41–52 (1994).

Li, S.T., Archibald, S.J., Krarup, C., and Madison, R.D., Peripheral nerve repair with collagen conduits, *Clin. Mater.*, **9** (3–4), 195–200 (1992).

Lindberg, K. and Badylak, S.F., Porcine small intestinal submucosa (SIS): a bioscaffold supporting in vitro primary human epidermal cell differentiation and synthesis of basement membrane proteins, *Burns*, **27** (3), 254–266 (2001).

Liu, S., Peulve, P., Jin, O., Boisset, N., Tiollier, J., Said, G., and Tadie, M., Axonal regrowth through collagen tubes bridging the spinal cord to nerve roots, *J. Neurosci. Res.*, **49**, 425–432 (1997).

Liu, S., Qu, Y., Stewart, T.J., Howard, M.J., Chakrabortty, S., Holekamp, T.F., and McDonald, J.W., Embryonic stem cells differentiate into oligodendrocytes and myelinate in culture and after spinal cord transplantation, *Proc. Natl. Acad. Sci.*, **97**, 6126–6131 (2000).

Liu, S., Said, G. and Tadie, M., Regrowth of the rostral spinal axons into the caudal ventral roots through a collagen tube implanted into hemisected adult rat spinal cord, *Neurosurgery*, **49** (1), 143–151 (2001).

Loh, N.K., Woerly, S., Bunt, S.M., Wilton, S.D., and Harvey, A.R., The regrowth of axons within tissue defects in the CNS is promoted by implanted hydrogel matrices that contain BDNF and CNTF producing fibroblasts, *Exp. Neurol.*, **170** (1), 72–84 (2001).

Lu, L., Stamatas, G.N., and Mikos, A.G., Controlled release of transforming growth factor beta-1 from biodegradable polymer microparticles, *J. Biomed. Mater. Res.*, **50**, 440–451 (2000).

Luciano, R.M., de Carvalho Zavaglia, C.A., and de Rezende Duek, E.A., Preparation of bioabsorbable nerve guide tubes, *Artif. Organs*, **24** (3), 206–208 (2000).

Lundborg, G., Dahlin, L.B., Danielsen, N., Gelberman, R.H., Longo, F.M., Powell, H.C., and Varon, S., Nerve regeneration in silicone chambers: influence of gap length and of distal stump components, *Exp. Neurol.*, **76** (2), 361–375 (1982).

Luo, J., Borgens, R., and Shi, R., Polyethylene glycol immediately repairs neuronal membranes and inhibits free radical production after acute spinal cord injury, *J. Neurochem.*, **83**, 471–480 (2002).

Madison, R.D., Da Silva, C.F., and Dikkes, P., Entubulation repair with protein additives increases the maximum nerve gap distance successfully bridged with tubular prostheses, *Brain Res.*, **447** (2), 325–334 (1988).

Madison, R.D., Da Silva, C.F., Dikkes, P., Sidman, R.L., and Chio, T.-H., Peripheral nerve regeneration with entubulation repair: comparison of biodegradable nerve guides versus polyethylene tubes and the effects of a laminin-containing gel, *Exp. Neurol.*, **95** (2), 378–390 (1987).

Maquet, V., Martin, D., Malgrange, B., Franzen, R., Schoenen, J., Moonen, G., and Jerome, R., Peripheral nerve regeneration using bioresorbable macroporous scaffolds, *J. Biomed. Mater. Res.*, **52** (4), 639–651 (2000).

McDonald, J.W. et al., Repair of the injured spinal cord and the potential of embryonic stem cell transplantation, *J. Neurotrauma*, **21** (4), 383–393 (2004).

McKerracher, L., Spinal cord repair: strategies to promote axon regeneration, *Neurobiol. Dis.*, **8**, 11–18 (2001).

Meek, M.F., Varejao, A.S., and Geuna, S., Muscle grafts and alternatives for nerve repair, *J. Oral Maxillofac. Surg.*, **60** (9), 1095–1096 (2002).

Meinel, L., Illi, O.E., Zapf, J., Malfanti, M., Merkle, H.P., and Gander, B., Stabilizing insulin-like growth factor-I in poly(D,L-lactide-co-glycolide) microspheres, *J. Controlled Rel.*, **70**, 193–202 (2001).

Monnier, D., Boutillier, A.L., Giraud, P., Chiu, R., Aunis, D., Feltz, P., Zwiller, J., and Loeffler, J.P., Insulin-like growth factor-I stimulates c-fos and c-jun transcription in PC12 cells, *Mol. Cell. Endocrinol.*, **104** (2), 139–145 (1994).

Mooney, D.J. et al., Localized delivery of epidermal growth factor improves the survival of transplanted hepatocytes, *Biotech. Bioeng.*, **50**, 422–429 (1996).

Navarro, X. et al., Peripheral nerve regeneration through bioresorbable and durable nerve guides, *J. Peripher. Nerv. Syst.*, **1** (1), 53–64 (1996).

Noback, N.L., Strominger, R.J., and Demarest, R.J., *Human Nervous System: Structure and Function*, 5th ed., Williams and Wilkins (1996).

Norenberg, M.D., Smith, J., and Marcillo, A., The pathology of human spinal cord injury: defining the problems, *J. Neurotrauma*, **21** (4), 429–440 (2004).

Novikov, L.N., Novikona, L.N., Mosahebi, A., Wiberg, M., Terenghi, G., and Kellerth, J.-O., A novel biodegradable implant for neuronal rescue and regeneration after spinal-cord injury, *Biomaterials*, **23**, 3369–3376 (2002).

Nugent, M.A., Chen, O.S., and Edelman, E.R., Controlled release of fibroblast growth factor: activity in cell culture, *Mater. Res. Soc. Symp. Proc.*, **252**, 273–284 (1992).

Oudega, M., Gautier, S.E., Chapon, P., Fragoso, M., Bates, M.L., Parel, J.-M., and Bunge, M.B., Axonal regeneration into Schwann cell grafts within resorbable poly(alpha-hydroxyacid) guidance channels in the adult rat spinal cord, *Biomaterials*, **22**, 1125–1136 (2001).

Oudega, M. and Hagg, T., Neurotrophins promote regeneration of sensory axons in the adult rat spinal cord, *Brain Res.*, **818**, 431–438 (1999).

Patist, C.M., Mulder, M.B., Gautier, S.E., Maquet, V., Jerome, R., and Oudega, M., Freeze-dried poly(D,L-lactic acid) macroporous guidance scaffolds impregnated with brain-derived neurotrophic factor in the transected adult rat thoracic spinal cord, *Biomaterials*, **25**, 1569–1582 (2004).

Pean, J.M., Menei, P., Morel, O., Montero-Menei, C., and Benoit, J.-P., Intraseptal implantation of NGF-releasing microspheres promote the survival of axotomized cholinergic neurons, *Biomaterials*, **21** (20), 2097–2101 (2000).

Pean, J.M., Venier-Julienne, M.C., Boury, F., Menei, P., Denizot, B., and Benoit, J.-P., NGF release from poly(D,L-lactide-co-glycolide) microspheres. Effect of some formulation parameters on encapsulated NGF stability, *J. Control. Rel.*, **56** (1–3), 175–187 (1998).

Pearse, D.D., Pereira, F.C., Marcillo, A.E., Bates, M.L., Berrocal, Y.A., Filbin, M.T., and Bunge, M.B., cAMP and Schwann cells promote axonal growth and functional recovery after spinal cord injury, *Nat. Med.*, **10** (6), 610–616 (2004).

Pego, A.P., Poot, A.A., Grijpma, D.W., and Feijen, J., Copolymers of trimethylene carbonate and epsilon-caprolactone for porous nerve guides: synthesis and properties, *J. Biomater. Sci. Polym. Ed.*, **12** (1), 35–53 (2001).

Peter, S.J., Lu, L., Kim, D.J., Stamatas, G.N., Miller, M.J., Yaszemski, M.J., and Mikos, A.G., Effects of transforming growth factor beta-1 released from biodegradable polymer microparticles on marrow stromal osteoblasts cultured on poly(propylene fumarate) substrates, *J. Biomed. Mater. Res.*, **50**, 452–462 (2000).

Porter, S., Clark, M.B., Glaser, L., and Bunge, R.P., Schwann cells stimulated to proliferate in the absence of neurons retain full functional capability, *J. Neurosci.*, **6**, 3070–3078 (1986).

Profyris, C., Cheema, S.S., Zang, D., Azari, M.F., Boyle, K., and Petratos, S., Degenerative and regenerative mechanisms governing spinal cord injury, *Neurobiol. Dis.*, **15**, 415–436 (2004).

Richardson, T.P., Peters, M.C., Ennet, A.B., and Mooney, D.J., Polymeric system for dual growth factor delivery, *Nat. Biotech.*, **19** (11), 1029–1034 (2001).

Robinson, P.H., van der Lei, B., Hoppen, H.J., Leenslag, J.W., Pennings, A.J., and Nieuwenhuis, P., Nerve regeneration through a two-ply biodegradable nerve guide in the rat and the influence of ACTH4-9 nerve growth factor, *Microsurgery*, **12** (6), 412–419 (1991).

Rodriguez, F.J., Gomez, N., Perego, G., and Navarro, X., Highly permeable polylactide–caprolactone nerve guides enhance peripheral nerve regeneration through long gaps, *Biomaterials*, **20** (16), 1489–1500 (1999).

Rodriguez, F.J., Verdu, E., Ceballos, D., and Navarro, X., Nerve guides seeded with autologous Schwann cells improve nerve regeneration, *Exp. Neurol.*, **161** (2), 571–584 (2000).

Rosner, B.I., Siegel, R.A., Grosberg, A., and Tranquillo, R.T., Rational design of contact guiding, neurotrophic matrices for peripheral nerve regeneration, *Ann. Biomed. Eng.*, **31** (11), 1383–1401 (2003).

Russell, J.W., Cheng, H.L., and Golovoy, D., Insulin-like growth factor-I promotes myelination of peripheral sensory axons, *J. Neuropathol. Exp. Neurol.*, **59** (7), 575–584 (2000).

Rutkowski, G.E. and Heath, C.A., Development of a bioartificial nerve graft I. Design based on a reaction-diffusion model, *Biotechnol. Progr.*, **18** (2), 362–372 (2002a).

Rutkowski, G.E. and Heath, C.A., Development of a bioartificial nerve graft II. Nerve regeneration in vitro, *Biotechnol. Progr.*, **18** (2), 373–379 (2002b).

Sayer, F.T., Oudega, M., and Hagg, T., Neurotrophins reduce degeneration of injured ascending sensory and corticospinal motor axons in adult rat spinal cord, *Exp. Neurol.*, **175**, 282–296 (2002).

Schmidt, C.E., Shastri, V.R., Vacanti, J.P., and Langer, R., Stimulation of neurite outgrowth using an electrically conducting polymer, *Proc. Natl. Acad. Sci. USA*, **94**, 8948–8953 (1997).

Shi, R. and Borgens, R., Acute repair of crushed guinea pig spinal cord by polyethylene glycol, *J. Neurophysiol.*, **81** (5), 2406–2414 (1999).

Shi, R. and Borgens, R., Anatomical repair of nerve membranes in crushed mammalian spinal cord with polyethylene glycol, *J. Neurocytol.*, **29**, 633–643 (2000).

Silver, J. and Miller, J.H., Regeneration beyond the glial scar, *Nature*, **5**, 146–156 (2004).

Stichel, C.C. and Muller, H.W., The CNS lesion scar: new vistas on an old regeneration barrier, *Cell Tissue Res.*, **294**, 1–9 (1998).

Stocum, D.L., Regenerative biology and engineering: strategies for tissue restoration, *Wound Repair Regen.*, **6** (4), 276–290 (1998).

Talac, R. et al., Animal models of spinal cord injury for evaluation of tissue engineering treatment strategies, *Biomaterials*, **25**, 1505–1510 (2004).

Tan, S.A., Deglon, N., Zurn, A.D., Baetge, E.E., Bamber, B., Kato, A.C., and Aebischer, P., Rescue of motoneurons from axotomy induced cell death by polymer encapsulated cells genetically engineered to release CNTF, *Cell Trans.*, **5**, 577–587 (1996).

Taylor, S.J. III, McDonald, J.W., and Sakiyama-Elbert, S.E., Controlled release of neurotrophin-3 from fibrin gels for spinal cord injury, *J. Controlled Rel.*, **98**, 281–294 (2004).

Terenghi, G., Peripheral nerve regeneration and neurotrophic factors, *J Anat.*, **194**, 1–14 (1999).

Timmer, M., Robben, S., Muller-Ostermeyer, F., Nikkhah, G., and Grothe, C., Axonal regeneration across long gaps in silicone chambers filled with Schwann cells overexpressing high molecular weight FGF-2, *Cell Transplant.*, **12** (3), 265–277 (2003).

Tobias, C.A., Dhoot, N.O., Wheatley, M.A., Tessler, A., Murray, M., and Fischer, I., Grafting of encapsulated BDNF-producing fibroblasts into the injured spinal cord without immune suppression in adult rats, *J. Neurotrauma*, **18** (3), 287–301 (2001).

Tom, V.J., Steinmetz, M.P., Miller, J.H., Doller, C.M., and Silver, J., Studies on the development and behavior of the dystrophic growth cone, the hallmark of regeneration failure, in an in vitro model of the glial scar and after spinal cord injury, *J. Neurosci.*, **24**, 6531–6539 (2004).

Tsai, E.C., Dalton, P.D., Shoichet, M.S., and Tator, C.H., Synthetic hydrogel guidance channels facilitate regeneration of adult rat brainstem motor axons after complete spinal cord transection, *J. Neurotrauma*, **21** (6), 789–804 (2004).

Valentini, R.F., Aebischer, P., Winn, S.R., and Galletti, P.M., Collagen- and laminin-containing gels impede peripheral nerve regeneration through semipermeable nerve guidance channels, *Exp. Neurol.*, **98** (2), 350–356 (1987).

Verdu, E., Labrador, R.O., Rodriguez, F.J., Ceballos, D., Fores, J., and Navarro, X., Alignment of collagen and laminin-containing gels improve nerve regeneration within silicone tubes, *Restor. Neurol. Neurosci.*, **20** (5), 169–179 (2002).

Verrijk, R., Smolders, I.J., McVie, J.G., and Begg, A.C., Polymer-coated albumin microspheres as carriers for intravascular tumour targeting of cisplatin, *Cancer. Chemother. Pharmacol.*, **29** (2), 117–121 (1991).

Voytik-Harbin, S.L., Brightman, A.O., Kraine, M.R., Waisner, B., and Badylak, S.F., Identification of extractractable growth factors from small intestinal submucosa, *J. Cell. Biochem.*, **67**, 478–491 (1997).

Waddell, R.L., Marra, K.G., Collins, K.L., Leung, J.T., and Doctor, J.S., Using PC12 cells to evaluate poly(caprolactone) and collagenous microcarriers for applications in nerve guide fabrication, *Biotechnol. Progr.*, **19** (6), 1767–1774 (2003).

Weber, R.A., Breidenbach, W.C., Brown, R.E., Jabaley, M.E., and Mass, D.P., A randomized prospective study of polyglycolic acid conduits for digital nerve reconstruction in humans, *Plast. Reconstr. Surg.*, **106** (5), 1036–1044 (2000).

Woerly, S., Doan, V.D., Sosa, N., Vellis, J.d., and Espinosa-Jeffrey, A., Prevention of gliotic scar formation by NeuroGel allows partial endogenous repair of transected cat spinal cord, *J. Neurosci. Res.*, **75**, 262–272 (2004).

Woerly, S., Pinet, E., Robertis, L.d., Diep, D.V., and Bousmina, M., Spinal cord repair with PHPMA hydrogel containing RGD peptides (NeuroGel™), *Biomaterials*, **22**, 1095–1111 (2001).

Woerly, S., Plant, G.W., and Harvey, A.R., Neural tissue engineering: from polymer to biohybrid organs, *Biomaterials*, **17** (3), 301–310 (1996).

Yaginuma, H., Tomita, M., Takashita, N., McKay, S.E., Cardwell, C., Yin, Q.W., and Oppenheim, R.W., A novel type of programmed neuronal death in the cervical spinal cord of the chick embryo, *J. Neurosci.*, **16** (11), 3685–3703 (1996).

Yakovchenko, E., Whalin, M., Movsesyan, V., and Guroff, G., Insulin-like growth factor I receptor expression and function in nerve growth factor-differentiated PC12 cells, *J. Neurochem.*, **67** (2), 540–548 (1996).

Zachor, D., Cherkes, J.K., Fay, C.T., and Ocrant, I., Cocaine differentially inhibits neuronal differentiation and proliferation in vitro, *J. Clin. Inv.*, **93** (3), 1179–1185 (1994).

# 24

## Cardiovascular Tissue Engineering

**Priya Ramaswami and William R. Wagner**

## CONTENTS

## 24.1 Introduction

The field of tissue engineering has utilized a variety of biomaterials to facilitate tissue repair and regeneration. These polymers range from naturally derived materials and acellular tissue matrices to synthetic polymers. Although synthetic biomaterials lack the biorecognition resulting from the use of native materials, they can usually be produced with minimal batch-to-batch variations in chemical and physical parameters. In addition, synthetic biomaterials provide a number of design variables that can be adjusted for optimal mechanical, chemical, and biological properties for a given application. Design criteria for these materials include: adequate mechanical strength, controllable biodegradation rates and lack of toxic degradation products, integration into surrounding tissue without extensive inflammatory response or support of infection, adequate support of cell proliferation, differentiation, and maturation, and the potential to deliver biological molecules.

Upon implantation, biomaterial scaffolds initially function as an artificial extracellular matrix (ECM) providing mechanical and biological support similar to that provided by native ECM (Putnam and Mooney, 1996). By aiding in the initiation of the tissue regeneration process, biomaterials provide cells with a surface for adhesion and with

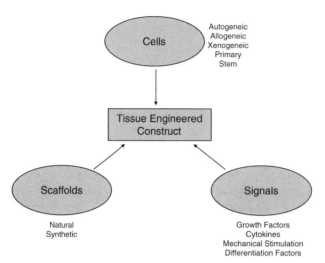

**FIGURE 24.1**
The building blocks of tissue-engineered constructs for tissue repair and regeneration.

mechanical support against *in vivo* stresses at the site of repair until the surrounding and/or new tissue can produce native ECM and take over the process of regeneration. Furthermore, while this process is occurring, the biomaterial may act to retain the delivered cells and/or factors in the defined three-dimensional space to which they were administered, thereby guiding new tissue growth at the site of injury (Kim et al., 2000a; Godbey and Atala, 2002; Tabata, 2003).

In recent years, tissue engineering research has focused on the application of growth factors, cytokines, and other molecules for the guidance of cell differentiation and growth. Progress has also been made towards the *ex vivo* mechanical stimulation of cells and constructs for improved tissue growth prior to implantation. Research in cardiovascular tissue engineering has placed special emphasis on the benefits of dynamic over static cell culture *in vitro* with the intent of subjecting cells to physical signals similar to those they will later encounter *in vivo*. The combined use of an optimal cell source, scaffold for cell delivery and physical support, and mechanical and biological signals may be a common pathway toward a viable tissue-engineered construct for cardiovascular tissue engineering (Figure 24.1). In this chapter, focus will be placed upon three areas of substantial research in cardiovascular tissue engineering: tissue engineered heart valves (TEHVs), blood vessels, and myocardium. Background on each application area will be provided together with discussion of cell sources, scaffolds, and conditioning techniques employed.

## 24.2   Tissue-Engineered Heart Valves

An estimated 87,000 heart valve replacements were performed in 2000 in the United States alone (American Heart Association: Dallas, 2005), while approximately 275,000 procedures are performed worldwide each year (Rabkin and Schoen, 2002). Heart valve disease occurs when one or more of the four heart valves cease to adequately perform their function, thereby failing to maintain unidirectional blood flow through the heart. The resultant burden on the heart leads to heart muscle dysfunction and eventual heart failure. Surgical valve repair is an accepted form of treatment, and in many cases, total valve replacement is necessary.

The first successful valve replacement procedure was performed in 1952 (Hufnagel, 1952). In the decades that have since passed, many designs for prosthetic heart valves have emerged, and valve replacement has proven to be clinically effective. Replacement devices currently include mechanical prostheses consisting of synthetic components, bioprostheses (derived from xenografts), and homografts from cadaveric tissues (Sodian et al., 2000a). Each of these valve replacements has limitations for clinical use. While mechanical valves have the advantage of durability and longevity, they are associated with a substantial risk of infection and thromboembolism (Hoerstrup et al., 2000). Therefore, patients receiving mechanical heart valve transplants are placed on anticoagulation therapy, which can result in complications such as hemorrhaging (Vongpatanasin et al., 1996). Patients receiving bioprosthetic devices generally do not require anticoagulation therapy. Furthermore, with primary valve structures derived from porcine or bovine tissue, the supply is not limited. Bioprosthestic valves, however, do exhibit structural dysfunction due to tissue deterioration over time (Schmidt and Baier, 2000). Homografts, which are derived from human cadavers, are considered more biocompatible than mechanical valves or xenografts; however, there is a limited supply of donor tissue and the possibility exists of foreign tissue rejection (Hogan and O'Brien, 2003). Furthermore, all current valve replacements lack the intrinsic ability to repair, remodel, and grow. This limit is of concern in pediatric patients who would require subsequent valve replacement with growth (Mayer, 2001).

In order to address the aforementioned shortcomings of current valve replacement technologies, researchers have turned to tissue engineering approaches to design a biocompatible, functional, living valve replacement. This replacement should have adequate mechanical and hemodynamic function, mature ECM, durability, and should not illicit immunogenic and/or inflammatory responses. The growth and remodeling capabilities of the construct should also mimic the native heart valve structure (Neuenschwander and Hoerstrup, 2004). Current efforts towards the development of a TEHV are directed toward the elucidation of the ideal cell types and scaffold materials as well as the signals necessary to guide proper cell development and tissue integration.

### 24.2.1 Cell Sources

Cardiovascular-derived autogeneic and allogeneic cells for TEHV development have been most commonly harvested from veins (e.g., saphenous vein) and arteries (e.g., femoral artery, carotid artery, mammary artery). Cell types commonly used include smooth muscle cells, fibroblasts, myofibroblasts, endothelial cells, valvular interstitial cells, and valvular endocardial cells (Kim et al., 2000b; Sodian et al., 2000a, 2000b; Stock et al., 2000a; Schnell et al., 2001; Hoerstrup et al., 2002). While the use of autologous cells is advantageous, expansion of cell numbers may be required *in vitro*, and their isolation often necessitates the disruption of an intact vascular structure.

Autogeneic and allogeneic ovine femoral artery-derived smooth muscle cells, endothelial cells, and fibroblasts were used in the first tissue-engineered valve leaflet construct and transplanted into ovines (Shinoka et al., 1995). Subsequent studies have also used femoral artery-derived cells for this application (Kim et al., 2000b). Autogeneic constructs performed better than their allogeneic counterparts; however, harvesting cells from the femoral artery is coupled with risks such as lower limb ischemia due to disrupted blood flow. Researchers have also used myofibroblasts and endothelial cells from carotid artery (Hoerstrup et al., 2000; Sodian et al., 2000a, 2000b; Stock et al., 2000a), but this also requires disruption of a major vessel, so the use of peripheral artery-derived cells may be a better option. The saphenous vein and jugular vein have been investigated as sources of myofibroblasts and endothelial cells, and the harvest of these cells requires a minimally invasive procedure (Schnell et al., 2001).

While vascular cells have shown promise in TEHV applications, they express a phenotype that can be considerably different from the native cells of the heart valve, valvular interstitial cells and valvular endocardial cells (Roy et al., 2000; Schnell et al., 2001). Furthermore, the ECM deposited by other cell types may not have the appropriate distribution and composition for heart valve replacement (Masters et al., 2004). There is thus interest in examining valvular interstitial cells and valvular endocardial cells for TEHV development. Preliminary studies using scaffolds seeded with valvular interstitial cells have been successful *in vitro* (Masters et al., 2004, 2005). However, autologous valvular interstitial cells may not yield an adequate cell population for clinical use depending on the age and medical condition of the donor.

In recent years, bone marrow-derived mesenchymal stem cells (MSCs) have emerged as an option for tissue repair and regeneration given their potential for differentiation to a number of cell types (Pittenger et al., 1999; Reyes et al., 2001). Compared to vascular and valvular cell sources, MSCs are easily collected from the donor via a bone marrow harvest. Being autologous, these cells demonstrate immunological characteristics allowing for their persistence *in vivo* (Hoerstrup et al., 2002). Scaffolds seeded with MSCs for use in TEHVs have shown excellent functional performance *in vitro* as well as the differentiation of MSCs to the intended cell phenotypes (Figure 24.2) (Hoerstrup et al., 2002; Perry et al., 2003). However promising, these results are preliminary, and further *in vitro* as well as *in vivo* work will be necessary for the clinical use of MSCs.

### 24.2.2  Scaffolds

As with other areas of tissue engineering, early work with TEHVs utilized scaffolds comprised of polyglycolic acid (PGA), polylactic acid (PLA), and composites of these polymers (PLGA) (Shinoka et al., 1995). Since then, many researchers have used PGA, PLA, and PLGA for TEHV applications (Hoerstrup et al., 2000, 2002; Perry et al., 2003; Engelmayr et al., 2003, 2005; Dvorin et al., 2003). PGA has a short lifespan *in vivo* due to

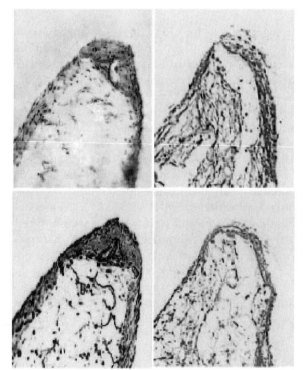

**FIGURE 24.2**

MSC-seeded TEHV leaflets stained positively for collagen type I (upper left), collagen type III (upper right), α-smooth muscle actin (bottom left), and vimentin (bottom right). These markers for myofibroblasts are also found in valvular interstitial cells. (*Source*: From Hoerstrup, S.P., *Circulation*, **106** (Suppl I), I-143 (2002). With permission.)

relatively rapid hydrolysis (2 to 4 weeks). Degradation products from this hydrolysis can create a locally acidic environment that triggers a significant local inflammatory response (Santavirta et al., 1990). While the inflammatory response is not of concern during *in vitro* development, local changes in pH may be. PLA has a longer resorption time (18 to 36 months). PLGAs exhibit a resorption time between the two polymers (8 to 12 weeks). It is noteworthy that PLGA degradation rate for a particular copolymer is not linearly dependent on the ratio of PGA:PLA (van der Giessen et al., 1996). While PGA, PLA, and PLGA scaffolds seeded with cardiovascular-derived cells showed cellular organization and structure similar to native valve leaflets, and while they produced elastin and collagen with mechanical properties similar to the ECM of valve leaflets, their initial compliance was inadequate for their function as flexible valve leaflets (Shinoka et al., 1996). The inadequate flexibility of PLGA scaffolds has led to the investigation of modified PLGA scaffolds as well as other biodegradable synthetic polymers for TEHV applications.

Other polymers investigated in lieu of PGA–PLA scaffolds include a class of naturally occurring polyesters, polyhydroxyalkanoates (PHAs). The PHA family includes poly-4-hydroxybutyrate (P4HB), a flexible, thermoplastic polymer which rapidly degrades *in vivo* (Stock, 2002), and medium chain length PHAs such as polyhydroxyoctanoates (PHOs) (Stock et al., 2000a). PHA scaffolds seeded with vascular cells were shown to open and close synchronously, and vascular cells seeded onto these constructs formed a confluent layer (Sodian et al., 2000a, 2000b). PHO scaffolds formed organized, fibrous tissue and persisted for up to 24 weeks *in vivo* (Stock et al., 2000a). While significant collagen and proteoglycan production was observed with both PHA and PHO scaffolds, no elastin production was evident. This may have significant implications for the adequate formation and function of ECM resembling native valve structure. Therefore, subsequent *in vitro* studies to improve these constructs are considered necessary before their use *in vivo* (Sodian et al., 2000a, 2000b; Stock et al., 2000a).

Researchers have also utilized PGA scaffolds coated with P4HB to successfully create TEHVs *in vitro* that were subsequently implanted in sheep and lamb models (Hoerstrup et al., 2000, 2002; Perry et al., 2003; Dvorin et al., 2003). PGA–P4HB scaffolds seeded with cardiovascular-derived cells have demonstrated well-developed ECM architecture as well as confluent, layered cellular architecture resembling native valves. Furthermore, these constructs remained thrombus free for up to 5 months *in vivo* (Hoerstrup et al., 2000). Researchers have also investigated the use of PGA–PLA–P4HB scaffolds for TEHVs (Engelmayr et al., 2003, 2005).

A number of naturally occurring biodegradable polymers have been investigated for use as TEHV scaffolds. These scaffolds offer a more native environment than synthetic scaffolds and are often lowly antigenic and immunogenic (Ramamurthi and Vesely, 2005). Several groups have investigated the use of hyaluronic acid (HA) and HA-derived hyaluronan gels for TEHVs due to their antigenic and immunogenic properties (Masters et al., 2004, 2005; Ramamurthi and Vesely, 2005). Another ECM and heart valve component investigated for use as a TEHV scaffold is collagen (Taylor et al., 2002). Fibrin gel has also been used for TEHV purposes as a natural scaffold readily derived from a patient's own blood (Ye et al., 2000).

An alternative approach to the use of synthetic or natural biodegradable scaffolds is the use of decellularized biological matrices. Researchers have utilized acellular small intestinal submucosa (SIS) for this purpose (Matheny et al., 2000). These matrices consist of either allogeneic or xenogeneic biological material that is decellularized by enzymatic digestion, detergent treatment, or the use of hypotonic conditions (Spina et al., 2003). The main challenge in creating an acellular biological matrix is to do so without disrupting the native ECM. Furthermore, adequate cell removal is necessary to avoid an immunologic response to the foreign tissue (Spina et al., 2003). Cross-linking of native ECM components

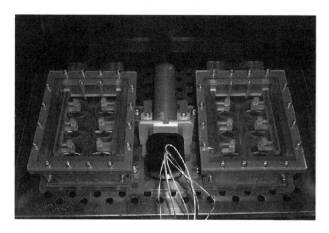

**FIGURE 24.3**
Novel bioreactor designed by Engelmayr et al. allowing for dynamic flexural stimulation of TEHV biomaterials. (*Source*: From Engelmayr, G.C., *Biomaterials*, **24**, 2523 (2003). With permission.)

may also occur to reduce immunogenicity. The decellularized scaffold then serves as a template for cell seeding and subsequent tissue growth. While the cellularization of such scaffolds is considered a tissue engineering approach, these scaffolds exhibit variable degradability based on their source and processing history. If a fixation chemistry is employed, specific concerns are raised about the impact of this technique on subsequent cytocompatibility.

### 24.2.3   Mechanical Conditioning

The anticipated benefits of *in vitro* mechanical stimulation of cells and constructs prior to implantation have led to the development of a number of bioreactor systems for the dynamic culture of TEHVs. Pulsatile flow systems with controllable parameters (e.g., pressure) have been constructed to condition trileaflet heart valve structures *in vitro* (Hoerstrup et al., 2000; Sodian et al., 2000b). A pulse duplicator system which gradually increases pressure and flow to mimic *in vivo* conditions resulted in increased ECM production and cellular organization and better mechanical properties of the tissue-engineered structure compared to constructs under static culture conditions (Hoerstrup et al., 2000, 2002; Perry et al., 2003).

While current bioreactor systems hold promise for use in TEHV development, they are limited by their capacity for only a small number of constructs and the use of coupled mechanical stimuli (preventing study of the individual effects of various mechanical stimulation modes) (Engelmayr et al., 2003). A bioreactor allowing for the independent study of the effects of cyclic three-point flexure on TEHV constructs has successfully incorporated a large sample size to study TEHV constructs *in vitro* while isolating the effects of flexure from other modes of stimulation (Figure 24.3) (Engelmayr et al., 2003, 2005). These results and others gathered from the use of bioreactors *in vitro* may prove increasingly successful in modifying the mechanical properties of TEHVs and improving their clinical suitability.

## 24.3   Tissue-Engineered Blood Vessels

Atherosclerosis, in the form of coronary artery disease results in over 515,000 coronary artery bypass graft procedures a year in the United States alone (American Heart Association: Dallas, 2005). Autologous vessels such as the internal mammary artery or saphenous vein are preferred for coronary bypass procedures. Synthetic coronary bypass vessels have not performed adequately to be employed to any significant degree. For peripheral bypass procedures, both autologous and synthetic materials are used. However, many patients do not have suitable vessels due to age, disease, or previous use. As such, researchers have turned to prosthetic grafts for the replacement of diseased arteries (Miller et al., 2004).

In the early 1950s, pioneers in the field developed vascular prostheses from materials such as silk, nylon, and polyethylene-terephthalate (PET, Dacron®, E.I. Du Pont de Nemours & Company, Inc., Wilmington, DE) (Chakfe et al., 1999; Sonoda et al., 2003). In the years since, synthetic materials such as PET and expanded polytetra-fluoroethylene (ePTFE, Teflon®, E.I. Du Pont de Nemours & Company, Inc., Wilmington, DE) have become common in replacing large arteries, but have failed in the successful repair of small diameter vessels (i.e., those with diameter <6 mm) (Cohen, 2000).

Small diameter vascular graft failure is often attributed to acute thrombosis or late-stage intimal hyperplasia (excessive tissue in-growth) at the anastomotic regions. These phenomena are hypothesized to be caused by compliance mismatch between the graft and the native artery (Sonoda et al., 2003), or excessive damage to the arterial wall (Hosono et al., 2000). Large diameter synthetic conduits are also affected by thrombosis (and thromboembolism) and some proliferative response. Yet thrombosis and intimal hyperplasia are far more detrimental in small diameter vascular grafts due to their smaller flow area (Sonoda et al., 2003). Failure of vascular prostheses may also be due to their inability to transmit dynamic arterial pressures and to be vasoresponsive (i.e., they must contract and recover in order to regulate blood flow) (Kaushal et al., 2001; Jeong et al., 2005). Most currently available vascular conduits lack the compliance necessary to transmit the pressures exerted on the native vessel (Sonoda et al., 2003). Furthermore, current vascular prostheses lack the ability to repair, remodel, and grow, thereby limiting their applicability to pediatric patients with certain congenital defects (Shum-Tim et al., 1999).

To address the aforementioned shortcomings of currently available vascular grafts, researchers have turned to tissue engineering approaches to design a biocompatible, living blood vessel. The first attempt at a tissue-engineered blood vessel (TEBV) arguably occurred in 1978 wherein a synthetic (nondegradable) matrix was seeded with endothelial cells (Herring et al., 1978). Since then, researchers have utilized a number of synthetic and natural materials, cell types, and conditioning methods in order to develop an arterial replacement with adequate mechanical function, nonthrombogenic behavior, mature ECM, and which does not illicit immunogenic and/or inflammatory responses. Research has also aimed to mimic the structure, growth, and remodeling capabilities of the native blood vessel structure (Figure 24.4).

## 24.3.1 Cell Sources

The intima, or internal layer, of a blood vessel is lined with a monolayer of endothelial cells that actively functions to prevent blood coagulation and platelet deposition (Vorp et al., 2005). Given the critical role of the endothelium in maintaining vessel patency, it is generally presumed that a successful TEBV will possess an inner cellular layer of viable, noninflammatory endothelial cells. Endothelial cells from human umbilical vein, ovine carotid artery, ovine peripheral limb vein, rat aorta, bovine aorta, and porcine aorta are amongst those used to line TEBVs under study (Shum-Tim et al., 1999; Stock et al., 2000b; Niklason et al., 2001; He and Matsuda, 2002; McKee et al., 2003; Cummings et al., 2004; Miller et al., 2004; Remy-Zolghadri et al., 2004). Endothelial cells seeded onto TEBV

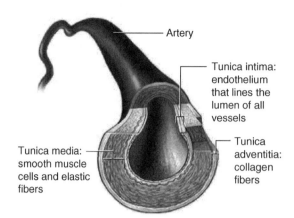

Artery

Tunica intima:
endothelium
that lines the
lumen of all
vessels

Tunica media:
smooth muscle
cells and elastic
fibers

Tunica
adventitia:
collagen
fibers

**FIGURE 24.4**
Arterial structure. (*Source*: From www.nlm.nih.
gov/medlineplus/ency/imagepages/19194.htm.)

constructs have been shown to form a confluent monolayer, to produce von Willebrand Factor (a marker of mature endothelial cells) in amounts similar to endothelial cells *in vivo*, to maintain levels of thrombomodulin (a major anticoagulant protein imparting thromboresistance) throughout the maturation process, and to lack overexpression of adhesion molecules associated with inflammation (Remy-Zolghadri et al., 2004). Furthermore, early thrombosis was not present in autologous endothelial cell-seeded grafts implanted into lambs, and no significant inflammatory response was evident after implantation (Shum-Tim et al., 1999).

The media, or middle layer, of blood vessels is composed of a dense population of smooth muscle cells while the adventitia, or outer layer, is composed of a collagenous ECM containing fibroblasts. For this reason, researchers have used smooth muscle cells and fibroblasts in conjunction with endothelial cells in their quest to engineer a vascular graft similar to a native vessel starting with the work of Weinberg and Bell in 1986 (Weinberg and Bell, 1986). Vascular smooth muscle cells, fibroblasts, and myofibroblasts derived from bovine, rat, and human aorta as well as porcine carotid artery and ovine and canine peripheral limb vein have been used with both natural and synthetic TEBV constructs (Stock et al., 2000b; Niklason et al., 2001; He and Matsuda, 2002; McKee et al., 2003; Prabhakar et al., 2003; Cummings et al., 2004; Miller et al., 2004). The first scaffold-free TEBV was constructed from monolayer sheets of fibroblasts and smooth muscle cells wrapped around a mandrel to form a distinct media and adventitia. The inner surfaces of these tubes were then seeded with endothelial cells to form a three-layered vessel similar to a native blood vessel (L'Heureux et al., 1998). Autologous fibroblasts can be obtained from a number of tissues, such as skin, with minimally invasive procedures. Endothelial cells grown on a layer of dermal fibroblasts have been shown to produce nitric oxide, an antiplatelet agent and vasodilator (Braddon et al., 2002). Furthermore, autologous myofibroblasts derived from human umbilical cord artery, umbilical cord vein, and whole umbilical cord have been used as an alternative to vascular cells (Kadner et al., 2004) since the harvest of autologous vascular cells often necessitates invasive surgery and disruption of an intact vessel.

Recently, genetically engineered cells have been explored as a means to manipulate cellular behavior in a TEBV. Regardless of cell type, terminally differentiated cells are limited in their proliferative capacity. Nonneonatal smooth muscle cells, for example, can proliferate for 10 to 30 population doublings *in vitro* before undergoing senescence. However, it has been shown that they must proliferate for at least 45 to 60 population doublings before a robust blood vessel is obtained *in vitro* (McKee et al., 2003). To alleviate this constraint, smooth muscle cell lifespan has been prolonged *in vitro* by genetic modification to express telomerase reverse transcriptase (TERT), an enzyme which prevents telomere shortening, thereby curtailing the mechanism of cell growth arrest (McKee et al., 2003). In addition, as an alternative to using endothelial cells directly, dermal fibroblasts have been genetically modified to express tissue factor pathway inhibitor, C-type natriuretic peptide, and vascular endothelial growth factor (VEGF) (Matsuda, 2004). While some of the preliminary reports have been promising, the potential additional regulatory burden in using genetically modified cells also needs to be considered when evaluating the potential benefits of such approaches.

The use of stem and progenitor cells has become increasingly common in TEBV applications in order to avoid some of the limitations associated with the use of terminally differentiated cells. Murine embryonic stem cells (ESCs) have been successfully differentiated into endothelial cells *in vitro* and further modified to express TERT (Shen et al., 2003). Endothelial progenitor cells isolated from ovine and canine blood have been seeded onto scaffolds and successfully implanted in an autologous fashion (Kaushal et al., 2001; He et al., 2003). MSCs have also been shown to differentiate to endothelial cell and smooth muscle cell phenotypes and have been used in a variety of approaches to a TEBV (Arakawa et al., 2000; Hamilton et al., 2004; Cho et al., 2005).

### 24.3.2 Scaffolds

The first tissue engineering efforts to endothelialize synthetic vascular grafts combined clinical materials such as PET and ePTFE with endothelial cells for large vessel repair (Herring et al., 1978; Graham et al., 1980). PET and ePTFE have since been modified in a number of ways to make them more suitable for the development of a functional endothelium. Both PET and ePTFE grafts have been coated with bioactive molecules such as collagen, gelatin, and heparin in order to maximize cell adhesion and tissue integration while minimizing thrombosis (Devine et al., 2001; Prager et al., 2001; Devine and McCollum, 2004). However, PET and ePTFE are relatively noncompliant materials, showing little inflation in physiological pressure regions. The resultant compliance mismatch between the native artery and TEBV may contribute to intimal hyperplasia, thrombus formation due to hemodynamic disturbances, and eventual graft failure, specifically in small vessel (i.e., diameter <6 mm) applications (Cohen, 2000; Tiwari et al., 2002; Sonoda et al., 2003; Miller et al., 2004).

As an alternative to PET and PTFE grafts, researchers have turned to a number of other synthetic, but biodegradable materials. PGA, PLA, and PLGA copolymers of the two have been repeatedly investigated for use as small diameter TEBVs. While PGA, PLA, and PLGA have been shown to elicit an inflammatory response *in vivo*, these scaffolds have been successfully used for the *in vitro* culture of a number of cell types for TEBVs (van der Giessen et al., 1996; Niklason et al., 2001; Braddon et al., 2002; McKee et al., 2003; Shen et al., 2003; Miller et al., 2004). PGA nonwoven fibers as tubular constructs were shown to be patent 6 to 8 weeks after implantation in nude mice and to support smooth muscle cell and EC proliferation and organization *in vitro* (Niklason et al., 2001; McKee et al., 2003; Shen et al., 2003). PGA scaffolds have been modified in order to increase their degradation while minimizing residual polymer fragments which lead to smooth muscle cell dedifferentiation in culture (Prabhakar et al., 2003). Furthermore, PGA–PHA copolymers have been investigated for aortic replacement and have been shown not to illicit a significant inflammatory response or thrombosis *in vivo* (Shum-Tim et al., 1999). PLGA scaffolds have also been surface modified to mimic the natural structural characteristics of the arterial wall to increase cell adhesion and growth (Miller et al., 2004). However, current PGA–PLA scaffolds have limited use as TEBVs due to their high porosity, stiffness, and relatively short degradation time, which can contribute to aneurysm formation *in vivo* (Shum-Tim et al., 1999).

In order to address the compliance mismatch issue between the vascular graft and native artery, researchers are developing grafts using elastic biomaterials often based on polyurethanes (PUs). PU can possess attractive physical properties for tissue engineering applications, with viscoelastic compliance stemming from hard domains dispersed in a soft domain matrix (Tiwari et al., 2002; Sonoda et al., 2003). Several PU types have been used as tissue engineering scaffolds, including poly(carbonate)urethanes, poly(ester)-urethanes, and poly(ether)urethanes. These may be specifically designed for degradation (e.g., through ester hydrolysis) or may be intended as permanent components providing mechanical support. A double-tubular PU consisting of a high-compliance inner tube inserted into a lower-compliance outer tube was able to mimic the pressure-dependent diameter change of a native artery *in vitro* (Figure 24.5). Furthermore, surface modifications of the PU lead to decreased thrombus formation and increased endothelialization of the luminal surface *in vivo* (He and Matsuda, 2002; Sonoda et al., 2003). A new generation of poly(carbonate) PUs that are more oxidatively stable and resistant to biodegradation has also been investigated for use in TEBVs. These grafts

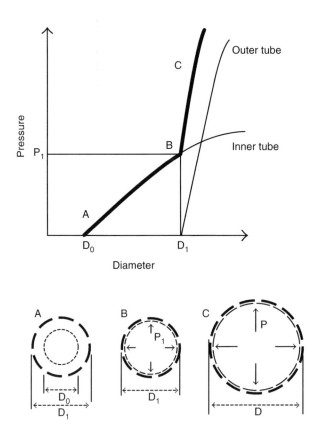

**FIGURE 24.5**
Coaxial double-tubular compliant graft for TEBV. Top: the pressure-diameter relationship of the coaxial double-tubular graft. This mimics the general J-curve pressure-diameter relationship of native artery. Bottom: the short-axis view of the graft. The inner tube inflates rapidly in the low-pressure regions (phase A and B). After the inner tube contacts the outer tube (phase B), both tubes inflate together gradually (phase C). (*Source*: From Sonoda, H., *J. Biomed. Mater. Res.*, **65A**, 170 (2003). With permission.)

exhibited more complete endothelialization and cell attachment while mimicking the compliance of native human artery (Tiwari et al., 2002; Salacinski et al., 2002).

Several other synthetic polymers have been investigated for use as TEBV scaffolds. These include P4HB, poly(lactide-*co*-caprolactone) (PLCL), and poly(glycolide-*co*-caprolactone) (PGCL). PGCL and PLCL scaffolds have exhibited good biocompatibility, cell proliferation and integration as well as adequate recovery after cyclic stretch *in vitro*, while P4HB scaffolds have demonstrated good biocompatibility and formation of organized and functional tissue *in vivo* (Stock et al., 2000b; Lee et al., 2003; Jeong et al., 2005). More studies are necessary, however, before the clinical use of these materials.

Naturally occurring materials have been used alone and in conjunction with synthetic polymers as TEBV scaffolds. The most common is collagen, a major component of the ECM and the arterial wall. The first TEBV without synthetic components consisted of collagen gel layers containing vascular cells (Weinberg and Bell, 1986). Since then, collagen gel-based methods have been used to create autologous grafts *in vitro* and *in vivo* (He et al., 2003; Berglund et al., 2004). Early collagen gel-based methods, however, produced grafts that were too mechanically weak to be implanted for study *in vivo*. To address this issue, researchers have tried incorporating other molecules, such as elastin, into the collagen matrix (Berglund et al., 2004; Boland et al., 2004). Long-term cyclic distension has also been shown to enhance the mechanical properties of collagen matrices (Isenberg and Tranquillo, 2003). Additional natural molecules investigated for use as TEBV scaffolds include fibrin gel- and HA-based constructs (Cummings et al., 2004; Remuzzi et al., 2004; Swartz et al., 2005). As with collagen-based conduits, while fibrin- and HA-based conduits exhibit good biocompatibility and cell growth and integration, they do not possess adequate mechanical strength to withstand *in vivo* stresses. Further research is necessary to make these conduits mechanically sound for clinical use.

Finally, as an alternative to synthetic and natural biodegradable materials, decellularized biological matrices have been investigated for use as TEBV scaffolds. These include allogeneic and autogeneic decellularized human cadaveric arteries and decellularized sheets of human dermal fibroblasts, respectively (Dahl et al., 2003; Remy-Zolghadri et al., 2004). Xenogeneic materials such as decellularized porcine SIS and iliac vessels have also been studied (Kim et al., 1999; Kaushal et al., 2001).

### 24.3.3 Mechanical and Biochemical Stimulation

*In vitro* mechanical stimulation of TEBV constructs has been shown to enhance their strength and functionality as well as to influence cell phenotype and function. Several bioreactor systems have been developed to precondition cells and constructs *in vitro* prior to *in vivo* implantation (Seliktar et al., 2000; Kaushal et al., 2001; Niklason et al., 2001; Braddon et al., 2002; Sodian et al., 2002; McKee et al., 2003; Prabhakar et al., 2003; Jeong et al., 2005). Biomimetic pulsatile perfusion systems, cyclic mechanical strain, and longitudinal strain have been applied to cell-seeded constructs *in vitro* to enhance collagen and ECM production by cells as well as the degree of gel compaction in gel-based constructs (Mironov et al., 2003; Solan et al., 2003; Cummings et al., 2004). Cell alignment and phenotype of bone marrow-derived MSCs have been shown to be modulated by mechanical strain (Hamilton et al., 2004). Furthermore, conditioned constructs have exhibited increased mechanical strength when subjected to pressures in the physiologic range (Seliktar et al., 2000; Niklason et al., 2001). *In vitro* mechanical conditioning regimens may prove instrumental in modifying the mechanical properties of TEBVs, making them more suitable for clinical use.

In conjunction with mechanical stimulation, biochemical signals help determine cell phenotype and ECM composition along with promoting angiogenesis *in vitro* and *in vivo*.

While many studies have been conducted on the use of various growth factors to direct stem cell differentiation, research has also demonstrated the various effects of these growth factors on smooth muscle cells, endothelial cells, and fibroblasts. Basic fibroblast growth factor (bFGF), platelet derived growth factor (PDGF), transforming growth factor beta (TGF-β), and VEGF are amongst the growth factors used for TEBV applications. These growth factors are not only mitogens for smooth muscle cells, endothelial cells, and fibroblasts, but also induce ECM production. Furthermore, these growth factors induce differentiation of MSCs and ESCs to the aforementioned cell phenotypes (Wang et al., 2004; Suzuki et al., 2005).

## 24.4  Tissue-Engineered Myocardium

Ischemic heart disease is one of the leading causes of morbidity and mortality in Western societies with 7,100,000 cases of myocardial infarction (MI) reported in 2002 in the United States alone (American Heart Association: Dallas, 2005). Heart failure after MI results from a loss of cardiomyocytes in the infarcted region of the heart. For many years, cardiomyocytes had been accepted as postmitotic, terminally differentiated cells incapable of self-renewal (Fukuda, 2001; Jackson et al., 2001; Shim et al., 2004) Although there is emerging evidence that a population of replicating cardiomyocytes and stem/progenitor cells may exist in the heart (Beltrami et al., 2001; Anversa and Nadal-Ginard, 2002; Deb et al., 2003), these cells appear to be few in number and have insignificant effect on regeneration after major injuries such as MI (Shim et al., 2004; Wu et al., 2004). Following MI, recruitment of fibroblasts, endothelial cells, and stem/progenitor cells leads to the formation of granulation tissue that is subsequently replaced by scar tissue (Jackson et al., 2001; Nian et al., 2004). Inadequate vascularization of this scar tissue leads to the apoptosis and necrosis of viable myocardium resulting in compensatory mechanisms such as hypertrophy of the remaining viable myocardium, activation of neurohumoral systems, and stimulation of various growth factors and cytokines. These events contribute to eventual total cardiac failure (Zimmermann and Eschenhagen, 2003; Nian et al., 2004). While cardiac transplantation remains the best solution for patients with end-stage heart failure, an inadequate supply of donor organs coupled with the need for life-long immunosuppression following transplantation (Kofidis et al., 2003a; Liu et al., 2003) drives the search for alternative treatments for heart failure after MI.

In recent years, research has concentrated on several strategies for repairing infarcted myocardium. These include the direct transplantation of cells into damaged myocardium, the use of tissue-engineered constructs to develop replacement tissues, and the therapeutic induction of the heart to regenerate damaged tissues. The last decade has witnessed the introduction of cellular therapies as a research protocol into the global clinical arena to putatively regenerate ischemic myocardium. This approach, however, is associated with significant questions concerning the appropriate cell type and delivery method, not to mention doubts regarding its efficacy and mechanisms prior to widespread clinical use. In the absence of successful cellular therapy treatment for heart failure, researchers continue to strive to develop a tissue-engineered myocardial patch (TEMP) capable of augmenting damaged myocardium. Efforts towards developing tissue-engineered myocardium are relatively new compared to TEHVs and TEBVs. As with other cardiovascular tissue engineering approaches, however, researchers have utilized a number of synthetic and natural materials, cell types, and conditioning methods to develop a myocardial patch with appropriate mechanical function that does not illicit significant immunogenic or inflammatory responses.

The design challenge for engineering myocardial tissue is multifaceted and difficult. Cardiac muscle is thick, compact, and highly vascularized, containing a high density of metabolically active, well-differentiated cells in a complex three-dimensional assembly of myocardial and collagen fibers in parallel. The metabolic demands require a high degree of vascularity. Cardiomyocytes contract synchronously with electrical stimulation, and myocardial fibers are therefore both electrically and mechanically anisotropic (Costa et al., 2003; Radisic et al., 2004). For this reason, cells implanted into infarcted myocardium (either through direct injection or via a scaffold) must not only survive and proliferate, but also become electrically coupled with the surrounding native myocardium and be able to withstand the mechanical loads imposed by contractile myocardium.

### 24.4.1 Cell Sources

Given the inadequate intrinsic repair mechanisms of native myocardium, the ideal cell type for cellular therapy or a TEMP would differentiate into functional, mature cardiomyocytes (and possibly supportive cell types) and regenerate damaged myocardium. A variety of cells, including progenitor cells, have been investigated. While many have shown promise *in vitro* and in animal models, all currently have limitations. Some of the cell types investigated include cardiomyocytes, cardiac progenitor cells, skeletal myoblasts, adult MSCs, smooth muscle cells, endothelial progenitor cells, and ESCs (Makino et al., 1999; Sakai et al., 1999; Tomita et al., 1999; Fukuda, 2001; Jackson et al., 2001; Kocher et al., 2001; Duan et al., 2003; Rangappa et al., 2003; Sachinidis et al., 2003; Zhou et al., 2003; Shim et al., 2004; Wu et al., 2004). For the purposes of this chapter, the focus of this section will be on those cells with possible use as part of a TEMP (as opposed to purely cellular therapies).

The early years of the 21st century have seen a flurry of activity with reports of the ability of rodent, murine, and human MSCs and ESCs to differentiate to the cardiac phenotype. While ESCs have been known to form spontaneously beating patches in culture, the conditions for this differentiation are poorly defined (Wu et al., 2004). Furthermore, differentiation is inefficient (i.e., limited to a small percentage of cells in a given culture) and is relatively nonselective (Wu et al., 2004). Methods resulting in more directed and efficient differentiation of these cells would clearly benefit cardiac tissue-engineering efforts. It has been demonstrated that cardiogenols A–D induce cardiomyogenesis in murine ESC cultures, with cardiogenol C being the most potent in a recent report (Wu et al., 2004). Here, differentiation was assessed by the presence of beating patches as well as the expression of cardiac specific markers, genes, and transcription factors including sarcomeric myosin heavy chain (MHC), GATA-4, MEF2, and Nkx2.5 (Wu et al., 2004). The downregulation of protein kinase-$\beta$ (PKC-$\beta$) and PKC-$\zeta$ as well as the upregulation of PKC-$\varepsilon$ has also proven successful in the *in vitro* differentiation of ESCs to cardiomyocytes. The PKCs are a major set of signal transduction components implicated in certain heart diseases in humans and mice (Zhou et al., 2003). Furthermore, ESCs maintained in serum-free medium have been shown to effectively differentiate to cardiomyocytes with the addition of insulin, transferrin, and PDGF-BB to the culture medium (Sachinidis et al., 2003).

Bone marrow-derived MSCs have also been shown to differentiate to the cardiac phenotype *in vitro*. Murine and rodent MSCs, when treated with 5-azacytidine, developed spontaneously beating patches and stained positively for markers of cardiac differentiation including atrial natriuretic peptide, brain natriuretic peptide, Nkx2.5, GATA-4, and MEF2 (Makino et al., 1999; Tomita et al., 1999; Fukuda, 2001). Murine cardiac progenitors isolated from adult myocardium also responded positively to 5-azacytidine treatment (Oh et al., 2003). Furthermore, treatment of MSCs with 5-azacytidine was augmented with overexpression of hepatocyte growth factor to induce neoangiogenesis *in vivo* (Duan et al., 2003). Human MSCs have been shown to differentiate to cardiac-like cells, expressing contractile and myofibrillar proteins, with culture in defined medium containing dexamethasone, insulin, and ascorbic acid (Shim et al., 2004). Human MSCs cultured in cardiomyocyte-conditioned media or cocultured with human cardiomyocytes also differentiated to a cardiac phenotype and expressed cardiac markers such as MHC and cardiac troponins (Rangappa et al., 2003). It should be noted, however, that the aforementioned results are still a topic of debate and some claim that reported differentiation with 5-azacytidine treatment is not reproducible (Liu et al., 2003). Furthermore, 5-azacytidine and coculturing treatments are not currently perceived to be clinically applicable due to their overall inefficiency and possible harmful side effects (Shim et al., 2004).

### 24.4.2  Scaffolds

Patches currently in use for ventricular or myocardial structural repair consist of synthetic materials such as Dacron and ePTFE. These materials, however, are not biodegradable, lack the ability to grow with the patient, and can be too stiff to comply with the contractions of the myocardial environment (Ozawa et al., 2002). These materials have been used for the repair of cardiovascular defects including congenital heart disorders. However, patches for myocardial regeneration need not only be biocompatible and mechanically robust, but also resorbable at a rate similar to the remodeling and repair process (Ozawa et al., 2002). A number of natural and synthetic polymers have emerged for use as a TEMP.

PCLA has been investigated for use as a myocardial patch. Consisting of a copolymer sponge of ε-caprolactone-*co*-L-lactide reinforced with poly-L-lactide fabric, these patches exhibit a biodegradation wherein the spongy component is resorbed within 2 months, whereas the fibrous portion persists for 1 to 2 years (Ozawa et al., 2002). Here acellular PCLA patches, due to their spongy structure, have been shown to foster cell adhesion and infiltration into the matrix more so than PGA matrices when implanted into rat heart (Ozawa et al., 2002). PCLA patches seeded with vascular smooth muscle cells prior to implantation in rat hearts result in elastic tissue formation and reduced abnormal chamber distensibility when compared to unseeded grafts 8 weeks post implantation (Matsubayashi et al., 2003). Furthermore, smooth muscle cell-seeded PCLA patches did not show evidence of dilation or produce a significant inflammatory response *in vivo* (Ozawa et al., 2002).

Electrospinning is a process that can produce fibers with diameters in the submicron range and forms fibers into a nonwoven mesh, resembling ECM topography. Neonatal rat cardiomyocytes have been successfully cultured on electrospun polycaprolactone (PCL) meshes extended over a wire ring acting as a passive load. Due to the high porosity of this particular scaffold, cells were able to be maintained throughout its thickness. Cells on this scaffold spontaneously contracted after 3 days in culture and expressed cardiac specific proteins (Shin et al., 2004).

Amorphous, elastomeric biomaterials made of poly(trimethylene carbonate) and D,L-lactide (TMC–DLLA) have also been evaluated as three-dimensional scaffolds for myocardial tissue engineering, as have elastomeric, SPUs. Rat cardiomyocytes have been shown to attach and proliferate well on TMC–DLLA scaffolds *in vitro*, and these scaffolds exhibit high strength at physiological conditions together with biodegradation rates of up to 3 years *in vitro* and *in vivo* (Pego et al., 2003). Rat neonatal cardiomyocytes cultured on biodegradable, segmented PU elastomers patterned with lanes of laminin responded to these spatial constraints by forming elongated, rod-shaped cells aligned parallel to the lanes. Patterned cardiomyocytes displayed a striking resemblance to intercalated disks. Furthermore, synchronously beating layers of patterned cardiomyocytes served as a suitable substrate for subsequent cardiomyocyte layers in order to build a three-dimensional, organized sheet of cardiomyocytes (McDevitt et al., 2002). Similar cell patterning was achieved on biodegradable PLGA (McDevitt et al., 2003). This patterning provides an increased ability to govern the morphology and architecture of cultured cardiomyocytes. It is important to note, however, that while neonatal rat cardiomyocytes have a known capacity to spontaneously beat *in vitro*, this has not been successfully demonstrated for cardiomyocytes that might be harvested from an adult population.

Several natural materials have been used as scaffolds for myocardial tissue repair. Commercially available collagen sponges (Tissue Fleece; Baxter Deutschland, Heidelberg, Germany) composed of type I bovine collagen seeded with rat neonatal cardiomyocytes have been shown to support spontaneous contraction of cells as well as homogeneous cell distribution. Electrical stimulation, stretching, and stimulation with $Ca^{2+}$, epinephrine, or adrenaline of these constructs resulted in increased force development with physiological beating patterns (Kofidis et al., 2002a, 2002b; Kofidis et al., 2003b). Collagen sponges seeded with neonatal rat ventricular myocytes were also induced to contract via application of a pulsatile electric field, resulting in enhanced contractile and conductive properties of cells within the scaffold, increased expression of cardiac-specific proteins, and differentiation comparable to that of native myocardium (Radisic et al., 2004).

Engineered heart tissue has been formed from a liquid cell–matrix mixture composed of collagen type I, ECM proteins (Matrigel™, Becton, Dickinson and Co., Franklin Lakes, NJ), and rat heart cells. Spontaneously and synchronously tissue formed this way and displayed morphological and functional characteristics of differentiated heart muscle. These constructs could be made in a variety of shapes and sizes for potential *in vivo* use (Zimmermann et al., 2002). Furthermore, alginate scaffolds have been used to culture high-density cardiomyocyte populations with a uniform distribution. Contractile cell clusters were found within these three-dimensional alginate constructs (Dar et al., 2002).

A novel approach to the formation of three-dimensional cardiac grafts has been developed in Japan without the use of a scaffold. The temperature-responsive polymer poly(N-isopropylacrylamide) was grafted on to tissue culture polystyrene. This slightly hydrophobic surface changed reversibly to become hydrophilic when the temperature was reduced from 37 to 32°C. Cultured cells detached spontaneously from the surface while maintaining cell–cell connections. Cardiomyocytes cultured on this surface could thus detach as cell sheets with intact electrical connections. Layering of these cardiomyocyte cell sheets allowed for the formation of three-dimensional cardiac constructs for use in myocardial tissue regeneration. It has been demonstrated that layered sheets formed electrical connections between the sheets and beat synchronously in culture. The application of mechanical loads to strengthen the tissue and inclusion of growth factors to stimulate vascularization allowed for the formation of three-dimensional, electrically coupled cardiac tissues without the need for a scaffold (Figure 24.6) (Shimizu et al., 2002a, 2002b; Itabashi et al., 2005).

### 24.4.3   Mechanical Stimulation

Since native myocardium is a dense tissue that is structurally and functionally governed by cell–cell interactions, it is essential that tissue-engineered myocardium possesses the same cell proximity and coupling. To facilitate obtaining effective structural and electrophysiological properties of tissue-engineered cardiac constructs, researchers have

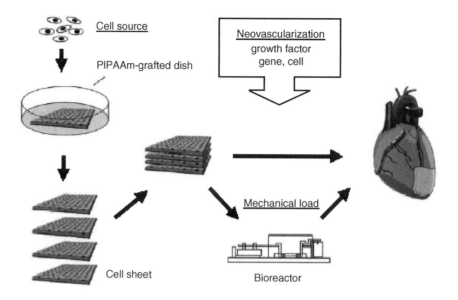

**FIGURE 24.6**
Myocardial regeneration based on cell sheet engineering. Cell sourcing and neovascularization for oxygen and nutrient supply are crucial issues for development of functional tissues. Mechanical loading should further strengthen constructs, which can then be implanted into infarcted myocardium for tissue repair and regeneration. (*Source*: From Shimizu, T., *Biomaterials*, **24**, 2309 (2003). With permission.)

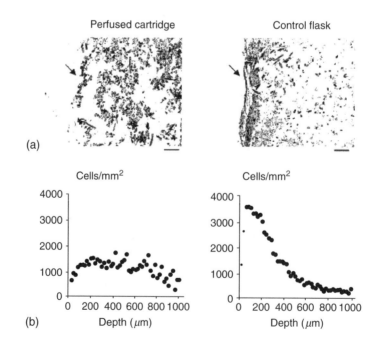

**FIGURE 24.7**
Cell distribution within perfused and stirred flask constructs (controls) after 10 days of culture in perfused cartridges at 0.6 ml/min or stirred flasks at 50 rpm. (a) Histomorphology. (Arrow denotes construct edge). (b) Two-dimensional cell density versus distance from the construct surface. Note that in perfused cultures, cells are more evenly distributed throughout the thickness of the construct. (*Source*: From Carrier, R.L., *Tissue Eng.*, **8**(2), 175 (2002). With permission.)

utilized rotating bioreactor systems *in vitro* to increase cell survival, density, metabolism, and expression of cardiac-specific markers. These bioreactor systems facilitate mass transfer of nutrients and oxygen to densely packed cells without the introduction of shear stresses (Gonen-Wadmany et al., 2004; Papadaki et al., 2001).

Although rotating bioreactor systems have been proven to augment cell density, this phenomenon is witnessed mainly at the surface of the construct (i.e., only to a depth of $\sim 100$ μm) due to mass transport limitations of oxygen and nutrients. In order to achieve a more spatially-consistent, high-density distribution of cells throughout the construct thickness, pulsatile perfusion systems have been used. Increased cell density, viability, and metabolism have been observed at the construct surface as well as the interior in these model systems (Figure 24.7) (Carrier et al., 2002a, 2002b; Kofidis et al., 2003a, 2003c; Radisic et al., 2003) Furthermore, the expression of cardiac-specific markers was enhanced in these constructs compared to those maintained in rotational bioreactors, and these patches demonstrated more synchronous contractions (Carrier et al., 2002b; Radisic et al., 2004). Scaffolds subjected to cyclic mechanical stretch regimens have also demonstrated increased cell proliferation and better spatial distribution than those statically cultured (Akhyari et al., 2002).

## Questions

1. List four design criteria for synthetic biomaterials used in cardiovascular tissue engineering.
   **Answer**: (1) adequate mechanical strength, (2) controllable biodegradation rates, (3) lack of toxic degradation products, (4) integration into surrounding tissue without extensive inflammatory response or support of infection, (5) adequate support of cell proliferation, differentiation, and maturation, and (6) the potential to deliver biological molecules.

2. What are the current alternatives to TEHVs? Briefly discuss the advantages and disadvantages of each of these alternatives.
   **Answer**: the alternatives to TEHVs are mechanical prostheses, bioprostheses (xenografts), and homografts. Mechanical valves have the advantage of durability and longevity, but they are associated with a substantial risk of infection and thromboembolism. Therefore, patients receiving mechanical valves require anticoagulation therapy. Bioprosthetic devices do not require anticoagulation therapy, and the supply is generally not limited. Bioprosthestic valves exhibit structural dysfunction due to tissue deterioration over time. Homografts are considered more biocompatible than mechanical valves or xenografts; however, there is a limited supply of donor tissue and the possibility exists of foreign tissue rejection. Furthermore, all current valve replacements lack the intrinsic ability to repair, remodel, and grow.

3. List five cell types investigated for use with TEHVs.
   **Answer**: (1) smooth muscle cells, (2) fibroblasts, (3) myofibroblasts, (4) endothelial cells, (5) valvular interstitial cells, (6) valvular endocardial cells, and (7) MSCs.

4. In general, why do small diameter vascular grafts fail more than large diameter grafts?

**Answer**: acute thrombosis and neointimal hyperplasia are often associated with small diameter graft failure. While these phenomena occur in large diameter grafts as well, they are far more detrimental in small diameter grafts due to the relative reduced effective flow area in small diameter grafts when compared to large diameter grafts with equal thrombus or intimal hyperplasia formation.

5. Why is endothelial cell seeding an essential component of TEBV success?
   **Answer**: endothelial cells actively prevent platelet activation and deposition as well as blood coagulation activation.

6. What is the advantage of genetically modifying cells to express TERT?
   **Answer**: TERT is an enzyme that prevents telomere shortening in cells. Telomere shortening has been linked with the mechanism of cell growth arrest. Therefore, modifying cells to express TERT effectively keeps cells from aging, allowing further expansion of cell numbers.

7. What mechanical and biochemical signals can be used to guide cell differentiation and cardiovascular construct development *in vitro*?
   **Answer**: mechanical stimulation including pulsatile perfusion, cyclic strain, and longitudinal strain can be used to condition constructs *in vitro* prior to *in vivo* implantation. Furthermore, chemical signals such as growth factors can be used to guide progenitor cell differentiation *in vitro*.

8. What are the current alternatives to a TEMP for the repair of damaged myocardium? Briefly discuss the obstacles to these alternatives.
   **Answer**: The alternatives to a TEMP include the direct transplantation of cells to the damaged myocardium and the therapeutic induction of the heart to regenerate the damaged tissue. However, there is a lack of knowledge regarding the "ideal" cell type to employ and the mechanisms that may contribute to clinical success. Furthermore, cells implanted into damaged myocardium must not only survive and proliferate, but must also become electrically and mechanically coupled to the cells of the surrounding native myocardium.

9. Briefly (and in your own words) discuss cell sheet engineering using a thermally responsive polymer such as poly(N-isopropylacrylamide).
   **Answer**: temperature-responsive polymer was grafted on to tissue culture polystyrene. The hydrophobic surface changed reversibly to hydrophilic when temperature was reduced from 37 to 32°C. Cultured cells detached spontaneously from the surface while maintaining cell–cell connections. Cardiomyocytes cultured on such a surface detached as cell sheets with intact electrical connections. Layering of these cell sheets allowed for the formation of three-dimensional cardiac constructs.

10. Why are dynamic cell culture systems proving more successful than static culture systems for cardiovascular construct development?
    **Answer**: a major limitation of three-dimensional constructs is the mass transport of oxygen and nutrients to the interior of the scaffold. Dynamic culture systems have proven more effective in augmenting cell density, viability, and metabolism not only at the surface of constructs, but also in the interior. Furthermore, a more spatially consistent distribution of cells throughout the construct thickness is achieved with dynamic culture. Finally, mechanical training has also been implicated in the commitment of progenitor cells to various phenotypes *in vitro*.

# References

Akhyari, P. et al., Mechanical stretch regimen enhances the formation of bioengineered autologous cardiac muscle grafts, *Circulation*, **106** (12 Suppl 1), I137–I142 (2002).

Anversa, P. and Nadal-Ginard, B., Myocyte renewal and ventricular remodelling, *Nature*, **415** (6868), 240–243 (2002).

Arakawa, E. et al., A mouse bone marrow stromal cell line, TBR-B, shows inducible expression of smooth muscle-specific genes, *FEBS Lett.*, **481** (2), 193–196 (2000).

Beltrami, A.P. et al., Evidence that human cardiac myocytes divide after myocardial infarction, *N. Engl. J. Med.*, **344** (23), 1750–1757 (2001).

Berglund, J.D., Nerem, R.M., and Sambanis, A., Incorporation of intact elastin scaffolds in tissue-engineered collagen-based vascular grafts, *Tissue Eng.*, **10** (9–10), 1526–1535 (2004).

Boland, E.D. et al., Electrospinning collagen and elastin: preliminary vascular tissue engineering, *Front. Biosci.*, **9**, 1422–1432 (2004).

Braddon, L.G. et al., Maintenance of a functional endothelial cell monolayer on a fibroblast/polymer substrate under physiologically relevant shear stress conditions, *Tissue Eng.*, **8** (4), 695–708 (2002).

Carrier, R.L. et al., Effects of oxygen on engineered cardiac muscle, *Biotechnol. Bioeng.*, **78** (6), 617–625 (2002a).

Carrier, R.L. et al., Perfusion improves tissue architecture of engineered cardiac muscle, *Tissue Eng.*, **8** (2), 175–188 (2002b).

Chakfe, N. et al., Impregnated polyester arterial prostheses: performance and prospects, *Ann. Vasc. Surg.*, **13** (5), 509–523 (1999).

Cho, S.W. et al., Vascular patches tissue-engineered with autologous bone marrow-derived cells and decellularized tissue matrices, *Biomaterials*, **26** (14), 1915–1924 (2005).

Cohen, J.R., Vascular surgery: research strategies for the new millennium, *1991, Austin, Tex.: R.G. Landes Co.*, **xiii**, 106 (2000).

Costa, K.D., Lee, E.J., and Holmes, J.W., Creating alignment and anisotropy in engineered heart tissue: role of boundary conditions in a model three-dimensional culture system, *Tissue Eng.*, **9** (4), 567–577 (2003).

Cummings, C.L. et al., Properties of engineered vascular constructs made from collagen, fibrin, and collagen–fibrin mixtures, *Biomaterials*, **25** (17), 3699–3706 (2004).

Dahl, S.L. et al., Decellularized native and engineered arterial scaffolds for transplantation, *Cell Transplant.*, **12** (6), 659–666 (2003).

Dar, A. et al., Optimization of cardiac cell seeding and distribution in 3D porous alginate scaffolds, *Biotechnol. Bioeng.*, **80** (3), 305–312 (2002).

Deb, A. et al., Bone marrow-derived cardiomyocytes are present in adult human heart: a study of gender-mismatched bone marrow transplantation patients, *Circulation*, **107** (9), 1247–1249 (2003).

Devine, C. and McCollum, C., Heparin-bonded Dacron or polytetrafluorethylene for femoropopliteal bypass: five-year results of a prospective randomized multicenter clinical trial, *J. Vasc. Surg.*, **40** (5), 924–931 (2004).

Devine, C., Hons, B., and McCollum, C., Heparin-bonded Dacron or polytetrafluoroethylene for femoropopliteal bypass grafting: a multicenter trial, *J. Vasc. Surg.*, **33** (3), 533–539 (2001).

Duan, H.F. et al., Treatment of myocardial ischemia with bone marrow-derived mesenchymal stem cells overexpressing hepatocyte growth factor, *Mol. Ther.*, **8** (3), 467–474 (2003).

Dvorin, E.L. et al., Quantitative evaluation of endothelial progenitors and cardiac valve endothelial cells: proliferation and differentiation on poly-glycolic acid/poly-4-hydroxybutyrate scaffold in response to vascular endothelial growth factor and transforming growth factor beta1, *Tissue Eng.*, **9** (3), 487–493 (2003).

Engelmayr, G.C., Jr. et al., A novel bioreactor for the dynamic flexural stimulation of tissue engineered heart valve biomaterials, *Biomaterials*, **24** (14), 2523–2532 (2003).

Engelmayr, G.C., Jr. et al., The independent role of cyclic flexure in the early in vitro development of an engineered heart valve tissue, *Biomaterials*, **26** (2), 175–187 (2005).

Fukuda, K., Development of regenerative cardiomyocytes from mesenchymal stem cells for cardiovascular tissue engineering, *Artif. Organs*, **25** (3), 187–193 (2001).

Godbey, W.T. and Atala, A., *In vitro* systems for tissue engineering, *Ann. NY Acad. Sci.*, **961**, 10–26 (2002).

Gonen-Wadmany, M., Gepstein, L., and Seliktar, D., Controlling the cellular organization of tissue-engineered cardiac constructs, *Ann. NY Acad. Sci.*, **1015**, 299–311 (2004).

Graham, L.M. et al., Endothelial cell seeding of prosthetic vascular grafts: early experimental studies with cultured autologous canine endothelium, *Arch. Surg.*, **115** (8), 929–933 (1980).

Hamilton, D.W., Maul, T.M., and Vorp, D.A., Characterization of the response of bone marrow-derived progenitor cells to cyclic strain: implications for vascular tissue-engineering applications, *Tissue Eng.*, **10** (3–4), 361–369 (2004).

He, H. and Matsuda, T., Arterial replacement with compliant hierarchic hybrid vascular graft: biomechanical adaptation and failure, *Tissue Eng.*, **8** (2), 213–224 (2002).

He, H. et al., Canine endothelial progenitor cell-lined hybrid vascular graft with nonthrombogenic potential, *J. Thorac. Cardiovasc. Surg.*, **126** (2), 455–464 (2003).

American Heart Association: Dallas, *Heart Disease and Stroke Statistics — 2005 Update*, American Heart Association: Dallas, Texas (2005).

Herring, M., Gardner, A., and Glover, J., A single-staged technique for seeding vascular grafts with autogenous endothelium, *Surgery*, **84** (4), 498–504 (1978).

Hoerstrup, S.P. et al., Functional living trileaflet heart valves grown in vitro, *Circulation*, **102** (19 Suppl 3), III44–III49 (2000).

Hoerstrup, S.P. et al., Tissue engineering of functional trileaflet heart valves from human marrow stromal cells, *Circulation*, **106** (12 Suppl 1), I143–I150 (2002).

Hogan, P.G. and O'Brien, M.F., Improving the allograft valve: does the immune response matter?, *J. Thorac. Cardiovasc. Surg.*, **126** (5), 1251–1253 (2003).

Hosono, M. et al., Neointimal formation at the sites of anastomosis of the internal thoracic artery grafts after coronary artery bypass grafting in human subjects: an immunohistochemical analysis, *J. Thorac. Cardiovasc. Surg.*, **120** (2), 319–328 (2000).

Hufnagel, C.S., [Method of preservation of arterial grafts by refrigeration.], *Arch. Med. Cuba*, **3** (3), 265–273 (1952).

Isenberg, B.C. and Tranquillo, R.T., Long-term cyclic distention enhances the mechanical properties of collagen-based media-equivalents, *Ann. Biomed. Eng.*, **31** (8), 937–949 (2003).

Itabashi, Y. et al., A new method for manufacturing cardiac cell sheets using fibrin-coated dishes and its electrophysiological studies by optical mapping, *Artif. Organs*, **29** (2), 95–103 (2005).

Jackson, K.A. et al., Regeneration of ischemic cardiac muscle and vascular endothelium by adult stem cells, *J. Clin. Invest.*, **107** (11), 1395–1402 (2001).

Jeong, S.I. et al., Mechano-active tissue engineering of vascular smooth muscle using pulsatile perfusion bioreactors and elastic PLCL scaffolds, *Biomaterials*, **26** (12), 1405–1411 (2005).

Kadner, A. et al., Human umbilical cord cells for cardiovascular tissue engineering: a comparative study, *Eur. J. Cardiothorac. Surg.*, **25** (4), 635–641 (2004).

Kaushal, S. et al., Functional small-diameter neovessels created using endothelial progenitor cells expanded ex vivo, *Nat. Med.*, **7** (9), 1035–1040 (2001).

Kim, S.S. et al., Small intestinal submucosa as a small-caliber venous graft: a novel model for hepatocyte transplantation on synthetic biodegradable polymer scaffolds with direct access to the portal venous system, *J. Pediatr. Surg.*, **34** (1), 124–128 (1999).

Kim, B.S., Baez, C.E., and Atala, A., Biomaterials for tissue engineering, *World J. Urol.*, **18** (1), 2–9 (2000a).

Kim, W.G. et al., Tissue-engineered heart valve leaflets: an effective method for seeding autologous cells on scaffolds, *Int. J. Artif. Organs*, **23** (9), 624–628 (2000b).

Kocher, A.A. et al., Neovascularization of ischemic myocardium by human bone-marrow-derived angioblasts prevents cardiomyocyte apoptosis, reduces remodeling and improves cardiac function, *Nat. Med.*, **7** (4), 430–436 (2001).

Kofidis, T. et al., In vitro engineering of heart muscle: artificial myocardial tissue, *J. Thorac. Cardiovasc. Surg.*, **124** (1), 63–69 (2002a).

Kofidis, T. et al., A novel bioartificial myocardial tissue and its prospective use in cardiac surgery, *Eur. J. Cardiothorac. Surg.*, **22** (2), 238–243 (2002b).

Kofidis, T. et al., Bioartificial grafts for transmural myocardial restoration: a new cardiovascular tissue culture concept, *Eur. J. Cardiothorac. Surg.*, **24** (6), 906–911 (2003a).

Kofidis, T. et al., Clinically established hemostatic scaffold (tissue fleece) as biomatrix in tissue- and organ-engineering research, *Tissue Eng.*, **9** (3), 517–523 (2003b).

Kofidis, T. et al., Pulsatile perfusion and cardiomyocyte viability in a solid three-dimensional matrix, *Biomaterials*, **24** (27), 5009–5014 (2003c).

L'Heureux, N. et al., A completely biological tissue-engineered human blood vessel, *FASEB J.*, **12** (1), 47–56 (1998).

Lee, S.H. et al., Elastic biodegradable poly(glycolide-*co*-caprolactone) scaffold for tissue engineering, *J. Biomed. Mater. Res. A*, **66** (1), 29–37 (2003).

Liu, Y. et al., Growth and differentiation of rat bone marrow stromal cells: does 5-azacytidine trigger their cardiomyogenic differentiation?, *Cardiovasc. Res.*, **58** (2), 460–468 (2003).

Makino, S. et al., Cardiomyocytes can be generated from marrow stromal cells in vitro, *J. Clin. Invest.*, **103** (5), 697–705 (1999).

Masters, K.S. et al., Designing scaffolds for valvular interstitial cells: cell adhesion and function on naturally derived materials, *J. Biomed. Mater. Res. A*, **71** (1), 172–180 (2004).

Masters, K.S. et al., Crosslinked hyaluronan scaffolds as a biologically active carrier for valvular interstitial cells, *Biomaterials*, **26** (15), 2517–2525 (2005).

Matheny, R.G. et al., Porcine small intestine submucosa as a pulmonary valve leaflet substitute, *J. Heart Valve Dis.*, **9** (6), 769–774, discussion 774–5 (2000).

Matsubayashi, K. et al., Improved left ventricular aneurysm repair with bioengineered vascular smooth muscle grafts, *Circulation*, **108** (Suppl 1), II219–II225 (2003).

Matsuda, T., Recent progress of vascular graft engineering in Japan, *Artif. Organs*, **28** (1), 64–71 (2004).

Mayer, J.E. Jr., In search of the ideal valve replacement device, *J. Thorac. Cardiovasc. Surg.*, **122** (1), 8–9 (2001).

McDevitt, T.C. et al., In vitro generation of differentiated cardiac myofibers on micropatterned laminin surfaces, *J. Biomed. Mater. Res.*, **60** (3), 472–479 (2002).

McDevitt, T.C. et al., Spatially organized layers of cardiomyocytes on biodegradable polyurethane films for myocardial repair, *J. Biomed. Mater. Res. A*, **66** (3), 586–595 (2003).

McKee, J.A. et al., Human arteries engineered in vitro, *EMBO Rep.*, **4** (6), 633–638 (2003).

Miller, D.C. et al., Endothelial and vascular smooth muscle cell function on poly(lactic-*co*-glycolic acid) with nano-structured surface features, *Biomaterials*, **25** (1), 53–61 (2004).

Mironov, V. et al., Perfusion bioreactor for vascular tissue engineering with capacities for longitudinal stretch, *J. Craniofac. Surg.*, **14** (3), 340–347 (2003).

Neuenschwander, S. and Hoerstrup, S.P., Heart valve tissue engineering, *Transpl. Immunol.*, **12** (3–4), 359–365 (2004).

Nian, M. et al., Inflammatory cytokines and postmyocardial infarction remodeling, *Circ. Res.*, **94** (12), 1543–1553 (2004).

Niklason, L.E. et al., Morphologic and mechanical characteristics of engineered bovine arteries, *J. Vasc. Surg.*, **33** (3), 628–638 (2001).

Oh, H. et al., Cardiac progenitor cells from adult myocardium: homing, differentiation, and fusion after infarction, *Proc. Natl Acad. Sci. USA*, **100** (21), 12313–12318 (2003).

Ozawa, T. et al., Histologic changes of nonbiodegradable and biodegradable biomaterials used to repair right ventricular heart defects in rats, *J. Thorac. Cardiovasc. Surg.*, **124** (6), 1157–1164 (2002a).

Ozawa, T. et al., Optimal biomaterial for creation of autologous cardiac grafts, *Circulation*, **106** (12 Suppl 1), I176–I182 (2002b).

Papadaki, M. et al., Tissue engineering of functional cardiac muscle: molecular, structural, and electrophysiological studies, *Am. J. Physiol. Heart Circ. Physiol.*, **280** (1), H168–H178 (2001).

Pego, A.P. et al., Preparation of degradable porous structures based on 1,3-trimethylene carbonate and D,L-lactide (*co*)polymers for heart tissue engineering, *Tissue Eng.*, **9** (5), 981–994 (2003).

Perry, T.E. et al., Thoracic Surgery Directors Association Award. Bone marrow as a cell source for tissue engineering heart valves, *Ann. Thorac. Surg.*, **75** (3), 767 (2003), discussion 767.

Pittenger, M.F. et al., Multilineage potential of adult human mesenchymal stem cells, *Science*, **284** (5411), 143–147 (1999).

Prabhakar, V. et al., Engineering porcine arteries: effects of scaffold modification, *J. Biomed. Mater. Res. A*, **67** (1), 303–311 (2003).

Prager, M. et al., Collagen versus gelatin-coated Dacron versus stretch polytetrafluoroethylene in abdominal aortic bifurcation graft surgery: results of a seven-year prospective, randomized multicenter trial, *Surgery*, **130** (3), 408–414 (2001).

Putnam, A.J. and Mooney, D.J., Tissue engineering using synthetic extracellular matrices, *Nat. Med.*, **2** (7), 824–826 (1996).

Rabkin, E. and Schoen, F.J., Cardiovascular tissue engineering, *Cardiovasc. Pathol.*, **11** (6), 305–317 (2002).

Radisic, M. et al., High-density seeding of myocyte cells for cardiac tissue engineering, *Biotechnol. Bioeng.*, **82** (4), 403–414 (2003).

Radisic, M. et al., Medium perfusion enables engineering of compact and contractile cardiac tissue, *Am. J. Physiol. Heart Circ. Physiol.*, **286** (2), H507–H516 (2004).

Radisic, M. et al., Functional assembly of engineered myocardium by electrical stimulation of cardiac myocytes cultured on scaffolds, *Proc. Natl Acad. Sci. USA*, **101** (52), 18129–18134 (2004).

Ramamurthi, A. and Vesely, I., Evaluation of the matrix-synthesis potential of crosslinked hyaluronan gels for tissue engineering of aortic heart valves, *Biomaterials*, **26** (9), 999–1010 (2005).

Rangappa, S. et al., Cardiomyocyte-mediated contact programs human mesenchymal stem cells to express cardiogenic phenotype, *J. Thorac. Cardiovasc. Surg.*, **126** (1), 124–132 (2003).

Remuzzi, A. et al., Vascular smooth muscle cells on hyaluronic acid: culture and mechanical characterization of an engineered vascular construct, *Tissue Eng.*, **10** (5–6), 699–710 (2004).

Remy-Zolghadri, M. et al., Endothelium properties of a tissue-engineered blood vessel for small-diameter vascular reconstruction, *J. Vasc. Surg.*, **39** (3), 613–620 (2004).

Reyes, M. et al., Purification and ex vivo expansion of postnatal human marrow mesodermal progenitor cells, *Blood*, **98** (9), 2615–2625 (2001).

Roy, A., Brand, N.J., and Yacoub, M.H., Molecular characterization of interstitial cells isolated from human heart valves, *J. Heart Valve Dis.*, **9** (3), 459–464 (2000), discussion 464–5.

Sachinidis, A. et al., Identification of plateled-derived growth factor-BB as cardiogenesis-inducing factor in mouse embryonic stem cells under serum-free conditions, *Cell Physiol. Biochem.*, **13** (6), 423–429 (2003).

Sakai, T. et al., Autologous heart cell transplantation improves cardiac function after myocardial injury, *Ann. Thorac. Surg.*, **68** (6), 2074–2080 (1999), discussion 2080–1.

Salacinski, H.J. et al., Thermo-mechanical analysis of a compliant poly(carbonate-urea)urethane after exposure to hydrolytic, oxidative, peroxidative and biological solutions, *Biomaterials*, **23** (10), 2231–2240 (2002).

Santavirta, S. et al., Immune response to polyglycolic acid implants, *J. Bone Joint Surg. Br.*, **72** (4), 597–600 (1990).

Schmidt, C.E. and Baier, J.M., Acellular vascular tissues: natural biomaterials for tissue repair and tissue engineering, *Biomaterials*, **21** (22), 2215–2231 (2000).

Schnell, A.M. et al., Optimal cell source for cardiovascular tissue engineering: venous vs. aortic human myofibroblasts, *Thorac. Cardiovasc. Surg.*, **49** (4), 221–225 (2001).

Seliktar, D. et al., Dynamic mechanical conditioning of collagen-gel blood vessel constructs induces remodeling in vitro, *Ann. Biomed. Eng.*, **28** (4), 351–362 (2000).

Shen, G. et al., Tissue engineering of blood vessels with endothelial cells differentiated from mouse embryonic stem cells, *Cell Res.*, **13** (5), 335–341 (2003).

Shim, W.S. et al., Ex vivo differentiation of human adult bone marrow stem cells into cardiomyocyte-like cells, *Biochem. Biophys. Res. Commun.*, **324** (2), 481–488 (2004).

Shimizu, T. et al., Electrically communicating three-dimensional cardiac tissue mimic fabricated by layered cultured cardiomyocyte sheets, *J. Biomed. Mater. Res.*, **60** (1), 110–117 (2002a).

Shimizu, T. et al., Fabrication of pulsatile cardiac tissue grafts using a novel 3-dimensional cell sheet manipulation technique and temperature-responsive cell culture surfaces, *Circ. Res.*, **90** (3), e40 (2002b).

Shin, M. et al., Contractile cardiac grafts using a novel nanofibrous mesh, *Biomaterials*, **25** (17), 3717–3723 (2004).

Shinoka, T. et al., Tissue engineering heart valves: valve leaflet replacement study in a lamb model, *Ann. Thorac. Surg.*, **60** (6 Suppl), S513–S516 (1995).

Shinoka, T. et al., Tissue-engineered heart valves. Autologous valve leaflet replacement study in a lamb model, *Circulation*, **94** (9 Suppl), II164–II168 (1996).

Shum-Tim, D. et al., Tissue engineering of autologous aorta using a new biodegradable polymer, *Ann. Thorac. Surg.*, **68** (6), 2298–2304 (1999), discussion 2305.

Sodian, R. et al., Tissue engineering of heart valves: in vitro experiences, *Ann. Thorac. Surg.*, **70** (1), 140–144 (2000a).

Sodian, R. et al., Fabrication of a trileaflet heart valve scaffold from a polyhydroxyalkanoate biopolyester for use in tissue engineering, *Tissue Eng.*, **6** (2), 183–188 (2000b).

Sodian, R. et al., Tissue-engineering bioreactors: a new combined cell-seeding and perfusion system for vascular tissue engineering, *Tissue Eng.*, **8** (5), 863–870 (2002).

Solan, A. et al., Effect of pulse rate on collagen deposition in the tissue-engineered blood vessel, *Tissue Eng.*, **9** (4), 579–586 (2003).

Sonoda, H. et al., Coaxial double-tubular compliant arterial graft prosthesis: time-dependent morphogenesis and compliance changes after implantation, *J. Biomed. Mater. Res. A*, **65** (2), 170–181 (2003).

Spina, M. et al., Isolation of intact aortic valve scaffolds for heart-valve bioprostheses: extracellular matrix structure, prevention from calcification, and cell repopulation features, *J. Biomed. Mater. Res. A*, **67** (4), 1338–1350 (2003).

Stock, U.A. et al., Tissue-engineered valved conduits in the pulmonary circulation, *J. Thorac. Cardiovasc. Surg.*, **119** (4 Pt 1), 732–740 (2000a).

Stock, U.A. et al., Patch augmentation of the pulmonary artery with bioabsorbable polymers and autologous cell seeding, *J. Thorac. Cardiovasc. Surg.*, **120** (6), 1158–1167 (2000b), discussion 1168.

Stock, U.A., Vacanti, J.P., Mayer, J.E. Jr., and Wahlers, T., Tissue engineering of heart valves—current aspects, *Thorac. Cardiovasc. Surg.*, **50** (3), 184–193 (2002).

Suzuki, H. et al., Roles of vascular endothelial growth factor receptor 3 signaling in differentiation of mouse embryonic stem cell-derived vascular progenitor cells into endothelial cells, *Blood*, **105** (6), 2372–2379 (2005).

Swartz, D.D., Russell, J.A., and Andreadis, S.T., Engineering of fibrin-based functional and implantable small-diameter blood vessels, *Am. J. Physiol. Heart Circ. Physiol.*, **288** (3), H1451–H1460 (2005).

Tabata, Y., Tissue regeneration based on growth factor release, *Tissue Eng.*, **9** (Suppl 1), S5–S15 (2003).

Taylor, P.M. et al., Human cardiac valve interstitial cells in collagen sponge: a biological three-dimensional matrix for tissue engineering, *J. Heart Valve Dis.*, **11** (3), 298–306 (2002), discussion 306–7.

Tiwari, A. et al., New prostheses for use in bypass grafts with special emphasis on polyurethanes, *Cardiovasc. Surg.*, **10** (3), 191–197 (2002).

Tomita, S. et al., Autologous transplantation of bone marrow cells improves damaged heart function, *Circulation*, **100** (19 Suppl), II247–II256 (1999).

van der Giessen, W.J. et al., Marked inflammatory sequelae to implantation of biodegradable and nonbiodegradable polymers in porcine coronary arteries, *Circulation*, **94** (7), 1690–1697 (1996).

Vongpatanasin, W., Hillis, L.D., and Lange, R.A., Prosthetic heart valves, *N. Engl. J. Med.*, **335** (6), 407–416 (1996).

Vorp, D.A., Maul, T., and Nieponice, A., Molecular aspects of vascular tissue engineering, *Front. Biosci.*, **10**, 768–789 (2005).

Wang, D. et al., Proteomic profiling of bone marrow mesenchymal stem cells upon transforming growth factor beta1 stimulation, *J. Biol. Chem.*, **279** (42), 43725–43734 (2004).

Weinberg, C.B. and Bell, E., A blood vessel model constructed from collagen and cultured vascular cells, *Science*, **231** (4736), 397–400 (1986).

Wu, X. et al., Small molecules that induce cardiomyogenesis in embryonic stem cells, *J. Am. Chem. Soc.*, **126** (6), 1590–1591 (2004).

Ye, Q. et al., Fibrin gel as a three dimensional matrix in cardiovascular tissue engineering, *Eur. J. Cardiothorac. Surg.*, **17** (5), 587–591 (2000).

Zhou, X., Quann, E., and Gallicano, G.I., Differentiation of nonbeating embryonic stem cells into beating cardiomyocytes is dependent on downregulation of PKC beta and zeta in concert with upregulation of PKC epsilon, *Dev. Biol.*, **255** (2), 407–422 (2003).

Zimmermann, W.H. and Eschenhagen, T., Cardiac tissue engineering for replacement therapy, *Heart Fail. Rev.*, **8** (3), 259–269 (2003).

Zimmermann, W.H. et al., Tissue engineering of a differentiated cardiac muscle construct, *Circ. Res.*, **90** (2), 223–230 (2002).

# 25

## Tissue Engineering — Skin

Jonathan Mansbridge

## CONTENTS

## 25.1 Introduction

The construction of skin substitutes was the first and simplest tissue engineering application undertaken (Bell et al., 1979). Skin substitutes also comprise the only commercialized products of this type, with both laboratory and therapeutic devices available. Since the construction of these entities is straightforward, much of this article will be devoted to questions that arise during their commercial development. The discussion cannot be comprehensive as the subject includes quality assurance and regulatory questions that are product specific and beyond the scope of this discussion.

Human skin consists of two major layers, the dermis forming a structurally robust component, formed by fibroblasts, which normally lie within the layer in a quiescent state, and the epidermis, which is almost entirely cellular, formed mainly of keratinocytes which provide an impermeable barrier and also support immune defence functions. In addition, there are a variety of other structures (adnexal), such as hair follicles, sweat and sebaceous glands and several other cell types that form blood vessels and lymphatics (endothelial cells, smooth muscle cells and pericytes), pigment cells (melanocytes), cells associated with the immune system (Langerhans cells, mast cells) and cells associated with nervous function (nerve fibers, Merckle cells). In general, tissue-engineered constructs have incorporated fibroblasts and/or keratinocytes, but recently have been extended to include melanocytes, Langerhans cells or endothelial cells and work is proceeding on hair follicles. The importance of the different cells types in tissue-engineered skin arises from their specific functions and paracrine interactions between them.

While normally quiescent in the adult, the cells of the skin generated the integument during embryogenesis and growth and are capable of recruiting cells of the immune system and repairing the structure following physical or microbiological injury. It is becoming evident that keratinocytes and fibroblasts, when activated, are capable of performing the basic repair of physical damage (Martin et al., 2003), without the intervention of inflammatory cells. However, the resident cells of the skin need to recruit other cells of the immune system (macrophages, neutrophils, lymphocytes) to destroy invading organisms and toxins.

## 25.2  Tissue-Engineered Skin Constructs

Tissue culture of skin cells started many decades ago. Fibroblasts were among the first cells grown and practical methods for growing keratinocytes have been available since the late seventies (Rheinwald and Green, 1975). In the case of keratinocytes, monoculture methods led to an epidermis-like structure that could be used as a skin model and for therapeutic purposes. It was recognized that keratinocytes are a rich source of cytokines and growth factors, which have been extensively studied. More recently, it has been realized that fibroblasts also produce a range of cytokines relevant to wound healing.

Fibroblasts are capable of three-dimensional growth in simple tissue culture in the presence of ascorbate, but have generally been grown as a monolayer. Currently, three-dimensional growth of fibroblasts is usually achieved using a support scaffold either of collagen or of a polymeric fabric or sponge. In either case, the fibroblasts detect the scaffold through surface receptors and respond appropriately. However, they will not grow in suspension, but undergo anoikis and die.

Keratinocytes can be grown on a fibroblast-derived, three-dimensional system to form a structurally faithful representation of the epidermis. Keratinocytes grown on scaffold-based or collagen-based fibroblast cultures have been used as skin models, wound models, for the testing of commercial skin products *in vitro* and for the treatment of wounds.

These skin culture systems have formed the basis for incorporating other cell types. The inclusion of melanocytes provides valuable models to investigate the effects of ultraviolet irradiation, testing of UV protective preparations, the study of the physiology of melanocytes and, in some cases, for experimental therapeutic purposes. Similar techniques have allowed the study of Langerhans cells in their normal environment. A goal of these models is to replicate the community of cells within the skin as completely as possible, as many cellular interactions involve paracrine signaling.

The inclusion of hair follicles and sebaceous glands in skin constructs is still in its infancy. It is known that hair follicles, provided with a suitable nutrient source, contain the elements required for their maintenance. Thus, they can be transplanted within the same host or between hosts. It has even been demonstrated that they can be transplanted to a tissue culture system (Michel et al., 1999), but at this point, this system has not been exploited. The understanding of the development of hair follicles, involving wnt, GATA3,

BMP FGFs, FOXe2 and hedgehog (Kishimoto et al., 2000; Jamora et al., 2003; Kaufman et al., 2003; Mill et al., 2003), is progressing steadily. It is possible to obtain hair growth *in vitro*. Recently, hair follicles have been reconstituted from dissociated cells, which represents a major advance in this field (Zheng et al., 2005).

### 25.2.1 Synthesis of an Artificial Dermis

The simplest dermal replacements consist of an acellular scaffold comprising collagen and chondroitin sulfate and treated so as to produce a sponge of defined porosity (Yannas et al., 1980). This material acts as a template for immigration of host fibroblasts and construction of a dermis.

Dermal structures are obtained from postnatal fibroblasts, which initially lay down a collagen-containing provisional matrix that can be remodeled into dermal tissue. Fibroblasts are generally obtained from a biopsy or surgical discard. In general, the cultures have to be expanded to produce sufficient cells. Stocks are cryopreserved at various stages of expansion to enable a consistent cell source over a long period and for convenience, using conventional liquid nitrogen storage systems. It may be noted that cryopreservation may cause DNA damage and also induce apoptosis and hence cell loss (Baust et al., 2000).

It is becoming evident that fibroblasts, during expansion, are susceptible to stress-induced premature senescence (SIPS) in addition to senescence due to telomere erosion (replicative senescence). Fibroblasts become unresponsive to growth factors, nonproliferative and change their metabolism in other ways when senescent and are unsatisfactory for skin models, testing or therapeutic purposes. Replicative senescence probably occurs at greater than 80 cell doublings. In the lab, 60 to 70 doublings can be achieved, but precautions should be taken to reduce oxidative stress to reduce SIPS. Experience indicates that cells at 25 to 35 doublings after isolation are suitable for tissue engineering.

### 25.2.2 Factors in the Selection of Dermal Support Systems

Collagen constructs have been used as the basis for fibroblast growth, including gels and sponges, with or without chondroitin sulfate. Emphasis in this technique has been placed on ensuring the optimal porosity, which is achieved by lyophilization, and acts as a dermal template for fibroblast growth. In the case of collagen gels, it was realized that fibroblasts cause gel contraction and the production of a relatively strong product.

The basis of many three-dimensional fibroblast culture systems involves suspending the cells in a collagen gel. Under these conditions, the fibroblasts bind to collagen mainly through integrin receptor $\alpha_2\beta_1$, with lesser contributions from integrin $\alpha_1\beta_1$ and discoidin domain receptors. This leads to a characteristic pattern of signal transduction pathway activation that involves protein kinase C$\zeta$ (Xu and Clark, 1997). Under these conditions, proliferation is reduced and there are changes in gene expression compared to monolayer culture. The cells become quiescent, proliferate slowly, reorganize and contract the gel, change their pattern of gene expression from that found in monolayer and express a diminished amount of collagen (Eckes et al., 1993). To reduce this effect, collagen gels are usually restrained within a ring, which prevents contraction in two dimensions and forms a "stressed" collagen gel (Kessler et al., 2001). In this case, fibroblast proliferation is increased and there is greater formation of extracellular matrices. Constructs of this type have been referred to as lattices.

The alternative approach to growing dermis from fibroblasts starts with a polymeric mesh, into which the cells are seeded. Under these conditions, since most tissue culture is still performed in serum, the polymer becomes coated with protein, notably fibronectin and the predominant initial binding of the cells to the scaffold is through integrin $\alpha_5\beta_1$, with some contribution from $\alpha_3\beta_1$. The outcome is cells very similar to monolayer culture. The cells proliferate rapidly, filling in the interstices of the scaffold, and subsequently laying down substantial quantities of extracellular matrix. The matrix, predominantly collagen type I but also containing types III, V and VI, fibronectin, tenascin, decorin, fibrillin, secreted protein, acidic and rich in cysteine (SPARC), glycosamino glycans (GA), particularly dermatan sulfate and other matricellular molecules, has many of the characteristics of the provisional matrix formed in granulation tissue during wound healing. The generation of an extracellular matrix is similar to the fibroblast component of foreign-body capsule formation. The proteins laid down by the cells lead to a complex pattern of cell adhesion, through both $\alpha_1\beta_1$, $\alpha_2\beta_1$, $\alpha_3\beta_1$ and $\alpha_5\beta_1$ and unidentified receptors that may include discoidin domain receptors and receptors for tenascin, thrombospondin and SPARC. The matrix is also capable of binding growth factors such as FGF-2 and FGF-7 and can thus transmit considerable information.

Porosity is also important in polymer scaffolds used for three-dimensional fibroblast growth. Material (Vicryl, nylon, polyglycolic acid, polyester, etc.) with quadrilateral pores with a diagonal of 200 $\mu$m has been found optimal.

Moreover, dermis can be grown without a scaffold in the presence of ascorbate to give extracellular matrix sheets that can be stacked to form a dermis or other structures (L'Heureux et al., 1998; Michel et al., 1999). These structures do not require nonhuman components, but demand labor-intensive manufacture.

Keratinocytes and fibroblasts, mixed together, are capable of spontaneously organizing themselves into dermis and epidermis (Wang et al., 2000). This strategy has been used as the basis of a commercial product. In addition, noncellular and cellular constructs have been developed, using collagen and chondroitin sulfate, based on porous collagen sponges that act as a template for *in vivo* or *in vitro* dermis formation.

### 25.2.3   Growth Medium for Skin Cells

The medium generally used for growing fibroblasts is serum-supplemented Dulbecco's minimal essential medium (DMEM). This also works well in three-dimensional systems. In this respect, calf serum is equivalent to fetal calf serum. Serum-free media are available for fibroblast growth, but these do not prevent senescence and have been unsatisfactory for three-dimensional growth. Serum-containing media, which include wound-healing growth factors derived from platelet degranulation, generate conditions that promote cell growth and differentiation characteristic of an acute injury site. Such conditions, while promoting cell proliferation, may not be suitable for the production of functional tissue-engineered constructs. In general, three-dimensional fibroblast growth medium is supplemented with ascorbic acid, which acts both as an antioxidant and as a requirement for collagen deposition (Fleischmajer et al., 1991). By contrast, serum-free media have been developed for keratinocytes and used successfully in three-dimensional cultures (Johnson et al., 1992).

### 25.2.4   Epidermal Construction

The ability of keratinocytes to proliferate and differentiate in culture has long been known (Green et al., 1977) and constructs comprising keratinocytes alone have been used commercially for both testing and treatment of severe burns (Compton et al., 1989). However, keratinocytes can also be seeded on to dermal lattices to make a bilayered construct. In general, the steps involve expansion of the keratinocytes in monolayer culture, followed by seeding on to the dermal structure. The monolayer expansion may be performed in a serum-free medium under conditions that support growth that is limited only by telomere erosion. However, under these conditions, stem cells tend to be lost from the keratinocyte population. On seeding on the dermal construct, the keratinocyte culture is comprised largely of transit-amplifying cells that terminally differentiate and do not persist. The resulting epidermis shows basal and spinous layers, a stratum corneum and frequently a granular layer similar to normal skin. However, the pathway of keratinocyte differentiation is related to wound healing, expressing keratins 6 and 16. In normal, unwounded skin, the basal layer is characterized by expression of keratins 5 and 14 (also seem in bilayered constructs) and the suprabasal layers by keratins 1, 2e and 10. Although the structure of a bilayered artificial skin may be generally excellent when examined by hematoxylin and eosin staining, its pathway of differentiation differs from normal interfollicular skin where keratins 6 and 16 are absent (Asselineau et al., 1986). Constructs of the noted type eventually develop a basement membrane, containing collagen IV, laminin and nidogen and subsequently type VII collagen (Fleischmajer et al., 1993; Fleischmajer et al., 1997).

### 25.2.5  Bioreactor Design for Skin Constructs

Experimental work using skin constructs can be performed in conventional tissue culture equipment (Petri dishes, flasks, roller bottles, multiwell plates). However commercial systems have generally been found to require specialized bioreactors. This is especially true of therapeutic products that are made under good manufacturing practices (GMP). Such devices have included bags, hard bioreactors and modified or unmodified tissue culture vessels. The importance of such devices lie in the maximal use of automation to reduce human error and the minimum of aseptic operations, as each such operation is an opportunity for contamination. In cases where the bioreactor is included in the final product, it should also be developed to provide maximal ease of application by the final user.

Skin substitutes have been grown under both flow and nonflow conditions, including conditions closely related to conventional tissue culture, e.g., in dishes. All systems have been batch-fed although the flow systems lend themselves to continuous replenishment. In a comparison of bioreactor systems, a flow rate of about 4 to 5 cm/min provides increased cell density over nonflow conditions. This approach allows reagents such as ascorbate to be added at various rates as well as enabling the monitoring of glucose utilization and lactate production.

Cell-related changes in glucose and lactate constitute the largest changes in metabolites during the growth of skin substitutes. Most of the metabolism of these nutrients is related to energy production. This can be used to monitor the progress of the culture. ATP is produced by the cells from glycolysis and the complete oxidation of glucose. Therefore, glucose utilization and lactate production have been combined to give a notional value for ATP turnover which reflects the energy consumed during culture and can be used to determine the time of harvest. In cases where a scaffold is used that hydrolyzes with the release of lactate (such as lactate polyesters, PLGA, PLLA), this method is not applicable, although glucose consumption alone can be used.

### 25.2.6  Growth Characteristics of Skin Cells in Three-Dimensional Culture

The growth of fibroblasts in dermal systems differs in gel and scaffold systems (Figure 25.1). Growth is slowest in unstressed gel systems, and fastest in scaffold-based systems. Proliferation analysis using PKH26 staining has revealed that fibroblast proliferation in collagen gels is heterogeneous, a substantial proportion of fibroblasts

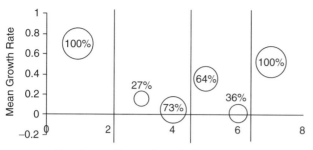

**FIGURE 25.1**
Comparison of growth fibroblast culture systems. The size of the population is given by the area of the circle and the proportion by accompanying number. The average growth rate in that population is given by the height of the center of the circle above the abscissa. The unit of growth rate is in day$^{-1}$.

barely dividing during the period of culture over 3 weeks. When the gel is stressed by mechanical constraint, a larger proportion proliferate. In monolayer and scaffold-based culture they behave as a single population.

Collagen gene expression is reduced in unstressed collagen gel culture; the reduction is less in stressed gels than in unstressed gels. These results suggest that fibroblasts reach a more quiescent state in collagen gels than on scaffolds. In clinical practice, it has been found worthwhile to activate the tissue by cutting or meshing. However, expression of chemokines and cytokine gene expression and secretion indicate that unmeshed collagen gel cultures are as active as scaffold-based cultures (Kessler–Becker et al., 2004).

The proliferation and deposition of extracellular matrix by fibroblasts in a scaffold-based culture is illustrated in Figure 25.2. Cell growth, based on DNA content is logistic reaching a maximal cell density after 10 to 12 days. The increase in cell density can be well described by the Verlhurst equation. MTT reductase (metabolic activity), fibronectin and GAG increase similarly. However, collagen, which forms the bulk of the extracellular matrix, initially increases exponentially. At an early stage, its secretion lags behind cell proliferation, but it continues to increase until day 25 or 30. Collagen production, therefore, does not fit easily into the Leudeking–Piret classification (Bailey and Ollis, 1986) of growth-associated and nongrowth-associated production. Collagen production can be well described on the basis that it is secreted in a logistic fashion by postmitotic fibroblasts (Mansbridge, 2001).

Cells in these systems produce a range of growth factors that are independent of extracellular matrix. A selection of genes expressed in a three-dimensional culture is listed in Table 25.1. Two prominent groups include angiogenic factors and inflammatory mediators. These factors impact the clinical efficacy of these products.

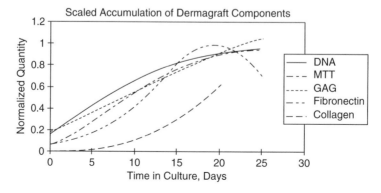

**FIGURE 25.2**
Accumulation of components in a three-dimensional fibroblast-based culture.

### 25.2.7  Quality Control

Quality control is critical for commercial products, including experimental and therapeutic systems.

The evaluation of tissue-engineered skin constructs has varied with their potential applications. In the case of skin models and testing applications, the major methods have focused on cell viability and cytokine secretion. Viability was determined using neutral red uptake or MTT reduction. An internal control was included in the experiment and comparison was made between untreated and treated samples. The product was qualified based on performance in the final protocols using either IL-1 or prostaglandin E2 secretion or viability (determined by metabolic activity by MTT reduction, neutral red uptake or lactate dehydrogenase release).

These approaches are a challenge for establishing the quality of therapeutic products. One reason is that positive controls are not readily available since there is no comparison of treated with untreated samples. Ideally, quality control tests should be related to the mode of action of the tissue-engineered device. In skin products this is both complex and elusive. Consequently, the quality of final skin products has been based on histology, collagen content, cellular density (by DNA determination) and metabolic activity (determined by MTT, XTT, Alamar Blue or other tetrazolium dye reduction). Cytokine determination (e.g., VEGF, IL-8) has been considered but it has been variable. Purportedly, the cells are responsive to minor environmental changes and the control systems frequently involve autocrine mechanisms.

In addition, sterility for mycoplasma, bacteria, moulds, yeasts and other organisms has to be established in the final product. Viral sterility is generally established once or twice for each fibroblast or keratinocyte culture used for master cell banks, as discussed below.

A critical factor in quality control is setting specifications. This issue is becoming more complex as the regulatory classification for tissue-engineered products develops and

### TABLE 25.1

Selected Growth Factors Detected in Scaffold-Based, Three-Dimensional Fibroblast Culture. All have been Detected on Expression Arrays. Those in Italics have also been Detected by ELISA

| Growth Factor | Autocrine and Paracrine Factors |
|---|---|
| IGF-II | *PDGF A chain* |
| IGFBP-4 | *KGF* |
| IGF-BP-5 | *TGF-b1* |
| IGFBP-6 | CTGF |
| **Inflammatory Mediators** | **Angiogenic Factors** |
| IL-1β | *VEGF* |
| *IL-6* | VEGF-B |
| *IL-8* | *HGF* |
| TNF-α | *PLGF* |
| *MCP-1* | *Basic FGF* |
| *MCP-3* | Cyr61 |
| *SDF-1* | FGF-5 |
| Interferon-β | *Angiopoietin-1* |
| *Gro-α* | |
| Gro-β | |
| Gro-γ | |
| *G-CSF* | |
| *GM-CSF* | |

becomes more closely related to the FDA definition of biologics than devices. One overall effect of these developments is to place more emphasis on testing. While specifications are ultimately set by clinical trial, initial specifications need to be set as widely as considered compatible with efficacy and within the capability of the production process. Three standard deviations from the mean performance of the synthetic system is generally a reasonable starting point. Ultimately, the specification will be set by values that are determined in a clinical trial to be safe and effective.

### 25.2.8  Stasis Preservation

Stasis is the ability to store a metabolically active material without change in properties or degradation. Such preservation in a commercial product is especially critical for sterility. Currently, a 4-week method recommended by the regulatory authorities for testing therapeutic products for mycoplasma. Requirements for test and diagnostic systems, where contaminated constructs can be replaced, are less stringent.

Many of the manufacturing processes take 2 to 4 months to complete, making demand forecasting difficult. Stasis preservation is, therefore, also desirable for inventory control.

Several methods of storage are possible, including refrigeration (useful for test systems), frozen (usable with nonliving systems), cryopreservation and vitrification. Test kits, where sterility testing is less critical, have generally been distributed at room temperature in medium gelled with agarose. To date, the best compromise for therapeutic products has been cryopreservation at $-70°C$ in a DMSO- or glycerol-based system, which can provide shelf-life of at least 6 months. However, the thawing process is an integral part of the preservation method since it is difficult to determine viability in the frozen state. It is critical to successful application of therapeutics that the tissue retain biological activity upon thawing. If it is intended that the product be shipped frozen, the thawing procedure must be easy enough to perform reliably in a physician's office. Details of these techniques are outside the scope of this article and the reader is referred to more specialized texts (Brockbank, 2002).

## 25.3   Regulation of Tissue-Engineered Skin

The regulation of tissue-engineered skin for clinical applications is complex and, currently, is not settled. Therefore, specific remarks about standards, guidelines and regulations are of limited value. In contrast, products for experimental testing are less rigorously regulated than therapeutic products.

Therapeutic products are regulated on the basis of clinical trials, which establish the safety and efficacy of the particular process and product. Any substantial alteration to the process may cause a change that the regulatory authorities consider may put the product outside the parameters of the original product and necessitate additional clinical trials. Since clinical trials are expensive, changing a process becomes more difficult as development proceeds. It is, therefore, wise to settle on the final process and to contact regulatory authorities as early as possible.

### 25.3.1   *In Vitro* Applications of Skin Models

Commercial and noncommercial tissue engineered skin products have been available for many years in a variety of formats. Some of the earliest commercial systems were scaffold-based dermis alone, or together with a single layer of keratinocytes; with multiple layers of keratinocytes (Slivka et al., 1993), or with fibroblast-loaded collagen gels with keratinocyte layers (Nelson and Gay, 1993). More recently, simpler systems such as EpiDerm (Monteiro-Riviere et al., 1997), consisting of keratinocytes alone, but still showing many of the properties of intact skin, have been developed. These systems have been used for testing corrosivity and irritation in commercial products, such as skin-care products and detergents that come into contact with human skin. In general, the assays have either determined the viability of the skin model following experimental treatment (using MTT reduction) or measured the secretion of inflammatory molecules such as IL-1 or prostaglandin E2. A comparison of the relative properties of several commercial kits has been reviewed (Faller and Bracher, 2002).

Skin models have been used to study the physiology of skin, particularly wound healing and the interaction between the dermal and epidermal components (Konstantinova et al., 1998). In several cases, these have involved transplanting models to mice. One example is the demonstration of the keratinocyte IL-1/fibroblast FGF-7/GM-CSF circuit in the skin (Szabowski et al., 2000). Another example focused on the development of the basement membrane (Fleischmajer et al., 1997).

Living skin equivalents have been applied to models of skin pathology and treatment as well as genetic disease (Briggaman, 1982; Bernerd et al., 2004) and the role of dermal–epidermal interactions (Saiag et al., 1985; Priestley and Lord, 1990; Coulomb and Dubertret, 1992). Tissue-engineered skin also has been used to test experimentally the therapeutic effects of drugs (Crooke et al., 1996) and gene therapy (Pfutzner et al., 1999).

Furthermore, experimental models of wound-healing skin constructs have been used to investigate the mechanism of cytokine changes (Falanga et al., 2002) and the mechanisms associated with the skin responses to external insults. While much of this is the function of cells derived from the immune system (mainly Langerhans cells), keratinocytes and fibroblasts are capable of activating the immunological responses and recruiting macrophages, neutrophils and lymphocytes.

Percutaneous penetration of drugs is a convenient mechanism for delivery and tissue-engineered constructs have been investigated as potential models (Kanikkannan et al., 2000). In normal skin, the molecular penetration is limited to molecules having a molecular weight of less than 500 (Bos and Meinardi, 2000) and a suitable partition coefficient (Wiechers, 1989). The use of tissue-engineered skin in this context has been limited since its permeability is about an order of magnitude higher than human skin. This is probably related to differences in keratinocyte between the model and normal skin (described above) and changes in the structure of the stratum corneum in the constructs.

### 25.3.2 Therapeutic Applications of Tissue-Engineered Skin Constructs

To date, tissue-engineered skin constructs have been used to treat acute and chronic wounds. Wound-treatment requirements differ in these two cases and, therefore, the skin substitutes must be tailored to address these issues.

Discussion of the therapeutic mode of action of artificial skin constructs has emphasized five major properties

1. provision of live cells
2. continuous and appropriate provision of growth factors, particularly angiogenic factors
3. provision of a substrate for keratinocyte proliferation
4. modification of the inflammatory process
5. provision of an epidermal barrier

Not all of these may be relevant in every application and discussion of their relative importance depends on understanding the mechanism of wound healing and its arrest in chronic wounds. Figure 25.3 gives a general scheme of these processes. In the case of chronic wounds, the progression of successive stages is interrupted. One concept to account for this is based on SIPS of the fibroblasts in chronic wounds, which proliferate slowly and respond poorly to growth factors. Senescent fibroblasts secrete diminished levels of cytokines in response to injury. Consequently, neutrophils are not attracted and activated in the wound site. Bacteria, therefore, colonize the wound bed, causing impaired reepithelialization. The comparatively young fibroblasts in skin constructs may supply functions differently from resident cells and persist for several months in the wound site. Fibroblasts have been detected for as long as 6 months after implant. Active fibroblasts in three-dimensional culture secrete 30 to 50 ng/$10^6$ cells/day IL-8 in response to IL-1 and TNF$\alpha$, and attract and activate of neutrophils.

Table 25.1 lists growth factors and cytokines that have been detected by analysis of mRNA on Affymetrix U95A expression arrays or by ELISA. Angiogenic and inflammatory factors form two prominent groups. Skin constructs are known to be angiogenic (Pinney et al., 2000), both through diffusible factors (VEGF$_{121}$) and matrix-bound factors (FGF-2). The angiogenic property of dermal substitutes has led to their investigation for conditions needing revascularization, such as ischemic heart and limbs.

Three-dimensional scaffold-based dermal replacements secrete factors that will support keratinocyte migration, including collagen type I and fibronectin. In addition, matricellular proteins have been identified by immunocytochemistry, including tenascin, SPARC, fibrillin and thrombospondin-2. These factors may modify cellular signal transduction systems and may cue keratinocyte migration.

By comparison with chronic wounds, acute wounds such as burns have different requirements. The provision of cells may not be appropriate, as there is no enhanced senescent phenotype among the resident cells of a young patient. Likewise, stimulation of inflammation may be inappropriate, contributing to autograft failure. However,

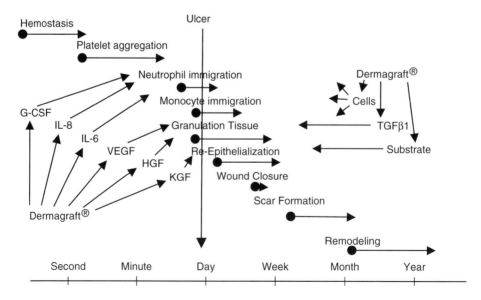

**FIGURE 25.3**
Scheme of action of a tissue engineered dermal implant (Dermagraft).

angiogenesis and a migration substrate for keratinocytes and leukocytes may be important. It has been found, in the case of severe burns, that nonviable material is superior to viable.

There are two fully approved therapeutic products on the market, a single layer dermal product and a bilayered material. In both products keratinocytes are important. Initially it was speculated that keratinocytes were the major source of cytokines and growth factors. Rather, both fibroblasts and keratinocytes secrete these factors, although in different patterns. The epidermal layer provides IL-1$\alpha$ and TGF-$\alpha$. Moreover, keratinocytes and fibroblasts have paracrine activating interactions. However, these characteristics seem to be less important to the efficacy of the bilayered material than originally thought and the major function of keratinocytes may be a temporary permeability barrier. The keratinocyte layer is lost from the construct after implantation, probably because the cells have a transit amplifying character and are terminally differentiated. However, chronic wounds have no lack of activated keratinocytes, which accumulate at the margins of the ulcer but do not migrate because of the migration-inhibitory properties of bacterial products. However, in other circumstances, such as epidermolysis simplex, where there is a genetic defect in keratin synthesis in the keratinocytes, provision of an epidermis is a real advantage (Fivenson et al., 2003).

## 25.4 Allogeneic vs. Autologous Tissue Engineering of Therapeutic Skin Constructs

Allogeneic cells are simpler to use for manufacturing than autologous, because there are several challenging regulatory requirements for autologous cell processing including more than temporary storage. Separate tissue culture suites are required for each patient, including separate air conditioning. Furthermore, a tissue-engineering process to expand autologous cells may take several weeks. This represents a large investment in fixed equipment. In addition, autologous tissue engineering is a service industry and does not provide benefits from increased scale of production, both in terms of equipment and of skilled operators. Autologous approaches are, however, possible for proof-of-principle experiments, where it is important to eliminate contributions from the immune system. Therefore, autologous approaches may be valuable in university and nonprofit settings, where economics are less pressing. The major advantage of using autologous tissue is that the regulatory requirements for testing are less stringent than for allogeneic approaches.

Manufacturing systems based on allogeneic cells can provide economies of scale. However, the requirements for testing are more burdensome than for autologous cells and include examination for adventitious viruses and tumorigenicity, for example. These tests must performed on new cell sources or master-cell banks. Tests are performed twice, once at construction of the master-cell bank and a second time on cells grown beyond the manufacturing requirement at the end of production. A master-cell bank may last 10 years or more. Consequently, this is an occasional incurred expense if production is sufficiently robust.

Immunogenicity and the use of allogeneic cells remain a concern. However, the clinical experience with tissue-engineered skin products is that immune rejection has not been problematic (Falanga, 1998). Of some tens of thousands of patients treated with allogeneic cells, immune rejection has never been observed. Moreover, no positive responses have been observed in direct tests for antibody production or T-cell activation. A possible reason for this is the absence of antigen presenting cells, such as endothelial cells or dendritic cells, which would activate acute rejection, in tissue-engineered skin substitutes. Chronic rejection cannot be eliminated, although fibroblasts have been found to persist in the wound site for 6 months. Further, no adverse clinical events have been attributed to chronic rejection.

The conclusion on the use of allogeneic or autologous cells is that immune rejection has not been observed. This result may also apply to other mesenchymal or epidermal cells provided antigen presenting cells are rigorously excluded.

## Questions

1. Briefly review the major structural elements of the skin with their respective functions. How far has tissue engineering succeeded in reproducing these properties *in vitro*?

2. What are the relative properties of different scaffold/matrix materials with respect to fibroblast and keratinocyte responses?

3. Tissue-engineered skin structures range from noncellular materials to structures containing multiple cell types. Briefly describe the salient increases in the complexity of tissue-engineered skin constructs.

4. Why should bioreactor design be undertaken in developing tissue-engineered skin production facilities? What features should such devices include?

5. What methods are available for determining the readiness of a tissue-engineered skin construct for harvesting?

6. Discuss available methods for setting specifications for test and therapeutic products.

7. What are the challenges facing tissue-engineered skin products in their acceptance as commercial products?

8. Discuss the applications of tissue-engineered skin devices as models of skin physiology.

9. What modes of action are believed to operate in the treatment of chronic wounds with tissue-engineered skin products? How do these differ from those thought to operate in acute wounds?

10. Compare the relative advantages on autologous and allogeneic approaches in the construction of tissue-engineered skin.

## References

Asselineau, D., Bernard, B.A., Bailly, C., Darmon, M., and Prunieras, M., Human epidermis reconstructed by culture: is it "normal"?, *J. Invest. Dermatol.*, **86**, 181 (1986).

Bailey, J.E. and Ollis, D.E., *Biochemical Engineering Fundamentals*, 2nd ed., McGraw-Hill, New York (1986).

Baust, J.M., Van, B., and Baust, J.G., Cell viability improves following inhibition of cryopreservation-induced apoptosis, *In Vitro Cell Dev. Biol. Anim.*, **36**, 262 (2000).

Bell, E., Ivarsson, G., and Merrill, C., Production of a tissue-like structure by contraction of collagen lattices by human fibroblasts of different proliferative potential in vitro, *Proc. Natl Acad. Sci. USA*, **76**, 1274 (1979).

Bernerd, F., Asselineau, D., Frechet, M., Sarasin, A., and Magnaldo, T., Reconstruction of DNA-repair deficient xeroderma pigmentosum skin in vitro: a model to study hypersensitivity to uv light, *Photochem. Photobiol.*, **1**, 1 (2004).

Bos, J.D. and Meinardi, M.M., The 500 dalton rule for the skin penetration of chemical compounds and drugs, *Exp. Dermatol.*, **9**, 165 (2000).

Briggaman, R.A., Epidermal–dermal interactions in adult skin, *J. Invest. Dermatol.*, **79**, 21s (1982).

Brockbank, K.G., Stabilization of tissue-engineered products for transportation and extended shelf-life, *Ann. NY Acad. Sci.*, **961**, 265 (2002).

Compton, C.C., Gill, J.M., Bradford, D.A., Regauer, S., Gallico, G.G., and O'Connor, N.E., Skin regenerated from cultured epithelial autografts on full-thickness burn wounds from 6 days to 5 years after grafting, *Lab. Invest.*, **60**, 600 (1989).

Coulomb, B. and Dubertret, L., [Dermo–epidermal interactions and skin pharmacology], *Pathol. Biol (Paris)*, **40**, 139 (1992).

Crooke, R.M., Crooke, S.T., Graham, M.J., and Cooke, M.E., Effect of antisense oligonucleotides on cytokine release from human keratinocytes in an in vitro model of skin, *Toxicol. Appl. Pharmacol.*, **140**, 85 (1996).

Eckes, B., Mauch, C., Huppe, G., and Krieg, T., Downregulation of collagen synthesis in fibroblasts within three-dimensional collagen lattices involves transcriptional and posttranscriptional mechanisms, *FEBS Lett.*, **318**, 129 (1993).

Falanga, V., Isaacs, D., Paquette, D., Downing, G., Kouttab, N., Butmarc, J., Bediavas, E., and Hardin-Young, J., Rapid healing of venous ulcers and lack of clinical rejection with an allogeneic cultured human skin equivalent. Human skin equivalent investigators group [see comments], *Arch. Dermatol.*, **134**, 293 (1998).

Falanga, V., Margolis, D., Alvarez, O., Auletta, M., Maggiacomo, F., Altman, M., Jensen, J., Sabolinski, M., and Hardin-Young, J., Wounding of bioengineered skin: cellular and molecular aspects after injury, *J. Invest. Dermatol.*, **119**, 653 (2002).

Faller, C. and Bracher, M., Reconstructed skin kits: reproducibility of cutaneous irritancy testing, *Skin Pharmacol. Appl. Skin Physiol.*, **15**, 74 (2002).

Fivenson, D.P., Scherschun, L., Choucair, M., Kukuruga, D., Young, J., and Shwayde, T., Graftskin therapy in epidermolysis bullosa, *J. Am. Acad. Dermatol.*, **48**, 886 (2003).

Fleischmajer, R., Contard, P., Schwartz, E., MacDonald, E.D., Jacos, L., and Sakai, L., Elastin-associated microfibrils (10 mm) in a three-dimensional fibroblast culture, *J. Invest. Dermatol.*, **97**, 638 (1991).

Fleischmajer, R., Kuhn, K., Sato, Y., Macdonald, E.D. II, Perlish, J.S., Pan, T.C., Chu, M.L., Kishiro, Y., Oohashi, T., Bernier, S.M., Yamada, Y., and Ninomiya, Y., Immunochemistry of a keratinocyte–fibroblast co-culture model for reconstruction of human skin, *J. Histochem. Cytochem.*, **441**, 1359 (1993).

Fleischmajer, R., Macdonald, E.D., Contard, P., and Perlish, J.S., There is temporal and spatial expression of alpha1 (iv), alpha2 (iv), alpha5 (iv), alpha6 (iv) collagen chains and beta1 integrins during the development of the basal lamina in an "in vitro" skin model, *J. Invest. Dermatol.*, **109**, 527 (1997).

Green, H., Rheinwald, J.G., and Sun, T.T., Properties of an epithelial cell type in culture: the epidermal keratinocyte and its dependence on products of the fibroblast, *Prog. Clin. Biol. Res.*, **17**, 493 (1977).

Jamora, C., DasGupta, R., Kocieniewski, P., and Fuchs, E., Links between signal transduction, transcription and adhesion in epithelial bud development, *Nature*, **422**, 317 (2003).

Johnson, E.W., Meunier, S.F., Roy, C.J., and Parenteau, N.L., Serial cultivation of normal human keratinocytes: a defined system for studying the regulation of growth and differentiation, *In Vitro Cell Dev. Biol.*, **28A**, 429 (1992).

Kanikkannan, N., Kandimalla, K., Lamba, S.S., and Singh, M., Structure–activity relationship of chemical penetration enhancers in transdermal drug delivery, *Curr. Med. Chem.*, **7**, 593 (2000).

Kaufman, C.K., Zhou, P., Pasolli, H.A., Rendl, M., Bolotin, D., Lim, K.C., Dai, X., Alegre, M.L., and Fuchs, E., Gata-3: an unexpected regulator of cell lineage determination in skin, *Genes Dev.*, **17**, 2108 (2003).

Kessler, D., Dethlefsen, S., Haase, I., Plomann, M., Hirche, F., Krieg, T., and Eckes, B., Fibroblasts in mechanically stressed collagen lattices assume a "synthetic" phenotype, *J. Biol. Chem.*, **276**, 36575 (2001).

Kessler-Becker, D., Krieg, T., and Eckes, B., Expression of pro-inflammatory markers by human dermal fibroblasts in a three-dimensional culture model is mediated by an autocrine interleukin-1 loop, *Biochem. J.*, **379**, 351 (2004).

Kishimoto, J., Burgeson, R.E., and Morgan, B.A., Wnt signaling maintains the hair-inducing activity of the dermal papilla, *Genes Dev.*, **14**, 1181 (2000).

Konstantinova, N.V., Lemak, N.A, Duong, D.M., Chuang, A.Z., Urso, R., and Duvic, M., Artificial skin equivalent differentiation depends on fibroblast donor site: use of eyelid fibroblasts, *Plast. Reconstr. Surg.*, **101**, 385 (1998).

L'Heureux, N., Páuet, S., Labbé, L., Germain, L., and Auger, F.A., A completely biological tissue-engineered human blood vessel, *FASEB J.*, **12**, 47 (1998).

Mansbridge, J.N., Dermal fibroblasts, In: *Primary Mesenchymal Cells*, Koller, M.N., Palsson, B.O., and Masters, J.R.W., Eds., Kluwer, Boston, pp. 125 (2001).

Martin, P., D'Souza, D., Martin, J., Grose, R., Cooper, L., Maki, R., and McKercher, S.R., Wound healing in the pu.1 null mouse — tissue repair is not dependent on inflammatory cells, *Curr. Biol.*, **13**, 1122 (2003).

Michel, M., L'Heureux, N., Pouliot, R., Xu, W., Auger, F.A., and Germain, L., Characterization of a new tissue-engineered human skin equivalent with hair, *In Vitro Cell Dev. Biol. Anim.*, **35**, 318 (1999).

Mill, P., Mo, R., Fu, H., Grachtchouk, M., Kim, P.C., Dlugosz, A.A., and Hui, C.C., Sonic hedgehog-dependent activation of gli2 is essential for embryonic hair follicle development, *Genes Dev.*, **17**, 282 (2003).

Monteiro-Riviere, N.A., Inman, A.O., Snider, T.H., Blank, J.A., and Hobson, D.W., Comparison of an in vitro skin model to normal human skin for dermatological research, *Microsc. Res. Tech.*, **37**, 172 (1997).

Nelson, D. and Gay, R.J., Effects of uv irradiation on a living skin equivalent, *Photochem. Photobiol.*, **57**, 830 (1993).

Pfutzner, W., Hengge, U.R., Joari, M.A., Foster, R.A., and Vogel, J.C., Selection of keratinocytes transduced with the multidrug resistance gene in an in vitro skin model presents a strategy for enhancing gene expression in vivo, *Hum. Gene Ther.*, **10**, 2811 (1999).

Pinney, E., Liu, K., Sheeman, B., and Mansbridge, J., Human three-dimensional fibroblast cultures express angiogenic activity, *J. Cell. Physiol.*, **183**, 74 (2000).

Priestley, G.C. and Lord, R., Fibroblast–keratinocyte interactions in psoriasis: failure of psoriatic fibroblasts to stimulate keratinocyte proliferation in vitro, *Br. J. Dermatol.*, **123**, 467 (1990).

Rheinwald, J.G. and Green, H., Formation of a keratinizing epithelium in culture by a cloned cell line derived from a teratoma, *Cell*, **6**, 317 (1975).

Saiag, P., Coulomb, B., Lebreton, C., Bell, E., and Dubertret, L., Psoriatic fibroblasts induce hyper-proliferation of normal keratinocytes in a skin equivalent model in vitro, *Science*, **230**, 669 (1985).

Slivka, S.R., Landeen, L.K., Zeigler, F., Zimber, M.P., and Bartel, R.L., Characterization, barrier function, and drug metabolism of an in vitro skin model, *J. Invest. Dermatol.*, **100**, 40 (1993).

Szabowski, A., Mass-Szabowski, N., Andrecht, S., Kolbus, A., Schorpp-Kistner, M., Fusenig, N.E., and Angel, P., C-jun and junb antagonistically control cytokine-regulated mesenchymal–epidermal interaction in skin, *Cell*, **103**, 745 (2000).

Wang, C.K., Nelson, C.F., Brinkman, A.M., Miller, A.C., and Hoeffler, W.K., Spontaneous cell sorting of fibroblasts and keratinocytes creates an organotypic human skin equivalent, *J. Invest. Dermatol.*, **114**, 674 (2000).

Wiechers, J.W., The barrier function of the skin in relation to percutaneous absorption of drugs, *Pharm. Weekbl. Sci.*, **11**, 185 (1989).

Xu, J. and Clark, R.A., A three-dimensional collagen lattice induces protein kinase c-zeta activity: role in alpha2 integrin and collagenase mrna expression, *J. Cell Biol.*, **136**, 473 (1997).

Yannas, I.V., Burke, J.F., Gordon, P.L., Huang, C., and Rubenstein, R.H., Design of an artificial skin. II. Control of chemical composition, *J. Biomed. Mater. Res.*, **14**, 107 (1980).

Zheng, Y., Du, X., Wang, W., Boucher, M., Parimoo, S., and Stenn, K., Organogenesis from dissociated cells: generation of mature cycling hair follicles from skin-derived cells. *J. Invest. Dermatol.*, **124** (5), 867 (2005).

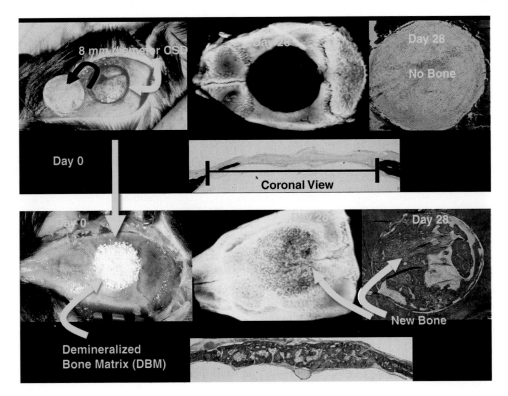

**FIGURE 6.2**
Rat Calvaria: bone gap model.

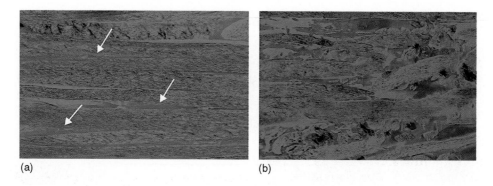
(a)                                                    (b)

**FIGURE 10.7**

Photomicrographs of rabbit knee joints implanted with poly(urethane urea) (PUUR) band. (a) 6 months post implantation. Arrows denote tissue in-growth between the PUUR fibers. (b) 18 months post implantation. Note the disruption of the fibers relative to 6-months post implantation. (*Source*: Adapted from Gisselfält, K. *Structure Dependent Chemical and Biological Interactions of Poly(urethane urea)s*, Ph.D. thesis, Chalmers University of Technology, Göteborg, Sweden (2002). With permission.)

# Tissue Engineering of Ligaments

## Gregory H. Altman and Rebecca L. Horan

## CONTENTS

## 26.1   Introduction

### 26.1.1   The Large Unmet Clinical Need

Within the field of ligament and tendon engineering, the majority of scientific and clinical efforts lie in the study, repair and regeneration of the anterior cruciate ligament (ACL). While most ligaments within the body possess the ability to self-repair and remodel following injury, the ACL is incapable of this due to its location in the intra-articular space of the knee joint. As a result, the ACL requires surgical replacement when torn. Over 200,000 Americans required ACL reconstructive surgery this year with a price tag exceeding 5 billion dollars (Weitzel et al., 2002; Vunjak-Novakovic et al., 2004). The ACL serves as a primary stabilizer of anterior tibial translation and as a secondary stabilizer of valgus–varus knee angulation, and is most often susceptible to rupture or tear resulting from a flexion–rotation–valgus force associated with sports injuries. Most ACL tears result from pivot and stop-jump motions. As a result, high ACL rupture rates are associated with sports such as football, soccer, basketball, skiing, and volleyball and are considered an epidemic among the young female athlete. Female athletes tear their ACLs at a rate of 5 to 7 times that of an equivalent male athlete (Ardent, 1999; Perrin, 1999). Ruptures or tears can result in severe limitations in mobility, pain, discomfort, and the loss of knee joint function leading to an inability to participate in sports and exercise (Arnoczky et al., 1993).

## 26.2   The Anterior Cruciate Ligament

### 26.2.1   ACL Structure–Function Relationship

The ACL has a unique helical fiber organization and structure to perform its stabilizing functions. The mode of attachment to bone and the need for the knee joint to rotate approximately 140° in extension/flexion results in a 90° twist of the major fiber bundles of the ACL resulting in a helical organization within the ligament structure, i.e., in full extension, individual fibers are attached anterior–posterior and posterior–anterior from the tibia to the femur. This helical geometry allows the individual ACL fiber bundles, during knee joint flexion, to remain isometric in length throughout the range of motion. As a result, fiber bundle isometry allows the ACL to equally distribute loads to all fiber bundles thereby maximizing its strength. It is this unique structure–function relationship that allows the ACL to sustain high loading through all degrees of knee joint extension and flexion. A prosthesis that does not account for the isometric nature of the ACL fibers (i.e., a 90° twist) would be prone to failure because as the degree of flexion increases, a fiber bundle attached anterior–anterior would dramatically increase in length and, as a result, be placed at a higher risk for rupture. The reverse is observed for a fiber bundle attached posterior–posterior, thus becoming lax unable to stabilize load.

The complex geometry and nature of ACL function in the knee is in part responsible for the difficulty encountered in developing suitable surgical replacements. Prosthesis design must consider not only the isometric issues described above, but also the ultimate tensile strength (UTS) of the ACL, and the properties of the ACL's entire stress–strain curve including its yield point, if the replacement ligament is to function successfully *in vivo* over the long term (Woo and Adams, 1990). The biomechanical basis for many of the synthetic ACL failures lies in the mismatches between synthetic and native ACL stress–strain curves. Of particular importance are the mismatches in prosthesis linear stiffness (e.g., prosthesis > ACL stiffness) that lead to "stress-shielding" of host tissue in-growth causing nondirected collagen fiber organization and alignment. As a result, host tissue incorporation contributes little to the mechanical integrity of a prosthesis. Therefore, stress-shielding places the majority of the physiological load on the prosthesis alone which is then limited by its inherent fatigue properties. The lack of directed collagenous in-growth due to stress-shielding shifts the natural biological phenomena of continuous ligament remodeling and degradation to degradation only. As a result, the timely resumption of physiological loading *in situ* of newly integrated graft tissue should be a top priority in ACL repair. This should be done by engineering tissue constructs to maintain joint stability and ACL mechanical properties, particularly load distribution, stiffness, UTS, and yield stress while at the same time transmitting relevant mechanical milieu to graft tissue.

### 26.2.2 ACL Graft Properties and Characteristics

The mechanical and viscoelastic properties of the human ACL are well documented (Table 26.1). Human ACLs range in length from 27 to 32 mm. The ACL's fiber crimp pattern allows for 7 to 16% of creep prior to permanent deformation and ligament damage. The ACL withstands cyclic loads of about 400 N in the region of 1 to 2 million times per year (Chen and Black, 1980). The ACL is regularly exposed to tensile forces ranging from 67 N (for ascending stairs) to 630 N (for jogging). The standards for ACL surgical replacement have been established at 1730 N for the tensile strength, linear stiffness of 182 N/mm, and energy absorbed at failure of 12.8 Nm (Table 26.1).

While ligaments are well profiled mechanically, no single unique biological marker for ACLs has yet been identified. The development of an accurately-defined, comprehensive biological template is critical as it is necessary for verification of success or failure in the generation of a tissue engineered ACL. As a result, combinations of (1) extracellular matrix (ECM) components (e.g., collagen types I and III, decorin and biglycan) (Amiel et al., 1984, 1990; Arnoczky et al., 1993; Lo et al., 1998), (2) the relative ratio of collagen type I to type III (~88% Type I: 12% Type III) (Amiel et al., 1990; Ross et al., 1990; Lo et al., 1998), (3) cell morphologies located within distinct regions of the ACL (Amiel et al., 1984; Murray and Spector, 1999), (4) type and percent of reducible cross-links (Amiel et al., 1984), (5) ligament tissue ultrastructure (e.g., crimp pattern, collagen fibril diameter) (Amiel et al., 1984; Arnoczky et al., 1993), and (6) tissue biomechanical properties are used to assess and characterize the ACL in comparison to other ligaments, tendons, and tissues.

### 26.2.3 The Intra-articular Environment

The rigors of the intra-articular environment include a demanding mechanical regime and limiting biochemical environment. The cruciate ligaments (anterior and posterior) within

**TABLE 26.1**

Mechanical Properties of the Human ACL

| Author | Age (mean) | Ultimate Load (N) | Linear Stiffness (N/mm) | Energy Absorbed (Nm) |
|---|---|---|---|---|
| Noyes and Grood, 1976 | 16–26 | 1725 ± 269 | 182 ± 33 | 12.8 ± 2.2 |
| Rauch et al. (1987) | 17–28 | 1716 ± 538 | 203 ± 34 | — |
| Woo (1991) | 22–35 (29) | 2160 ± 157 | 242 ± 28 | 11.6 ± 1.7 |
| Woo and Adams (1990) | 22–49 (34) | 1954 ± 187 | 292 ± 28 | 8.5 ± 1.0 |

intra-articular space are encapsulated by synovium containing synovial fluid designed to lubricate the joint and prevent clots. Due to a lack of blood flow within the space, long-term nourishment of the cruciates is provided by a vascular network extending from the femoral and tibial bone attachment sites through the ligament. Immediately following ACL reconstruction and prior to angiogenesis, which typically occurs within ~ 12 weeks following implantation(Arnoczky et al., 1982), the graft is dependent on the synovial fluid for nutrient and metabolite supply and transport. As a result of the mass transfer limitations associated with dense tendon grafts, the interior of these collagenous tissues is rendered necrotic, leading to alterations in mechanical properties (Jackson et al., 1996).

## 26.3   Current Reconstructive Techniques

At present, four options are utilized for repair or replacement of a damaged ACL: (1) auto-grafts, (2) allografts, (3) xenografts, and (4) synthetic prostheses. Currently, none of these ACL grafts recreates the isometric nature and geometry of the ACL, and/or matches the ACL's stress–strain curve. These limitations translate into an absence of a truly successful reconstructive technique for restoration of knee joint function without debilitating side effects. Of the options available, the most commonly selected is the autograft as it is considered the "gold standard" for purposes of comparison with tissue-engineered grafts.

### 26.3.1   Autografts

Autografts typically utilize the middle third of the patellar tendon harvested with bony attachments (B-PT-B) or two of four hamstring tendons (gracilis and semitendinosus). Surgical replacements utilizing B-PT-B grafts have produced the most satisfactory long-term results, likely due to anchoring methods available for the bony graft ends. B-PT-B harvest, mismatches in tendon geometry and structural features result in long graft remodeling times, preventing ~ 15% of all surgical patients from returning to pretrauma activity levels (Weitzel et al., 2002). Hamstring reconstructions have gained popularity as tendon anchoring techniques to reduce graft laxity have improved (no bony attachments are harvested with the hamstring tendons). However, tendon creep prior to the healing of the grafts to bone within the tunnels (i.e., the first 12 weeks) is still a major potential surgical problem.

   In both cases, donor-site morbidity (DSM) associated with the loss of autologous tissue, leads to the most significant complications. Pain, muscle atrophy, and tendonitis associated with DSM often result in prolonged rehabilitation periods (3 to 6 months), and a return to pretrauma activity levels is typically delayed for 12 to 18 months post reconstruction; 15 to 30% of autologously reconstructed patients never regain pretrauma IKDC activity levels (Otto et al., 1998; Fu et al., 2000; Tsuda et al., 2001; Weitzel et al., 2002). Approximately 30% of all patients who tear their ACL do not undergo ACL reconstruction as a result of age (poor tendon integrity) and graft limitations. Currently, these outcomes are associated with the best available reconstructive techniques on the market.

### 26.3.2   Synthetic Prostheses

Synthetic polymers evaluated for use as prosthetic devices include: (a) carbon fiber-based materials, e.g., Versigraft, (b) Dacron, (c) ultra high molecular weight polyethylene (UHMWPE), (d) Gore-Tex (polytetrafluoroethylene), (e) polyester (Leeds-Keio), (f) polypropylene (Kennedy Ligament-Augmentation Device), and (g) stents, such as the Carbon Integraft (Weitzel et al., 2002). However, stress-shielding limiting prosthesis fatigue life (e.g., Dacron), lack of biological incorporation (Gore-Tex), and debris particle formation (UHMWPE) have been reported as problems (Richmond et al., 1992). The shortcomings of each reconstructive option have guided a tissue-engineering approach and requirements for the engineered graft have been established. Due to these imperfections within the currently available synthetic grafts as well as a general inability to interact favorably with host tissue, alternatives remain necessary. In fact, the flaws exhibited as limiting in each of these approaches to graft design have provided additional design inputs for a successful tissue-engineered ligament.

## 26.4 Ligament Tissue Engineering

### 26.4.1 Advantage of a Tissue Engineered Ligament

There exists a substantial margin for improvement compared to both autograft and prosthetic options. A tissue-engineered ACL developed from a patient's own bone marrow-derived stem cells would: (1) eliminate DSM, thus increasing the rate and degree of rehabilitation leading to dramatically shortened periods of disability (potentially from 6 months for ligament remodeling to 6 weeks for bone tunnel ingrowth), (2) create an "unlimited" amount of autologous ligament tissue (for instance, 25 ml of marrow provides enough first-passage adult stem cells to grow approximately 30 ligaments), and (3) potentially avail patients over the age of 40 (a major portion of the torn ACL population) with autologous graft options for ACL reconstruction. In addition, the tissue-engineering strategy proposed here should increase the rates of ligament remodeling by: (1) better approximating the geometry and structure of the native ACL through matrix design (e.g., multi-bundle isometric graft), (2) initiating collagenous organization that better supports *in vivo* function by preexposure to physiologically relevant environment *in vitro* in an *in vitro* bioreactor system, and (3) providing increased and improved anchor options (compared to the hamstring).

Tissue engineering can potentially provide improved clinical options in orthopedic medicine through the generation of biologically based functional tissues *in vitro* for transplantation at the time of injury or disease. A tissue-engineered ACL with the appropriate biological and mechanical properties available at the time of reconstruction would eliminate the limitations associated with present-day surgical techniques.

The problems associated with the use of synthetic ACL replacements, along with the limited availability of donor tissue, motivated research towards the development of functional equivalents of native tissues (Altman et al., 2002a–c, 2003; Chen et al., 2003, 2005; Horan et al., 2005; Lu et al., 2005; Moreau et al., 2005). The shift from synthetic to biologically-based ACL replacements has been seen in early studies in which collagenous composite ACL prostheses were prepared consisting of reconstituted type I collagen fibers in a collagen I matrix with polymethylmethacrylate bone fixation plugs, and used as ACL replacement tissues in rabbits (Dunn et al., 1992). Subsequent studies have involved ligament analogs based on ligament fibroblasts seeded on cross-linked collagen fiber scaffolds (Dunn et al., 1995; Dunn, 1996), and suggested that structures approximating native ligaments can be generated. A tendon-gap model, based on prestressed collagen sutures seeded with mesenchymal stem cells provided improved repair of large tendon defects (Young et al., 1998). Goulet et al. (1997) modified the collagen-fibroblast system by using ligament fibroblasts in noncross-linked collagen, with bone anchors to prestress the tissue and facilitate surgical implantation. Passive tension produced by growing the new ligament in a vertical position attached to the two ends of the culture vessel induced fibroblast elongation and the alignment of the cells and surrounding extracellular matrix (Goulet et al., 1997). More recently, cyclic mechanical strain promoted collagen I synthesis by ACL fibroblasts (Toyoda et al., 1998).

However, to date, no human clinical trials have been reported with tissue-engineered ACLs. This may be due to many issues including: (1) the lack of a readily-available ligament cell or tissue source, (2) the unique complex structure and mechanical function of the ACL (crimp pattern, peripheral helical pattern, and isometric fiber organization), and (3) the necessary remodeling time *in vivo* for progenitor cells to differentiate and/or autologous cells to infiltrate the graft.

## 26.4.2   Healing Strategy

An alternative approach to ACL repair with replacement graft tissue currently being explored is the possibility of enhancing the ability of the damaged native ligament to heal itself through application of tissue engineering strategies. Previous studies on the healing of extra-articular ligaments such as the MCL have shown that a blood clot functions as the scaffold allowing fibroblasts to migrate and heal the defect (Lo et al., 1998; Murray and Spector, 2001). It has also been shown that no blood clot forms within the intra-articular environment of the ruptured ACL, which would normally provide a scaffold for repair (Harris et al., 1997). Even with macroscopic reapproximation of the ligament, the lack of a blood clot scaffold inhibits the ability of the ACL to heal itself. It is thought that implantation of an engineered scaffold which could hold the ligament ends in microscopic proximity, resist synovial degradation, and stimulate cell invasion and regeneration could provide for success with primary repair of the ACL (Lo et al., 1998). Research into scaffolds and optimization of the intra-articular environment with growth factors or gene delivery are directions that are actively being pursued (Murray and Spector, 2001).

## 26.4.3   ACL Marker Baseline

In engineering ACL tissue for healing or replacement, a concise quantitative molecular baseline of selected markers in ACL is essential in assessing the ligaments' own healing capacity or stem cell progression towards the ligament lineage. Biochemical and molecular markers indicative of different states of ACL tissue function and repair, including variables of age, gender, trauma, associated intra-articular conditions such as torn or arthritic cartilage and inflammation, require further examination in order to provide enhanced understanding of ACL regulation and function.

It is believed that matrix metalloproteinases (MMPs) play a large role in remodeling native tissue structures. In order to better understand the healing mechanism of the ACL, the transcript expression of MMPs and ECM components in 33 ruptured human ACLs have been characterized using the sensitive and accurate quantitative real-time RT-PCR method (Bramono et al., 2005). Marker expressions were correlated to several predictors such as age, gender, post-injury period, and site of ACL tissue scarring (e.g., to the posterior cruciate ligament or tibia). The relationship between markers and the predictors were analyzed utilizing univariate and multivariate statistical methods. The ECM of ACL tissue consists mainly of collagen type I and III; mRNA levels were highly correlated to each other with an average collagen type I to collagen type III transcript ratio of $2.28 \pm 0.81$. MMP-2 and TIMP-1 were expressed at much greater levels compared to MMP-1 and MMP-9. All of the MMPs analyzed had significant correlation to collagen type I and III after logarithmic transformation of the normalized mRNA amount (Bramono et al., 2005).

**TABLE 26.2**

Correlation Table Illustrating the Relationship Between Patient Demographics and Marker mRNA Expressions Represented by R-value ($p$-value)

| | Age | Post-Injury | Col 1 | Col 3 | Bgn | Dcn | MMP-1 | MMP-2 | MMP-9 | TIMP-1 |
|---|---|---|---|---|---|---|---|---|---|---|
| Age | 1 | | | | | | | | | |
| Post-Injury | | 1 | | | | | | | | |
| Col 1 | −0.20 | −0.67 | | | | | | | | |
| | (0.2714) | (0.0000) | 1 | | | | | | | |
| Col 3 | −0.29 | −0.56 | 0.93 | | | | | | | |
| | (0.1002) | (0.0007) | (0.0000) | 1 | | | | | | |
| Bgn | −0.19 | −0.18 | 0.65 | 0.69 | | | | | | |
| | (0.2861) | (0.3070) | (0.0000) | (0.0000) | 1 | | | | | |
| Dcn | −0.14 | 0.53 | −0.36 | −0.24 | 0.10 | | | | | |
| | (0.4138) | (0.0016) | (0.0420) | (0.1740) | (0.5782) | 1 | | | | |
| MMP-1 | −0.092 | −0.40 | 0.44 | 0.44 | 0.17 | −0.13 | | | | |
| | (0.6112) | (0.0221) | (0.0100) | (0.0098) | (0.3568) | (0.4714) | 1 | | | |
| MMP-2 | −0.025 | −0.31 | 0.58 | 0.62 | 0.57 | 0.036 | 0.41 | | | |
| | (0.8923) | (0.0758) | (0.0004) | (0.0001) | (0.0005) | (0.8403) | (0.0188) | 1 | | |
| MMP−9 | 0.080 | −0.43 | 0.49 | 0.40 | 0.28 | −0.57 | 0.49 | 0.23 | | |
| | (0.6595) | (0.0126) | (0.0034) | (0.0212) | (0.1146) | (0.0006) | (0.0034) | (0.1906) | 1 | |
| TIMP-1 | 0.15 | 0.031 | −0.088 | −0.076 | 0.093 | 0.34 | 0.24 | 0.20 | −0.24 | |
| | (0.3963) | (0.8653) | (0.6247) | (0.6730) | (0.6086) | (0.0493) | (0.1836) | (0.2536) | (0.1837) | 1 |

Significant correlations evaluated at $p < 0.05$ are shadowed in grey. Taken from Bramono, D. et al., *Connect. Tissue Res.*, (2005), in press. With permission.

Hence, collagenases and gelatinases may play a significant role in the remodeling and healing of this tissue as well as in the development of viable and functional tissue-engineered ACL constructs. Univariate analysis showed no significant differences in most marker expressions between the two types of scar attachment conditions, confirming previous results (Lo et al., 1998). However, through multivariate analysis, scar attachment significantly contributed in predicting the outcome of collagen type I, collagen type III, biglycan, and MMP-2. Post-injury period was also found to contribute significantly to these predictions using both univariate and multivariate analysis (Table 26.2). Such findings may support future studies that lead to the identification of specific stages associated with ligament development *in vitro* or healing *in vivo*, or may serve to better identify donor tissue candidates with which to extract healing ACL cells still capable of remodeling for use in tissue engineering.

### 26.4.4  Clinical Requirements of Matrix Design for Tissue Engineering

Tissue-engineered ligaments with appropriate biological and mechanical properties already established at the time of implantation would eliminate the limitations associated with present-day surgical techniques. The following requirements for clinically relevant tissue engineering of ligaments have been identified (Weitzel et al., 2002)

- *Minimal patient morbidity* does not require tendon graft harvest for use in ACL reconstruction.
- *Surgically simple to insert* and has reliable methods of fixation which will withstand aggressive rehabilitation.

- *Produce and maintain immediate stabilization* of the knee without tissue-fixation device creep to allow patients to rapidly return to their preinjury level of function.
- *Minimal risk* for infection or disease transmission.
- *Biocompatible* (i) non-antigenic and (ii) minimal foreign body response.
- *Support host tissue in-growth* through matrix geometry design, void volume, and porosity.
- *Direct host tissue in-growth* without causing stress-shielding, i.e., the device must adequately communicate environmental signals (both mechanical and biochemical) to the developing host tissue such that in-growth is properly directed and organized.
- *Biodegrade*, i.e., capable of being metabolized by the host at a rate that provides adequate mechanical stability during replacement by new ECM.
- *Maintain mechanical integrity prior to degrading*, either *in vitro* or *in vivo*, for a duration sufficient to allow host tissue in-growth and organization to eventually maintain the mechanical integrity of the ACL over the lifetime of the patient.

## 26.5   Ligament Engineering Approach

Development of a fully functional ACL *in vitro* requires a multifaceted approach in order to address the large clinical need. Such an approach has utilized (i) pluripotent bone marrow stromal cells (BMSCs), capable of directed differentiation and development into multiple lineages, (ii) a mechanically robust, long-term degradable silk fiber matrix, (iii) directed stimulation using an advanced bioreactor system capable of mimicking physiologically relevant multidimensional strains as well as timely and appropriate biochemical supplementation, and (iv) quantitative methods of ligament characterization *in vitro* and *in vivo* including molecular, structural, and histomorphological, which are required to support the multifaceted approach.

### 26.5.1   Cell Source

Often in tissue engineering there is a need to rapidly engineer tissue *ex vivo* for immediate implantation *in vivo*; such is the case in engineering ACL replacements. Considering that, on average, patients typically wait 8 weeks from the time of injury to the time of ACL reconstruction, it is critical to rapidly induce differentiation and autologous ligament tissue development *ex vivo*. This might be accomplished through introduction of specific growth factors and/or dynamic mechanical stimulation to mature ACL fibroblasts which have been shown to be responsive to such stimuli (Goulet et al., 1997; Toyoda et al., 1998; Murray and Spector, 2001). Unfortunately, as previously described, a reliable source of autologous ACL fibroblasts remains to be identified, leaving a need for an alternative autologous cell supply.

One candidate source of cells for engineering skeletal tissues is adult human bone marrow, which maintains a pool of BMSCs capable of both self-renewal and differentiation into cells of various mesenchymal lineages. BMSCs are very intriguing as a cell source as they are free from the ethical worry of embryonic stem cells, easy to collect, and isolate (Bruder et al., 1997; Caplan and Bruder, 1997; Jaiswal et al., 1997; Ohgushi and Caplan, 1999), and their differentiation may be directed into multiple phenotypes including osteoblasts, chondrocytes, adipocytes, and fibroblasts (Caplan, 1991; Bruder and Jaiswal,

1996; Prockop, 1997; Young et al., 1998; Dennis et al., 1999). Additionally, while their numbers in the bone marrow decrease with age, (Bruder et al., 1997), BMSCs retain the ability to proliferate and differentiate (Caplan et al., 1998; Turgeman et al., 2001). Of particular relevance here, BMSCs can be directed into a fibroblastic lineage to produce ACL autografts capable of being implanted in a timely fashion without the risk of immune reaction.

### 26.5.2 Matrix Design

In addition to providing initial mechanical integrity to functional tissue-engineered grafts, biomaterial scaffolds provide a structural template for cell attachment and tissue development biodegrading in parallel with the accumulation of tissue components. Most studies suggest that a properly designed scaffold is essential for promoting orderly tissue repair (Freed et al., 1994; Chu et al., 1995; Caplan and Bruder, 1997; Hunziker, 1999; Schaefer et al., 2002). Scaffold structure plays a role in mass-transfer dynamics relating to nutrients, metabolites, and regulatory molecules, while simultaneously its mechanical properties determine mechanotransduction at cellular and tissue levels. Ideally, a scaffold should be made of biocompatible, biodegradable material, and degrade at a rate matching that of new tissue deposition (Yannas, 2001).

Specifically, matrix design should consider: (1) mechanical properties, (2) potential for stress-shielding, (3) void volume, and (4) implant size. ACL scaffolds must meet typical native tissue strength requirements not only at failure, but also at yield due to the permanent deformation which will occur after this point limiting the function of the graft. Grafts designed with a stiffness greater than that of the native tissue have resulted in stress-shielding and therefore limited the graft to its fatigue life (Woo and Adams, 1990). Grafts must fit within the size limitations of the native tissue as well as address mass-transfer limitations into the graft which may hinder in-growth. The correct geometry will encourage organized in-growth within the graft as the distribution and transmission of mechanical stimuli may direct the growth of connective tissue in the direction of applied load (Chu et al., 1995). Furthermore, an appropriate geometry will address the porosity and directionality needed to promote functional tissue formation.

The majority of ligament prosthetics at the present time rely upon fibrous yarn-like constructs, favored because of their tensile loadbearing characteristics, resistance to complete failure, and large void area conducive to tissue in-growth. These stand in contrast to alternative matrices formed from gels or sponges which tend to lack the mechanical and structural integrity necessary for such an environment. Techniques including braiding, twisting, cabling, texturing, and plying have been explored to generate yarn scaffolds for use as grafts or as the building blocks of grafts (i.e., as a component of a mesh, weave, or nonwoven structure) (Chu et al., 1995; Wintermantel et al., 1996; Altman et al., 2002; Cosson et al., 2003; Lu et al., 2005). An infinite number of possible geometries demand an understanding of how each structure behaves mechanically relative to each other. The ability to predict changes in mechanics on the basis of changes in geometry (e.g., increasing the number of turns per inch or the number of fibers per yarn) and changes in processing (e.g., surface modification or environment) will decrease the need for significant trial-and-error testing. Yarn design has been shown to be a major factor in tensile and burst strength, as well as flexure rigidity, of higher order structures such as meshes and superstructures and should be considered during matrix design (Chu and Welch, 1985; Wintermantel et al., 1996; Cosson et al., 2003).

### 26.5.3   Matrix Mechanical Analysis

Just as important as matrix design are the methods of analysis used to characterize potential biomaterial scaffolds for ligament tissue engineering. Single-pull-to-failure and fatigue analysis will largely describe the mechanical behavior of a ligament replacement material (whether linear or nonlinear) and will serve as a solid foundation on which to determine if additional testing is warranted (Figure 26.1). Yarns with promising initial properties should be further characterized to determine tensile and fatigue properties as a function of loading conditions and viscoelastic characteristics through creep and stress relaxation testing. The graft should be characterized according to: (1) ultimate tensile strength (N), (2) stiffness over the effective graft length (N/mm), (3) percentage elongation at break (%), (4) energy at break (N mm), (5) yield strength (N), (6) yield elongation (mm), (7) creep characteristics, and (8) stress-relaxation characteristics.

Terms which describe critical properties are often used interchangeably and can lead to confusion when comparing data reported in the literature. For example, *elastic modulus* is defined as the slope of the linear portion of a stress–strain curve, while *stiffness* is defined as the slope of the linear portion of a force-elongation curve (Trencer and Johnson, 1994). If stiffness is reported and the data is not normalized to cross-sectional area, comparison is difficult. Care should be taken to clarify any ambiguous terminology. The critical mechanical properties listed above are defined as such

- *Tensile strength* is determined during tensile loading methods as the ultimate load prior to scaffold failure.

- *Stiffness* is determined as the slope of the linear portion of the load-elongation curves.

- *Percent elongation at break* is determined as the percent strain observed at failure during tensile loading.

- *Energy to break* (i.e., work) is determined as the area under the curve of the load-deformation curve.

- *Yield strength* and *yield elongation* are established by generating a line parallel to the linear portion of the load-elongation curve and offset by a 0.2% strain. The point

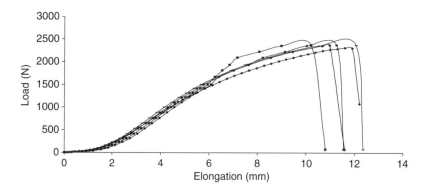

**FIGURE 26.1**
Histogram of silk ligament matrices illustrates typical plots of load vs. elongation data obtained during single-pull-to-failure analysis from which graft tensile properties including ultimate tensile strength (N) and yield point (N) may be derived (Altman et al., 2002).

where the offset line and the load-elongation curve intersect is defined as the yield
strength and elongation.

- *Creep* is defined as the change in scaffold length under a static load over time.
- *Stress-relaxation* is defined as the reduction in load with time under a static displacement.
- *Failure* can be defined by yield or fracture (ASTM, 2003) and is classified as brittle or ductile. In addition, it should be noted whether a complete mechanical failure or permanent deformation was observed.

It is a combination of these mechanical characteristics which will result in a clinically functional ligament replacement. When feasible, theoretical calculations should be performed to estimate the mechanical properties under ideal loading conditions. Tensile strength and stiffness will provide insight into the maximum load-carrying capabilities of the ligament under typical loading conditions. However, the yield characteristics will provide a more functional measure of the loads which can be withstood prior to permanent deformation. Stress and strain should be calculated with the measurements taken prior to testing and the stress–strain curve plotted. Despite the value of stress–strain curves for normalizing data to cross-sectional area and length, the significance of load-deformation curves in calculating energy to break should not be overlooked. Modeling and calculations can provide an estimate of expected properties and should serve as an "order of magnitude check" for empirical data. Response time to loading (i.e., viscoelastic behavior) and graft creep or relaxation must be examined to gain an understanding of the scaffold behavior in the dynamic and static *in vivo* loading environment. A graft which relaxes during static loading may experience decreased functionality when ligaments are loaded for extended periods of time in daily life. Ligament graft remodeling occurs within a complex *in vivo* environment; the scaffold must survive multiple cycles *in vivo* until tissue in-growth and remodeling can support the loading regimes, therefore cyclic testing must be performed. At the onset of the biological response, the scaffold structural integrity will weaken and the load burden will be gradually transferred to the newly-formed extracellular ligament matrix. An understanding of this transfer rate is critical to determining the graft's success as the rate of decrease in scaffold mechanics must not exceed the rate of increase in tissue load-carrying capabilities.

### 26.5.4 Bioreactor System

Our recent studies support the notion that advanced bioreactors providing physiologic loading are essential for meeting the complex requirements of *in vitro* engineering of functional skeletal tissues (Altman et al., 2002). An advanced bioreactor system with medium perfusion and mechanical loading has been described in detail and used to engineer ligaments starting from BMSCs (Figure 26.2) (Altman et al., 2002a–c). The bioreactor was specifically designed for ligament tissue engineering to provide the application of multidimensional mechanical strains (axial tension/compression and torsion) to BMSCs cultured in a hydrogel or on a fibrous scaffold. The bioreactor is computer controlled and consists of (a) 12 individual cartridges containing one engineered ligament apiece, each within a separate perfusion loop, (b) a gas exchanger to control medium pH and oxygen levels, (c) a 12-channel peristaltic pump, and (d) a strain control system for mechanical stimulation of cultured constructs. Two bioreactors are operated in parallel, allowing concurrent cultivation of 24 ligaments, e.g., 12 with loading and 12 with unloaded controls.

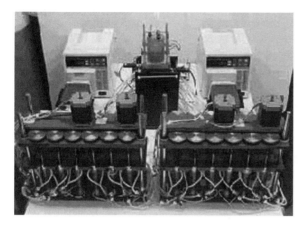

**FIGURE 26.2**
Image showing an advanced bench-top bio-reactor system developed for ligament tissue engineering (Altman et al., 2003). Two banks for bioreactors, each containing 12 reactor vessels with ligaments being cultured within, can be seen on the bottom portion of the image with a communal environmental chamber with gas inlets shown in the center.

## 26.6   Regulatory Factors

### 26.6.1   Biochemical Factors

As mentioned previously, rapid development of functional tissue within a tissue-engineered ligament graft is critical and, as a result, an understanding of relevant biochemical factors which may be used to enhance such in-growth is as well. Research has shown that such milieu are essential for inducing and/or supporting the differentiation of BMSCs toward ligament-specific tissue formation. Proper identification of factors is critical, even aspects of the environment as rudimentary as oxygen can markedly affect ECM synthesis rates and the *in vitro* development of engineered tissues (Carrier et al., 1999; Obradovic et al., 1999). Little is known about the effects of oxygen on stem cell differentiation into ligament fibroblasts. Fermor et al. (1998) showed that high oxygen tensions (21%) supported optimal ACL fibroblast proliferation, whereas lower tensions (10%) enhanced ECM collagen synthesis. Ascorbate-2-phosphate, a long-acting derivative of vitamin C, enhanced cell growth *in vitro* and supported the maintenance of connective tissues (Fermor et al., 1998; Murray et al., 2003). Epidermal growth factor (EGF) and transforming growth factor beta-1 (TGF-β) have been implemented for the induction of proliferation and differentiation of mesenchymal progenitor cell lines, in addition to native ACL tissue cultured *in vitro* (Deie et al., 1997; Marui et al., 1997; Sakai et al., 2002). TGF-β has also demonstrated the capacity to increase expression of ECM proteins in soft connective tissues (Attisano and Wrana, 2002). Basic fibroblast growth factor (bFGF) is required to prevent BMSC differentiation during cell expansion for tissue engineering applications, in addition to its role as a potent mitogen *in vivo* (Takayama et al., 1997; Murakami et al., 1999). Our previous studies have assessed the effects of these selected growth factors on BMSC in two-dimensional culture, assessing their influence on cell activity, morphology, and collagen type I production as correlated to native ACL fibroblasts (Moreau et al., 2005). After screening numerous growth factors, serum percentages and combinations thereof, bFGF, EGF and TGF-β in 5% supplemented serum were identified as the most efficacious factors in fibroblast differentiation and collagen type I accumulation as shown by immunohistochemistry (Figure 26.3) (Moreau et al., 2005).

In addition to enhancing BMSC growth *in vitro* through biochemical factor supplementation, it is believed that sequential administration of growth factors to BMSCs may provide improved tissue outcomes. It is known that *in vitro* BMSC growth may be enhanced through culture medium supplementation, mimicking the biochemical environment in

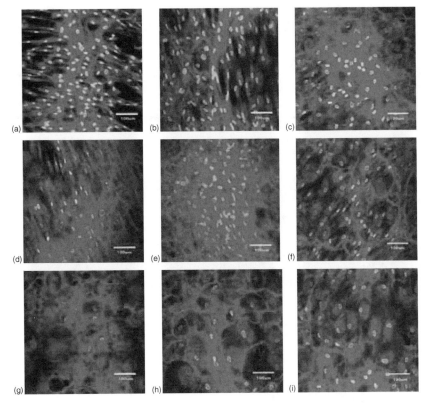

**FIGURE 26.3**

Collagen type I immunostaining of BMSC exhibiting enhanced collagen deposition, characteristic of fibroblasts, induced through sequential application of growth factors to culture medium. Cells on tissue culture plastic after 14 days of culture were stained using antibodies (red) against collagen type I, and Picogreen (green) to locate cell nuclei (Moreau, 2005). Images arranged as follows — a: bFGF only, b: bFGF followed by TGF-β1, c: control; d: EGF, e: EGF followed by TGF-β1, f: IGF-II; g: insulin, h: TGF-β1, i: bFGF followed by TGF-β1 and insulin.

which cells optimally proliferate and differentiate. Our group postulates that the sequential and "on-time" administration of growth factors to first proliferate and then differentiate BMSCs cultured on silk fiber matrices will support the enhanced development of ligament tissue *in vitro*. In a study performed to validate this theory confluent BMSCs obtained from purified bone marrow aspirates were seeded on surface-modified silk matrices (Moreau, 2005). Seeded matrices were divided into three groups for 5 days of static culture, with medium supplements of basic fibroblast growth factor (B) (1 ng/mL), epidermal growth factor (E) (1 ug/mL), or growth-factor-free control (C). After day 5, medium supplementation was changed to transforming growth factor beta 1 (T) (5 ng/mL) or (C) for nine additional days of culture. Real-time RT-PCR, SEM, cell-viability analysis, histology, and protein quantification for collagen type I of all sample groups were performed.

Results indicated that bFGF followed by TGF after 5 days in culture supported the greatest cell in-growth after 14 days in addition to the greatest cumulative collagen type I expression measured by ELISA. Sequential growth-factor application promoted significant increases in collagen type I transcript expression from day 5 of culture to day 14, for 5 of 6 groups tested. All TGF sequentially-supplemented samples surpassed their respective control samples in both cell in-growth and collagen deposition (Figure 26.4). All samples supported spindle-shaped, fibroblast cell morphology, aligning with the direction of silk fibers. These findings indicate significant *in vitro* ligament development after 14 days of

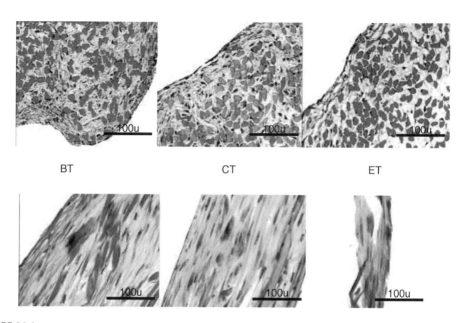

**FIGURE 26.4**
Trichrome staining of BMSC-seeded matrices harvested after 14 days of culture with mitogen supplementation imaged in cross-section (top) and longitudinal section (bottom). Groups pictured are bFGF followed by TGF-β (BT), control medium followed by TGF-β (CT), and EGF followed by TGF-β (ET) (Moreau, 2005).

culture with the sequential addition of growth factors (Moreau et al., 2005). The ability to improve tissue outcomes on a short time scale may prove beneficial not only to ligament tissue engineering but also to other tissue types, though further research is still necessary on a case-by-case basis.

In addition to serving as a tool for characterizing cells, biochemical baselines are also being considered strongly as potential effectors of the intra-articular *in vivo* environment. Properly selected molecules such as growth factors or genes delivered via a tissue-engineering scaffold may be able to provide or impose a desired biochemical *in situ* (Toyoda et al., 1998). While typically introduced to cells through culture-medium supplementation (Lecanda et al., 1997; Martin et al., 1998, 2001; Gooch et al., 2001; Pei et al., 2002), various regulatory molecules have also been incorporated into biomaterial scaffolds to provide localized delivery (Ito et al., 1991; Massia and Hubbell, 1991; Liu et al., 1992; Zheng et al., 1994; Kuhl and Griffith-Cima, 1996; Laffargue et al., 2000; Lam et al., 2000; Mann et al., 2001). Research in bone tissue engineering has already begun to address the possibility of bioinductive molecules coupled to tissue engineering scaffolds (Callen et al., 1993; Gomi and Davies, 1993; Locklin et al., 1995; Reddi, 1995; Rogers et al., 1995; Honda et al., 1997; Jaiswal et al., 1997; Mason et al., 1998; Reddi, 1998). Ligament tissue engineering might greatly benefit from the new generation of bioinductive biomaterial scaffolds including improved collagens and silk (Minoura et al., 1990; Inouye et al., 1998; Santin et al., 1999; Sofia et al., 2001; Altman et al., 2002, 2003), materials capable of delivering multiple growth factors (Richardson et al., 2001), and even materials capable of releasing growth factors in response to mechanical loading (Lee et al., 2000).

## 26.6.2 Mechanical Stimulation

Mechanical signals that affect the growth and development of native ligaments *in vivo* are likely to play similar roles during the *in vitro* cultivation of engineered ligaments.

The application of loading can affect tissue development in at least two ways, by (i) enhanced mass transport, and (ii) direct stimulation of the cells. Mechanical stimulation of cultured ligament fibroblasts has been shown to upregulate the expression of collagens type I and type III, fibronectin, and tenascin-C (Chiquet-Ehrismann et al., 1994; Chiquet et al., 1996; Toyoda et al., 1998; Trachslin et al., 1999). Human BMSCs, in the absence of specific ligament growth and regulatory factors, might directed to differentiate into ligament-like cells through the application of physiologically relevant cyclic strain (Altman et al., 2002a,b). Loading can cause changes to the extracellular environment both in native and engineered ligaments by direct effects on cell shape and interfibrillar spacing or by fluid flow that can enhance the rate of mass transport to and from the cells.

Cells are known to rebuild ECM under dynamic culture conditions in order to adapt to the environmental stress (Chiquet-Ehrismann et al., 1994). Consistent with our own collagen gel system, dynamic three-dimensional culture on fibrous silk scaffolds upregulated collagen type I transcript levels (Altman et al., 2002a). Correspondingly, cells upregulated the expression of biglycan and decorin, which are small leucine-rich proteoglycans that play important roles in modifying the kinetics of collagen fibril formation and affect the morphology of collagen fibrils (San Martin and Zorn, 2003). The type (nonpulsatile or pulsatile), rate (from 0 to 2.5 mL/min) and duration (continuous or 1 h per 24 h) of the medium flow and a multitude of regimes with translational strains (from $-10$ to 10% and rotational strains 0 to 25%) in combination with strain rates (between $1.67 \times 10^{-2}$ and $6.9 \times 10^{-5}$ Hz [as well as a true static environment]) were studied. BMSCs cultured on the silk matrices positively responded to the dynamic stimulation as compared with static control samples in the bioreactor when introduced immediately following 5 days of culture under static conditions which allowed attainment of peak activity, cell density, and ECM expression levels before stimulation (Figure 26.5). Given that the same mechanical regimes were shown to have detrimental effects to the matrices after 1 and 3 days post seeded, results indicate that the accumulation of ECM, the

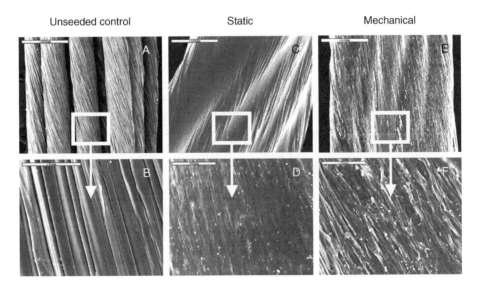

**FIGURE 26.5**
Scanning electron micrographs showing nonseeded silk fiber matrix at different magnifications (A, B), BMSC-seeded bioreactor static control (C, D) and seeded mechanically-stimulated matrix (E, F) after 15 days of culture (Chen et al., 2005). Scale bars for A, C, E = 500 μm; for B,D, F = 50 μm. Images E and F clearly depict a distinct fibroblast morphology induced as a result of dynamic mechanical stimulation as compared to the static controls (C, D) where the cell sheet appears as a drape covering the matrix.

establishment of cell-ECM interactions (through integrins), and peak cell activity is a prerequisite for the utilization of ligament-like mechanical stimulation (Chen et al., 2005). The results further validate the need for the on-time application of a chosen stimulus.

## 26.7   Functional Model to Prove Efficacy

### 26.7.1   Goat Model and Properties

Bench-top or *in vitro* simulation are not entirely representative of the intra-articular environment of the knee joint or the bone tunnels created during ACL reconstructive surgery. Once successfully engineered *in vitro*, a potential tissue engineered ligament requires additional evaluation *in vivo* to demonstrate safety and efficacy prior to human clinical studies. The applicable *in vivo* model requires a knee joint that is skeletally mature, substantial in size, and that has an ACL which functions similarly to that of the human ACL. The goat model, above most other models, including that of the rabbit or canine, meets these criteria and has been well established in the literature as a good model for ACL reconstruction (Table 26.3 and Table 26.4) (Jackson et al., 1993). Additionally, the soft tissue healing response in goats is similar to that of humans (Ng et al., 1996).

### 26.7.2   *In Vivo* Evaluation Periods

The times at which evaluations occur are critical in capture graft-host interactions and should be carefully chosen; here we propose evaluation at 3, 6, and 12 months. The 3-month period is proposed for several reasons: (i) bone-tunnel in-growth and resultant ligament mechanical properties can be evaluated within this time frame (bone in-growth in the femoral and tibial tunnels will have taken place between 6 and 10 weeks); (ii) initiation of tissue in-growth into the ligament (at both the ligament mid-substance and in the bone tunnels) will have occurred; (iii) early initiation of angiogenesis may be evaluated histologically; (iv) matrix abrasion, if a problem, will be apparent; (v) problems (graft creep, joint laxity) with fixation would be apparent. The 6-month evaluation is of particular importance as: (i) angiogenesis will have been initiated in earnest providing an indication of the graft's developmental potential as a function of newly formed and remodeling tissue, (ii) the presence of biologically viable ligament tissue and the extent of matrix degradation will be apparent through histology and may be assessed histomorphometrically, (iii) the adoption of biologically functional ligament tissue can be observed through mechanical testing of the joint (in combination with histology), and (iv) it is at this time point that patients are typically allowed to return to pretrauma activity levels. The latter establishes firm criteria for the degree of graft success or failure on physiologically relevant biomechanical and biological baselines. The 12-month *in vivo* period will provide information regarding the adoption of a biologically viable ligament tissue by the host and demonstrate the ability of the ligament to serve the patient in the long term.

### 26.7.3   Potential Device Failure Modes

Several potential failure modes exist given the intra-articular environment of both the goat and human joints. However, given the anatomy and rigors of the goat joint, several additional factors exist that place the graft at a higher risk of failure, potentially producing false negatives within an *in vivo* goat study.

**TABLE 26.3**

Goat ACL Mechanical Data Found in the Literature

| Reference | Study Goal | Goat Gender | # of Animals | Weight (kg) | Age (yrs) | Graft Type | Time Point |
|---|---|---|---|---|---|---|---|
| Roth et al. (1988) | Study effect of 6 weeks immobilization | | 6 | | | B-PT-B w/LAD | 3 mo |
| Jackson et al. (1987) | Evaluate freeze-dried allografts in the goat | Female | 7 | 35–50 | Skeletally mature | ACL allograft | 12 mo |
| Jackson et al. (1987) | Evaluate freeze-dried allografts and 3M LAD in goats | Female | 7 | 35–50 | Skeletally mature | ACL allograft + LAD | 12 mo |
| Holden et al. (1988) | Investigate soft-tissue fixation, and examine sources of early increases in AP translation | Both | 50 | 51 ± 2 | Adult | Fascia lata autograft | 0, 2, 4, 8 wks |
| Jackson et al. (1988) | Determine the effects of freeze drying and EO sterilization | | 12 | | Adult (cadaver) | Femur-ACL-tibia graft | |
| Jackson et al. (1991) | Effect of freezing *in situ* models, a graft in perfect tension and alignment | Female | 33 | 35–50 | Skeletally mature | *In situ* frozen ACL | 0, 6 wks, 6 mo |
| Gibbons et al. (1991) | Effect of gamma irradiation on patellar tendon allografts | | 48 grafts | 34–76 | 4–6 yrs (cadaver) | B-PT-B irradiated grafts | Cadaver |
| Drez et al. (1991) | Determine the effects of freeze-dried, EO-sterilized B-PT-B allografts | | 28 | 22–32 | 2–3 yrs (7 of 12 failed thru plate) | Freeze-dried B-PT-B allografts | 6, 12 mo |
| Jackson et al. (1993) | Compare autografts and allografts | Female | 46 | >25 | 4–5 yrs | B-PT-B allograft and autografts | 6 wks, 6 mo |
| Chvapil et al. (1993) | Evaluate collagen fibers as an ACL replacement scaffold | Both | 14 | | 1.5–3 + | Collagen fiber scaffolds | 2.5 – 6 mo |
| Ng et al. (1996) | Study repair of ACL after hemitransection | Female | 12 | 24–51 | adult | ACL control | |
| Smith et al. (1996) | Evaluate intraoperative set force on the mechanics of an autograft augmented with a synthetic | | 7 | 40–60 | Skeletally mature | LAD + B-PT-B autograft | 3 mo |
| Badylak et al. (1999) | Evaluate SIS as a potential ACL substitute | Female | 60 | 38–46 | 1-yr-old (right leg only) | B-PT-B autograft or SIS graft | 0, 3, 12 mo |

**TABLE 26.4**

Goat Mechanical Data in the Literature

| Reference | Sample | Time | Total Laxity (mm) | Stiffness (N/mm) | Anterior Stiffness (N/mm) | Graft Length (mm) | Max Load (N) | Stiffness (N/mm) | Elong (mm) |
|---|---|---|---|---|---|---|---|---|---|
| Jackson et al. (1987a) | ACL control | | 1.0 ± 0.1 | 36 ± 5 | 80 ± 5 | 18.9 ± 0.4 | 2301 ± 155 | 686 ± 47 | 4.7 ± 0.3 |
| Jackson et al. (1987b) | ACL control | | 1.0 ± 0.1 | 43.1 ± 9.2 | 93.2 ± 5.6 | 19.9 ± 0.6 | 2448 ± 144 | 691 ± 51 | 4.9 ± 0.2 |
| Jackson et al. (1988) | ACL control | | | | | | 2403 ± 133 | 692 ± 37 | 4.85 ± 0.16 |
| Harris et al. (1997) | ACL control | | 1.9 ± 0.1 | | 99 ± 11 | | 2748 ± 128 | 804 ± 65 | |
| Jackson et al. (1993) | ACL control | | 0.9 ± 0.1 | 88.45.8 | | 15.6 ± 0.3 | 2192 ± 119 | 352 ± 21 | |
| Ng et al. (1996) | ACL control | | | | | | 1167.2 ± 54.4 | 258.7 ± 7.1 | |
| Jackson et al. (1993) | ACL cut | 0 | 8.6 ± 1.0 | 15.6 ± 4.3 | | | | | |
| Jackson et al. (1993) | ACL cut (cut at 0) | 6 mo | 5.4 ± 0.5 | 25.4 ± 1.9 | | | | | |
| Jackson et al. (1987b) | ACL_LAD graft | 1 yr | 3.1 ± 0.5 | 9.4 ± 3.3 | 32.4 ± 3.3 | 18.8 ± 1.5 | 1052 ± 145 | 364 ± 49 | 4.8 ± 0.2 |
| Jackson et al. (1988) | Freeze-dried + EO | 0 | | | | | 2059 ± 273 | 718 ± 60 | 4.00 ± 0.3 |
| Jackson et al. (1988) | Freeze-dried ACL | 0 | | | | | 2023 ± 214 | 680 ± 65 | 4.3 ± .3 |
| Jackson et al. (1991) | ACL control | 6 wks | 0.5 ± 0.1 | | 101.9 ± 11.8 | 18.1 ± 1.2 | 2274 ± 116 | 521 ± 45 | 6.0 ± 0.7 |
| | | | 0.6 ± 0.1 | | 104.4 ± 6.3 | | | | |
| Jackson et al. (1991) | ACL control | 6 mo | 0.6 ± 0.2 | | 106.4 ± 11.5 | 18.1 ± 0.6 | 2603 ± 213 | 524 ± 22 | 5.3 ± 0.4 |
| | | | 0.5 ± 0.1 | | 130.4 ± 10.2 | | | | |
| Jackson et al. (1991) | ACL-frozen in place | 0 | 0.7 ± 0.1 | | 92.8 ± 12.0 | 18.4 ± -.6 | 2366 ± 125 | 481 ± 35 | 5.3 ± 0.6 |
| | | | 0.7 ± 0.1 | | 89.4 ± 8.0 | | | | |
| Jackson et al. (1991) | ACL-frozen in place | 6 wks | 0.6 ± 0.1 | | 107.5 ± 9.7 | 18.2 ± 0.3 | 1915 ± 110 | 548 ± 31 | 5.8 ± 0.4 |
| | | | 0.7 ± 0.1 | | 115.5 ± 11.3 | | | | |
| Jackson et al. (1991) | ACL-frozen in place | 6 mo | 0.8 ± 0.1 | | 86.7 ± 12.2 | 18.1 ± 0.2 | 2380 ± 184 | 550 ± 40 | 5.3 ± 0.5 |
| | | | 0.8 ± 0.1 | | 107.1 ± 8.7 | | | | |
| Drez et al. (1991) | ACL control | 0 | 1.1 ± 0.1 | | 75 ± 5 | | 1704 ± 110 | 681 ± 49 | |
| Drez et al. (1991) | B-PT-B allograft | 6 mo | 5.1 ± 1.2 | | 29 ± 4 | | 751 ± 191 | 203 ± 59 | |

| Study | Graft | Time | | | | | | |
|---|---|---|---|---|---|---|---|---|
| Drez et al. (1991) | B-PT-B allograft | 12 mo | 3.4 ± 1.1 | 58.1 ± 32.4 | 30 ± 5 | | 731 ± 191 | 187 ± 43 |
| Jackson et al. (1993) | B-PT-B Autograft | 6 wks | 6.3 ± 1.3 | 32.0 ± 3.1 | | 17.0 ± 0.7 | 265 ± 81 | 116 ± 10 |
| Jackson et al. (1993) | B-PT-B allograft | 6 wks | 6.2 ± 0.9 | 35.6 ± 5.0 | | 16.9 ± 1.3 | 241 ± 54 | 134 ± 42 |
| Jackson et al. (1993) | B-PT-B Autograft | 6 mo | 3.4 ± 0.5 | 35.1 ± 10.0 | | 15.2 ± 1.2 | 1337 ± 313 | 327 ± 50 |
| Jackson et al. (1993) | B-PT-B allograft | 6 mo | 5.3 ± 1.0 | 0 | | 15.9 ± 0.7 | 578 ± 91 | 166 ± 20 |
| Feder, 1993 | B-PT-B allograft | 6 mo | | | 35.8 ± 10.4 | | | |
| Ng et al. (1995) | Control ACL | | 0.6 ± 0.3 | | | | 1546.7 ± 464.4 | 305.8 ± 67.4 |
| Ng et al. (1995) | B-PT-B Autograft | 0 | 1.6 ± 1.0 | | | | 165.3 ± 68.2 | 36.3 ± 15.3 |
| Ng et al. (1995) | B-PT-B Autograft | 6 wks | 4.8 ± 2.5 | | | | 268.1 ± 76.6 | 39.4 ± 18.2 |
| Ng et al. (1995) | B-PT-B Autograft | 3 mo | 4.8 ± 1.3 | | | | 268.8 ± 175.8 | 37.2 ± 22.0 |
| Ng et al. (1995) | B-PT-B Autograft | 6 mo | 2.8 ± .5 | | | | 259.7 ± 71.1 | 65.5 ± 24.2 |
| Ng et al. (1995) | B-PT-B Autograft | 12 mo | 3.6 ± 2.5 | | | | 486.0 ± 236.1 | 108.2 ± 50.8 |
| Ng et al. (1995) | B-PT-B Autograft | 3 yrs | 1.1 ± 0.6 | | | | 677.3 ± 185.1 | 149.7 ± 5.4 |
| Badylak et al. (1999) | SIS | 0 | 1.6 ± 0.5 | | | | 721 ± 68 | 50 ± 4 |
| Badylak et al. (1999) | SIS | 3 mo | 1.3 ± 0.2 | | | | 293 ± 254 | 92 ± 73 |
| Badylak et al. (1999) | SIS | 12 mo | 1.3 ± 0.1 | | | | 706 ± 544 | 180 ± 113 |
| Badylak et al. (1999) | B-PT-B autograft | 0 | 1.5 ± 0.3 | | | | 253 ± 55 | 51 ± 12 |
| Badylak et al. (1999) | B-PT-B autograft | 3 mo | 1.1 ± 0.1 | | | | 611 ± 138 | 47 ± 54 |
| Badylak et al. (1999) | B-PT-B autograft | 12 mo | 1.1 ± 0.1 | | | | 879 ± 145 | 217 ± 64 |
| Cummings et al. (2002) | 4 mm wide B-PT-B auto | 6 mo | 4.12 | 8.02 | 58 | 22.3 | 847.7 | 245.4 |
| Cummings et al. (2002) | 7 mm wide B-PT-B auto | 6 mo | 5.11 | 5.83 | 50.5 | 22.1 | 784.2 | 210.4 |

1. Graft abrasion at the aperture of the femoral tunnel. Abrasion will lead to (a) complete rupture of the matrix, (b) a partially torn graft, and/or (c) particulate debris generation

2. Incorrect tunnel and graft placement leading to a destabilized joint, loss of isometry, articular cartilage damage or an increase in abrasion

3. Anchor choice limitation (compared to those available for humans)

4. Anchor pull-out (prior to bone healing within 6 weeks of implantation due to 3 above)

5. Anchor-matrix abrasion as a result of 3 and anatomic size limitations

6. Engineered tissue rejection resulting from (a) rejection of biomaterial and (b) the production and reaction to particulate debris (debris particles result from graft abrasion)

### 26.7.4  *In Situ* ACL Mechanical Analysis

Site-specific testing (i.e., testing the scaffold in its intended location) most closely mimics *in vivo* loading conditions and provides for design of an implant to mimic native properties *in situ*. Properties to be determined should include: (1) anterior-posterior (AP) laxity of the intact knee, (2) UTS of the bone-ligament-bone construct, (3) stiffness of the bone-ligament-bone construct, (4) failure stress, (5) failure strain, and (6) anchor pull-out strength (Table 26.3 and Table 26.4). Variables including surgical implant method, anchor type, and graft-host interactions will impact the mechanical properties of the bone-ligament-bone construct. The ability to rigidly anchor the ligament *in vivo* following implantation is required for ensuring the mechanical environment of the knee joint is communicated to the ligament tissue. Graft creep as a function of poor anchoring can detrimentally affect the ability to regain normal joint functionality and will appear during proper *in situ* joint analysis.

## 26.8  Conclusion

Tissue engineering of functional ligaments and tendons requires a comprehensive multidisciplinary approach and integrated analytical scheme in order to address a challenging problem in orthopaedic medicine and unmet clinical needs. Multiple beneficial outcomes should result from the diligent efforts of ligament tissue engineers in the near future as the field continues to advance along three paths: (i) the development of engineered biological tissue that may serve as functional tissue at the time of surgical replacement; (ii) the development of novel model systems utilizing cells, bioreactors and biochemical/biomechanical stimuli that may reveal or direct the development of a unique bioinductive matrix that may possess the potential to serve as an ACL replacement without additional cellular manipulation or components *in vitro*, and (iii) the development of unique *in vitro* reactor and model systems that can be used to provide a controlled environment for the study of environmental cues on stem cell differentiation. This system might also be used for the study of tissue disease/repair/ healing states, alleviating the need for animal models and improving the safety of human trials.

## Acknowledgments

The authors thank Adam Collette and Laura Geuss for their valuable contributions during the preparation of this article and Dr. Jingsong Chen, Dr. Jodie Moreau, and Dr. Diah Bramono for their contributions of ligament engineering data. Funding for the authors' studies of ligament tissue engineering has been provided by the NIH, NASA, NSF, and Tissue Regeneration, Inc.

## References

Altman, G.H. et al., Cell differentiation by mechanical stress, *FASEB J.*, **16** (2), 270–272 (2002a).

Altman, G.H. et al., Silk matrix for tissue engineered anterior cruciate ligaments, *Biomaterials*, **23** (20), 4131–4141 (2002b).

Altman, G.H. et al., Advanced bioreactor with controlled application of multi-dimensional strain for tissue engineering, *J. Biomech. Eng.*, **124** (6), 742–749 (2002c).

Altman, G.H. et al., Silk-based biomaterials, *Biomaterials*, **24** (3), 401–416 (2003).

Amiel, D. et al., Tendons and ligaments: a morphological and biochemical comparison, *J. Orthop. Res.*, **1** (3), 257–265 (1984).

Amiel, D. et al. Ligament structure, chemistry, and physiology, In: *Knee Ligaments: Structure, Function, Injury, and Repair*, Daniel, D. et al., Eds., Raven, New York, pp. 77–91 (1990).

Ardent, E. et al., Anterior cruciate ligament injury patterns among collegiate men and women, *J. Athl. Training*, **34** (2), 86–92 (1999).

Arnoczky, S. et al., Anterior cruciate ligament replacement using patellar tendon, *J. Bone Joint Surg.*, **64A**, 217–224 (1982).

Arnoczky, S. et al. Anatomy of the ACL, In: *The Anterior Cruciate Ligament: Current and Future Concepts*, Jackson, D.W., Ed., Raven, New York, pp. 5–22 (1993).

Attisano, L. and Wrana, J.L., Signal transduction by the TGF-beta superfamily, *Science*, **296** (5573), 1646–1647 (2002).

Badylak, S. et al., Naturally occurring extracellular matrix as a scaffold for musculoskeletal repair, *Clin. Orthop. Related Res.*, (367 Suppl), S333–S343 (1999).

Bramono, D. et al., Characterization of transcript levels for matrix molecules and proteases in ruptured human anterior cruciate ligaments, *Connect. Tissue Res.*, (2005), in press.

Bruder, S.P. and Jaiswal, N., The osteogenic potential of human mesenchymal stem cells is not diminished after one billion-fold expansion in vitro, *Trans. Orthop. Res. Soc.*, **21**, 580 (1996).

Bruder, S.P. et al., Growth kinetics, self-renewal, and the osteogenic potential of purified human mesenchymal stem cells during extensive subcultivation and following cryopreservation, *J. Cell. Biochem.*, **64** (2), 278–294 (1997).

Callen, B.W. et al., Behavior of primary bone cells on characterized polystyrene surfaces, *J. Biomed. Mater. Res.*, **27** (7), 851–859 (1993).

Caplan, A.I. and Bruder, S.P., Cell and molecular engineering of bone regeneration, In: *Principles of Tissue Engineering*, Lanza, R. et al., Eds., Landes/Academic, Austin, TX, pp. 603–617 (1997).

Caplan, A.I., Mesenchymal stem cells, *J. Orthop. Res.*, **9** (5), 641–650 (1991).

Caplan, A.I. et al., Cell-based tissue engineering therapies: the influence of whole body physiology, *Adv. Drug Deliv. Rev.*, **33** (1–2), 3–14 (1998).

Carrier, R. et al., Cardiac tissue engineering: cell seeding, cultivation parameters and tissue construct characterization, *Biotechnol. Bioeng.*, **64**, 580–589 (1999).

Chen, E. and Black, J., Materials design analysis of the prosthetic anterior cruciate ligament, *J.Biomed. Mat. Res*, **14**, 567–586 (1980).

Chen, J. et al., Human bone marrow stromal cell and ligament fibroblast responses on RGD-modified silk fibers, *Journal of Biomedical Materials Research. Part A*, **67** (2), 559–570 (2003).

Chen, J. et al., Ligament tissue engineering by directed regulation of mesenchymal stem cell (MSC) responses under dynamic culture conditions, (2005), in preparation.

Chiquet, M. et al., Regulation of extracellular matrix synthesis by mechanical stress, *Biochem. Cell. Biol.*, **74** (6), 737–744 (1996).

Chiquet-Ehrismann, R. et al., Tenascin-C expression by fibroblasts is elevated in stressed collagen gels, *J. Cell. Biol.*, **127** (6 Pt 2), 2093–2101 (1994).

Chu, C.C. and Welch, L., Characterization of morphologic and mechanical properties of surgical mesh fabrics, *J. Biomed. Mater. Res.*, **19**, 903–916 (1985).

Chu, C.R. et al., Articular cartilage repair using allogeneic perichondrocyte-seeded biodegradable porous polylactic acid (PLA): a tissue-engineering study, *J. Biomed. Mater. Res.*, **29** (9), 1147–1154 (1995).

Chvapil, M. et al., Collagen fibers as a temporary scaffold for replacement of ACL in goats, *J. Biomed. Mater. Res.*, **27** (3), 313–325 (1993).

Cosson, M. et al., Mechanical properties of synthetic implants used in the repair of prolapse and urinary incontinence in women: which is the ideal material?, *Int. Uro-gynecol. J.*, **14**, 169–178 (2003).

Cummings, J.F. et al., The effects of graft width and graft laxity on the outcome of caprine anterior cruciate ligament reconstruction, *J. Orthop. Res.*, **20** (2), 338–345 (2002).

Deie, M. et al., The effects of age on rabbit MCL fibroblast matrix synthesis in response to TGF-beta 1 or EGF, *Mech. Ageing Dev.*, **97** (2), 121–130 (1997).

Dennis, J.E. et al., A quadripotential mesenchymal progenitor cell isolated from the marrow of an adult mouse, *J. Bone Miner. Res.*, **14** (5), 700–709 (1999).

Drez, D.J. Jr. et al., Anterior cruciate ligament reconstruction using bone-patellar tendon-bone allografts. A biological and biomechanical evaluation in goats, *Am. J. Sports Med.*, **19** (3), 256–263 (1991).

Dunn, M.G., Tissue-engineering strategies for ligament reconstruction, *Mater. Res. Soc. Bull.*, **21** (11), 43–46 (1996).

Dunn, M.G. et al., Anterior cruciate ligament reconstruction using a composite collagenous prosthesis. A biomechanical and histologic study in rabbits, *Am. J. Sports Med.*, **20** (5), 507–515 (1992).

Dunn, M.G. et al., Development of fibroblast-seeded ligament analogs for ACL reconstruction, *J. Biomed. Mater. Res.*, **29** (11), 1363–1371 (1995).

Fermor, B. et al., Proliferation and collagen synthesis of human anterior cruciate ligament cells in vitro: effects of ascorbate-2-phosphate, dexamethasone and oxygen tension, *Cell. Biol. Int.*, **22** (9–10), 635–640 (1998).

Freed, L.E. et al., Biodegradable polymer scaffolds for tissue engineering, *Biotechnology (NY)*, **12** (7), 689–693 (1994).

Fu, F.H. et al., Current trends in anterior cruciate ligament reconstruction. Part II. Operative procedures and clinical correlations, *Am. J. Sports Med.*, **28** (1), 124–130 (2000).

Gibbons, M.J. et al., Effects of gamma irradiation on the initial mechanical and material properties of goat bone-patellar tendon-bone allografts, *J. Orthop. Res.*, **9** (2), 209–218 (1991).

Gomi, K. and Davies, J.E., Guided bone tissue elaboration by osteogenic cells in vitro, *J. Biomed. Mater. Res.*, **27** (4), 429–431 (1993).

Gooch, K.J. et al., IGF-I and mechanical environment interact to modulate engineered cartilage development, *Biochem. Biophys. Res. Commun.*, **286** (5), 909–915 (2001).

Goulet, F. et al. Tendons and ligaments, In: *Principles of Tissue Engineering*, Lanza, R. et al., Eds., Landes/Academic, Austin, TX, pp. 633–643 (1997).

Harris, N. et al., Central quadriceps tendon for anterior cruciate ligament reconstruction. Part I. Morphometric and biomechanical evaluation, *Am. J. Sports Med.*, **25**, 23–28 (1997).

Holden, J.P. et al., Biomechanics of fascia lata ligament replacements: early postoperative changes in the goat, *J. Orthop. Res.*, **6** (5), 639–647 (1988).

Honda, Y. et al., Osteogenic protein-1 stimulates mRNA levels of BMP-6 and decreases mRNA levels of BMP-2 and -4 in human osteosarcoma cells, *Calcif. Tissue Int.*, **60** (3), 297–301 (1997).

Horan, R.L. et al., In vitro degradation of silk fibroin, *Biomaterials*, **26**, 3385–3393 (2005).

Hunziker, E.B., Biologic repair of articular cartilage. Defect models in experimental animals and matrix requirements, *Clin. Orthop. Relat. Res.*, (367), S135–S146 (1999).

Inouye, K. et al., Use of Bombyx mori silk fibroin as a substratum for cultivation of animal cells, *J. Biochem. Biophys. Methods*, **37** (3), 159–164 (1998).

Ito, Y. et al., Enhancement of cell growth on growth factor-immobilized polymer film, *Biomaterials*, **12** (5), 449–453 (1991).

Jackson, D.W. et al., Freeze dried anterior cruciate ligament allografts. Preliminary studies in a goat model, *Am. J. Sports Med.*, **15** (4), 295–303 (1987), erratum appears in *Am. J. Sports Med.*, **15** (5), 482, September–October.

Jackson, D.W. et al., Cruciate reconstruction using freeze dried anterior cruciate ligament allograft and a ligament augmentation device (LAD). An experimental study in a goat model, *Am. J. Sports Med.*, **15** (6), 528–538 (1987).

Jackson, D.W. et al., The effects of processing techniques on the mechanical properties of bone-anterior cruciate ligament-bone allografts. An experimental study in goats, *Am. J. Sports Med.*, **16** (2), 101–105 (1988).

Jackson, D.W. et al., The effects of in situ freezing on the anterior cruciate ligament. An experimental study in goats, *J. Bone Joint Surg. Am. Volume*, **73** (2), 201–213 (1991).

Jackson, D.W. et al., A comparison of patellar tendon autograft and allograft used for anterior cruciate ligament reconstruction in the goat model, *Am. J. Sports Med.*, **21** (2), 176–185 (1993).

Jackson, D.W. et al., A comparison of patellar tendon autograft and allograft used for anterior cruciate ligament reconstruction in the goat model, *Am. J. Sports Med.*, **21** (2), 176–185 (1993).

Jackson, D.W. et al., Assessment of donor cell and matrix survival in fresh articular cartilage allografts in a goat model, *J. Orthop. Res.*, **14** (2), 255–264 (1996).

Jaiswal, N. et al., Osteogenic differentiation of purified, culture-expanded human mesenchymal stem cells in vitro, *J. Cell. Biochem.*, **64** (2), 295–312 (1997).

Kuhl, P.R. and Griffith-Cima, L.G., Tethered epidermal growth factor as a paradigm for growth factor-induced stimulation from the solid phase, *Nat. Med.*, **2** (9), 1022–1027 (1996).

Laffargue, P. et al., Adsorption and release of insulin-like growth factor-I on porous tricalcium phosphate implant, *J. Biomed. Mater. Res.*, **49** (3), 415–421 (2000).

Lam, X.M. et al., Sustained release of recombinant human insulin-like growth factor-I for treatment of diabetes, *J. Controlled Release*, **67** (2–3), 281–292 (2000).

Lecanda, F. et al., Regulation of bone matrix protein expression and induction of differentiation of human osteoblasts and human bone marrow stromal cells by bone morphogenetic protein-2, *J. Cell. Biochem.*, **67** (3), 386–396 (1997).

Lee, K.Y. et al., Controlled growth factor release from synthetic extracellular matrices, *Nature*, **408** (6815), 998–1000 (2000).

Liu, S.Q. et al., Cell growth on immobilized cell-growth factor; 4: interaction of fibroblast cells with insulin immobilized on poly(methyl methacrylate) membrane, *J. Biochem. Biophys. Methods*, **25** (2–3), 139–148 (1992).

Lo, Y.Y. et al., Interleukin-1 beta induction of c-fos and collagenase expression in articular chondrocytes: involvement of reactive oxygen species, *J. Cell. Biochem.*, **69** (1), 19–29 (1998).

Lo, I.K. et al., Comparison of mRNA levels for matrix molecules in normal and disrupted human anterior cruciate ligaments using reverse transcription-polymerase chain reaction, *J. Orthop. Res.*, **16** (4), 421–428 (1998).

Locklin, R.M. et al., In vitro effects of growth factors and dexamethasone on rat marrow stromal cells, *Clin. Orthop. Relat. Res.*, (313), 27–35 (1995).

Lu, H.H. et al., Anterior cruciate ligament regeneration using braided biodegradable scaffolds: in vitro optimization studies, *Biomaterials*, **26** (23), 4805–4816 (2005).

Mann, B.K. et al., Tethered-TGF-beta increases extracellular matrix production of vascular smooth muscle cells, *Biomaterials*, **22** (5), 439–444 (2001).

Martin, I. et al., In vitro differentiation of chick embryo bone marrow stromal cells into cartilaginous and bone-like tissues, *J. Orthop. Res.*, **16** (2), 181–189 (1998).

Martin, I. et al., Selective differentiation of mammalian bone marrow stromal cells cultured on three-dimensional polymer foams, *J. Biomed. Mater. Res.*, **55** (2), 229–235 (2001).

Marui, T. et al., Effect of growth factors on matrix synthesis by ligament fibroblasts, *J. Orthop. Res.*, **15** (1), 18–23 (1997).

Mason, J.M. et al., Expression of human bone morphogenic protein 7 in primary rabbit periosteal cells: potential utility in gene therapy for osteochondral repair, *Gene Ther.*, **5** (8), 1098–1104 (1998).

Massia, S.P. and Hubbell, J.A., Human endothelial cell interactions with surface-coupled adhesion peptides on a nonadhesive glass substrate and two polymeric biomaterials, *J. Biomed. Mater. Res.*, **25** (2), 223–242 (1991).

ASTM, *Medical Surgical Materials and Devices*, ASTM International 13.01, (2003).

Minoura, N. et al., Physico-chemical properties of silk fibroin membrane as a biomaterial, *Biomaterials*, **11** (6), 430–434 (1990).

Moreau, J.E. et al., Growth factor induced fibroblast differentiation from human bone marrow stromal cells in vitro, *J. Orthop. Res.*, **23** (1), 164–174 (2005).

Moreau, J., Sequential growth factor application in bone marrow stem cell ligament engineering, *Tissue Eng.*, (2005), unpublished data.

Murakami, S. et al., Regeneration of periodontal tissues by basic fibroblast growth factor, *J. Periodontal Res.*, **34** (7), 425–430 (1999).

Murray, M.M. and Spector, M., Fibroblast distribution in the anteromedial bundle of the human anterior cruciate ligament: the presence of alpha-smooth muscle actin-positive cells, *J. Orthop. Res.*, **17** (1), 18–27 (1999).

Murray, M.M. and Spector, M., The migration of cells from the ruptured human anterior cruciate ligament into collagen-glycosaminoglycan regeneration templates in vitro, *Biomaterials*, **22** (17), 2393–2402 (2001).

Murray, M. et al., The effect of selected growth factors on human anterior cruciate ligament cell interactions with a three-dimensional collagen-GAG scaffold, *J. Orthop. Res.*, **21**, 238–244 (2003).

Ng, G.Y. et al., Biomechanics of patellar tendon autograft for reconstruction of the anterior cruciate ligament in the goat — 3-year study, *J. Orthop. Res.*, **13** (4), 602–608 (1995).

Ng, G.Y. et al., The long-term biomechanical and viscoelastic performance of repairing anterior cruciate ligament after hemitransection injury in a goat model, *Am. J. Sports Med.*, **24** (1), 109–117 (1996).

Noyes, F.R. and Grood, E.S., The strength of the anterior cruciate ligament in humans and Rhesus monkeys, *J. Bone Joint Surg. Am.*, **58** (8), 1074–1082 (1976).

Obradovic, B. et al., Gas exchange is essential for bioreactor cultivation of tissue engineered cartilage, *Biotechnol. Bioeng.*, **63**, 197–205 (1999).

Ohgushi, H. and Caplan, A.I., Stem cell technology and bioceramics: from cell to gene engineering, *J. Biomed. Mater. Res.*, **48** (6), 913–927 (1999).

Otto, D. et al., Five-year results of single-incision arthroscopic anterior cruciate ligament reconstruction with patellar tendon autograft, *Am. J. Sports Med.*, **26** (2), 181–188 (1998).

Pei, M. et al., Growth factors for sequential cellular de- and re-differentiation in tissue engineering, *Biochem. Biophys. Res. Commun.*, **294** (1), 149–154 (2002).

Perrin, D., Anterior cruciate ligament injury in the female athlete, *J. Athl. Training*, **34** (2), 86 (1999).

Prockop, D.J., Marrow stromal cells as stem cells for nonhematopoietic tissues, *Science*, **276** (5309), 71–74 (1997).

Rauch, G. et al., Tensile strength of the anterior cruciate ligament in dependence on age. Biomechanics of human knee ligaments, *Proc. Eur. Soc. Biomech.*, **24** (1987).

Reddi, A.H., Bone morphogenetic proteins, bone marrow stromal cells, and mesenchymal stem cells. Maureen Owen revisited, *Clin. Orthop. Relat. Res.*, (313), 115–119 (1995).

Reddi, A.H., Role of morphogenetic proteins in skeletal tissue engineering and regeneration, *Nat. Biotechnol.*, **16** (3), 247–252 (1998).

Richardson, T.P. et al., Polymeric system for dual growth factor delivery, *Nat. Biotechnol.*, **19** (11), 1029–1034 (2001).

Richmond, J.C. et al., Anterior cruciate reconstruction using a dacron ligament prosthesis, *Am. J. Sports Med.*, **20** (1), 24–28 (1992).

Rogers, J.J. et al., Differentiation factors induce expression of muscle, fat, cartilage, and bone in a clone of mouse pluripotent mesenchymal stem cells, *Am. Surg.*, **61** (3), 231–236 (1995).

Ross, S.M. et al., Establishment and comparison of fibroblast cell lines from the medial collateral and anterior cruciate ligaments of the rabbit, *In Vitro Cell. Dev. Biol.*, **26** (6), 579–584 (1990).

Roth, J.H. et al., The effect of immobilization on goat knees following reconstruction of the anterior cruciate ligament, *Clin. Orthop. Relat. Res.*, (229), 278–282 (1988).

Sakai, T. et al., Effects of combined administration of transforming growth factor-beta1 and epidermal growth factor on properties of the in situ frozen anterior cruciate ligament in rabbits, *J. Orthop. Res.*, **20** (6), 1345–1351 (2002).

San Martin, S. and Zorn, T.M., The small proteoglycan biglycan is associated with thick collagen fibrils in the mouse decidua, *Cell. Mol. Biol (Noisy-le-grand)*, **49**, 673–678 (2003).

Santin, M. et al., In vitro evaluation of the inflammatory potential of the silk fibroin, *J. Biomed. Mater. Res.*, **46** (3), 382–389 (1999).

Schaefer, D. et al., Tissue-engineered composites for the repair of large osteochondral defects, *Arthritis Rheum.*, **46** (9), 2524–2534 (2002).

Smith, J.J. et al., Intraoperative force-setting did not improve the mechanical properties of an augmented bone-tendon-bone anterior cruciate ligament graft in a goat model, *J. Orthop. Res.*, **14** (2), 209–215 (1996).

Sofia, S. et al., Functionalized silk-based biomaterials for bone formation, *J. Biomed. Mater. Res.*, **54** (1), 139–148 (2001).

Takayama, S. et al., Effects of basic fibroblast growth factor on human periodontal ligament cells, *J. Periodontal Res.*, **32** (8), 667–675 (1997).

Toyoda, T. et al., Tensile load and the metabolism of anterior cruciate ligament cells, *Clin. Orthop. Relat. Res.*, (353), 247–255 (1998).

Trachslin, J. et al., Rapid and reversible regulation of collagen XII expression by changes in tensile stress, *Exp. Cell. Res.*, **247** (2), 320–328 (1999).

Trencer, A.F. and Johnson, K.D., *Biomechanics in Orthopaedic Trauma*, Martin Dunitz, London (1994).

Tsuda, E. et al., Techniques for reducing anterior knee symptoms after anterior cruciate ligament reconstruction using a bone-patellar tendon-bone autograft, *Am. J. Sports Med.*, **29** (4), 450–456 (2001).

Turgeman, G. et al., Engineered human mesenchymal stem cells: a novel platform for skeletal cell mediated gene therapy, *J. Gene Med.*, **3** (3), 240–251 (2001).

Vunjak-Novakovic, G. et al., Tissue Engineering of Ligaments, *Annu. Rev. Biomed. Eng.*, **6**, 131–156 (2004).

Weitzel, P.P. et al., Future direction of the treatment of ACL ruptures, *Orthop. Clin. North Am.*, **33** (4), 653–661 (2002).

Wintermantel, E. et al., Tissue engineering scaffolds using superstructures, *Biomaterials*, **17**, 83–91 (1996).

Woo, S.-Y. and Adams, D., The tensile properties of human anterior cruciate ligament (ACL) and ACL graft tissues, In: *Knee Ligaments: Structure, Function, Injury and Repair*, D.D.e, Ed., Raven Press, New York, 279–289, (1990).

Woo, S.L. et al., Tensile properties of the human femur-anterior cruciate ligament-tibia complex. The effects of specimen age and orientation, *Am. J. Sports Med.*, **19** (3), 217–225 (1991).

Yannas, I., *Tissue and Organ Regeneration in Adults*, Springer, Berlin (2001).

Young, R.G. et al., Use of mesenchymal stem cells in a collagen matrix for Achilles tendon repair, *J. Orthop. Res.*, **16** (4), 406–413 (1998).

Zheng, J. et al., Cell growth on immobilized cell-growth factor. 10. Insulin and polyallylamine co-immobilized materials, *Biomaterials*, **15** (12), 963–968 (1994).

# 27

## Tissue Engineering of Articular Cartilage

**James W. Larson III and Constance R. Chu**

## CONTENTS

## 27.1   Introduction

Traumatic and degenerative lesions of articular cartilage are leading causes of disability (Lawrence et al., 1998; Cooper et al., 2000). Articular cartilage, however, is a thick, avascular tissue with limited intrinsic healing capacity. In the larger weight-bearing joints of the body, the cartilage may be up to 3 to 4 mm thick. This limited repair capacity has been attributed in part to the absence of a blood supply. Without a vascular response to injury, there is no fibrin clot scaffold, there are no growth factors, and there is no migration of repair cells into the defect (Shapiro et al., 1993). The problem of cartilage regeneration, however, is more complex than simply restoring blood flow. It therefore poses an ideal challenge for the multidisciplinary field of tissue engineering.

The unique ability of articular cartilage to provide a near frictionless bearing surface for a lifetime of pain-free motion depends on a complex interplay between cells and matrix (Chu, 2001). Articular cartilage is composed of relatively few cells within a dense, extracellular matrix (ECM). The main components of this ECM are type II collagen (Col II) and proteoglycans. While this composition may appear trivial, these three basic components are arrayed in an exquisite functional architecture that provides articular cartilage with mechanical properties far superior to any man-made material. Restoration of the unique functional relationship between cartilage cells and matrix does not readily occur and poses the greatest scientific challenge.

There are two general approaches to tissue engineering of articular cartilage. The first approach is that of *ex vivo* tissue regeneration in which functional cartilage is created in the laboratory. Strategies used in this approach include encapsulation of repair cells into scaffolds for culture within sophisticated bioreactors delivering growth factors, nutrients, and mechanical forces. The second approach to cartilage regeneration focuses on enhancing intrinsic repair processes. As such, the emphasis is on augmenting and modulating the *in vivo* response to injury through the addition of scaffolds, cells and growth factors.

*Ex vivo* and *in vivo* approaches differ mainly with respect to whether neocartilage formation occurs within a bioreactor or *in situ* within the cartilage defect. While the approaches differ in perspective, the basic science similarly focuses on the repair cell and its response to local biochemical and biomechanical factors. Recent research using both approaches support the use of cells, growth factors and scaffolds to enhance articular cartilage repair (Chu et al., 1995; Chu et al., 1997; Fortier et al., 1997; Freed and Vunjak-Novakovic, 1997).

## 27.2   Cells

The cartilage wound has a paucity of repair cells for several reasons. Normal adult articular cartilage is a hypocellular tissue with chondrocytes composing only approximately 10% of the tissue. The chondrocytes are encapsulated within a dense matrix that prevents migration to the repair site (Figure 27.1). The matrix similarly impedes entry of reparative cells from the synovial fluid. As noted previously, the avascular nature of articular cartilage effectively eliminates the bloodstream as a source of repair cells. Clinical treatments have therefore focused on the introduction of chondrogenic repair cells into the cartilage defect .

Current cell-based clinical treatments include implantation of chondrocytes cultured *ex vivo*, and *in situ* marrow stimulation procedures where systematic violation of the subchondral bone plate allows entry of reparative cells from the bone marrow into the cartilage defect (Bert and Maschka, 1989; Frisbie et al., 2003). Bone marrow stimulation procedures include subchondral drilling, abrasion arthroplasty and microfracture. These procedures are simple to perform and can regenerate a clinically useful scar cartilage that

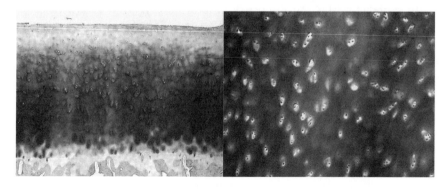

**FIGURE 27.1**

Cross sectional images of normal human articular cartilage. (Left) Notice the transition from the smooth joint surface (top) through the more randomly aligned middle zone and into the deep zone where the cartilage anchors into subchondral bone. (Right) Higher magnification of the middle zone reveals chondrocytes within spaces called lacunae surrounded by extracellular matrix.

is thought to originate from multipotential cells from the bone marrow (Frisbie et al., 2003; Steadman et al., 2003). Several studies show, however, that *in situ* marrow cell-based repairs produce a type 1 collagen dominant and low aggrecan fibrocartilaginous repair tissue of uncertain durability (Mitchell and Shepard, 1976; Robinson and Nevo, 2001; Frisbie et al., 2003). Despite the long clinical history, repair quality is unpredictable and improving the *in vivo* chondrogenic potential of bone marrow-derived cells remains a major therapeutic goal.

Chondrocyte transplantation proposes to introduce the fully differentiated cell as the putative repair cell (Brittberg et al., 1994; Grande et al., 1989). However, the current technique requires the patient to undergo an arthroscopic biopsy followed by a second more invasive arthrotomy to implant the cultured chondrocytes. While chondrocytes can be expected to produce a type II collagen dominant hyaline repair tissue (Freed and Vunjak-Novakovic, 1997), whether chondrocytes can revert to a chondroblastic state and regenerate articular cartilage is less certain (Benya and Shaffer, 1982; Dell'Accio et al., 2001). A randomized clinical trial comparing autologous chondrocyte implantation with microfracture failed to demonstrate significant differences by clinical criteria or histology (Knutsen et al., 2004).

For these reasons, there is intense interest in developing the chondrogenic potential of mesenchymal stem cells (Johnstone and Yoo, 1999). Descended from embryonic mesoderm, MSC are progenitors of the connective tissues of the body and may be induced to differentiate into bone, cartilage, tendon, muscle, fat, and dermis. While the multipotentiality of embryonic cells is undisputed, the use of multipotential cells isolated from adult tissues has advantages for potential autologous use and reduction of ethical concerns. MSC may be harvested from mesodermal tissues such as muscle, fat, and bone marrow using minimally invasive techniques.

The chondrogenic potential of bone marrow-derived cells has been well characterized (Caplan, 1991; Prockop, 1997; Johnstone et al., 1998; Pittenger et al., 1999; Barry et al., 2001; Sekiya et al., 2002). Numerous investigators have shown it is possible to isolate pluripotential cells from the bone marrow and to expand these cells *in vitro* to form cartilage (Caplan, 1991; Prockop, 1997; Pittenger et al., 1999; Barry et al., 2001). High-density suspension cultures and the use of chondrogenic growth factors such as transforming growth factor-β1 (TGF-β1) facilitate expression of the cartilage phenotype *in vitro* (Johnstone et al., 1998; Naumann et al., 2004). Bone marrow is relatively easily obtained by needle aspiration of a bone near the skin, such as the iliac crest or the greater trochanter of the femur.

Similarly, a skeletal muscle biopsy can be obtained with minimal trauma for use in tissue engineering applications. In recent years, muscle derived cells have been shown to be pluripotential. A population of skeletal muscle cells isolated from mice using a preplate technique (Qu et al., 1998) has been capable of regenerating several musculoskeletal tissues to include bone, muscle, tendon, ligament, and cartilage (Lee et al., 2001).

Ease of access to excess body fat has led to enthusiasm for development of the regenerative potential of adipose-derived stem cells (Erickson et al., 2002; Awad et al., 2004). Because the knee is frequently affected by symptomatic chondral injuries, the infrapatellar fat pad of the knee is being studied as a potential donor site for cells suitable for cartilage repair and regeneration. Adipocytes derived from the infrapatellar fat pad have been induced towards chondrogenesis and show potential for use in cartilage tissue engineering (Wickham et al., 2003).

While the introduction of chondrogenic cells alone has been shown to enhance articular cartilage repair, the resulting neocartilage is variable. All too frequently, a mixed or fibrocartilaginous repair predominates. Efforts to enhance the chondrogenic potential of chondrocytes, chondroblasts, and mesenchymal stem cells through manipulation of the cellular microenvironment therefore represent areas of intense study in the field of cartilage tissue engineering.

---

## 27.3 Factors Affecting the Growth of Engineered Cartilage

Because of the difficulty in regenerating functional articular cartilage, increasingly sophisticated methods for *ex vivo* creation of tissue-engineered cartilage are being pursued. Several groups are creating multilayered cartilaginous and osteochondral tissues *in vitro* (Klein et al., 2003; Tuli et al., 2004). Chondrogenesis of multipotential mesenchymal cells can be induced *ex vivo* using growth factors and three-dimensional suspension culture (Fortier et al., 2002a). For longer term *ex vivo* culture, bioreactors are being developed with particular attention to simulation of *in vivo* biochemical and mechanical environments (Freed and Vunjak-Novakovic, 1997; Hunter et al., 2004; Hunter and Levenston, 2004; Seidel et al., 2004). Factors affecting chondrogenesis may include growth factors, mechanical forces, oxygen tension, and cell-culture technique.

### 27.3.1 Growth Factors

The transforming growth factor (TGF) family of growth factors includes TGF-β and the bone morphogenetic proteins (BMP). Members of this family of growth factors have consistently demonstrated the ability to induce chondrogenesis from a variety of pluripotential mesenchymal cells. TGF-β was at one time known as cartilage growth factor and is known to increase the amount and proportion of type II collagen, promote cartilage phenotype differentiation, and increase proteoglycan synthesis in chondrocyte and stem-cell cultures.

Transforming growth factor-β (TGF-β) exists as three isoforms (TGF-β1, TGF-β2, TGF-β3), and TGF-β1 is of particular interest because multiple studies show it predictably induces chondrogenesis of human BMSC *in vitro* (Caplan, 1991; Prockop, 1997; Pittenger et al., 1999; Barry et al., 2001; Tuli et al., 2003). Transforming growth factor-β (TGF-β) is also extremely important to cartilage homeostasis and morphogenesis (Morales and Roberts, 1988; van der Kraan et al., 2002). TGF-β is very abundant in articular cartilage and TGF-β1 is the predominant isoform (Morales and Roberts, 1988; Morales et al., 1991). Using transgenic mice expressing a dominant-negative inhibitor of TGF-β receptor signaling, it has been determined that TGF-β plays crucial roles in both cartilage differentiation and in maintaining the articular surface (Serra et al., 1997). During embryological development, the expression patterns of TGF-β appears to be associated with the proliferative or nonterminally differentiated state of articular chondrocytes (Hayes et al., 2001).

The importance of TGF-β1 to the prevention of terminal differentiation is of special interest in the use of growth factors to enhance articular cartilage repair. The process of bone formation through endochondral ossification means that bone forms by replacing a cartilage anlagen after the chondrocytes undergo a process of hypertrophy, calcification and apoptosis know as chondrocyte terminal differentiation. As such, potent osteogenic growth factors such as bone morphogenetic proteins (BMP) can be expected to also be chondrogenic (Chubinskaya and Kuettner, 2003; Kim et al., 2005). However, the cartilage formed during endochondral ossification is destined for replacement by bone, an undesirable outcome for articular cartilage repair. BMP signaling has been shown to be necessary for chondrocyte terminal differentiation (Enomoto-Iwamoto et al., 1998; Li et al., 2003). In contrast, numerous studies by O'Keefe and others show that TGF-β1 inhibits the terminal differentiation of chondrocytes and that TGF-β1 acts to preserve the chondrocyte phenotype (Kato et al., 1988; Serra et al., 1997; Ionescu et al., 1999; Serra et al., 1999; Ferguson et al., 2000; Hayes et al., 2001; Pateder et al., 2001; Zhang et al., 2004). These qualities support efforts to study the chondrogenic effects of TGF-β1 in cartilage repair, especially when used with cells of known osteogenic potential such as BMSC.

Insulin-like growth factor-1 (IGF-1) has been also shown to be chondrogenic and to increase glycosaminoglycan (GAG) and type II collagen production *in vitro* (Fortier et al., 2002a, 2002b; Chu et al., 2004). IGF-1 increases proteoglycan synthesis when used alone and in combination with dynamic compression applied to chondrocyte cultures (Bonassar et al., 2001). Additionally, it has been shown that TGF-β and IGF-1 may depend on each other to produce their anabolic actions (Fukumoto et al., 2003; Yaeger et al., 1997). This finding underscores the coregulatory importance of growth factors for tissue engineering.

Because of their chondrogenic effects, there is intense interest in the cartilage repair potential of growth factors such as TGF-β1, BMP and IGF-1. The effects of growth factors, however, are dose-, time-, and cell-dependent. For example, uncontrolled dosing of TGF-β1 has been reported to result in unpredictable and adverse effects (Fortier et al., 1997; Mi et al., 2003). For *ex vivo* approaches, precise dosing regimens can be readily achieved. However, the potential for unintended *in vivo* effects highlight the need for methods to control and contain *in vivo* dosing of growth factors. As such, safe use and delivery of growth factors is a major consideration for tissue engineering strategies to enhance *in vivo* cartilage repair.

## 27.3.2 Mechanical Forces

Mechanical loading is critical to the development and maintenance of articular cartilage. Cartilage is subjected to active motion and compression during growth and development. Without motion, joints fail to develop. The use of continuous passive motion to improve cartilage repair is supported by basic studies demonstrating chondroprotective properties of cyclic loading within physiological ranges. Excess loading, however, leads to cartilage degeneration. Optimizing the loading of tissue engineered cartilage will be important to improving cartilage repair and regeneration.

Loading parameters include type of stress, applied forces and the frequency of loading. When a low static load was applied to a culture of chondrocytes in agarose, an 11% increase in GAG levels was seen; whereas, a 1-Hz cyclic load produced no difference in GAG levels (Toyoda et al., 2003; Awad et al., 2004). Other studies show that both the length of the cycle and the scaffold material affect chondrogenic responses when cyclical loading is applied (Hunter et al., 2004). For example, chondrocyte cultures under constant strain showed decreased proteoglycan production, while a 0.1-Hz dynamic compression applied to a mildly statically compressed culture showed increased total biosynthesis of protein and proteoglycan (Lee et al., 2003). These studies highlight that specific frequencies and load levels may be required for optimal neocartilage formation.

## 27.3.3 Hypoxia

Oxygen tension is another environmental factor that can influence the growth of articular cartilage. Hypoxia is the physiological state of chondrocytes within the deeper layers of articular cartilage. It has been shown that the surface and deep tissues have an approximate $O_2$ tension of 6 and $<1\%$, respectively (Silver, 1975). The positive influence of hypoxia on the chondroid phenotype has been also demonstrated *in vitro* with studies showing that culture in low $O_2$ tension (5% or less) facilitated chondrogenesis as determined by increased type II collagen and aggrecan production (Murphy and Sambanis, 2001).

The mechanism of adaptation to hypoxia appears to be highly dependant on a class of proteins known as hypoxia-inducible factors (HIF). HIF-1α in particular appears to be vital in chondrogenesis. HIF-1α appears to increase glycolitic enzymes and angiogenic factors, enabling chondrocytes to survive in low oxygen tensions (Semenza, 1998; Semenza, 2001). HIF-1α may also be important in the expression of cartilaginous extracellular matrix in chondrocytes. In a study of chondrocytes lacking the HIF-1α gene cultured under hypoxic conditions, there was greatly decreased production of aggrecan and type II collagen when compared to normal chondrocytes grown in hypoxia (Pfander et al., 2003). Collagen prolyl-hydroxylase alpha, an enzyme involved in cross-linking of collagen in the ECM, also shows an increased transcription in response to HIF-1α (Takahashi et al., 2000). As such, opportunities may exist for the use of growth factors within a hypoxic environment to improve cartilage regeneration.

### 27.3.4   Three-Dimensional (3D) Culture

Three-dimensional culture systems have been recognized as important for cartilage tissue engineering. When chondrocytes and their precursors are grown in standard monolayer cultures, the chondrocyte phenotype is lost after a few passages and the chondrocytes are known to "dedifferentiate" and exhibit a fibroblastic phenotype (Figure 27.2). However in 3D, or suspension culture, the cartilage phenotype can be restored (Murphy and Sambanis, 2001).

There are several methods by which chondrocytes can be grown in 3D culture. One of the simplest methods is through pellet or micromass cultures (Johnstone et al., 1998). Another option is to suspend the chondrocytes in hydrogels such as alginate or agarose. The use of both natural and polymer scaffolds can also provide the necessary 3D structure for cartilage differentiation. A bioreactor may additionally promote suspension culture due to turning and rolling of the cultured cells, thereby preventing them from forming a monolayer.

A recently-described scaffold-free method to produce cartilage occurs through maintenance of the 3D environment through use of alginate-recovered chondrocytes (ARC) (Masuda et al., 2003). In this method, chondrocytes are isolated and resuspended in alginate for 3D culture. This permits the cells to maintain their chondrocytic phenotype and to reform a pericellular matrix. Once the pericellular matrix has reformed, the beads

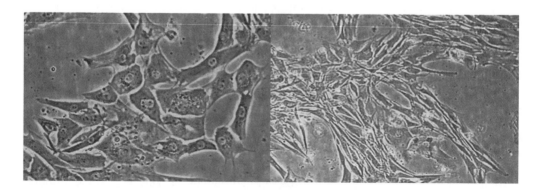

**FIGURE 27.2**
Chondrocytes in cell culture either maintain their chondrocytic morphology or dedifferentiate into fibroblasts. (Left) Round and icosahedral cells with few appendages have retained chondrocyte morphology. (Right) Thin spindle shaped cells indicate that the chondrocytes have dedifferentiated into a fibroblastic morphology.

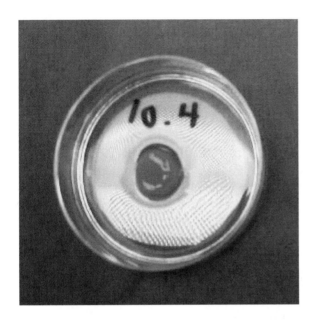

**FIGURE 27.3**
Tissue engineered cartilage. Cartilage-like tissue was grown in tissue culture using the alginate-recovered-chondrocyte method in chondrogenic media. Deposition of extracellular matrix resulted in formation of a thick neocartilage that could be handled with instruments.

are digested and the resulting cells surrounded by cell-associated matrix are plated on to a membrane. A thick, cartilage tissue can be reliably produced using this method without the use of scaffolds (Figure 27.3).

### 27.3.5  Bioreactors

Bioreactors are designed to replicate a defined environment for optimal culture of the cell-type of interest (Martin et al., 2004). A basic bioreactor consists of spinning drums that gently rotate the culture media and cultured cartilage constructs (Freed and Vunjak-Novakovic, 1997). A motor rotates the drum at a speed that results in a steady state of free fall, thereby eliminating the effect of gravity on the cultures. More sophisticated bioreactors can provide cyclic compression in a preprogrammed fashion. As an *ex vivo* culture chamber, nutrients, growth factors, and oxygen tension can be potentially added in combinations suitable for optimal chondrogenesis. As such, bioreactors have been shown to improve the chondrogenic responses of three-dimensional constructs, including the ratio of type II to type I collagen, the amount of collagen, and the amount of GAG when compared to monolayer. Moreover, the morphology of the cartilage grown in a bioreactor more closely resembles natural cartilage (Pei et al., 2002). Information from basic research into the use of growth factors, oxygen tension, biomechanical factors and stem cells to optimize chondrogenesis will be important to improving bioreactor design for the production of tissue-engineered cartilage.

### 27.4  Scaffolds

The concept of the cell–polymer construct is a basic tissue engineering principle where a polymer scaffold supports desired cell growth and differentiation. Scaffolds may be composed of biocompatible polymers, natural substances or a combination of materials. Examples of polymers widely used for biodegradable matrices include polylactic acid and polyglycolic acid. Natural scaffolds include collagen gels or sponges as well as hyaluronic acid and its derivatives. Scaffolds can be designed to support and direct cellular in-growth, to deliver growth factors, and to enhance the formation of engineered tissues. Growth factors and other substances can be encapsulated within scaffolds for controlled release over defined periods of time. Essential features for a scaffold suitable for cartilage tissue engineering include the ability to support chondrogenesis, biocompatibility and ease of use. Biodegradation at a rate compatible with that of anticipated cellular in-growth is important. Clinically, scaffolds must offer ease of sterilization, handling and cell implantation.

Poly(lactic acid) (PLA) and poly(glycolic acid) are FDA-approved materials that can be used singly or in combination to form a variety of biodegradable implants ranging from screws, meshes, and suture, to porous sponges. Both materials have been shown to support chondrogenesis. Other biocompatible/biodegradable materials that have been used for cartilage repair include polyurethane and poly(ethylene glycol) (PEG).

Among natural materials, hyaluronic acid and collagens are frequently used for cartilage tissue engineering. Hyaluronic acid has been used both as a filling agent and as a chondrogenic scaffold. Hyaluronic acid is a natural component of hyaline cartilage and is easily and safely incorporated into the repair site. Chondrocyte seeded hyaloronic-acid-based scaffolds are being studied clinically in the repair of chondral defects (Pavesio et al., 2003; Dickinson et al., 2005).

Type II Collagen is also a natural part of the chondral surface. Several studies have shown that type II collagen repair of chondral defects. Col II scaffolds seeded with cells were incubated in chondrocyte-inducing media and then implanted into defects in the cartilage of animal knees to improve defect filling and hyaline cartilage production (Lee et al., 2003). Type I collagen and gelatin scaffolds have also been used for cartilage repair. Chondrocytes seeded into collagen based scaffolds are also being studied in the clinical repair of chondral and osteochondral defects (Bartlett et al., 2005a, 2005b).

Natural hydrogels such as alginate and agarose approximate the dense matrix of articular cartilage and are known to support the cartilage phenotype. Polymer hydrogels appear equally promising. Hydrogels are comprised of water-soluble chains that can be cross-linked to form insoluble gels. While many biocompatible polymers can form hydrogels via chemical or physical cross-linking, poly(ethylene glycol) (PEG) is one of the most widely investigated systems (Sawhney et al., 1993a, 1993b). PEG can be photopolymerized into a stable hydrogel that supports chondrocyte survival and matrix deposition (Elisseeff et al., 2000). In order to obtain biodegradable hydrogels, PEG has been copolymerized with degradable polymers such as poly(lactic acid), (PLA), poly(glycolic acid) and poly(propylene fumarate) (Metters et al., 1999; Behravesh et al., 2003; Holland et al., 2004). It has recently been shown that genipin, a naturally derived cross-linking agent found in the gardenia fruit, can be used to produce PEG–genipin hydrogels that can be tailored to biodegrade at defined time periods (Moffat and Marra, 2004). It has also been shown that growth factors can be incorporated into PLA–PGA microspheres for sustained release (Royce et al., 2004). Controlled release of growth factors from biodegradable hydrogels lend further promise for cartilage tissue engineering applications (Lu et al., 2000; Meese et al., 2002; Parker et al., 2002).

Use of cross-linked polymers can provide highly reproducible delivery of growth factors. It has been reported that the release of TGF-β1 from cross-linked gelatin microspheres incorporated in PEG-fumarate hydrogels can be controlled by altering the degree of cross-linking (Holland et al., 2004). As such, TGF-β1 release may be tailored using cross-linked PEG to optimize cartilage repair (Holland et al., 2004). Engineering growth-factor releasing scaffolds will be critical to tissue-engineering strategies to enhance *in vivo* cartilage repair.

## 27.5 Conclusion

Articular cartilage injury and degeneration is a leading cause of disability (Lawrence et al., 1998; Cooper et al., 2000). It is well established that human articular cartilage has limited healing capacity (Hunter, 1995; Akeson et al., 2001).

The prevalence of chondral defects in the symptomatic knee is high (Curl et al., 1997; Lewandrowski et al., 1997). Untreated, cartilage defects are thought to progress to degenerative arthritis in the majority of patients (Messner and Maletius, 1996). It is estimated that over 40 million Americans currently suffer from osteoarthritis (Lawrence et al., 1998). Methods to improve cartilage repair and regeneration will therefore have high clinical impact.

The two basic strategies of cartilage tissue engineering both require study of chondrogenic cells, biomaterials, and biomechanics. To achieve the goal of producing an implantable biological construct that adequately replaces the function of the damaged articular cartilage, repair cells are encapsulated into scaffolds and cultured within bioreactors delivering an optimal program of nutrients, mechanical stress, growth-factor supplementation and oxygen tension. To enhance intrinsic cartilage repair processes, scaffolds are used primarily as vehicles to deliver growth factors and repair cells to the cartilage wound. Mechanical stimuli in the form of controlled passive motion of the injured joint may be used. While the approaches differ, the basic science similarly focuses on the repair cell and its response to local biochemical and biomechanical factors.

As highlighted in this chapter, the challenging problem of articular cartilage repair and regeneration is ideally suited for a multidisciplinary tissue-engineering team. The ability to modulate cellular responses to growth factors and mechanical stimuli to effect cartilage repair and regeneration will require collaboration between cell biologists, molecular biologists, polymer scientists and bioengineers. In order to remain focused on solving the clinical problem, clinician input and involvement in all stages of the process will be critical.

## References

Akeson, W.H. et al., Differences in mesenchymal tissue repair, *Clin. Orthop.*, **391** (Suppl), S124–S141 (2001).

Awad, H.A. et al., Chondrogenic differentiation of adipose-derived adult stem cells in agarose, alginate, and gelatin scaffolds, *Biomaterials*, **25** (16), 3211–3222 (2004).

Barry, F. et al., Chondrogenic differentiation of mesenchymal stem cells from bone marrow: differentiation-dependent gene expression of matrix components, *Exp. Cell Res.*, **268** (2), 189–200 (2001).

Bartlett, W. et al., Autologous chondrocyte implantation versus matrix-induced autologous chondrocyte implantation for osteochondral defects of the knee: a prospective, randomised study, *J. Bone Joint Surg. Br.*, **87** (5), 640–645 (2005a).

Bartlett, W. et al., Autologous chondrocyte implantation at the knee using a bilayer collagen membrane with bone graft. A preliminary report, *J. Bone Joint Surg. Br.*, **87** (3), 330–332 (2005b).

Behravesh, E., Sikavitsas, V.I., and Mikos, A.G., Quantification of ligand surface concentration of bulk-modified biomimetic hydrogels, *Biomaterials*, **24** (24), 4365–4374 (2003).

Benya, P.D. and Shaffer, J.D., Dedifferentiated chondrocytes reexpress the differentiated collagen phenotype when cultured in agarose gels, *Cell*, **30** (1), 215–224 (1982).

Bert, J.M. and Maschka, K., The arthroscopic treatment of unicompartmental gonarthrosis: a five-year follow-up study of abrasion arthroplasty plus arthroscopic debridement and arthroscopic debridement alone, *Arthroscopy*, **5** (1), 25–32 (1989).

Bonassar, L.J. et al., The effect of dynamic compression on the response of articular cartilage to insulin-like growth factor-I, *J. Orthop. Res.*, **19** (1), 11–17 (2001).

Brittberg, M. et al., Treatment of deep cartilage defects in the knee with autologous chondrocyte transplantation, *N. Engl. J. Med.*, **331** (14), 889–895 (1994).

Caplan, A.I., Mesenchymal stem cells, *J. Orthop. Res.*, **9** (5), 641–650 (1991).

Chu, C.R., Chondral and osteochondral injuries: mechanisms of injury and repair responses, *Oper. Tech. Orthop.*, **11** (2), 70–75 (2001).

Chu, C.R. et al., Articular cartilage repair using allogeneic perichondrocyte-seeded biodegradable porous polylactic acid (PLA): a tissue-engineering study, *J. Biomed. Mater. Res.*, **29** (9), 1147–1154 (1995).

Chu, C.R. et al., Osteochondral repair using perichondrial cells. A 1-year study in rabbits, *Clin. Orthop.*, (340), 220–229 (1997).

Chu, C.R. et al., Recovery of articular cartilage metabolism following thermal stress is facilitated by IGF-1 and JNK inhibitor, *Am. J. Sports Med.*, **32** (1), 191–196 (2004).

Chubinskaya, S. and Kuettner, K.E., Regulation of osteogenic proteins by chondrocytes, *Int. J. Biochem. Cell Biol.*, **35** (9), 1323–1340 (2003).

Cooper, C. et al., Risk factors for the incidence and progression of radiographic knee osteoarthritis, *Arthritis Rheum.*, **43** (5), 995–1000 (2000).

Curl, W.W. et al., Cartilage injuries: a review of 31,516 knee arthroscopies, *Arthroscopy*, **13** (4), 456–460 (1997).

Dell'Accio, F., De Bari, C., and Luyten, F.P., Molecular markers predictive of the capacity of expanded human articular chondrocytes to form stable cartilage in vivo, *Arthritis Rheum*, **44** (7), 1608–1619 (2001).

Dickinson, S.C. et al., Quantitative outcome measures of cartilage repair in patients treated by tissue engineering, *Tissue Eng.*, **11** (1–2), 277–287 (2005).

Elisseeff, J. et al., Photoencapsulation of chondrocytes in poly(ethylene oxide)-based semi-interpenetrating networks, *J. Biomed. Mater. Res.*, **51** (2), 164–171 (2000).

Enomoto-Iwamoto, M. et al., Bone morphogenetic protein signaling is required for maintenance of differentiated phenotype, control of proliferation, and hypertrophy in chondrocytes, *J. Cell Biol.*, **140** (2), 409–418 (1998).

Erickson, G.R. et al., Chondrogenic potential of adipose tissue-derived stromal cells *in vitro* and *in vivo*, *Biochem. Biophys. Res. Commun.*, **290** (2), 763–769 (2002).

Ferguson, C.M. et al., Smad2 and 3 mediate transforming growth factor-beta1-induced inhibition of chondrocyte maturation, *Endocrinology*, **141** (12), 4728–4735 (2000).

Fortier, L.A. et al., Altered biological activity of equine chondrocytes cultured in a three-dimensional fibrin matrix and supplemented with transforming growth factor beta-1, *Am. J. Vet. Res.*, **58** (1), 66–70 (1997).

Fortier, L.A., Nixon, A.J., and Lust, G., Phenotypic expression of equine articular chondrocytes grown in three-dimensional cultures supplemented with supraphysiologic concentrations of insulin-like growth factor-1, *Am. J. Vet. Res.*, **63** (2), 301–305 (2002a).

Fortier, L.A. et al., Insulin-like growth factor-I enhances cell-based repair of articular cartilage, *J. Bone Joint Surg. Br.*, **84** (2), 276–288 (2002b).

Freed, L.E. and Vunjak-Novakovic, G., Microgravity tissue engineering, *In Vitro Cell. Dev. Biol. Anim.*, **33** (5), 381–385 (1997).

Frisbie, D.D. et al., Early events in cartilage repair after subchondral bone microfracture, *Clin. Orthop.*, (407), 215–227 (2003).

Fukumoto, T. et al., Combined effects of insulin-like growth factor-1 and transforming growth factor-beta1 on periosteal mesenchymal cells during chondrogenesis *in vitro*, *Osteoarthr. Cartilage*, **11** (1), 55–64 (2003).

Grande, D.A. et al., The repair of experimentally produced defects in rabbit articular cartilage by autologous chondrocyte transplantation, *J. Orthop. Res.*, **7** (2), 208–218 (1989).

Hayes, A.J. et al., The development of articular cartilage: evidence for an appositional growth mechanism, *Anat. Embryol. (Berl.)*, **203** (6), 469–479 (2001).

Holland, T.A. et al., Transforming growth factor-beta 1 release from oligo(poly(ethylene glycol)fumarate) hydrogels, *J. Control. Release*, **94** (1), 101–114 (2004).

Hunter, W., Of the structure and disease of articulating cartilages, *Clin. Orthop.*, **1743** (317), 3–6 (1995).

Hunter, C.J. and Levenston, M.E., Maturation and integration of tissue-engineered cartilages within an in vitro defect repair model, *Tissue Eng.*, **10** (5–6), 736–746 (2004).

Hunter, C.J., Mouw, J.K., and Levenston, M.E., Dynamic compression of chondrocyte-seeded fibrin gels: effects on matrix accumulation and mechanical stiffness, *Osteoarthr. Cartilage*, **12** (2), 117–130 (2004).

Ionescu, A.M. et al., ATF-2 cooperates with Smad3 to mediate TGF-beta effects on chondrocyte maturation, *Exp. Cell Res.*, **288** (1), 198–207 (1999).

Johnstone, B. and Yoo, J.U., Autologous mesenchymal progenitor cells in articular cartilage repair, *Clin. Orthop.*, **367** (Suppl), S156–S162 (1999).

Johnstone, B. et al., In vitro chondrogenesis of bone marrow-derived mesenchymal progenitor cells, *Exp. Cell Res.*, **238** (1), 265–272 (1998).

Kato, Y. et al., Terminal differentiation and calcification in rabbit chondrocyte cultures grown in centrifuge tubes: regulation by transforming growth factor beta and serum factors, *Proc. Natl. Acad. Sci. USA*, **85** (24), 9552–9556 (1988).

Kim, M.S. et al., Musculoskeletal differentiation of cells derived from human embryonic germ cells, *Stem Cells*, **23** (1), 113–123 (2005).

Klein, T.J. et al., Tissue engineering of stratified articular cartilage from chondrocyte subpopulations, *Osteoarthr. Cartilage*, **11** (8), 595–602 (2003).

Knutsen, G. et al., Autologous chondrocyte implantation compared with microfracture in the knee. A randomized trial, *J. Bone Joint Surg. Am.*, **86-A** (3), 455–464 (2004).

Lawrence, R.C. et al., Estimates of the prevalence of arthritis and selected musculoskeletal disorders in the United States, *Arthritis Rheum.*, **41** (5), 778–799 (1998).

Lee, C.R., Grodzinsky, A.J., and Spector, M., Biosynthetic response of passaged chondrocytes in a type II collagen scaffold to mechanical compression, *J. Biomed. Mater. Res.*, **64A** (3), 560–569 (2003).

Lee, J.Y. et al., Effect of bone morphogenetic protein-2-expressing muscle-derived cells on healing of critical-sized bone defects in mice, *J. Bone Joint Surg. Am.*, **83-A** (7), 1032–1039 (2001).

Lee, C.R. et al., Effects of a cultured autologous chondrocyte-seeded type II collagen scaffold on the healing of a chondral defect in a canine model, *J. Orthop. Res.*, **21** (2), 272–281 (2003).

Lewandrowski, K.U., Muller, J., and Schollmeier, G., Concomitant meniscal and articular cartilage lesions in the femorotibial joint, *Am. J. Sports Med.*, **25** (4), 486–494 (1997).

Li, X. et al., Smad6 is induced by BMP-2 and modulates chondrocyte differentiation, *J. Orthop. Res.*, **21** (5), 908–913 (2003).

Lu, L., Stamatas, G.N., and Mikos, A.G., Controlled release of transforming growth factor beta1 from biodegradable polymer microparticles, *J. Biomed. Mater. Res.*, **50** (3), 440–451 (2000).

Martin, I., Wendt, D., and Heberer, M., The role of bioreactors in tissue engineering, *Trends Biotechnol.*, **22** (2), 80–86 (2004).

Masuda, K. et al., A novel two-step method for the formation of tissue-engineered cartilage by mature bovine chondrocytes: the alginate-recovered-chondrocyte (ARC) method, *J. Orthop. Res.*, **21** (1), 139–148 (2003).

Meese, T.M. et al., Surface studies of coated polymer microspheres and protein release from tissue-engineered scaffolds, *J. Biomater. Sci. Polym. Ed.*, **13** (2), 141–151 (2002).

Messner, K. and Maletius, W., The long-term prognosis for severe damage to weight-bearing cartilage in the knee: a 14-year clinical and radiographic follow-up in 28 young athletes, *Acta Orthop. Scand.*, **67** (2), 165–168 (1996).

Metters, A.T., Anseth, K.S., and Bowman, C.N., Fundamental studies of biodegradable hydrogels as cartilage replacement materials, *Biomed. Sci. Instrum.*, **35**, 33–38 (1999).

Mi, Z. et al., Adverse effects of adenovirus-mediated gene transfer of human transforming growth factor beta 1 into rabbit knees, *Arthritis Res. Ther.*, **5** (3), R132–R139 (2003).

Mitchell, N. and Shepard, N., The resurfacing of adult rabbit articular cartilage by multiple perforations through the subchondral bone, *J. Bone Joint Surg. Am.*, **58** (2), 230–233 (1976).

Moffat, K.L. and Marra, K.G., Biodegradable poly(ethylene glycol) hydrogels crosslinked with genipin for tissue engineering applications, *J. Biomed. Mater. Res.*, **71B** (1), 181–187 (2004).

Morales, T.I. and Roberts, A.B., Transforming growth factor beta regulates the metabolism of proteoglycans in bovine cartilage organ cultures, *J. Biol. Chem.*, **263** (26), 12828–12831 (1988).

Morales, T.I. et al., Transforming growth factor-beta in calf articular cartilage organ cultures: synthesis and distribution, *Arch. Biochem. Biophys.*, **288** (2), 397–405 (1991).

Murphy, C.L. and Sambanis, A., Effect of oxygen tension and alginate encapsulation on restoration of the differentiated phenotype of passaged chondrocytes, *Tissue Eng.*, **7** (6), 791–803 (2001).

Naumann, A. et al., Tissue engineering of autologous cartilage grafts in three-dimensional *in vitro* macroaggregate culture system, *Tissue Eng.*, **10** (11/12), 1695–1706 (2004).

Parker, J.A. et al., Release of bioactive transforming growth factor beta(3) from microtextured polymer surfaces *in vitro* and *in vivo*, *Tissue Eng.*, **8** (5), 853–861 (2002).

Pateder, D.B. et al., PTHrP expression in chick sternal chondrocytes is regulated by TGF-beta through Smad-mediated signaling, *J. Cell Physiol.*, **188** (3), 343–351 (2001).

Pavesio, A. et al., Hyaluronan-based scaffolds (Hyalograft C) in the treatment of knee cartilage defects: preliminary clinical findings, *Novartis Found. Symp.*, **249**, 203–217 (2003), discussion 229–233, 234–238, 239–241.

Pei, M. et al., Bioreactors mediate the effectiveness of tissue engineering scaffolds, *Faseb. J.*, **16** (12), 1691–1694 (2002).

Pfander, D. et al., HIF-1alpha controls extracellular matrix synthesis by epiphyseal chondrocytes, *J. Cell Sci.*, **116** (Pt9), 1819–1826 (2003).

Pittenger, M.F. et al., Multilineage potential of adult human mesenchymal stem cells, *Science*, **284** (5411), 143–147 (1999).

Prockop, D.J., Marrow stromal cells as stem cells for nonhematopoietic tissues, *Science*, **276** (5309), 71–74 (1997).

Qu, Z. et al., Development of approaches to improve cell survival in myoblast transfer therapy, *J. Cell Biol.*, **142** (5), 1257–1267 (1998).

Robinson, D. and Nevo, Z., Articular cartilage chondrocytes are more advantageous for generating hyaline-like cartilage than mesenchymal cells isolated from microfracture repairs, *Cell Tissue Bank*, **2** (1), 23–30 (2001).

Royce, S.M., Askari, M., and Marra, K.G., Incorporation of polymer microspheres within fibrin scaffolds for the controlled delivery of FGF-1, *J. Biomater. Sci. Polym. Ed.*, **15** (10), 1327–1336 (2004).

Sawhney, A.S., Pathak, C.P., and Hubbell, J.A., Interfacial photopolymerization of poly(ethylene glycol)-based hydrogels upon alginate-poly(l-lysine) microcapsules for enhanced biocompatibility, *Biomaterials*, **14** (13), 1008–1016 (1993a).

Sawhney, A.S., Pathak, C.P., and Hubbell, J.A., Bioreadible hydrogels based on photopolymerized poly(ethylene glycol)-co-poly(a-hydroxy acid) diacrylate macromers, *Macromolecules*, **26**, 581–587 (1993b).

Seidel, J.O. et al., Long-term culture of tissue engineered cartilage in a perfused chamber with mechanical stimulation, *Biorheology*, **41** (3–4), 445–458 (2004).

Sekiya, I. et al., Expansion of human adult stem cells from bone marrow stroma: conditions that maximize the yields of early progenitors and evaluate their quality, *Stem Cells*, **20** (6), 530–541 (2002).

Semenza, G.L., Hypoxia-inducible factor 1: master regulator of $O_2$ homeostasis, *Curr. Opin. Genet. Dev.*, **8** (5), 588–594 (1998).

Semenza, G.L., Hypoxia-inducible factor 1: oxygen homeostasis and disease pathophysiology, *Trends Mol. Med.*, **7** (8), 345–350 (2001).

Serra, R. et al., Expression of a truncated, kinase-defective TGF-beta type II receptor in mouse skeletal tissue promotes terminal chondrocyte differentiation and osteoarthritis, *J. Cell Biol.*, **139** (2), 541–552 (1997).

Serra, R., Karaplis, A., and Sohn, P., Parathyroid hormone-related peptide (PTHrP)-dependent and -independent effects of transforming growth factor beta (TGF-beta) on endochondral bone formation, *J. Cell Biol.*, **145** (4), 783–794 (1999).

Shapiro, F., Koide, S., and Glimcher, M.J., Cell origin and differentiation in the repair of full-thickness defects of articular cartilage, *J. Bone Joint Surg. Am.*, **75** (4), 532–553 (1993).

Silver, I., Measurements of pH and ionic composition of pericellular sites, *Philos. Trans. R. Soc. London Biol. Sci.*, **271**, 261–272 (1975).

Steadman, J.R. et al., Outcomes of microfracture for traumatic chondral defects of the knee: average 11-year follow-up, *Arthroscopy*, **19** (5), 477–484 (2003).

Takahashi, Y. et al., Hypoxic induction of prolyl 4-hydroxylase alpha (I) in cultured cells, *J. Biol. Chem.*, **275** (19), 14139–14146 (2000).

Toyoda, T. et al., Hydrostatic pressure modulates proteoglycan metabolism in chondrocytes seeded in agarose, *Arthritis Rheum.*, **48** (10), 2865–2872 (2003).

Tuli, R. et al., Transforming growth factor-beta-mediated chondrogenesis of human mesenchymal progenitor cells involves N-cadherin and mitogen-activated protein kinase and Wnt signaling cross-talk, *J. Biol. Chem.*, **278** (42), 41227–41236 (2003).

Tuli, R. et al., Human mesenchymal progenitor cell-based tissue engineering of a single-unit osteochondral construct, *Tissue Eng.*, **10** (7–8), 1169–1179 (2004).

van der Kraan, P.M. et al., Interaction of chondrocytes, extracellular matrix and growth factors: relevance for articular cartilage tissue engineering, *Osteoarthr. Cartilage*, **10** (8), 631–637 (2002).

Wickham, M.Q. et al., Multipotent stromal cells derived from the infrapatellar fat pad of the knee, *Clin. Orthop. Relat. Res.*, **412**, 196–212 (2003).

Yaeger, P.C. et al., Synergistic action of transforming growth factor-beta and insulin-like growth factor-I induces expression of type II collagen and aggrecan genes in adult human articular chondrocytes, *Exp. Cell Res.*, **237** (2), 318–325 (1997).

Zhang, X. et al., Primary murine limb bud mesenchymal cells in long-term culture complete chondrocyte differentiation: TGF-beta delays hypertrophy and PGE2 inhibits terminal differentiation, *Bone*, **34** (5), 809–817 (2004).

# Index

## A

# Related Titles

*Biodegradable Systems in Tissue Engineering and Regenerative Medicine*
Rui L. Reis, University of Minho, Braga, Portugal
Julio San Roma, Instituto de Ciencia y Tecnolo, Madrid, Spain
ISBN: 0849319366

*Bioengineering of the Skin: Water and the Stratum Corneum, 2nd Edition*
Joachim Fluhr, Friedrich Schiler University, Jena, Germany
Peter Elsner, Friedrich Schiler University, Jena, Germany
Enzo Berardesca, Instituto Dermatologico San Gallico, Rome, Italy
Howard I. Maibach, University of California, San Francisco, CA
ISBN: 0849314437

*Bio-Implant Interface: Improving Biomaterials and Tissue Reactions*
J.E. Ellison, University of Oslo, Oslo, Norway
S.P. Lyngstadaas, University of Oslo, Oslo, Norway
ISBN: 0849314747

*Biomaterials, Artificial Organs and Tissue Engineering*
L. Hench, Woodhead Publishing, Cambridge, United Kingdom
Julian R. Jones, Imperial College of London, London, United Kingdom
ISBN: 0849325773